MEDICAL RADIOLOGY
Radiation Oncology

Editors:
L.W. Brady, Philadelphia
H.-P. Heilmann, Hamburg
M. Molls, Munich
C. Nieder, Bodø

P. M. Harari · N. P. Connor · C. Grau (Eds.)

Functional Preservation and Quality of Life in Head and Neck Radiotherapy

With Contributions by

R. J. Amdur · A. Argiris · H. P. Bijl · T. C. Campbell · S. Chaiet · A. W. Chan · H. Chen
J. F. Cleary · N. P. Connor · A. Eisbruch · U. V. Elstroem · E. Filion · X. Geets
M. K. Gibson · C. Grau · V. Grégoire · P. M. Harari · G. Hartig · J. Herrstedt
R. W. Hinerman · T. Hoang · J. Irish · K. Jensen · J. Johansen · D. E. Jorenby · R. Kammer
M. V. Karamouzis · W. (Ken) Zhen · M. Knigge · C. A. Kristensen · J. A. Langendijk
Q.-T. Le · A. W. M. Lee · P.C. Levendag · N. Liebsch · M. A. List · W. M. Mendenhall
W. T. Ng L. Ning · I. Noever · B. O'Sullivan · G. M. Richards · P. Sandow
P. I. M. Schmitz · R. S. Sippel D. N. Teguh · C. Terhaard · W. A. Tomé · A. Trofimov
R. Tsang · H. van der Est · P. van Rooij · M. Vaysberg · P. Voet · J. W. Werning
D. L. Wheeler · P. A. Wiederholt · R. M. W. Yeung

Foreword by
L. W. Brady, H.-P. Heilmann, M. Molls, and C. Nieder

With 78 Figures in 105 Separate Illustrations, 54 in Color and 60 Tables

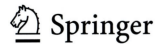

PAUL M. HARARI, MD
Jack Fowler Professor and Chairman
Department of Human Oncology
University of Wisconsin School of Medicine
600 Highland Ave K4/332
Madison, Wisconsin 53792
USA

CAI GRAU MD
Department of Oncology
Aarhus University Hospital
44 Norrebrogade
8000 Aarhus C
Denmark

NADINE P. CONNOR PhD
Associate Professor, Division of Otolaryngology
Head and Neck Surgery
University of Wisconsin
600 Highland Avenue K4/711
Madison, WI 53792-7375
USA

MEDICAL RADIOLOGY · Diagnostic Imaging and Radiation Oncology
Series Editors:
A. L. Baert · L. W. Brady · H.-P. Heilmann · M. Knauth · M. Molls · C. Nieder

Continuation of Handbuch der medizinischen Radiologie
Encyclopedia of Medical Radiology

ISBN: 978-3-540-73231-0   e-ISBN: 978-3-540-73232-7

DOI: 10.1007/978-3-540-73232-7

Medical Radiology · Diagnostic Imaging and Radiation Oncology ISSN 0942-5373

Library of Congress Control Number: 2008942722

© 2009 Springer-Verlag Berlin Heidelberg

This work is subject to copyright. All rights are reserved, whether the whole or part of the material is concerned, specifically the rights of translation, reprinting, reuse of illustrations, recitation, broadcasting, reproduction on microfilms or in any other way, and storage in data banks. Duplication of this publication or parts thereof is permitted only under the provisions of the German Copyright Law of September 9, 1965, in its current version, and permission for use must always be obtained from Springer-Verlag. Violations are liable for prosecution under the German Copyright Law.

The use of general descriptive names, registered names, trademarks, etc. in this publication does not imply, even in the absence of a specific statement, that such names are exempt from the relevant protective laws and regulations and therefore free for general use.

Product liability: The publishers cannot guarantee the accuracy of any information about dosage and application contained in this book. In every individual case the user must check such information by consulting the relevant literature.

Cover design: Publishing Services Teichmann, 69256 Mauer, Germany

The middle image on the cover (see also Fig. 23.1) was originally published in: Jensen K, Lambertsen K, Grau C (2008) Late swallowing dysfunction and dysphagia after radiotherapy for pharynx cancer: Frequency, intensity and correlation with dose and volume parameters. Radiotherapy and Oncology 85:74--82. The image is reproduced here by kind permission of Elsevier.

Printed on acid-free paper

9 8 7 6 5 4 3 2 1

springer.com

Dedication

To our Families and our Patients

Foreword

The emphasis on cancer management in the past was based primarily on control rates from multidisciplinary input in management. There has always been a recognition that one would like to achieve the best result with the least complication, but never has there been any major emphasis on evidence-based outcome studies, nor on functional preservation and quality of life. The authors of this book have dealt very effectively with the various tumor types in head and neck cancer with the experts in the field of management. The contents range from epidemiology and treatment outcome, treatment techniques with the potential impact on the quality of life such as dysphagia, to the various options relative to high technology radiation therapy programs for management. The potential for improving form and function through surgical care as an integrated part of the program is dealt with very effectively as well as the potentials for chemotherapy and the use of targeted agents have on quality of life issues.

The volume also addresses toxicity, quality of life, and techniques for prevention of adverse effects, as well as the potentials for rehabilitation and supportive care.

The authors have clearly done an extraordinarily good job in addressing the multiplicity of problems that impact upon the functional preservation and quality of life in head and neck radiation therapy.

Philadelphia	Luther W. Brady
Hamburg	Hans-Peter Heilmann
Munich	Michael Molls
Bodø	Carsten Nieder

Preface

Treating head and neck cancer involves the treatment of tumors within a highly complex anatomical and physiological environment. Because end organs for critical sensorimotor functions such as breathing, speaking, swallowing, seeing, and hearing are found within the head and neck, the eradication of the disease is particularly challenging. Life-threatening diseases must be approached in a manner that not only maximizes survival, but also maximizes functional outcome.

While the overall goal is generally cure or palliation, a variety of treatment options exists. Treatment approaches must be balanced with planning for toxicity reduction and functional preservation. A major objective of this book is to emphasize that the evaluation of treatment methods for head and neck cancer can transcend simple measurement of survival by also considering how particular treatments affect the life of the individual patient. That is, the manner in which function is preserved must be evaluated in conjunction with more traditional measures of health and disease. Measures of function are important clinical endpoints and can serve to evaluate the extent to which a treatment affects a patient's overall health and well-being. Chapters in this volume examine this concept from the perspective of sites of disease within the head and neck as well as treatment methodology.

Measures that take into account the patient's perspective are particularly useful for dimensions of health in which the individual is the only person who can truly appreciate the condition. Variables such as pain and fatigue fit into this category, as do assessments of "quality of life." As a field of study, health-related quality of life (HR-QOL) research and measurement has expanded greatly over the last 30 years. To date, there are over 125,000 articles indexed in Medline (PubMed) with the heading of "quality of life" and over 2700 of these articles are concerned with head and neck cancer. This great interest in HR-QOL with regard to head and neck cancer not only reflects the importance of including concepts of quality of life in our research but it also shows that quality of life is an important factor influencing our treatment selection in the care of individual patients.

The contributors to this volume are renowned international experts in the field of head and neck cancer. Their outstanding contributions cover a wide range of topics including epidemiological issues associated with different tumor sites, treatment outcomes and toxicities associated with different treatment techniques, and the support of quality of life and the prevention of its decrements associated with therapy. The incorporation of quality of life themes into this framework offers a patient-centered perspective to the treatment of head and neck cancer and is geared toward functional preservation.

Our goal is to have an accessible volume with state-of-the-art content focused on preservation of function in head and neck cancer patients. All chapters in this volume begin with a list of key points providing readers a synopsis of core information concerning each of the major content areas discussed. Thus, it is possible for the busy clinician to gain an appreciation of the subject matter and to follow with more in depth study as time allows.

We are grateful for the opportunity to work on this rewarding project and thank all of the contributors for their outstanding chapters. It is our hope that this book will provide a foundation for exploration of patient-centered functional outcomes for individuals with head and neck cancer across the full range of sites and stages. For this field, our ultimate goals include a decrease in cancer incidence, increase in cancer cure, and, importantly, preservation of function. Much work has been done to this end, and there is more work to do. Perhaps the information presented in this book will inspire new directions related to the treatment of this complex disease.

Thanks to Ms. Ursula Davis and the production team at Springer for their superb collaborative work on this project.

Madison   PAUL M. HARARI
Madison   NADINE P. CONNOR
Aarhus   CAI GRAU

Contents

Epidemiology and Treatment Outcome 1

1 Oral Cavity Cancer 3
WEINING (KEN) ZHEN

2 Oropharynx: Epidemiology and Treatment Outcome..................... 15
EDITH FILION and QUYNH-THU LE

3 Hypopharynx... 31
GREGORY M. RICHARDS and PAUL M. HARARI

4 Laryngeal Cancer: Epidemiology and Treatment Outcomes 43
WILLIAM M. MENDENHALL, RUSSELL W. HINERMAN,
ROBERT J. AMDUR, MIKAHAIL VAYSBERG,
and JOHN W. WERNING

5 Nasopharynx 57
ANNE W. M. LEE, REBECCA M. W. YEUNG,
and WAI TONG NG

6 Paranasal Sinus and Nasal Cavity.................................... 75
CLAUS ANDRUP KRISTENSEN

7 Salivary Glands and Quality of Life 89
CHRIS TERHAARD

8 Head and Neck Sarcomas and Lymphomas 103
BRIAN O'SULLIVAN, JONATHAN IRISH,
and RICHARD TSANG

9 Thyroid Cancer 117
LI NING, HERBERT CHEN, and REBECCA S. SIPPEL

10 Cervical Lymph Node Metastases
from Unknown Primary Tumors 125
CAI GRAU

Treatment Techniques with Potential Impact on QOL 133

11 Dysphagia-Related Quality of Life of Patients with Cancer in the Oropharynx: An Advantage for Brachytherapy? 135
PETER C. LEVENDAG, PETER VAN ROOIJ, DAVID N. TEGUH, INGE NOEVER, PETER VOET, HENRIE VAN DER EST, and PAUL I. M. SCHMITZ

12 Improving the Quality of Life of Patients with Head and Neck Cancer by Highly Conformal Radiotherapy 145
AVRAHAM EISBRUCH

13 Advantages of Proton Beam Therapy in Functional Preservation and Quality of Life in Head and Neck Radiotherapy 155
ANNIE W. CHAN, NORBERT LIEBSCH, and ALEXEI TROFIMOV

14 Target Definition and Delineation CT/MRI/ PET-Guided Targets 163
XAVIER GEETS and VINCENT GRÉGOIRE

15 Advanced Techniques for Setup Precision and Tracking 175
WOLFGANG A. TOMÉ

16 Adaptive Image-Guided Radiotherapy for Head and Neck Cancer 183
ULRIK VINDELEV ELSTROEM, and CAI GRAU

17 Improving Form and Function Through Surgical Care in Head and Neck Squamous Cell Carcinoma 191
GREG HARTIG and SCOTT CHAIET

18 The Contribution of Chemotherapy 203
MICHALIS V. KARAMOUZIS, MICHAEL K. GIBSON, and ATHANASSIOS ARGIRIS

19 Contributions of Targeted Agents 215
DERIC L. WHEELER, TIEN HOANG, and PAUL M. HARARI

Toxicity, Quality of Life, Prevention, Rehabilitation, Supportive Care 225

20 Late Radiation-Induced Side Effects 227
JOHANNES A. LANGENDIJK and HENDRICUS P. BIJL

21 Head and Neck Cancer Quality of Life Instruments 243
MARCY A. LIST

22 Measuring and Reporting Toxicity 251
KENNETH JENSEN and CAI GRAU

23 Effects of Radiotherapy on Swallowing Function: Evaluation, Treatment and Patient-Reported Outcomes 259
MOLLY KNIGGE, RACHAEL KAMMER, and NADINE P. CONNOR

24 Dental Prophylaxis and Care 269
PAMELA SANDOW

25 Smoking Cessation 277
DOUGLAS E. JORENBY

26 Supportive Therapy Including Nutrition 287
JØRGEN JOHANSEN and JØRN HERRSTEDT

27 Communication and Palliative Care in Head and Neck Cancer 299
TOBY C. CAMPBELL and JAMES F. CLEARY

28 Organized Head and Neck Cancer Care 307
PEGGY A. WIEDERHOLT

Subject Index 317

List of Contributors 321

Epidemiology and Treatment Outcome

Oral Cavity Cancer

1

WEINING (KEN) ZHEN

CONTENTS

1.1   Epidemiology and Treatment Outcome   *3*
1.1.1   Oral Cavity Cancer   *3*
1.1.1.1   Epidemiology of Oral Cavity Cancer   *3*
1.1.1.2   Treatment Outcome for Oral Cavity
         Cancer   *8*

References   *13*

KEY POINTS

- Oral cavity cancer is relatively uncommon, which consists of 1.6% of all cancers diagnosed in the United State annually.
- Tobacco exposure is a major risk factor.
- Oral tongue cancer is the most common site for oral cavity cancer and has the highest risk of regional and distant metastasis.
- Lip cancer has the best and oral tongue has the worst prognosis.
- Increasing tumor thickness correlates with the disease control and survival.
- Surgery alone is the most commonly used treatment modality for oral cavity cancer, followed by combined surgery and radiotherapy.
- Radiotherapy alone is used in less than 15% of patients.
- Either surgery or radiotherapy alone can achieve excellent local control for early-stage disease.
- For locally advanced-stage cancer combined surgery and radiotherapy offers the best chance of local and regional control of the disease.

WEINING (KEN) ZHEN, MD
987521 Nebraska Medical Center, Omaha, NE 68198, USA

1.1
Epidemiology and Treatment Outcome

1.1.1
Oral Cavity Cancer

1.1.1.1
Epidemiology of Oral Cavity Cancer

1.1.1.1.1
Overall Incidence

The oral cavity is the most anterior subdivision of the head and neck, which involves the mucosal lip anteriorly to the junction of the hard and soft palates superiorly and to the circumvallate papillae inferiorly. It is further divided into several anatomical subsites, including mucosal lip from the junction of the skin–vermillion border, buccal mucosa, lower alveolar ridge, retromolar trigone, upper alveolar ridge, hard palate, floor of the mouth, and oral tongue (anterior two thirds of the tongue). According to the National Cancer Institute SEER (Surveillance, Epidemiology, and End Results) Program, the oral tongue is the most common site for oral cavity cancer in both American men and women, which consists of 38% of all oral cavity cancers diagnosed in the USA between 1988 and 2004. The second most common site is the floor of mouth (26%), followed by all other sites of mouth (18%) and lip (18%) (RIES et al. 2007).

Oral cavity cancer is relatively uncommon in the USA and developed countries. According to the American Cancer Society (ACS 2008), an estimated 22,900 new cases of oral cancer (excluding oropharynx) are expected in 2008 in the USA, which represents 1.6% (2.0% for men and 1.1% for women) of all cancer cases. Among all head and neck cancers (295,022) collected between 1985 and 1994 in the USA by the National Cancer Data Base (NCDB), 17.5% were oral cavity cancers, including lip cancers and 14.1% when lip cancers were not included (HOFFMAN et al. 1998). The incidence rates are more than twice as high in men (15,250 cases) as in women (7,650 cases). An estimated 5,390 deaths (3,590 in men and 1,800 in women) from oral cavity cancer are expected in 2008, which represents about 1% of all cancer mortality (565,650 deaths) in the USA (ACS 2008).

Worldwide, cancers of the oral cavity accounted for 274,000 cases in 2002. The region of the world with the highest incidence is Melanesia (31.5/100,000 in men and 20.2/100,000 in women). Rates in men are high in Western Europe (11.3/100,000), southern Europe (9.2/100,000), south Asia (12.7/100,000), southern Africa (11.1/100,000), and Australia/New Zealand (10.2/100,000). In females, incidence is relatively high in southern Asia (8.3/100,000; PARKIN et al. 2005). Oral cavity cancer is also more common in developing countries with estimated cases of 129,356 in men (3.6% of all cancers in men) and 84,840 in women (2.7% of all cancers in women) in 2007. It represents the seventh most common malignancy for men in developing countries with an estimated mortality rate of 2.6% (GARCIA et al. 2007).

In the last few decades it has been suggested that the incidence of oral cancer in all age groups has been rising worldwide (BOYLE et al. 1990). The similar trend has also been observed in the USA, especially among African American men (CANTO and DEVESA 2002) and in young adults, a group with less tobacco and/or alcohol exposure. Despite the decline in incidence rates for the majority of oral cancer sites for the period 1973–2001 among White American men and women between ages 20 and 44, the incidence of oral tongue cancer has continued to rise by 1.7% per year during this time period as reported by SHIBOSKI et al. (2005). Furthermore, oral tongue cancer incidence in this age group grew more rapidly at an annual rate of 6.7% from 1975 to1985 before reaching a plateau. However, despite a plateau in oral tongue cancer incidence rates in the late 1970s and early 1980s, the incidence of base of tongue and tonsil cancers continued to increase by 2.1 and 3.9% per year through 1998, predominantly among African American and White men younger than 60 years in the USA (FRISCH et al. 2000). The age-standardized incidence rates for oral cancers, including oral cavity and oropharyngeal carcinomas, are strongly influenced by age, sex, race, primary site, year of birth, and geographic region.

1.1.1.1.2
Major Risk Factors for Oral Cancer

Tobacco Smoking
Tobacco exposure is clearly a major risk factor for oral cancer in adults. Tobacco contains at least 55 known carcinogens, which can be grouped into three classes: polycyclic aromatic hydrocarbons, *N*-nitrosamines, and Asz-arenes (HECHT 1999). The risk of oral cancer is definitely increased in smokers of all tobacco products, whether smoked, chewed, or taken as snuff, although the risk is reported to be higher in smokers who consume cigarettes without filters. Furthermore, there is a strong association of oral cancer and unfiltered tobacco products, namely pipes or cigars (FRANCESCHI et al. 1990; ZHENG et al. 2004).

The risk of oral cancer increases with amount and duration of smoking, with duration of smoking having a greater impact on risk than amount. In addition, the risk of oral cancer is higher in current smokers than in ex-smokers and is higher in people who start smoking at an early age than in people who start smoking at a later age (IARC 2004). The relative risks (RRs) for oral cancer were 5.3 for people who smoked less than 15 cigarettes/day and 14.3 for people who smoked 25 or more cigarettes/day compared with people who never smoked. Likewise, the RRs were 5.9 for people who had smoked for less than 30 years, which increased to 18.0 if he or she had smoked at least 40 years. The age of exposure also has a significant impact on the risk of oral cancer, with RRs of 13.6 for people who had started smoking before age 17 (DAVIS and SEVERSON 1987). DEPUE (1986) reported that the rising mortality and increasing incidence of oral tongue cancer among young males in the USA has been linked to the use of smokeless tobacco products as one of the possible etiological factors. Additionally, environmental tobacco smoke exposure, also known as second-hand smoking, may be an important risk factor for oral cancer in both individuals with a history of tobacco smoking and among never smokers (ZHANG et al. 2000).

Despite overwhelming evidence of the strong association of tobacco and oral cancer, only a minority of the overall smoker population actually develop cancer. Studies have suggested a possible link between genetic polymorphisms and risk of oral cancer (GEISLER and OLSHAN 2001). Certain polymorphisms of carcinogen-metabolizing enzymes are known to be involved in the metabolism of carcinogens found in tobacco smoke. The enzymes have important roles in both converting tobacco-related carcinogens to reactive intermediates capable of forming adducts with DNA and those that subsequently detoxify these intermediates. In certain genetic polymorphisms, the expression and function of those so-called tobacco-carcinogen-detoxifying enzymes can be altered or deleted. A study by OLSHAN et al. (2000) reported that heavy smokers (more than 40 pack years) with a gene polymorphism in which a detoxifying enzyme is not expressed (glutathione *S*-transferase, GSTT1 null) appeared to have a higher risk of oral cancer (OR 13.5; 95% CI, 3.6–50.4) than those with the gene present (OR 5.4; 95% CI, 2.1–14.2). A similar study showed a significant association between oral and laryngeal cancer and predicted activity of UDP-glucuronosyltransferase, a tobacco-detoxifying gene among smokers, but not among nonsmokers. Heavy smokers with the genotype that expresses a low level of UDP-glucuronsyltransferase activity had a higher risk (OR 44; 95% CI, 5.3–373) for cancer than those with high levels of enzyme activity (OR 5.3; 95% CI, 1.9–15) (ZHENG et al. 2001).

Alcohol Use and Tobacco Smoking

The risk of developing oral cancer multiplies in people who use both tobacco and alcohol because of a synergistic effect from combined exposure to both products (CASTELLSAGUE et al. 2004). Attributable risk estimates indicate that tobacco smoking and alcohol account for approximately three-fourths of all oral and pharyngeal cancers in the USA. There is a strong association between the risk of oral cancer and the amount of alcohol consumed and the length of habitual consumption of alcohol and tobacco. The risk may increase directly with alcohol concentration, even after adjustment for total alcohol consumed. It has been demonstrated that the combined use of alcohol and tobacco increased the risk above that expected with either exposure alone. In a case–control study in Spain, heavy smokers and drinkers were estimated to have an ~50-fold of increased risk of oral cancer (CASTELLSAGUE et al. 2004).

Alcohol by itself has not been proved to be directly carcinogenic. The actual mechanism by which alcohol consumption leads to an increased risk of oral cancer remains unclear. Alcohol may cause local irritation to the area or it may act as a solvent to enhance mucosal exposure to carcinogens, or to facilitate the passage of carcinogens through cellular membranes. It is also possible that alcohol may enhance liver metabolism, and therefore, may activate carcinogenic substances (WIGHT and OGDEN 1998). Another possible mechanism may be the alteration of intracellular metabolism of the epithelial cells at the target site by ethanol, which may also be aggravated by nutritional deficiencies. Alcohol is metabolized to acetaldehyde by alcohol dehydrogenase (ADH) and subsequently to acetate. Acetaldehyde can form DNA adducts that interfere with DNA synthesis and repair. It is unclear whether there is any association between the ADH genotype and risk of oral cancer.

Smokeless Tobacco

Smokeless tobacco, also known as spit tobacco, has been implicated as a risk factor for oral cancer and is speculated to be a contributing factor for the increase in oral tongue cancer incidence rates among young men in the USA, although there is little US-based data to substantiate the claim. The relationship between the use of smokeless tobacco products and oral cancer is also complicated by significant variations in smokeless tobacco products by region, culture, and time period. However, in a study conducted among women in North Carolina who used predominantly fire-cured dry snuff, a strong dose–response relationship was observed between duration of smokeless tobacco use and risk of buccal and gingival cancer among nonsmokers, with an OR 47.5 (95% CI, 9.1–249.5) for 50 years or longer of use (WINN et al. 1986).

Betel Quid Chewing

Betel quid chewing has long been identified as a major risk factor for oral cancer (THOMAS and WILSON 1993). It is commonly consumed among older Asians, especially in India. Fifty percent of oral cancers in India occur in the buccal mucosa in contrast to less than 5% in many Western countries.

Viral Infection

Human papillomavirus (HPV) is a relatively widespread virus and has been detected more frequently in oral dysplastic and carcinomatous epithelium when compared with normal oral mucosa. The role of HPV in oral cancer continues to evolve. By contrast with cervical cancer, a pathogenic role for high-risk HPV viruses in nonanogenital cancers has been unclear until recently. Epidemiological and laboratory evidence now warrant the conclusion that, in addition to tobacco and alcohol, HPV is a causative agent or cofactor for head and neck squamous cell carcinoma (HNSCC). The recognition that HPV is causative for some HNSCCs may have important implications for their prognosis, prevention, and therapy. The IARC study reported by HERRERO et al. (2003) provides some evidence that HPV may contribute to the development of a small proportion of oral cavity carcinomas. HPV16 DNA was found in around 3.9% (95% CI, 2.5–5.3) of these carcinomas, compared with around 18% of oropharyngeal tumors. Seroreactivity for HPV 16 to viral capsid proteins and to viral oncoproteins was associated with increased risk of oral cavity carcinoma (OR 1.5; 95% CI, 1.1–2.1), although this has not been observed by other studies. These HPV-associated HNSCCs are characterized clinically by their location within the lingual and palatine tonsils of the oropharynx, their poorly differentiated histopathology, and they are more frequently found in nonsmoker nondrinker and in younger patients than in HNSCC not associated with HPV (GUILLISON and LOWY 2004).

Diet

There is strong evidence in the literature to demonstrate the relationship between diet and risk of oral cancer. Case–controlled studies have consistently shown an inverse association between the risk of oral cancer and consumption of fruits and vegetables after adjusting for smoking and alcohol intake (MARSHALL and BOYLE 1996). Frequent consumption of vegetables, citrus fruits, fish, and vegetable oil are the major features of a low-risk diet for cancer of the oral cavity. Patients with the highest quartile of intake of fruits and vegetables had significantly lower risk for oral cancer (OR 0.4; 95% CI, 0.4–0.8) than those in the lowest quartile of intakes as shown in the IARC multinational case–control study (KREIMER et al. 2006). On the other hand, diets high in meat and dairy products and low in fruits and vegetables jointly increased the risk for oral cancers (OR 12; 95% CI, 4.1–34.6), after controlling for the effects of alcohol and tobacco use (DE STEFANI et al. 2005). The protective effect of a diet high in fruits and vegetables may be modified by other risk factors as some studies have shown the protective function of diet was only relevant to ever-smoker ever-drinker (KREIMER et al. 2006), although other studies indicated that protective effect extended to nonsmoker nondrinker, including former smokers and light to moderate drinkers (SANCHEZ et al. 2003).

Oral Hygiene

Poor oral health such as chronic mucosal irritation or chronic inflammatory state (gingivitis and periodontitis), dental caries, tooth loss (a surrogate for poor oral hygiene), and tartar has been linked to an increased risk for oral cancer. Although both smoking and alcohol consumption have a significant impact on oral health and hygiene, poor oral hygiene may increase the risk of oral cancer by two- to fourfold after adjustment for gender, age, diet, alcohol, and tobacco use (TALAMINI et al. 2000). Furthermore, an independent role for oral hygiene was supported by significant elevations in oral cancer risk among nonsmoker nondrinker, suggesting that poor oral hygiene may be an independent risk factor for oral cancer.

Genetic and Familial Factors

There are indications that there is at least a contributing component related to a genetic susceptibility of the individual exposed to carcinogens and a potential for malignant transformation of the oral tissues. In general, the risk of all HNSCCs is increased by two- to fourfold among individuals with a positive family history (defined as one or more first-degree relatives with the disease), after adjusting for age, sex, alcohol, and tobacco exposure of the index case. The risk is greater (~8–14-fold) if the affected family member is a sibling. A case–control study from Canada has demonstrated a role for inherent genetic factors in the etiology of head and neck cancer with an adjusted relative risk for developing head and neck cancer of 3.79 (95% CI, 1.11–13.0), which doubles to 7.89 (RR, 1.5–41.6) in first-degree relatives of patients with multiple primary head and neck tumors (FOULKES et al. 1996).

1.1.1.1.3
Patient and Tumor Characteristics for Oral Cavity Cancer in the USA

The most common type of oral cancer is squamous cell carcinoma (SCC). According to NCDB, 86.3% of 58,976 oral cavity cancers diagnosed between 1985 and 1995 are SCC, although in much younger patients (younger than 35 years) SCC only comprises 48% (FUNK et al. 2002). The second most prevalent histologic type is adenocarcinoma (5.9%), which is slightly higher in women (8.6%). The tongue and floor of mouth are the most common sites of tumor origin overall (32 and 28%), which also have the highest percentage of SCC tumors (94.3 and 94.2%, respectively), whereas only 43% of palatal cancers are SCC. Adenocarcinoma is more commonly found in the palate (31.6%) (Table 1.1).

In the NCDB study, over half (55%) of all oral SCCs are early stage (0–II). Women had a higher proportion of stage I disease than that of men (31.9 and 27.7%), whereas men had a larger proportion of stage IV cancer than did women (32.7 and 27.3%). The SEER data, a population-based study also demonstrated a similar trend in stage distribution during the years of 1996–2004 (Ries et al. 2008). This showed that only 29% of men had localized disease

compared with 41% of women who had tumors confined to the primary. The overall rates of lymph node metastasis for men and women were 55 and 45%, respectively. The risk of distant metastasis was similar, about 10% (11 and 9%). Among the cases of oral cancers accumulated between 2001 and 2005, the lip primary has the highest rate for localized disease and lowest for distant disease (79 and 1%). On the other hand, oral tongue has the lowest rate for locally confined cancer and the highest risk for distant metastasis at presentation (34 and 13%).

Histologically low-grade (grades 1–2) tumors represent the majority of oral cancers. In the NCDB

Table 1.1. Patient characteristics by histologic type and anatomic subsite for all oral cavity cancer (Source: Adapted from Funk et al. (2002))

	Histologic type (%)									
	SCC	Adeno	Verruc	Carc NOS	Lymph	Sarc	Other	Total	Cases	Percentage of all cases
All cases	86.3	5.9	2.0	1.5	1.5	1.5	1.3	100	58,976	
Age										
<35	48.1	19.6	0.2	1.2	4.1	21.7	4.9	100	2,148	3.6
36–45	75.3	11.1	0.4	1.4	2.6	7.7	1.5	100	4,224	7.2
46–55	88.4	6.2	0.7	1.6	0.9	1.0	1.2	100	9,550	16.2
56–65	90.5	4.8	1.2	1.5	0.8	0.1	1.1	100	15,786	26.8
66–75	89.1	4.8	2.2	1.3	1.5	<0.1	1.1	100	16,011	27.1
76–85	86.2	4.5	4.4	1.5	2.1	0.1	1.2	100	8,799	14.9
>86	84.5	3.4	5.9	1.8	2.8	<0.1	1.4	100	2,406	4.1
Unknown	75	1.9	1.9	5.8	5.8	1.9	7.7	100	52	0.1
Subsite										
Tongue	94.3	1.1	1.2	1.5	0.6	0.5	0.8	100	18,809	31.9
Upper gum	77.4	3.2	5.7	0.8	4.8	4.0	4.1	100	1,684	2.8
Lower gum	89.0	2.4	4.2	0.9	1.6	0.4	1.5	100	3,581	6.1
FOM	94.2	2.2	0.9	1.6	0.3	<0.1	0.8	100	16,742	28.4
Palate	43.0	31.6	2.8	1.5	6.9	10.8	3.4	100	4,555	7.7
BM	74.6	11.8	6.0	1.4	3.6	0.6	2.0	100	3,928	6.7
RMT	92.5	4.5	0.9	1.0	0.2	0.1	0.8	100	5,502	9.3
MV	74.7	11.7	4.3	0.5	4.6	1.1	3.1	100	368	0.6
Other parts	68.6	15.0	2.8	2.6	3.1	5.3	2.6	100	3,807	6.5

Adeno adenocarcinoma; *Verruc* verrucous carcinoma; *Carc NOS* carcinoma otherwise not specified; *Lymph* lymphoma; *Sarc* sarcoma; *FOM* floor of mouth; *BM* buccal mucosa; *MV* mouth vestibule study, low-grade was identified in 83.1% of the oral SCC cases; this percentage of low-grade disease was much higher than that for all head and neck cases in which 70% were reported to be low-grade (HOFFMAN et al. 1998). Grade 3 tumors only comprised 16.2% of cases, and grade 4 oral cavity SCCs were found in less than 1% of all cases. There was a clear correlation between the degree of differentiation and the stage for the disease. Among stage I oral cavity SCC, 37.9% were identified as grade 1 and 15.5% as grade 2. Conversely, only 23.4% of all stage IV SCCs were grade 1, and 46.9% were grade 4.

1.1.1.2
Treatment Outcome for Oral Cavity Cancer

There are multiple factors that influence the prognosis and treatment outcome for oral cavity cancer.

1.1.1.2.1
Patient Factors

Age
The age at diagnosis has influence on the prognosis. The SEER data on 42,748 cases of oral cavity cancer collected between 1996 and 2004 demonstrated the best 5-year survival rate of 76.6% in patients younger than 45 years compared with 51.4% of survival rate in the age group over 65 years. This trend was also observed in the NCDB data pool, which contained 41,875 cases of oral cavity SCC. For all stages combined, the 5-year survival advantage for younger patients was significant (95% CI) across all three age groups (younger than 35, 36–65, and 66 years and older). When broken down by stage, a trend toward greater survival in the younger age groups remained for all stages although the statistical significance was maintained only for stage I oral cavity SCC.

Race
The survival differences in different ethnic groups have been observed. The NCDB data showed the 5-year survival difference between African Americans and the other two racial groups (Caucasians and Non-African American, Non-Caucasians). For all stages combined, African Americans had significantly lower 5-year survival rates (35.5%) than did Caucasians (51.1%) and other minorities (50.1%). When broken down by stage of oral cavity SCC, the difference between the Whites and the African Americans remained statistically significant for stages I, III, and IV. The poor survival for the African Americans was also demonstrated in the SEER program. For all oral cancers diagnosed between 1996 and 2004, the 5-year survival rate for Caucasians was 62.6% and for the African Americans was 43.7%. This discrepancy was even more profound in males (61.7 vs. 36%).

Gender
In general, men with HNSCC have a worse prognosis than that of women, which is also true for the oral cavity SCC. In the NCDB series for all stages combined, men had a significantly worse 5-year survival (47.1%) than did women (54%). This superior 5-year survival for women was evident for each stage, but remained statistically significant only for stages I and II when each stage was analyzed separately. The SEER data (1996–2004, which also included some nontonsil pharynx cases) also showed a better overall 5-year survival rate for women (64.4%) than for men (59.3%).

1.1.1.2.2
Tumor Factors

Histologic Type
Histologic type may have prognostic implications. The NCDB data demonstrated the best 5-year survival rate of 85.6% for adenocarcinoma, followed by carcinoma NOS (55.1%), lymphoma (52.8%), and SCC (49.8%). Oral cavity sarcoma has the worst prognosis and only 5% survived for 5 years.

Anatomic Subsite of the Oral Cavity
The overall survival rates of oral cavity cancer vary by anatomic subsites. According to the SEER data, the lip primary has the best prognosis with a 10-year survival rate of 87.3%, followed by gum/other mouth, and the floor of mouth with 10-year survival rates of 69.7 and 48.4%, respectively. The oral tongue cancer has the worst survival rate of 44.8% at 10 years (Fig. 1.1). The survival differences by site are also observed in the same stage of each subsite. For localized disease, the lip cancer has a 5-year survival rate of 97%, followed by gum/other mouth (94.7%), floor of mouth (81.4%), and tongue (74.1%). The prognosis for lip cancer even with lymph node metastasis remains good with the 5-year relative survival rate of 80.7%. The prognosis for other sites is much worse, around 50% of 5-year survival, when the cancer has spread to the regional lymph nodes (Fig. 1.2).

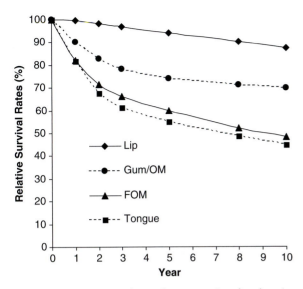

Fig. 1.1. Relative survival rates by cancer site of oral cavity among 22,415 cases. SEER 1988–2004. *OM* other mouth; *FOM* floor of mouth. Source: Adapted from Reis et al. (2007)

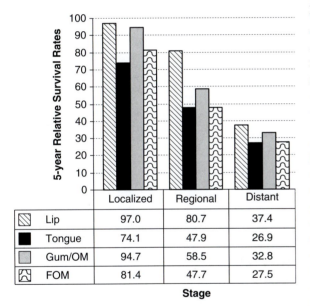

Fig. 1.2. Five-year relative survival rates by stage and site of oral cavity cancer. SEER 1988–2004. *OM* other mouth; *FOM* floor of mouth. Source: Adapted from Reis et al. (2007)

Stage

With the exception of lip cancer, regional lymph node metastasis decreases the survival rates by 40% as demonstrated by the SEER data. Distant metastasis further reduces the survival to about 30% ranging from 26.9% for tongue to 37.4% for lip cancer (Fig. 1.2). The overall 5-year relative survival rates by AJCC stage for oral cavity SCC are 68.1, 52.9, 41.3, and 26.5% for stages I, II, III and IV, respectively (Frederick et al. 2002). When broken down by TNM stage, the survival rate falls significantly with increasing clinical T stage from 50% for T1 and 45% for pT2 down to 25% for T3 as demonstrated in 524 patients with oral cavity SCC reported by Jones (1994). Similarly, the prognosis is also significantly influenced by N stage. In Jones' series, the observed 5-year survival fell from 44% for cN0 tumor to 29% for cN1, 18% for cN2, and 11% for cN3 disease, respectively. The survival also fell significantly with increasing number of positive nodes with survival rates of 46% if only one node was involved, down to 27% for two nodes, and 11% if more than three nodes were positive.

The Depth of Invasive Carcinoma

It has been demonstrated by a number of studies that tumor thickness and depth of invasion are important prognostic indicators in upper aerodigestive neoplasms, especially for oral cavity tumors such as tongue and floor of the mouth. The depth of invasion correlates with the risk for regional metastasis and survival. The overall incidence of nodal metastasis for T1 or T2 SCC of the oral tongue and floor of mouth with tumor thickness less than 2 mm was 13% as reported by Shah (2007), which increased to 65% for 8 mm or thicker disease (46% for thickness 3–8 mm). The depth of invasion was also found to correlate to disease-free survival; 97% for thickness less than 2-mm tumors, 83% for 2–8 mm, and 65% if the tumor thickness was greater than 8 mm, respectively. Sprio et al. (1986a) reviewed 105 consecutive patients who underwent operation for N0 SCC of the oral tongue and floor of the mouth. They observed that the disease-related death was less common when oral tumors were thin (2 mm or less), regardless of the tumor stage. A multivariate analysis in that study confirmed that increasing tumor thickness, rather than tumor stage, had the best correlation with the disease control and survival.

1.1.1.2.3
Treatment Factors

At present, a cancer registry does not exist to collect all cancer cases in the entire USA. However, it is estimated that the NCDB currently captures over 70% of new cancers occurring in the USA. Therefore, patterns of cancer care reported by the NCDB should present a broad spectrum of hospitals and

Table 1.2. Historical review of treatment outcomes for oral cavity SCC

Study period	References	N	Site of oral cavity	Stage	Close/+ margin (%)	Treatment modality (%)		
						Surgery only	RT alone	S + RT
1964–1974	Byers (1978)	82	All	All	12.1	100	0	0
1964–1977	Shaha (1984)	320	FOM	All		77	4	19
1970–1990	Eicher et al. (1996)	155	Lower gingival	All		84.5	0	15.5
1970–1979	Scholl et al. (1986)	268	Tongue	All	79.9 (IM−) 15.3 (IM + UM−) 4.9 (UM+)	58.6	0	41.4
1970–1992	Kowalski (2002)	513	Excluding lip	All		55.6	0	44.4
1973–1986	Pernot et al. (1992)	147	Tongue	T2N0		0	47.6 BT 54.4 XRT + BT	0
1974–1983	Lefebvre (1994)	579	Excluding lip	Early		15.9		74.1 BT 6 XRT + BT 4 XRT only
1977–1981	Spiro et al. (1986b)	105	Tongue	T1/2 N0	16.2	100	0	0
1979–1983	Lapreyre et al. (2004)	82	All	All 62% I/II	30.5 + 69.5 close	0	0	56 XRT + BT 44 BT (N0)
1979–1983	Loree (1990)	398	All	All	32	73.4	0	26.4
1980–1987	Turner (1996)	333	Excluding lip	All 85% N0		6 (ND only)	76	18 (RT + CT only)
1985–1982	Oliver et al. (1996)	92	All	All		73	0	27
1987–1993	Spiro et al. (1999)	146	Tongue	All	24.1	66	0	34
1989–2002	Brandwein-Gensler et al. (2005)	168	All	All	29.2	37.5	0	62.5
1990–1994	Carvalho et al. (2004)	238	All	All 63% I/II	21.2 14.9 for I/II 32.5 for III/IV	60.3 80.4 I/II 24.4 III/IV	2.5 0.7 5.7	37.2 18.9 69.9
1990–1994	Carvalho et al. (2004)	364	All	All 26.6% I/II	20.1 14.4 for I/II 22.6 for III/IV	21.6 62.6 I/II 4.6 III/IV	19.2 8.2 23.2	59.2 29.2 72.2

| Patterns of failure (%) | | | | 5-year survival rate (%) | Complication/ mortality (%) |
Local	Regional	L + R	Distant		
20.7				70.7 (2-year)	
21	37	29	13	65	20/2.5
				72	
13 aft S; 7 aft S + RT 22 aft S 0 aft S + RT				49 31	
20.3	16	3.7	2.9		
10.2 49.4	22.2 5.9	32.4 43.5		51.1 33.3	1.4 grade 3 3.5 grade 3
19.5 aft S; 11 aft sal S 18 (23 for T3); 9 aft salvage S 49; 40 aft salvage S 52, 43.5 aft salvage S	14 aft S; 12 aft sal S 18; 11 aft salvage S		5.4 3.5 8.8 0	42 52 14 0	19 overall 5 ORN, 11 MN
12	20.7	2.2	2.2	82 (2-year)	
19 overall 12 for BT 24 for XRT + BT (8 for T1/2N0)	14.6		5	68 overall 72 for N0 30 for N+	17.1 >grade 2
18 if margin (−) 36 if margin (+)	21.6 26.4		7.4 11.6	60 52	
39 35 if init N0 56 if init N+	40 overall 15.7 init N0	15.7 Init N0		55	5.9 ORN
5 (2-year)		5 (2-year)		68 (2-year)	
20.4 12 if margin − 36 if margin +	19	3.6	4.4	60	
17	14	5	7		
22.7 (overall recurrence rate) 22.8 for stage I/II 36 for stage III/IV	61 74 38	17.7/1.3 10.1/0 31.3/3.6			
34.6 (overall recurrence rate) 22.7 for stage I/I 39 for stage III/IV	43 68 for I/II 33 for III/IV	36.6/3.4 25.6 (3.4) 41.3/3.4			

N number of patients; *S* surgery; *RT* radiotherapy; *L* local; *R* regional; *IM* initial margin; *UM* ultimate margin; *BT* brachytherapy; *XRT* external beam radiotherapy; *ND* neck dissection; *CT* chemotherapy; *aft* after; *init* initial; *ORN* osteoradionecrosis; *MN* mucosal necrosis closely reflect a contemporary representation of the management and outcome of patients with certain cancer diagnosed within a given period of time in the USA. According to the NCDB, for cases of oral cavity SCC (total of 41,875 cases) diagnosed between 1985 and 1996, 45.7% of cases were treated primarily with surgery alone. Surgery with radiotherapy (RT) was the second most commonly used strategy (26.0%), followed by radiation therapy alone (13.6%). Tumors arising in the retromolar area (31.5%) and the palate (37.6%) were treated least frequently with surgical resection alone. A large proportion of retromolar primary tumors received surgery with RT (31.7%) or RT alone (19.9%). A large percentage of palatal tumors received RT only (21.5%). Tumors of the palate also had the highest percentage of cases (6.9%) managed with combined RT and chemotherapy.

The selection of treatment modality varies among different institutions. Table 1.2 summarizes a number of reported studies on the treatment outcome of oral cavity SCC. Either surgery or RT alone can achieve excellent local control for early-stage disease. LEFEBVRE et al. (1994) reported their experience of 579 patients with early-stage oral-cavity SCC. Among 92 patients treated with surgery alone, the initial local control rate was 80.5%, with an ultimate local control rate of 89% after salvage resurgery. A total of 429 patients were treated with brachytherapy (BT) to the primary, with or without elective neck dissection. The local control was achieved with BT alone in 352 patients (82%), although the control rate was poor for T3 tumors (63%). After successful salvage surgery, the final local control rates were 90% for the entire group: 96% for T1, 91% for T2, and 73% for T3 disease, respectively. Fourteen percent of T1-2N0 patients were found to have neck disease by elective neck dissection. The subsequent nodal failure rate for the BT patients without elective neck dissection was 17%. With salvage neck dissection, the final control of the neck was achieved in 89% of patients, suggesting BT alone may be appropriate for this cohort of patients. TURNER et al. (1996) analyzed a series of 268 clinically node-negative patients treated with RT to primary only and found an overall neck failure rate of 31%. The risk of subsequent neck failure varied between the sites of oral cavity and was as high as 40% for oral tongue (Fig. 1.3). There was a numerical trend toward more cancer deaths in the "watched" group. Therefore, the authors had concluded that elective neck irradiation should be given for T2-4N0 oral cavity SCC if RT were the primary treatment modality. Although BT has the advantage over external beam RT of delivering a high dose to the tumor with a relatively low dose to surrounding tissues, and the radiobiologic advantage of a short overall treatment time, BT alone is not adequate for neck disease.

For more advanced-stage disease or for patients who had an inadequate resection, combined surgery and RT is the most commonly used treatment strategy. Positive nodes or margins clearly increase the risk of local recurrence. Postoperative RT is frequently used in an attempt to decrease the risk of local recurrence and improve survival in the setting of positive margins. LOREE and STRONG (1990) demonstrated that

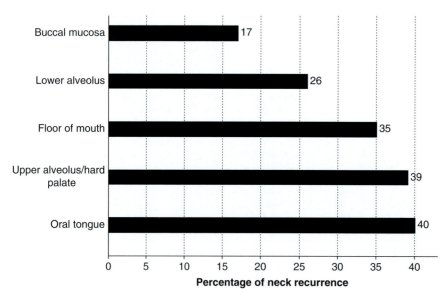

Fig. 1.3. Neck node recurrence in clinically N0 neck by site of oral cavity. All patients did not receive prophylactic nodal treatment. Source: Adapted from TURNER et al. (1996)

the overall local recurrence rate doubled (36 vs. 18%) and the 5-year survival rate was also statistically inferior (52 vs. 60%, $p < 0.025$) for patients with positive margin(s). Although the lack of statistical power and patient selection bias prevented the study to show a statistical significance, there was a consistent trend toward lower rates of local recurrence and regional metastases in patients treated with postoperative RT. The local failure rate after surgery alone for T1–2N0 patients with positive margins was 28%, but none of the patients had local failure when postoperative RT was given. The difference was more profound for T3–4 or N+ disease with local recurrence rates of 80 and 60% without RT compared with 38 and 43% with RT, respectively. SCHOLL et al. (1986) analyzed the significance of initially positive, but ultimately negative, margins on the treatment outcome. When the initial margin(s) was negative, the local failure rate was 13% without and 7% with postoperative RT. However, when the initial margin(s) was positive, but final margin (s) was negative, the local recurrence was 22% without and 0% with RT.

It is hoped that with advancement in surgical techniques and RT technology such as intensity-modulated RT (IMRT) and image-guided RT (IGRT) augmented by more effective systemic therapy such as targeted therapy, the treatment outcome for oral cancer will continue to improve with less treatment-related toxicities.

References

American Cancer Society (2008) Cancer Facts & Figures 2008. American Cancer Society, Atlanta

Boyle P, Macfarlane GJ, Maisonneuve P et al. (1990) Epidemiology of mouth cancer in 1989: a review. J R Soc Med 83:724–730

Brandwein-Gensler M, Teixeira MS, Lweis CM et al. (2005) Oral squamous cell carcinoma-Histologic risk assessment, but not margin status, is strongly predictive of local disease-free and overall survival. Am J Surg Pathol 29:167–178

Byers RM, Bland KI, Borlase B et al. (1978) The prognostic and therapeutic value of frozen section determinations in the surgical treatment of squamous cell carcinoma of the head and neck. Am J Surg 136:525–528

Canto MT, Devesa SS (2002) Oral cavity and pharynx cancer incidence rates in the United States, 1975–1998. Oral Oncol 38:610–617

Carvlho AL, Singh B, Spiro RH et al. (2004) Cancer of the oral cavity: a comparison between institutions in a developing and a developed nation. Head Neck 26:31–38

Castellsague X, Quintana MJ, Martinez MC et al. (2004) The role of type of tobacco and type of alcoholic beverage in oral carcinogenesis. Int J Cancer 108:741–749

Davis S, Severson RK (1987) Increasing incidence of cancer of the tongue in the United States among young adults. Lancet 2:910–911

Depue RH (1986) Rising mortality from cancer of the tongue in young white males. N Engl J M315:647

De Stefani E, Boffetta P, Ronco AL et al. (2005) Dietary patterns and risk of cancer of the oral cavity and pharynx in Uruguay. Nutr Cancer 51:132–139

Eicher SA, Overholt M, El-Naggar AK et al. (1996) Lower gingival carcinoma – clinical and pathologic determinations of regional metastases. Arch Otolaryngol Head Neck Surg 122:634–638

Foulkes W, Brunet JS, Sieh W et al. (1996) Familial risks of squamous cell carcinoma of the head and neck: retrospective case–control study. BMJ 313:716–721

Franceschi S, Talamini R, Barra S et al. (1990) Smoking and drinking in relation to cancers of the oral cavity, pharynx, larynx, and esophagus in northern Italy. Cancer Res 50:6502–6507

Frederick GL, Greene FL, Page DL et al. (2002) AJCC cancer staging manual, 6th edn. Springer, New York, p 28.

Frisch M, Hjalgrim J, Jaeger AB et al. (2000) Changing patterns of tonsillar squamous cell carcinoma in the United States. Cancer Causes Control 11:489–495

Funk GF, Karnell LH, Robinson RA et al. (2002) Presentation, treatment, and outcome of oral cavity cancer: a national cancer data base report. Head Neck 24:165–180

Garcia M, Jemal A, Ward EM et al. (2007) Global cancer facts & figures 2007. American Cancer Society, Atlanta

Geisler SA, Olshan AF (2001) GSTM1, GSTT1, and the risk of squamous cell carcinoma of the head and neck: a Mini-HuGE review. Am J Epidemiol 154:95–195

Guillison ML, Lowy DR (2004) A causal role for human papillomavirus in head and neck cancer. Lancet 363:1488–9.

Hecht S (1999) Tobacco smoke carcinogens and lung cancer. J Natl Cancer Inst 91:1194–1210

Herrero R, Castellsague X, Pawlita M et al. (2003) Human papillomavirus and oral cancer: the International Agency for Research on Cancer multicenter study. J Natl Cancer Inst 95:1772–1783.

Hoffman HT, Karnell LH, Funk GF et al. (1998) The National Cancer Data Base report on cancer of the head and neck. Arch Otolarngol Head Neck Surg 124:951–962

International Agency for Research on Cancer (IARC) (2004). Tobacco smoking and involuntary smoking. IARC monographs on the evaluation of carcinogenic risks to humans, vol 83. IARC, Lyon

Jones AS (1994) Prognosis in mouth cancer: tumor factors. Oral Oncol Eur J Cancer 30B:8–15

Kowalski LP (2002) Results of salvage treatment of the neck in patients with oral cancer. Arch Otolaryngol Head Neck Surg 128:58–62

Kreimer AR, Randi G, Herrero R et al. (2006) Diet and body mass, and oral and oropharyngeal squamous cell carcinomas: analysis from the IARC multinational case–control study. Int J Cancer 118:2293–2297

Lapeyre M, Bollet MA, Racadot S et al. (2004) Postoperative brachytherapy alone and combined postoperative radiotherapy and brachytherapy boost for squamous cell carcinoma of the oral cavity, with positive or close margins. Head Neck 26:216–223

Lefebvre JL, Dequeant BC, Buisseet E et al. (1994) Management of early oral cavity cancer. Experience of Centre Oscar Lambret. Eur J Cancer 30B 216–220

Loree TR and Strong EW (1990) Significance of positive margins in oral cavity squamous carcinoma. Am J Surg 160:410–414

Marshall JR, Boyle P (1996) Nutrition and oral cancer. Cancer Causes Control 7:101–111

Oliver AJ, Helfrick JF, Gard D (1996) Primary oral squamous cell carcinoma – a review of 92 cases. J Oral Maxillofac Surg 54:949–954

Olshan AF, Weissler MC, Watson MA et al. (2000). GSTM1, GSTT1, GSTP1, CYP1A1, and NAT1 polymorphisms, tobacco use, and the risk of head and neck cancer. Cancer Epidemiol Biomarkers Prev 9:185–191

Parkin DM, Bray F, Ferlay J et al. (2005) Global cancer statistics, 2002. CA Cancer J Clin 55:74–108

Pernot M, Malissard L, Aletti P et al. (1992) P Iridium-192 brachytherapy in the management of 147 T2N0 oral tongue carcinomas treated with irradiation alone: comparison of two treatment techniques. Radiother Oncol 23: 223–228

Ries LAG, Melbert D, Krapcho M et al. (eds) (2007) SEER cancer statistics review, 1975–2005. National Cancer Institute, Bethesda

Ries LAG, Melbert D, Krapcho M et al. (eds) (2008) SEER Cancer Statistics Review, 1975–2005, National Cancer Institute. Bethesda, MD, http://seer.cancer.gov/csr/1975_2005/, based on November 2007 SEER data submission, posted to the SEER web site

Sanchez MJ, Martinez C, Neito A et al. (2003) Oral and oropharyngeal cancer in Spain: influence of dietary patterns. Eur J Cancer Prev 12:49–56

Scholl P, Byers RM, Batsakis JG et al. (1986) Microscopic cut-through of cancer in the surgical treatment of squamous cell carcinoma of the tongue. Am J Surg 152:354–360

Shah JP (2007) Surgical approaches to the oral cavity primary and neck. Int J Radiat Oncol Biol Phys 69(2):S15–18

Shaha AR, Spiro RH, Shah JP et al. (1984) Squamous carcinoma of the floor of the mouth. Am J Surg 148:455–459

Shiboski CH, Schmidt BL, Jordan RC (2005) Tongue and tonsil carcinoma: increasing trends in the U.S. population ages 20–44 years. Cancer 103:1843–1849

Spiro RH, Hovos AG, Wong GY et al. (1986a) Predictive value of tumor thickness in squamous cell carcinoma confined to the tongue and floor of the mouth. Am J Surg 152: 345–350

Spiro RH, Guillamondegui O, Paulino AF et al. (1999) Pattern of invasion and margin assessment in patients with oral tongue cancer. Head Neck 21:408–413

Spiro RH, Spiro JD, Strong EW (1986b) Surgical approach to squamous carcinoma confined to the tongue and the floor of the mouth. Head Neck Surg 9:27–31

Talamini R, Vaccarella S, Barbone F et al. (2000) Oral hygiene, dentition, sexual hatbits and risk of oral cancer. Br J Cancer 83:1238–1242

Thomas S, Wilson A (1993) A quantitative evaluation of the aetiological role of betel-quid in oral carcinogenesis. Oral Oncol Eur J of Cancer 29B:265–271

Turner SL, Slevin NJ, Gupta NK et al. (1996) Radical external beam radiotherapy for 333 squamous cell carcinomas of the oral cavity-evaluation of morbidity and a watch policy for the clinically negative neck. Radiother Oncol 41:21–29

Wight AJ, Ogden GR (1998) Possible mechanisms by which alcohol may influence the development of oral cancer – a review. Oral Oncol 34:441–447

Winn DM, Blot WJ, Shy CM et al. (1986) Snuff dipping and oral cancer among women in the southern United States. N Engl J Med 304:745–749

Zhang ZF, Morgenstern H, Spitz MR et al. (2000) Environmental tobacco smoking, mutagen sensitivity, and head and neck squamous cell carcinoma. Cancer Epidemiol Biomarkers Prev 9:1043–1049

Zheng A, Park JY, Guillemette C et al. (2001) Tobaccocarcinogen-detoxifying enzyme UGT1A7 and its association with orolaryngeal cancer risk. J Natl Cancer Inst 93:1411–1418

Zheng T, Boyle P, Zhang B (2004) Tobacco use and risk of oral cancer. In: Boyle P, Gray N, Henningfield J, Seffrin J, and Zatonski W (eds) Tobacco science, policy and public health. Oxford University Press, Oxford, pp 399–432

Oropharynx:
Epidemiology and Treatment Outcome

2

EDITH FILION and QUYNH-THU LE

CONTENTS

2.1 Introduction *16*

2.2 Epidemiology *16*

2.3 Staging *17*
2.3.1 The Role of ^{18}Fluoro Deoxy-Glucose Positron Emission Topography in OPSCC Management *17*

2.4 Treatment by Stages *18*
2.4.1 Early Stage (Stages I–II) *18*
2.4.2 Locally Advanced Stage (Stages III–IV) *19*
2.4.2.1 Surgery and Adjuvant Radiotherapy vs. Radiotherapy or Chemoradiotherapy *19*
2.4.2.2 Radiation Fractionation *19*
2.4.2.3 Chemotherapy and Radiation Therapy *19*
2.4.2.4 Targeted Therapy *20*
2.4.2.5 Postoperative Treatment: Radiation and Chemoradiation *20*

2.5 Radiation Therapy Technique: Three-Dimensional Conformal Radiation Therapy vs. Intensity-Modulated Radiotherapy *21*

2.6 Treatment-Related Toxicities *22*
2.6.1 Acute Toxicities *22*
2.6.2 Late Toxicities *23*

2.7 Conclusion *26*

Abbreviations *26*

References *26*

> ### KEY POINTS
>
> - Oropharyngeal (OP) carcinoma comprises over half of all head and neck cancers in the United States.
> - While the incidence of squamous cell carcinoma (SCC) in the other head and neck sites has been steadily declining in association with smoking cessation, the incidence of SCC in the OP is rising, especially in younger patients and has been linked to the exposure of the human papillomavirus (HPV).
> - The treatment of OP carcinoma is complex because of the intricate anatomy of the involved organs, their rich lymphatic networks, and their critical function in the activities of daily living. Such treatment therefore requires a multidisciplinary approach.
> - This chapter focuses on the epidemiology of OP squamous cell carcinoma, specifically looking at the emerging role of HPV virus in their development.
> - It also describes the different treatment options for these tumors with a focus on those for organ preservation.
> - Finally, it highlights recent advances in treatment using molecularly targeted therapies and modern radiation delivery using intensity-modulated approach with the goal to minimize treatment-related toxicity in these highly curable patients.

EDITH FILION, MD
Department of Radiation Oncology, Stanford University Cancer Center, 875 Blake Wilbur Drive, Stanford, CA 94305-5847, USA
QUYNH-THU LE, MD
Department of Radiation Oncology, Stanford University Cancer Center, 875 Blake Wilbur Drive, Stanford, CA 94305-5847, USA

2.1 Introduction

Oropharynx squamous cell carcinoma (OPSCC) has emerged as one of the most common malignancies in the head and neck (HN) sites. Around 123,000 new cases of oropharyngeal (OP) cancers are estimated to occur annually worldwide, resulting in 79,000 annual deaths (Parkin et al. 2001). In the United States, the incidence of OP cancers in 2008 is estimated to be 35,310 new cases, from which 7,590 deaths will occur (Jemal et al. 2008). The oropharynx, which comprises of the soft palate, uvula, tonsillar fossa and pillars, glossotonsillar sulci, lateral and posterior pharyngeal wall, vallecula, and base of tongue, harbors a rich lymphatic network. Therefore, tumors arising from this region are likely to have early nodal involvement and ~60% of these patients present with stage III–IV tumors at diagnosis (Greene et al. 2002). The treatment of OP cancers has evolved over time. Although either surgery or radiation therapy (RT) remains the main treatment modality for early-stage OP cancers, concurrent chemoradiation therapy (CRT) has largely replaced RT alone for locally advanced neoplasms. Recent advances in RT techniques and molecular technologies have ushered in a new age of novel therapy for OP cancers, which holds promise for a better outcome with potentially less normal tissue toxicity. In this chapter, we will focus on the new developments in epidemiology and treatment approaches for OPSCC.

2.2 Epidemiology

The most common histology for OP tumors is squamous cell carcinoma (SCC). Established risk factors for these tumors include tobacco exposure (either directly or indirectly), alcohol consumption, genetic and environmental factors such as diet, poor oral hygiene, and RT exposure (Rosenquist 2005). A synergism between smoking and alcohol abuse has been described and could increase the relative risk of these cancers as much as 30-fold (Castellsague et al. 2004). Marijuana consumption has also been linked to the development of OPSCC (Zhang et al. 1999).

While the overall incidence of other HNSCC has been declining since the early 1980s because of smoking cessation, the incidence of OPSCC has either been stable or rising, especially in younger populations (Ernster et al. 2007; Sturgis and Cinciripini 2007) This is due to the increasing number of OPSCC associated with human papillomavirus (HPV). Reports indicated that up to 50–60% of OPSCC might harbor HPV DNA, depending on the detection method used (Gillison et al. 2000; Gillison and Shah 2001; Mork et al. 2001; Dai et al. 2004). HPV is most commonly found in tonsillar and base of tongue tumors, with HPV16 being found in the vast majority (>90%) (Gillison et al. 2000; Dahlgren et al. 2003). Evidence for the causal relationship between the presence of HPV and HNSCC incidence comes from prospective studies, indicating increased risk for developing HNSCC in patients who are seropositive for anti-HPV antibodies. In a large, nested case–control study from a Scandinavian cohort of almost 900,000 individuals, HPV-16 seropositivity was observed on the average of 9.4 years prior to the onset of disease and was associated with a 14-fold increased risk of OPSCC (Mork et al. 2001). Recent case–control studies suggest that HPV(+) and (−) tumors have distinct risk factor profile. While HPV(−) tumors had the traditional association with tobacco and alcohol use and poor oral hygiene, HPV(+) HNSCC was independently associated with marijuana exposure and several measures of sexual behavior (such as increasing numbers of lifetime vaginal or oral sex partners, casual sex participation, no barrier use during vaginal or oral sex, and history of a sexually transmitted disease) but not with tobacco or alcohol consumption (D'Souza et al. 2007; Gillison et al. 2008).

Some studies have suggested that HPV-related OPSCC not only represents a molecularly distinct disease but is also associated with a better prognosis (Gillison et al. 2000; Fakhry et al. 2008; Weinberger et al. 2006; Licitra et al. 2006). Figure 2.1 shows the disease-specific survival (DSS) curves for HPV(+) and (−) patients treated at our institution. A recent meta-analysis confirmed that HPV(+) OPSCC patients had a 28% lower risk of death than their negative counterparts (Ragin and Taioli 2007). The reason for this difference in prognosis is unclear but could be related to the distinct molecular and epidemiologic profiles of these tumors. HPV(+) tumors are more likely to be undifferentiated, have basaloid histology, and more frequent nodal metastasis (Fakhry and Gillison 2006). At the molecular level, they

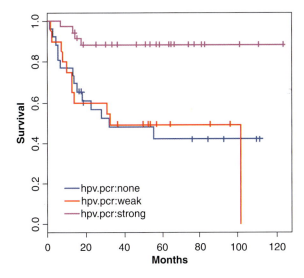

Fig. 2.1. Disease-specific survival for 82 HNSCC patients by HPV status as assessed by pyrosequencing at Stanford University. "HPV PCR none" reflects negative PCR amplification signal for HPV L1 gene ($n = 26$); "HPV PCR weak," very weak PCR amplification signal ($n = 20$); "HPV PCR strong," strong PCR amplification signal ($n = 36$); $p = 0.0005$

are more likely to be p53 wildtype and p16INK4a-positive (Weinberger et al. 2006; Licitra et al. 2006; Fakhry and Gillison 2006). The intact apoptotic response to chemoradiation due to less p53 mutations and functional p16INK4a may explain the improved outcomes for HPV(+) tumors. Other hypotheses for improved outcomes include the lack of field cancerization and enhanced immune surveillance (Fakhry and Gillison 2006). Regardless of the underlying mechanism for improved outcome, such favorable prognosis would have significant implications for therapeutic management and posttreatment surveillance in patients with HPV(+) tumors.

2.3
Staging

Clinical staging is used for OPSCC. Evaluation is based on inspection/palpation of the tumor and neck nodes as well as nasopharyngoscopy. Radiologic assessment of the tumor should include at least a contrast enhanced computed tomography (CT) scan. Magnetic resonance imaging (MRI), which is often less sensitive to dental artefact than is CT, is useful for assessment of the base of tongue, pterygoid muscles, skull base, and mandibular bone marrow. Panendoscopy is routinely done to determine the tumor extent and to rule out a synchronous second primary cancer. The American Joint Committee on Cancer cancer staging system is used worldwide to stage OPSCC for prognosis and treatment recommendations (Greene et al. 2002).

2.3.1
The Role of [18]Fluoro Deoxy-Glucose Positron Emission Topography in OPSCC Management

[18]Fluoro deoxy-glucose positron emission topography (FDG PET)/CT has become a widely used imaging modality for a variety of common malignancies, including OPSCC. The primary utility of FDG PET in OPSCC is for the detection of regional nodal and distant metastases. Several studies have established that FDG PET is superior to physical examination, and CT and MRI scans in determining the extent of involved nodes in patients with clinically enlarged nodes at diagnosis (Adams et al. 1998; Stuckensen et al. 2000; Quon et al. 2007; Branstetter et al. 2005). In general, PET does not play a significant role in the characterization of the primary tumor except for aiding in the detection of the primary tumor site in patients presenting with nodal metastases from an unknown primary site (Hanasono et al. 1999; Menda and Graham 2005). In patients with clinically negative nodal (N0) involvement by clinical examination and CT or MRI, the role of PET in guiding elective neck treatment is uncertain because of its limited resolution and its unacceptably low sensitivity in detecting occult nodal metastases (Hyde et al. 2003; Stoeckli et al. 2002; Schoder et al. 2006). In patients with more advanced tumors, PET is useful and superior to CT for detecting distant spread as well as synchronous tumors (Schwartz et al. 2003; Schmid et al. 2003; Wax et al. 2002). PET is also useful in determining response to chemotherapy and RT. However, several authors have described diminishing specificity in PET scans when performed within 3 months of RT (Andrade et al. 2006; Porceddu et al. 2005). Long-term surveillance may also be accomplished by FDG PET, where it has a higher sensitivity than CT alone.

Integrated FDG PET/CT imaging has provided a logical bridge between anatomical and functional imaging that appears ideally suited not only for

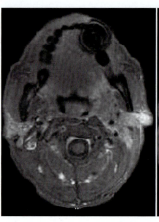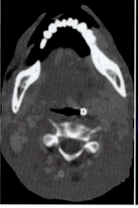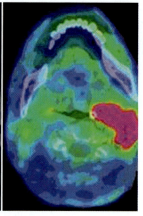

Fig. 2.2. An example of a treatment planning PET-CT scan with contrast in a patient with a T4aN2bM0 left tonsillar squamous cell carcinoma. The figure shows an axial slice across the tumor on a T1-weighted MRI scan with gadolinium, CT scan with contrast and merged PET-CT

diagnostic purposes but also for radiotherapy (RT) planning. PET data can be imported into workstations specific to RT treatment planning. Further, immobilization devices can be used during the acquisition of PET/CT scan in a similar fashion as when performed on dedicated CT scanners and can improve the registration of PET and CT images. Figure 2.2 shows an example of a treatment planning PET-CT scan. Several reports have noted that target volumes may be modified in as many as 20% of cases when using FDG PET/CT vs. CT alone (Ciernik et al. 2003; Ahn and Garg 2008). The target volume may increase in some cases, where the viable tumor fraction is larger than previously noted or smaller, particularly in bulky tumors where the fraction of necrosis may be quite large. These changes in RT planning are in addition to the changes already brought on by the detection of unexpected metastatic disease using PET. Accordingly, PET/CT is commonly used as an adjunctive examination for radiation treatment planning for HN cancers at our institution. Preliminary outcome data from a series of 42 HNSCC patients suggested that the use of FDG PET for RT treatment planning resulted in a high level of disease control combined with favorable toxicity profiles (Vernon et al. 2008). A study from our institution with 82 HNSCC, of which 45 were from the oropharynx, indicated that high metabolic tumor burden as measured by total metabolic tumor volume (MTV, semi-automatically delineated on pretreatment PET scans using a custom software) or total tumor burden (defined as the product of MTV and median standard uptake value) is an adverse prognostic factor for disease recurrence and death in these patients (La et al. 2008) However, since there is still scant outcome data and nonstandardization of contouring methods, PET/CT is not recommended as a prime means of treatment planning, but as an adjunct to contrast enhanced CT and/or MRI.

2.4
Treatment by Stages

Treatment of OPSCC is complex and requires participation of a multidisciplinary team. The extent of the cancer, TNM stages, pathologic findings, and the overall condition of the patient dictate the appropriate therapeutic plan. The main treatment modalities for OPSCC are surgery, radiotherapy, and chemotherapy. More recently, biologically targeted therapy has also emerged as an effective therapy for OPSCC.

2.4.1
Early Stage (Stages I–II)

Either surgery or definitive RT can effectively manage stages I–II OPSCC. The choice of treatment is dictated by functional and cosmetic considerations and the medical team expertise. Several reports have compared the results of surgery and RT and none have found any difference in outcomes between the two modalities (Kramer et al. 1987; Mendenhall et al. 2000a, b). Traditional surgical treatment consists of a wide local excision, followed by a selective neck dissection. The gettec group showed that surgery alone yielded a 5-year locoregional control (LRC) rate of 89%, DSS of 100%, and overall survival (OS) of 73% in 53 T1–2 N0 OPSCC (Cosmidis et al. 2004). Similar results were achieved with definitive RT with a 5-year local control rate of 88% for T1 and 84% for T2 tonsillar carcinomas, and a 5-year DSS of 100% for stage I and 86% for stage

II tumors (MENDENHALL et al. 2006a). Analogous excellent results were also achieved with RT alone for early-stage base-of-tongue cancer with less functional morbidity (MENDENHALL et al. 2006a).

Patients with T1–2N0 tonsillar carcinoma with minimal base of tongue and soft palate involvement can be safely irradiated to the tumor bed and ipsilateral neck alone, thereby sparing the contralateral neck and parotid gland. O'Sullivan et al. reported a 3-year LRC rate of 77% and a contralateral neck failure rate of only 3.5% in 228 tonsillar carcinoma patients treated with ipsilateral neck irradiation alone. Specifically there was no contralateral neck failure in 118 patients with T1–2N0 tumor in that series (O'SULLIVAN et al. 2001). In patients with base-of-tongue, vallecula, or soft palate tumors that require bilateral neck treatment, intensity-modulated radiotherapy (IMRT, discussed in details below) can provide favorable outcomes with less xerostomia. GARDEN et al. (2007) reported a 2-year LRC, recurrence-free, and OS rates of 94, 88, and 94%, respectively, for 51 patients receiving IMRT treatment for T1–2 OPSCC. More important, they were able to achieve a mean dose of <30 Gy to at least one parotid gland in 95% of their patients, thereby preserving some salivary function.

2.4.2
Locally Advanced Stage (Stages III–IV)

2.4.2.1
Surgery and Adjuvant Radiotherapy vs. Radiotherapy or Chemoradiotherapy

Stages III–IV OPSCC can be treated with either surgery and RT or concurrent chemoradiation therapy (CRT). RTOG 73-03 randomized 129 patients with oropharynx and oral cavity SCC to (1) preoperative RT (50 Gy) followed by surgery, (2) surgery followed by postoperative RT (60 Gy), or definitive RT alone (65–70 Gy). There was no significant difference in between the three arms in terms of LRC or OS; however, the study was significantly underpowered to address that question (TUPCHONG et al. 1991). More recently, SOO et al. reported on a phase III randomized study, comparing cisplatin and 5-fluorouracil (5-FU) based CRT vs. surgery and postoperative RT in 119 patients with locally advanced but resectable HNSCC, among whom 21% had OP primaries. The trial was closed prematurely before the targeted accrual of 200 patients because of poor enrolment.

There was no significant difference in survival between the two groups and organ preservation was achieved in 55% of the OPSCC group (SOO et al. 2005).

2.4.2.2
Radiation Fractionation

For many years, RT alone was the main treatment modality for the majority of these patients, mainly for organ preservation. RT treatment intensification with altered fractionation such as accelerated fractionation or hyperfractionation has resulted in improved LRC and disease-free survival. EORTC 22791 randomized 325 patients with T2–3 N0–1 OPSCC to either conventional fractionation (70, 2 Gy/fraction/day over 7 weeks) or hyperfractionation (80.5, 1.15 Gy twice daily [b.i.d] over 7 weeks) (HORIOT et al. 1992). There was a significant improvement in 5-year LRC rate (40 vs. 60%, $p = 0.02$). Specifically, patients with T3 tumors had a trend for higher 5-year survival (30 vs. 40%, $p = 0.08$) if treated with hyperfractionation. RTOG 90-03 randomized 1,113 patients with locally advanced HNSCC, of whom 60% had OP primaries, to (1) standard fractionation (70 Gy/35 fractions/7 weeks), (2) hyperfractionation (81.6 Gy/68 fractions/7 weeks), (3) split-course accelerated fractionation (67.2 Gy/42 fractions/6 weeks), and (4) concomitant boost accelerated fractionation (72 Gy/42 fractions/6 weeks) (FU et al. 2000). Patients treated with hyperfractionation or concomitant boost accelerated fractionation had significantly higher LRC than those treated with conventional fractionation; however, there was no difference in OS. Although most randomized studies did not find a survival advantage with altered fractionation, a meta-analysis using individual patient data found an absolute 5-year survival benefit of 3.4% (hazard ratio, 0.92; 95% CI, 0.86–0.97; $p = 0.003$), favoring altered fractionation, with the largest survival advantage noted for hyperfractionation (8% at 5 years) (BOURHIS et al. 2006).

2.4.2.3
Chemotherapy and Radiation Therapy

Within the last decade, chemoradiation therapy (CRT) has become the main treatment for locally advanced OPSCC. GORTEC 94-01 randomized 226 patients with stages III–IV OPSCC to either conventional RT (70 Gy/7 weeks) or the same RT plus concurrent carboplatin and 5-FU chemotherapy. There was a significant improvement in LRC, disease-free, and overall survival, favoring the chemotherapy arm (CALAIS et al. 1999). The 5-year OS, disease-free survival (DFS), and LRC rates were 22 vs. 16% ($p = 0.05$), 27 vs. 15% ($p = 0.01$), and 48 vs. 25% ($p = 0.002$) for CRT vs. RT arm, respectively (DENIS et al. 2004). Several other randomized studies that included all HNSCC, of which a large proportion of patient had OP primaries, also found a survival advantage with the addition of concurrent chemotherapy (BRIZEL et al. 1998; ADELSTEIN et al. 2003; JEREMIC et al. 1997; BUDACH et al. 2005). A meta-analysis of 10,826 patients with individual data confirmed an absolute 8% survival benefit with the addition of concurrent chemotherapy, with the largest benefit noted for cisplatin-based chemotherapy (PIGNON et al. 2000). These data established the role of CRT as the standard of care for locally advanced OPSCC.

As LRC improves with the addition of concurrent chemotherapy and more refined RT delivery techniques, a higher rate of distant metastasis has been observed in recent series (ARGIRIS et al. 2003). This provides a rationale for re-investigating induction chemotherapy in these patients. Phase 2 studies have shown that the addition of a taxane to a cisplatin/5-FU (PF) platform yielded promising results in unresectable HNSCC (PIGNON et al. 2004). Two large phase III studies in the USA and Europe, both included OPSCC patients and both using a taxane-platinum-5-FU (TPF) platform prior to definitive RT, reported positive survival results in comparison to induction PF. EORTC 24971/TAX 323 randomized 358 patients with unresectable pharyngeal cancer (46% OP) to either TPF or PF every 3 weeks for four cycles followed by RT alone in nonprogressing patients (VERMORKEN et al. 2007). The TPF group had a statistically superior progression-free and overall survival (11 vs. 8 months, 18.8 vs. 14.5 months). TAX 324 randomized 501 patients with HNSCC (52% OP) to three cycles of TPF or PF induction chemotherapy followed by CRT (weekly carboplatin) (POSNER et al. 2007). The estimated 3-year OS was 62 vs. 48%, favoring the TPF group. Patterns of failure study showed superior LRC for the TPF arm without any improvement in distant metastases. TPF was also better tolerated than PF in both studies. However, between 10 & 15% of TAX 323 and 21 & 25% of TAX 324 patients never completed RT as specified in the protocols. Therefore, the role of TPF induction chemotherapy in addition to CRT needs to be further tested in randomized studies and this question is presently being addressed in two international randomized trials.

2.4.2.4
Targeted Therapy

The area of targeted therapy in HNSCC is rapidly growing. A correlative study of RTOG 90-03 showed that overexpression of the epidermal growth factor receptor (EGFR) was an independent predictor of poorer LCR and OS after conventionally fractionated RT (ANG et al. 2002). This preclinical data provided the rationale for a phase III randomized study, comparing RT alone to RT plus cetuximab, an anti-EGFR antibody in 424 patients with locally advanced HNSCC (BONNER et al. 2006). The addition of cetuximab to RT resulted in superior 2-year LCR (50 vs. 41%, $p = 0.005$), progression-free survival (46 vs. 37%, $p = 0.006$) and OS (55 vs. 45%, $p = 0.03$). Subset analysis revealed that patients with OPSCC had the most survival benefit (hazard ratio of 0.62) compared with other sites. Based on these positive findings and the fact that CRT is the currently most accepted treatment approach for patients with stage III–IV HNSCC, a large randomized study (RTOG 0522) has been mounted comparing cisplatin-based CRT alone to the same regimen with cetuximab. This study will address the role of adding cetuximab to standard CRT in HNSCC.

2.4.2.5
Postoperative Treatment: Radiation and Chemoradiation

Well-accepted indications for postoperative radiation therapy (PORT) in patients with OPSCC include T3–4 tumor, multiple pathological nodal involvement (≥ 2 nodes), extracapsular nodal extension (ECE), involved surgical margins, perineural invasion, dermal involvement, and lymphovascular involvement (ANG et al. 2001). A small percentage of patients with clinical stage I–II and most patients with stage III–IV OPSCC will therefore require PORT for these high-risk features if they receive surgery as the initial treatment. It is strongly recommended that PORT be started within 3–6 weeks of surgery. Two large studies indicated that the package time, defined as the time from surgery to the date of PORT completion, should be kept as short as possible in patients with high-risk features (ANG et al. 2001; SANGUINETI et al. 2005). The best LCR and survival was observed for patients with package time <11 weeks, intermediate for 11–13 weeks, and worst for >13 weeks (ANG et al. 2001).

A retrospective analysis of patients treated with PORT on 2 RTOG studies suggests that those who had one or more of the following features: (1) involved surgical margin, (2) ECE, or (3) ≥2 involved node, fared poorly despite appropriate PORT treatment (AL-SARRAF et al. 1998). A small randomized study from France showed that the addition of weekly cisplatin to PORT in patients with ECE resulted in improved disease-free and overall survival (BACHAUD et al. 1996). This data prompted two large randomized studies from the USA (RTOG 95-01) and Europe (EORTC-22931), evaluating the role of cisplatin chemotherapy delivered concurrently with PORT in high-risk patients (COOPER et al. 2004; BERNIER et al. 2004). Although the treatment regimens are identical in both studies, the eligibility criteria were different, resulting in different patient profiles. Both studies showed a significant improvement in LRC and DFS with the addition of cisplatin to PORT in high-risk patients. However, only EORTC found a significant improvement in OS. Pooled analysis of patients in both studies showed that the patients who benefited the most from PORT and chemotherapy were those with ECE and/or involved surgical margins (BERNIER et al. 2005).

2.5 Radiation Therapy Technique: Three-Dimensional Conformal Radiation Therapy vs. Intensity-Modulated Radiotherapy

Intensity-modulated radiotherapy (IMRT) is a refinement of three-dimensional conformal radiation therapy. It utilizes a computerized treatment planning system along with sophisticated delivery machinery to tailor the radiation dose to the tumor target. By subdividing a broad radiation beam into smaller pencil beams and by varying the intensities of these pencil beams, a conformal dose distribution is generated. Tumor coverage is improved and more normal tissue sparing is achieved. Although LRC rates for OPSCC treated with non-IMRT techniques are excellent, both parotid glands are almost always included in the RT portal. As a result, patients suffer from permanent xerostomia, which has a negative impact on nutrition, dentition, communication, and emotional well-being. With parotid-sparing IMRT, patients' quality of life has improved when compared with conventional RT (LIN et al. 2003). CHAO et al. (2001) showed that IMRT significantly reduced the rate of G2–3 xerostomia when compared with conventional RT in patients treated either definitively or postoperatively for OPSCC. We also evaluated the role of IMRT in improving salivary function by administering a validated xerostomia questionnaire to 29 representative IMRT-treated patients and 75 matched conventional-treated patients at the same institution. We found that IMRT-treated patients had less xerostomia (lower score) with the largest difference noted for patients with oral cavity and OP cancers (Fig. 2.3) (DALY et al. 2007).

Dose sculpting and parotid sparing raise a general concern for possible tumor misses with IMRT. However, no clinical reports to date have shown any compromise in local control for OP cancers treated with IMRT. With a median follow-up of 32 months, EISBRUCH et al. (2004) reported a 3-year LRC rate of 94% in 80 OP cancer patients. Over 90% of the patients had stage III or IV disease. CHAO et al.

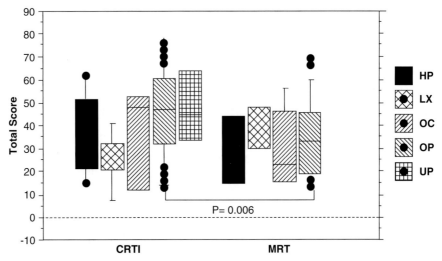

Fig. 2.3. Average xerostomia scores based on a validated xerostomia questionnaire in 29 representative IMRT-treated patients and 75 matched conventionally treated patients at the same institution. *HP* hypopharynx; *LX* larynx; *OC* oral cavity; *OP* oropharynx; *UP* unknown primary

Table 2.1. Results of IMRT for oropharyngeal carcinomas

References	N	Stage	Follow-up (months)	2-Year locoregional control (%)
CHAO et al. (2003)	74	I–IV	33	87
EISBRUCH et al. (2004)	80	I–IV	32	94
DE ARRUDA et al. (2006)	50	I–IV	24	92
HODGE et al. (2007)	52	I–IV	24	96
GARDEN et al. (2007)	51	I–IV[a]	45	93

[a]Primary tumor ≥ 4 cm in maximal dimension

Table 2.2. Dose constraint guidelines for target volume and organ at risk (Adapted and modified from RTOG protocols)

Organ/volume	Constraints	Mean dose
Brachial plexus	≥60 Gy to any point	NS
Brainstem	<54 Gy	NS
Larynx	NS	<45 Gy
Mandible	<70 Gy if no possible then no more than 1 cm³ to exceed 75 Gy	NS
Oral cavity	NS	<40 Gy
Parotid	At least 20 cm³ of the combined volume of both parotid <20 Gy or at least 50% of the volume of one parotid <30 Gy	≥26 Gy (at least one gland)
Postcricoid pharynx	NS	<45 Gy
Spinal cord	<48 Gy to any volume larger than 0.03 cm³	NS
Unspecified tissue outside the target volume	≥5% can receive greater than the dose to CTV[a]	NS
PTV[b]	No more than 20% will receive > 100% of the prescribed dose	NS
	No more than 1% will receive < 93% of the prescribed dose	
	No more than 1% or 1 cm³ of the tissue outside the PTV will receive > 110% of the prescribed dose	

NS not specified
[a]Clinical target volume
[b]Planning target volume

(2004) reported a local control rate of 87% using IMRT in 74 patients with OP cancer. In this report, 46% had T3/T4 tumors and 76% of the patients had stage III/IV disease. Other centers also reported excellent LRC rates. De Arruda et al. (2006) noted a 100% tumor control rate at a median follow-up of 24 months. An update with a median follow-up of 31 months continues to show excellent local control in this patient cohort (LEE et al. 2006). Table 2.1 shows a summary of IMRT results for OPSCC. A multi-institutional RTOG study, H-0022, using IMRT for early-stage OP cancer has completed accrual. The protocol tests the transportability of IMRT to multiple institutions. Preliminary results have been presented at an American Society of Therapeutic Radiation Oncology (ASTRO) meeting showing low IMRT violation rates and reduced xerostomia when compared with historical controls (EISBRUCH et al. 2006). This protocol also provides useful dose constraint guidelines for target volume and organ (Table 2.2). Figure 2.4 shows an example of an IMRT plan for an OP cancer.

2.6
Treatment-Related Toxicities

2.6.1
Acute Toxicities

The most common acute RT-related toxicities include dermatitis, taste impairment, pain, weight loss, and fatigue, with mucositis being perhaps the most debilitating side effect. The addition of concurrent chemotherapy has been shown to enhance mucositis (CALAIS et al. 1999). Care must be taken to minimize these incapacitating side effects. Smoking cessation is a must as studies have shown that cigarette smoking can increase the severity and the duration of the mucosal reactions and interfere with oncologic outcome if continued during RT (BROWMAN et al. 1993). Clinical practice guidelines exist for the prevention and management of oral mucositis (KEEFE et al. 2007). These include meticulous, systematic oral care hygiene with brushing, flossing, bland rinses and moisturizer, regular assessment of oral pain, early intervention with topical and systemic analgesics to promote oral comfort and involvement of a multidisciplinary team (nurses, physician, dentist, nutritionist).

Several agents have been shown to be promising in reducing mucositis in small phase II or observational studies, only to be negated in large randomized phase III trials. These include sucralfate (Dodd et al. 2003), antimicrobial lozenges (Trotti et al. 2004; El-Sayed et al. 2002), amifostine (Buentzel et al. 2006; Brizel et al. 2000), GMCSF (Ryu et al. 2007), pilocarpine (Scarantino et al. 2006; Warde et al. 2002) and aloe vera (Su et al. 2004). The use of zinc sulfate during RT may reduce severe mucositis as suggested by two small trials, but needs to be confirmed in a larger setting (Ertekin et al. 2004; Lin et al. 2006). A comprehensive review of the oral mucositis trials has been performed by the Cochrane Group (Worthington et al. 2007).

Recently, palifermin (@Kepivance), a recombinant human keratinocyte growth factor, has been shown to reduce the duration and severity of oral mucositis after intensive chemotherapy and RT in preparation for autologous hematopoietic stem cell transplantation in patients with hematologic malignancies (Spielberger et al. 2004). It has also been shown to reduce the incidence of WHO II or higher oral mucositis in patients with metastatic colorectal cancer treated with 5-FU-based chemotherapy in a small randomized study (Rosen et al. 2006). These results prompted a few randomized trials in HNSCC, two for patients receiving definitive CRT and one for patients receiving postoperative CRT for high-risk features. Two studies have been completed and one is still accruing patients. The results of these studies will define the role of palifermin in the management of oral mucositis in HNSCC.

2.6.2
Late Toxicities

Late toxicities, though less common, can be irreversible and unpredictable; therefore application of preventive measures and vigilant surveillance for these toxicities are critical. A higher incidence of aspiration has been noted with treatment intensification. Between a third to half of the patients treated for locally advanced OPSCC develop silent aspiration and up to a third have severe dysphagia after therapy (Nguyen et al. 2007, 2008). Swallowing therapy during and after treatment can be effective in minimizing dysphagia and reduce the need for tube feedings (Nguyen et al. 2007). Dose distribution studies have suggested a correlation between aspiration/dysphagia symptoms and RT dose to the pharyngeal constrictors and supraglottic larynx (Feng et al. 2007; Eisbruch et al. 2007). These observed dose–response relationships suggest that reducing the doses to these structures with either IMRT or brachytherapy may help to minimize the development of long-term dysphagia.

A common late toxicity is xerostomia due to RT damages to the salivary gland tissues. As indicated above, IMRT has been shown to be superior to conventional therapy in preserving salivary function in OPSCC patients without compromising tumor curability. Since parotid function has been shown to substantially decrease after a mean dose of >26 Gy, the recommendation is to limit the mean dose of one gland to <26 Gy for preservation of stimulated saliva (Eisbruch et al. 1999, 2003). As the submandibular glands are responsible for basal saliva secretion, there is increasing interest to also minimize the dose to these glands. Murdoch-Kinch et al. (2008) showed that above a mean dose of 39 Gy, there is no recovery in submandibular gland function, whereas recovery over time was noted when mean dose was kept below 39 Gy. These results have identified a threshold dose for submandibular glands; however, extreme caution must be exercised when sparing the submandibular gland to ensure no tumor misses due to the gland's proximity to the level II nodes.

In addition to IMRT, the addition of intravenous amifostine to conventional RT has been shown to reduce acute side effects and xerostomia in a large randomized study of 315 HNSCC (Brizel et al. 2000). However, the inconvenient route of administration, high cost of the drug, and daily IV infusion procedure, as well as associated side effects of nausea/vomiting, have limited its use.

An emerging late RT complication is carotid stenosis from neck irradiation. In a study of 40 patients treated with unilateral neck irradiation, ultrasound and CT angiography revealed more carotid stenosis and more high-grade stenosis in the irradiated neck compared with the untreated neck, especially for doses ≥50 Gy (Martin et al. 2005). These findings were substantiated in another study, which found that neck dissection also contributed to the increased risk of carotid stenosis (Brown et al. 2005). Therefore, for long-term survivors after RT, especially for those who also had neck dissection, RT dose >50 Gy and/or symptomatic, ultrasonographic carotid artery screening should be considered.

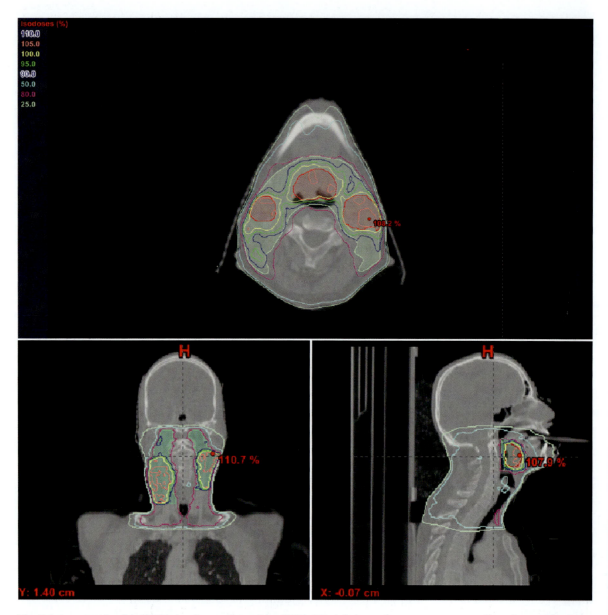

Fig. 2.4. An example of an IMRT plan for a patient with a T1N2cM0 right base of tongue squamous cell carcinoma. The figure shows an axial, coronal, and sagittal view of the plan. Dose–volume histogram and dose statistics are also included

Oropharynx: Epidemiology and Treatment Outcome

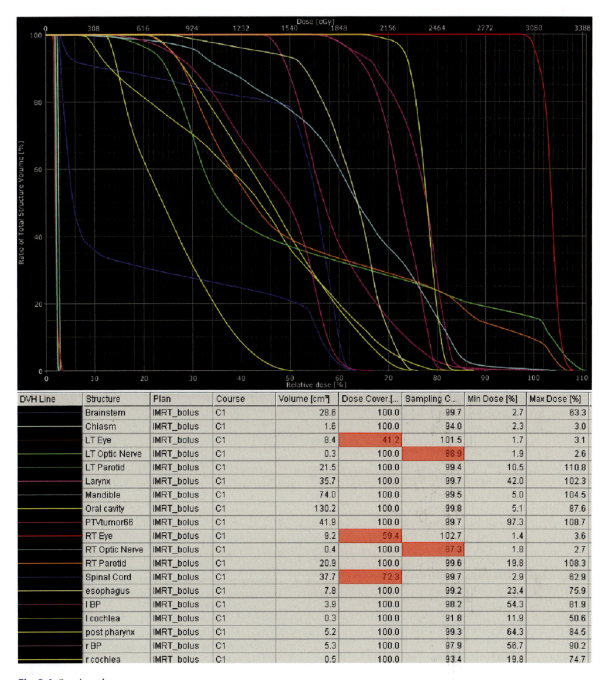

Fig. 2.4. Continued.

2.7 Conclusion

OPSCC is a highly curable cancer. The therapeutic options are expanding as more is learned about the molecular profiles ans prognosis. Although standard treatments of OPSCC still consist of traditional therapeutic approaches such as surgery, RT, and chemotherapy, molecularly targeted therapy is becoming prominent in their management. Major advances in radiation delivery also hold promises of decreasing late toxicity and improving quality of life in these patients. Since HPV-related OPSCC is emerging as a new entity with distinct pathogenesis, molecular profile, and highly favorable prognosis, it is now time to conduct separate clinical trials for these tumors to avoid overtreating many of these patients.

Abbreviations

AJCC	American Joint Committee on Cancer
ASTRO	American Society of Therapeutic Radiation Oncology
CRT	Chemoradiation therapy
CT	Computed tomography scan
DFS	Disease-free survival
DSS	Disease-specific survival
ECE	Extracapsular nodal extension
EGFR	Epidermal growth factor receptor
FDG PET	Fluoro deoxy glucose positron emission tomography
HN	Head and neck
HPV	Human papillomavirus
IMRT	Intensity modulated radiotherapy
LRC	Locoregional control
MRI	Magnetic resonance imaging
MTV	Metabolic tumor volume
OP	Oropharynx
OS	Overall survival
OPSCC	Oropharynx squamous cell carcinoma
PF	Cisplatin/5-FU
PORT	Postoperative radiation therapy
RT	Radiation therapy
SCC	Squamous cell carcinoma
SUV	Standard uptake value
TPF	Taxane-platinum-5-FU
WHO	World health organization
3DCRT	3-Dimensional conformal radiation therapy
5-FU	5-Fluoruracil

References

Adams S, Baum RP, Stuckensen T et al. (1998) Prospective comparison of 18F-FDG PET with conventional imaging modalities (CT, MRI, US) in lymph node staging of head and neck cancer. Eur J Nucl Med 25:1255–1260

Adelstein DJ, Li Y, Adams GL et al. (2003) An intergroup phase III comparison of standard radiation therapy and two schedules of concurrent chemoradiotherapy in patients with unresectable squamous cell head and neck cancer. J Clin Oncol 21:92–98

Ahn PH, Garg MK (2008) Positron emission tomography/computed tomography for target delineation in head and neck cancers. Semin Nucl Med 38:141–148

Al-Sarraf M, LeBlanc M, Giri PG et al. (1998) Chemoradiotherapy versus radiotherapy in patients with advanced nasopharyngeal cancer: a phase III randomized intergroup study 0099. J Clin Oncol 16:1310–1317

Andrade RS, Heron DE, Degirmenci B et al. (2006) Posttreatment assessment of response using FDG-PET/CT for patients treated with definitive radiation therapy for head and neck cancers. Int J Radiat Oncol Biol Phys 65:1315–1322

Ang KK, Berkey BA, Tu X et al. (2002) Impact of epidermal growth factor receptor expression on survival and pattern of relapse in patients with advanced head and neck carcinoma. Cancer Res 62:7350–7356

Ang KK, Trotti A, Brown BW et al. (2001) Randomized trial addressing risk features and time factors of surgery plus radiotherapy in advanced head-and-neck cancer. Int J Radiat Oncol Biol Phys 51(3):571–578

Argiris A, Haraf DJ, Kies MS et al. (2003) Intensive concurrent chemoradiotherapy for head and neck cancer with 5-Fluorouracil- and hydroxyurea-based regimens: reversing a pattern of failure. Oncologist 8:350–360

Bachaud JM, Cohen-Jonathan E, Alzieu C et al. (1996) Combined postoperative radiotherapy and weekly cisplatin infusion for locally advanced head and neck carcinoma: final report of a randomized trial. Int J Radiat Oncol Biol Phys 36:999–1004

Bernier J, Cooper JS, Pajak TF et al. (2005) Defining risk levels in locally advanced head and neck cancers: a comparative analysis of concurrent postoperative radiation plus chemotherapy trials of the EORTC (#22931) and RTOG (# 9501). Head Neck 27:843–850

Bernier J, Domenge C, Ozsahin M et al. (2004) Postoperative irradiation with or without concomitant chemotherapy for locally advanced head and neck cancer. N Engl J Med 350:1945–1952

Bonner JA, Harari PM, Giralt J et al. (2006) Radiotherapy plus cetuximab for squamous-cell carcinoma of the head and neck. N Engl J Med 354:567–578

Bourhis J, Overgaard J, Audry H et al. (2006) Hyperfractionated or accelerated radiotherapy in head and neck cancer: a meta-analysis. Lancet 368:843–854

Branstetter BFt, Blodgett TM, Zimmer LA et al. (2005) Head and neck malignancy: is PET/CT more accurate than PET or CT alone? Radiology 235:580–586

Brizel DM, Albers ME, Fisher SR et al. (1998) Hyperfractionated irradiation with or without concurrent chemotherapy for locally advanced head and neck cancer. N Engl J Med 338:1798–1804

Brizel DM, Wasserman TH, Henke M et al. (2000) Phase III randomized trial of amifostine as a radioprotector in head and neck cancer. J Clin Oncol 18:3339–3345

Browman GP, Wong G, Hodson I et al. (1993) Influence of cigarette smoking on the efficacy of radiation therapy in head and neck cancer. N Engl J Med 328:159–163

Brown PD, Foote RL, McLaughlin MP et al. (2005) A historical prospective cohort study of carotid artery stenosis after radiotherapy for head and neck malignancies. Int J Radiat Oncol Biol Phys 63:1361–1367

Budach V, Stuschke M, Budach W et al. (2005) Hyperfractionated accelerated chemoradiation with concurrent fluorouracil-mitomycin is more effective than dose-escalated hyperfractionated accelerated radiation therapy alone in locally advanced head and neck cancer: final results of the radiotherapy cooperative clinical trials group of the German Cancer Society 95-06 Prospective Randomized Trial. J Clin Oncol 23:1125–1135

Buentzel J, Micke O, Adamietz IA et al. (2006) Intravenous amifostine during chemoradiotherapy for head-and-neck cancer: a randomized placebo-controlled phase III study. Int J Radiat Oncol Biol Phys 64:684–691

Calais G, Alfonsi M, Bardet E et al. (1999) Randomized trial of radiation therapy versus concomitant chemotherapy and radiation therapy for advanced-stage oropharynx carcinoma. J Natl Cancer Inst 91:2081–2086

Castellsague X, Quintana MJ, Martinez MC et al. (2004) The role of type of tobacco and type of alcoholic beverage in oral carcinogenesis. Int J Cancer 108:741–749

Chao KS, Majhail N, Huang CJ et al. (2001) Intensity-modulated radiation therapy reduces late salivary toxicity without compromising tumor control in patients with oropharyngeal carcinoma: a comparison with conventional techniques. Radiat Oncol 61:275–280

Chao KS, Ozyigit G, Blanco AI et al. (2004) Intensity-modulated radiation therapy for oropharyngeal carcinoma: impact of tumor volume. Int J Radiat Oncol Biol Phys 59:43–50

Chao KS, Ozyigit G, Tran BN et al. (2003) Patterns of failure in patients receiving definitive and postoperative IMRT for head-and-neck cancer. Int J Radiat Oncol Biol Phys 55:312–321

Ciernik IF, Dizendorf E, Baumert BG et al. (2003) Radiation treatment planning with an integrated positron emission and computer tomography (PET/CT): a feasibility study. Int J Radiat Oncol Biol Phys 57:853–863

Cooper JS, Pajak TF, Forastiere AA et al. (2004) Postoperative concurrent radiotherapy and chemotherapy for high-risk squamous-cell carcinoma of the head and neck. N Engl J Med 350:1937–1944

Cosmidis A, Rame JP, Dassonville O et al. (2004) T1-T2 N0 oropharyngeal cancers treated with surgery alone. A GETTEC study. Eur Arch Otorhinolaryngol 261:276–281

D'Souza G, Kreimer AR, Viscidi R et al. (2007) Case–control study of human papillomavirus and oropharyngeal cancer. N Engl J Med 356:1944–1956

Dahlgren L, Mellin H, Wangsa D et al. (2003) Comparative genomic hybridization analysis of tonsillar cancer reveals a different pattern of genomic imbalances in human papillomavirus-positive and negative tumors. Int J Cancer 107:244–249

Dai M, Clifford GM, le Calvez F et al. (2004) Human papillomavirus type 16 and TP53 mutation in oral cancer: matched analysis of the IARC multicenter study. Cancer Res 64:468–471

Daly ME, Lieskovsky Y, Pawlicki T et al. (2007) Evaluation of patterns of failure and subjective salivary function in patients treated with intensity modulated radiotherapy for head and neck squamous cell carcinoma. Head Neck 29:211–220

de Arruda FF, Puri DR, Zhung J et al. (2006) Intensity-modulated radiation therapy for the treatment of oropharyngeal carcinoma: the Memorial Sloan-Kettering Cancer Center experience. Int J Radiat Oncol Biol Phys 64:363–373

Denis F, Garaud P, Bardet E et al. (2004) Final results of the 94-01 French Head and Neck Oncology and Radiotherapy Group randomized trial comparing radiotherapy alone with concomitant radiochemotherapy in advanced-stage oropharynx carcinoma. J Clin Oncol 22:69–76

Dodd MJ, Miaskowski C, Greenspan D et al. (2003) Radiation-induced mucositis: a randomized clinical trial of micronized sucralfate versus salt & soda mouthwashes. Cancer Invest 21:21–33

Eisbruch A, Dawson LA, Kim HM et al. (1999) Conformal and intensity modulated irradiation of head and neck cancer: the potential for improved target irradiation, salivary gland function, and quality of life. Acta Otorhinolaryngol Belg 53 271–275

Eisbruch A, Harris J, Garden A et al. (2006) Phase II Muti-Institutional Study of IMRT for oropharyngeal cancer (RTOG 00-22): early results. American Society of Therapeutic Radiology and Oncology, PA. Int J Radiat Oncol Biol Phys 66:S46–S47; Abstract 79

Eisbruch A, Levendag PC, Feng FY et al. (2007) Can IMRT or brachytherapy reduce dysphagia associated with chemoradiotherapy of head and neck cancer? The Michigan and Rotterdam experiences. Int J Radiat Oncol Biol Phys 69:S40–S42

Eisbruch A, Marsh LH, Dawson LA et al. (2004) Recurrences near base of skull after IMRT for head-and-neck cancer: implications for target delineation in high neck and for parotid gland sparing. Int J Radiat Oncol Biol Phys 59:28–42

Eisbruch A, Ship JA, Dawson LA et al. (2003) Salivary gland sparing and improved target irradiation by conformal and intensity modulated irradiation of head and neck cancer. World J Surg 27:832–837

El-Sayed S, Nabid A, Shelley W et al. (2002) Prophylaxis of radiation-associated mucositis in conventionally treated patients with head and neck cancer: a double-blind, phase III, randomized, controlled trial evaluating the clinical efficacy of an antimicrobial lozenge using a validated mucositis scoring system. J Clin Oncol 20:3956–3963

Ernster JA, Sciotto CG, O'Brien MM et al. (2007) Rising incidence of oropharyngeal cancer and the role of oncogenic human papilloma virus. Laryngoscope 117:2115–2128

Ertekin MV, Koc M, Karslioglu I et al. (2004) Zinc sulfate in the prevention of radiation-induced oropharyngeal mucositis: a prospective, placebo-controlled, randomized study. Int J Radiat Oncol Biol Phys 58:167–174

Fakhry C, Gillison ML (2006) Clinical implications of human papillomavirus in head and neck cancers. J Clin Oncol 24:2606–2611

Fakhry C, Westra WH, Li S et al. (2008) Improved survival of patients with human papillomavirus-positive head and neck squamous cell carcinoma in a prospective clinical trial. J Natl Cancer Inst 100:261–269

Feng FY, Kim HM, Lyden TH et al. (2007) Intensity-modulated radiotherapy of head and neck cancer aiming to reduce dysphagia: early dose-effect relationships for the swallowing structures. Int J Radiat Oncol Biol Phys 68:1289–1298

Fu KK, Pajak TF, Trotti A et al. (2000) A Radiation Therapy Oncology Group (RTOG) phase III randomized study to compare hyperfractionation and two variants of accelerated fractionation to standard fractionation radiotherapy for head and neck squamous cell carcinomas: first report of RTOG 9003. Int J Radiat Oncol Biol Phys 48:7–16

Garden AS, Morrison WH, Wong PF et al. (2007) Disease-control rates following intensity-modulated radiation therapy for small primary oropharyngeal carcinoma. Int J Radiat Oncol Biol Phys 67:438–444

Gillison ML, D'Souza G, Westra W et al. (2008) Distinct risk factor profiles for human papillomavirus type 16-positive and human papillomavirus type 16-negative head and neck cancers. J Natl Cancer Inst 100:407–420

Gillison ML, Koch WM, Capone RB et al. (2000) Evidence for a causal association between human papillomavirus and a subset of head and neck cancers. J Natl Cancer Inst 92:709–720

Gillison ML, Shah KV (2001) Human papillomavirus-associated head and neck squamous cell carcinoma: mounting evidence for an etiologic role for human papillomavirus in a subset of head and neck cancers. Curr Opin Oncol 13:183–188

Greene FL, Page DL, Fleming ID (2002) AJCC cancer staging manual, 6th edn. Springer, New York

Hanasono MM, Kunda LD, Segall GM et al. (1999) Uses and limitations of FDG positron emission tomography in patients with head and neck cancer. Laryngoscope 109:880–885

Hodge CW, Bentzen SM, Wong G et al. (2007) Are we influencing outcome in oropharynx cancer with intensity-modulated radiotherapy? an inter-era comparison. Int J Radiat Oncol Biol Phys 69:1032–1041

Horiot JC, Le Fur R, N'Guyen T et al. (1992) Hyperfractionation versus conventional fractionation in oropharyngeal carcinoma: final analysis of a randomized trial of the EORTC cooperative group of radiotherapy. Radiother Oncol 25:231–241

Hyde NC, Prvulovich E, Newman L et al. (2003) A new approach to pre-treatment assessment of the N0 neck in oral squamous cell carcinoma: the role of sentinel node biopsy and positron emission tomography. Oral Oncol 39:350–360

Jemal A, Siegel R, Ward E, et al. (2008) Cancer statistics, 2008. CA Cancer J Clin 58:71–96

Jeremic B, Shibamoto Y, Stanisavljevic B et al. (1997) Radiation therapy alone or with concurrent low-dose daily either cisplatin or carboplatin in locally advanced unresectable squamous cell carcinoma of the head and neck: a prospective randomized trial. Radiother Oncol 43:29–37

Keefe DM, Schubert MM, Elting LS et al. (2007) Updated clinical practice guidelines for the prevention and treatment of mucositis. Cancer 109:820–831

Kramer S, Gelber RD, Snow JB et al. (1987) Combined radiation therapy and surgery in the management of advanced head and neck cancer: final report of study 73–03 of the Radiation Therapy Oncology Group. Head Neck Surg 10:19–30

La TH, Filion EJ, Turnbull BB et al. (2008) Metabolic tumor burden predicts for recurrence and death in head and neck cancer. American Society of Therapeutic Radiology and Oncology, Boston

Lee NY, de Arruda FF, Puri DR et al. (2006) A comparison of intensity-modulated radiation therapy and concomitant boost radiotherapy in the setting of concurrent chemotherapy for locally advanced oropharyngeal carcinoma. Int J Radiat Oncol Biol Phys 66:966–974

Licitra L, Perrone F, Bossi P et al. (2006) High-risk human papillomavirus affects prognosis in patients with surgically treated oropharyngeal squamous cell carcinoma. J Clin Oncol 24:5630–5636

Lin A, Kim HM, Terrell JE et al. (2003) Quality of life after parotid-sparing IMRT for head-and-neck cancer: a prospective longitudinal study. Int J Radiat Oncol Biol Phys 57:61–70

Lin LC, Que J, Lin LK et al. (2006) Zinc supplementation to improve mucositis and dermatitis in patients after radiotherapy for head-and-neck cancers: a double-blind, randomized study. Int J Radiat Oncol Biol Phys 65:745–750

Martin JD, Buckley AR, Graeb D et al. (2005) Carotid artery stenosis in asymptomatic patients who have received unilateral head-and-neck irradiation. Int J Radiat Oncol Biol Phys 63:1197–1205

Menda Y, Graham MM (2005) Update on 18F-fluorodeoxyglucose/positron emission tomography and positron emission tomography/computed tomography imaging of squamous head and neck cancers. Semin Nucl Med 35:214–219

Mendenhall WM, Amdur RJ, Stringer SP et al. (2000a) Radiation therapy for squamous cell carcinoma of the tonsillar region: a preferred alternative to surgery? J Clin Oncol 18:2219–2225

Mendenhall WM, Stringer SP, Amdur RJ et al. (2000b) Is radiation therapy a preferred alternative to surgery for squamous cell carcinoma of the base of tongue? J Clin Oncol 18: 35–42

Mendenhall WM, Morris CG, Amdur RJ et al. (2006a) Definitive radiotherapy for tonsillar squamous cell carcinoma. Am J Clin Oncol 29:290–297

Mork J, Lie AK, Glattre E et al. (2001) Human papillomavirus infection as a risk factor for squamous-cell carcinoma of the head and neck. N Engl J Med 344:1125–1131

Murdoch-Kinch CA, Kim HM, Vineberg KA et al. (2008) Dose-effect relationships for the submandibular salivary glands and implications for their sparing by intensity modulated radiotherapy. Int J Radiat Oncol Biol Phys 72(2):373–382

Nguyen NP, Frank C, Moltz CC et al. (2008) Dysphagia severity and aspiration following postoperative radiation for locally advanced oropharyngeal cancer. Anticancer Res 28: 431–434

Nguyen NP, Moltz CC, Frank C et al. (2007) Impact of swallowing therapy on aspiration rate following treatment for locally advanced head and neck cancer. Oral Oncol 43: 352–357

O'Sullivan B, Warde P, Grice B et al. (2001) The benefits and pitfalls of ipsilateral radiotherapy in carcinoma of the tonsillar region. Int J Radiat Oncol Biol Phys 51:332–343

Parkin DM, Bray F, Ferlay J et al. (2001) Estimating the world cancer burden: globocan 2000. Int J Cancer 94:153–156

Pignon JP, Bourhis J, Domenge C et al. (2000) Chemotherapy added to locoregional treatment for head and neck squamous-cell carcinoma: three meta-analyses of updated individual data. MACH-NC Collaborative Group. Meta-analysis of chemotherapy on head and neck cancer. Lancet 355: 949–955

Pignon JP, Syz N, Posner M et al. (2004) Adjusting for patient selection suggests the addition of docetaxel to 5-fluorouracil-cisplatin induction therapy may offer survival benefit in squamous cell cancer of the head and neck. Anticancer Drugs 15:331–340

Porceddu SV, Jarmolowski E, Hicks RJ et al. (2005) Utility of positron emission tomography for the detection of disease in residual neck nodes after (chemo)radiotherapy in head and neck cancer. Head Neck 27:175–181

Posner MR, Hershock DM, Blajman CR et al. (2007) Cisplatin and fluorouracil alone or with docetaxel in head and neck cancer. N Engl J Med 357:1705–1715

Quon A, Fischbein NJ, McDougall IR et al. (2007) Clinical role of 18F-FDG PET/CT in the management of squamous cell carcinoma of the head and neck and thyroid carcinoma. J Nucl Med 48(Suppl 1):58S–67S

Ragin CC, Taioli E (2007) Survival of squamous cell carcinoma of the head and neck in relation to human papillomavirus infection: review and meta-analysis. Int J Cancer 121:1813–1820

Rosen LS, Abdi E, Davis ID et al. (2006) Palifermin reduces the incidence of oral mucositis in patients with metastatic colorectal cancer treated with fluorouracil-based chemotherapy. J Clin Oncol 24:5194–5200

Rosenquist K (2005) Risk factors in oral and oropharyngeal squamous cell carcinoma: a population-based case–control study in southern Sweden. Swed Dent J Suppl (179):1–66

Ryu JK, Swann S, LeVeque F et al. (2007) The impact of concurrent granulocyte macrophage-colony stimulating factor on radiation-induced mucositis in head and neck cancer patients: a double-blind placebo-controlled prospective phase III study by Radiation Therapy Oncology Group 9901. Int J Radiat Oncol Biol Phys 67:643–650

Sanguineti G, Richetti A, Bignardi M et al. (2005) Accelerated versus conventional fractionated postoperative radiotherapy for advanced head and neck cancer: results of a multicenter Phase III study. Int J Radiat Oncol Biol Phys 61:762–771

Scarantino C, LeVeque F, Swann RS et al. (2006) Effect of pilocarpine during radiation therapy: results of RTOG 97-09, a phase III randomized study in head and neck cancer patients. J Support Oncol 4:252–258

Schmid DT, Stoeckli SJ, Bandhauer F et al. (2003) Impact of positron emission tomography on the initial staging and therapy in locoregional advanced squamous cell carcinoma of the head and neck. Laryngoscope 113:888–891

Schoder H, Carlson DL, Kraus DH et al. (2006) 18F-FDG PET/CT for detecting nodal metastases in patients with oral cancer staged N0 by clinical examination and CT/MRI. J Nucl Med 47:755–762

Schwartz DL, Rajendran J, Yueh B et al. (2003) Staging of head and neck squamous cell cancer with extended-field FDG-PET. Arch Otolaryngol Head Neck Surg 129:1173–1178

Soo KC, Tan EH, Wee J et al. (2005) Surgery and adjuvant radiotherapy vs concurrent chemoradiotherapy in stage III/IV nonmetastatic squamous cell head and neck cancer: a randomised comparison. Br J Cancer 93:279–286

Spielberger R, Stiff P, Bensinger W et al. (2004) Palifermin for oral mucositis after intensive therapy for hematologic cancers. N Engl J Med 351:2590–2598

Stoeckli SJ, Steinert H, Pfaltz M et al. (2002) Is there a role for positron emission tomography with 18F-fluorodeoxyglucose in the initial staging of nodal negative oral and oropharyngeal squamous cell carcinoma. Head Neck 24:345–349

Stuckensen T, Kovacs AF, Adams S et al. (2000) Staging of the neck in patients with oral cavity squamous cell carcinomas: a prospective comparison of PET, ultrasound, CT and MRI. J Craniomaxillofac Surg 28:319–324

Sturgis EM, Cinciripini PM (2007) Trends in head and neck cancer incidence in relation to smoking prevalence: an emerging epidemic of human papillomavirus-associated cancers? Cancer 110:1429–1435

Su CK, Mehta V, Ravikumar L et al. (2004) Phase II double-blind randomized study comparing oral aloe vera versus placebo to prevent radiation-related mucositis in patients with head-and-neck neoplasms. Int J Radiat Oncol Biol Phys 60:171–177

Trotti A, Garden A, Warde P et al. (2004) A multinational, randomized phase III trial of iseganan HCl oral solution for reducing the severity of oral mucositis in patients receiving radiotherapy for head-and-neck malignancy. Int J Radiat Oncol Biol Phys 58:674–681

Tupchong L, Scott CB, Blitzer PH et al. (1991) Randomized study of preoperative versus postoperative radiation therapy in advanced head and neck carcinoma: long-term follow-up of RTOG study 73-03. Int J Radiat Oncol Biol Phys 20:21–28

Vermorken JB, Remenar E, van Herpen C et al. (2007) Cisplatin, fluorouracil, and docetaxel in unresectable head and neck cancer. N Engl J Med 357:1695–1704

Vernon MR, Maheshwari M, Schultz CJ et al. (2008) Clinical outcomes of patients receiving integrated PET/CT-guided radiotherapy for head and neck carcinoma. Int J Radiat Oncol Biol Phys 70:678–684

Warde P, O'Sullivan B, Aslanidis J et al. (2002) A phase III placebo-controlled trial of oral pilocarpine in patients undergoing radiotherapy for head-and-neck cancer. Int J Radiat Oncol Biol Phys 54:9–13

Wax MK, Myers LL, Gabalski EC et al. (2002) Positron emission tomography in the evaluation of synchronous lung lesions in patients with untreated head and neck cancer. Arch Otolaryngol Head Neck Surg 128:703–707

Weinberger PM, Yu Z, Haffty BG et al. (2006) Molecular classification identifies a subset of human papillomavirus–associated oropharyngeal cancers with favorable prognosis. J Clin Oncol 24:736–747

Worthington HV, Clarkson JE, Eden OB (2007) Interventions for preventing oral mucositis for patients with cancer receiving treatment. Cochrane Database Syst Rev:CD000978

Zhang ZF, Morgenstern H, Spitz MR et al. (1999) Marijuana use and increased risk of squamous cell carcinoma of the head and neck. Cancer Epidemiol Biomarkers Prev 8:1071–1078

Hypopharynx

3

GREGORY M. RICHARDS and PAUL M. HARARI

C O N T E N T S

3.1 Introduction *31*

3.2 Epidemiology and Etiology *32*

3.3 Staging *32*

3.4 Patterns of Spread *33*

3.5 Clinical Presentation *33*

3.6 Treatment Strategies *33*
3.6.1 Primary Surgical Therapy *33*
3.6.2 Definitive Radiation or Chemoradiation Therapy *33*
3.6.3 Radiation Therapy with Molecular Targeted Agents *34*
3.6.4 Induction Chemotherapy *34*
3.6.5 Postoperative Adjuvant Radiation or Chemoradiation Therapy *34*
3.6.6 Neck Dissection Following Definitive Radiation of Chemoradiation *35*

3.7 Quality of Life *35*
3.7.1 Quality Of Life in Head and Neck Trials With Regard to Larynx Preservation *36*
3.7.2 Altered Fractionation Regimens and Quality Of Life *37*
3.7.3 Evolution of Quality of Life from Diagnosis to Long-Term Follow-up *37*
3.7.4 Relative Health-Related Quality of Life in Hypopharyngeal Squamous Cell Carcinoma Compared with Other Head and Neck Sites *38*
3.7.5 The Impact of Intensity-Modulated Radiotherapy on Quality of Life *38*

3.8 Conclusion *39*

References *39*

GREGORY M. RICHARDS, MD
Department of Human Oncology, University of Wisconsin School of Medicine, 600 Highland Avenue, Madison, WI 53792, USA
PAUL M. HARARI, MD
Department of Human Oncology, University of Wisconsin School of Medicine, 600 Highland Avenue, Madison, WI 53792, USA

KEY POINTS

- Hypopharyngeal cancer is a relatively infrequent subset of head and neck cancer.
- Hypopharynx tumors generally present at advanced stage and have a poor prognosis relative to other head and neck cancer subsites.
- Single modality therapy can be considered for early-stage disease whereas multimodality therapy is generally recommended for advanced stage disease.
- Five-year overall survival ranges from 50 to 70% for stage I, 35–60% for stage II, 25–40% for stage III, and 5–30% for stage IV disease.
- Overall quality of life can be significantly affected by hypopharyngeal cancer, with profound impact on speech, swallowing, and social interactions.
- Modern radiation, surgical, and systemic therapy strategies hold promise to improve quality of life.

3.1
Introduction

Hypopharyngeal cancer is a relatively uncommon subset of head and neck (HN) cancer that includes primary tumors originating in the pyriform sinus, postcricoid region, and posterior pharyngeal wall. Patients with hypopharyngeal cancer tend to have a worse prognosis than do patients with cancer at other subsites within the HN. They commonly present with locoregionally advanced disease requiring multimodality therapy with associated morbidity that can significantly influence patient quality of life

(QOL). In light of close proximity to or direct involvement of the larynx, hypopharyngeal cancer, and the treatment required, often compromises speech and swallow functions. In this chapter we focus primarily on squamous cell carcinoma of the hypopharynx and specific QOL issues that impact these patients.

3.2
Epidemiology and Etiology

Approximately 2,500–3,000 cases of hypopharyngeal cancer are diagnosed annually in the USA, making this a relatively uncommon entity. The pyriform sinus is the most common subsite of origin, comprising 65–75% of hypopharynx cases (CARPENTER and DESANTO 1977), followed by the posterior pharyngeal wall (10–20%) and the postcricoid region (5–15%) (BARNES and JOHNSON 1986). A relative absence of symptoms until the primary tumor becomes locally advanced, coupled with rich local lymphatics, results in a 50% clinically positive cervical lymph node rate at the time of diagnosis (KEANE 1982). The jugular chain and retropharyngeal lymph nodes are at high risk for regional metastases, with levels II and III most commonly the first involved. However, the retropharyngeal nodes are occasionally the first site of spread, similar to nasopharyngeal cancer. Postcricoid tumors may spread directly to pre- and paratracheal nodal basins. Because of these characteristics, the vast majority of hypopharyngeal cancer patients present with stage III and IV disease.

There is a strong association between tobacco use and the development of hypopharyngeal cancer (SPITZ 1994; BRUGERE et al. 1986). Alcohol in isolation is not clearly associated with an increased risk of developing hypopharyngeal cancer; however, it appears to potentiate the carcinogenic effects of tobacco. Smoking cessation can enhance treatment tolerance and diminish the risk of developing subsequent cancers of the upper aerodigestive tract. In fact, there has been an ~35% decline in the rate of hypopharyngeal cancer since 1975, possibly the result of smoking cessation efforts (DAVIES and WELCH 2006).

The relationship and clinical implications of human papillomavirus (HPV) infection and hypopharyngeal cancer is yet to be well defined. Studies reveal that ~20–25% of patients with hypopharyngeal cancer test positive for HPV DNA (KLUSSMANN et al. 2001; MINETA et al. 1998). A higher rate of cancers of the postcricoid region has been documented in patients with Plummer Vinson Syndrome, characterized by iron-deficiency anemia, hypopharyngeal webbing, weight loss, and dysphagia (LARSSON et al. 1975). Favorable changes in the epidemiology of hypopharyngeal cancer have resulted from changes in nutrition, including the addition of iron to flour.

3.3
Staging

The AJCC staging system, based on clinical and radiographic data, is most commonly used. Table 3.1 contains the AJCC 2002 T stage for hypopharyngeal cancer (GREENE et al. 2002). The nodal and group staging is similar to other laryngopharyngeal sites, with the exception of nasopharynx.

Table 3.1. 2002 AJCC T staging

T Stage	
T1	Limited to one subsite of the hypopharynx and ≤ 2 cm in greatest dimension
T2	Tumor invades more than one subsite of the hypopharynx or an adjacent site, or measures >2 cm but ≤ 4 cm in greatest diameter without fixation of hemilarynx
T3	Tumor measures >4 cm in greatest dimension or with fixation of hemilarynx
T4a	Invades thyroid/cricoid cartilage, hyoid bone, thyroid gland, esophagus, or central compartment soft tissue, which includes prelaryngeal strap muscles and subcutaneous fat
T4b	Tumor invades prevertebral fascia, encases carotid artery, or involves mediastinal structures

3.4
Patterns of Spread

Hypopharynx tumors often spread via local extension to the paraglottic and pre-epiglottic space, including the thyroid cartilage, lateral compartment of the neck, the intrinsic muscles of the larynx resulting in vocal cord fixation, and the thyroid gland itself. Late presenting disease can involve the trachea, esophagus, prevertebral fascia, and retropharyngeal space posteriorly. These tumors have a propensity for submucosal spread, making it difficult to accurately quantify disease extent on examination (Ho et al. 1993).

Lymphatics of the pyriform sinus drain primarily into the level II and III jugular chain nodes. Posterior pharyngeal wall can involve the retropharyngeal nodes (Rouviere's nodes), extending to the base of skull. There is a significant risk of bilateral cervical adenopathy because of rich cross-draining lymphatics (MUKHERJI et al. 2001). The most common site for distant metastasis is the lung. Approximately 25% of patients will either present with or develop distant metastasis at some time during the course of their disease (MERINO et al. 1977).

3.5
Clinical Presentation

The majority of patients present with advanced locoregional disease, after experiencing nonspecific symptoms or undergoing management for presumed infectious etiology. Symptoms are usually related to local tumor spread and include dysphagia, odynophagia, sore throat, hoarseness, weight loss >10lb, and neck mass. Unilateral ear pain, representing referred otalgia due to involvement of the nerve of Arnold, a branch of the superior laryngeal nerve, is occasionally the presenting symptom.

A comprehensive work-up should include a detailed history, thorough physical examination, direct laryngoscopy under general anesthesia with panendoscopy and biopsy confirmation of the primary tumor site, mapping of its extent, and surveying for synchronous primary tumors. Imaging should include a HN CT or MRI and a chest X-ray or CT. [18]FDG-PET can be valuable in assessing locoregional and distant disease as well as complimenting CT or MRI in the radiation treatment planning process. A formal swallow evaluation should be performed

prior to primary therapy to establish the patient's baseline functional swallow capacity.

3.6
Treatment Strategies

3.6.1
Primary Surgical Therapy

Primary surgical management of patients with early cancers of the hypopharynx is indicated in those with a history of previous HN radiation, those in whom organ-conserving surgery is possible, and those refusing radiation. Relative contraindications to surgical organ conservation include transglottic tumor extension, deep pyriform sinus invasion, postcricoid invasion, vocal fold paralysis, cartilage invasion, and extension beyond the larynx.

Options for organ preservation in more advanced tumors are limited and total laryngectomy is often necessary if primary surgical therapy is pursued. However, favorable T3 tumors in the superior aspect of the pyriform sinus occasionally permit resection by either an extended supraglottic laryngectomy or extended vertical partial laryngopharyngectomy with free flap reconstruction. Most T3 and T4 tumors require total laryngectomy with either preservation of a 3–3.5-cm-wide posterior strip spanning from the oropharynx to the esophagus to tube on itself, or reconstruction of the anterior and lateral walls of the remaining hypopharynx with either a pedicled or a free flap. Bulkier tumors can require total laryngopharyngectomy with removal of the larynx and the entire hypopharynx, thus creating a gap between the oropharynx and esophagus. Reconstruction is typically performed with either a tubed fascio-cutaneous flap such as the radial forearm free flap or lateral thigh flap, or a free jejunum or tubed pedicled myocutaneous flap. If the tumor extends inferiorly to the cricopharyngeus, a laryngopharyngectomy with esophagectomy and gastric pull-up or colonic interposition may be performed to ensure a negative inferior margin.

3.6.2
Definitive Radiation or Chemoradiation Therapy

Definitive radiation therapy for patients with stage I or II disease affords good potential for organ preservation without compromise in clinical outcome and is typically the preferred treatment option. A common fractionation regimen for early-stage disease delivers 70 Gy to gross disease in 35 daily 2 Gy fractions over 7 weeks with either a conformal shrinking field technique or IMRT to minimize toxicity to neighboring normal tissue. Radiation is delivered comprehensively from skull base to clavicle, encompassing even N0 nodal regions to a dose of 50–56 Gy because of the high likelihood of occult nodal metastases. Patients may achieve 5-year disease-specific survival (DSS) on the order of 90% with T1N0 lesions, while T2N0 lesions may achieve DSS of greater than 70% (NAKAMURA et al. 2006).

For stage III and IV disease the use of altered fractionation regimens (FU et al. 2000; OVERGAARD et al. 2003; SKLADOWSKI et al. 2006; BOURHIS et al. 2006) and/or concomitant chemotherapy (PIGNON et al. 2000; BRIZEL et al. 1998; HUGUENIN et al. 2004; JEREMIC et al. 2000; ADELSTEIN et al. 2003; PIGNON et al. 2007) improves locoregional control and survival. Patients with primary hypopharynx tumors comprised up to 25% of all patients on these trials.

3.6.3
Radiation Therapy with Molecular Targeted Agents

There is considerable interest in the use of molecular targeted therapies in the treatment of HN cancer patients. A phase III trial compared radiation alone vs. radiation plus cetuximab in advanced HN cancer patients, 15% of whom had a hypopharyngeal primary tumor, revealing significant improvement in locoregional control, progression-free survival, and overall survival with the addition of cetuximab (BONNER et al. 2006). However, subset analysis of patients with hypopharyngeal cancer did not demonstrate a clear advantage with use of cetuximab. RTOG 0522 is currently investigating whether there is added benefit of using cisplatin with or without cetuximab in this patient population.

3.6.4
Induction Chemotherapy

Historically, surgery followed by postoperative radiation therapy was the most common treatment strategy for patients with locoregionally advanced

hypopharyngeal cancer. However, the development of active chemotherapy regimens opened a new era of HN cancer research in the 1980s, which included exploration of larynx-preserving strategies using induction chemotherapy for patients with hypopharyngeal cancer. EORTC 24981 analyzed 194 patients with stage II to stage IV hypopharyngeal cancer (94% stage III or IV) that were randomized to either definitive laryngopharyngectomy with neck dissection followed by postoperative RT (50–70 Gy) vs. induction chemotherapy with bolus cisplatin (100 mg m^{-2}) on day 1 and infusion 5-FU (1,000 mg m^{-2} day^{-1}) on days 1–5, with endoscopic assessment of response after each cycle for up to three cycles. Patients with a complete response after two or three cycles then underwent 70 Gy of RT; all others underwent conventional surgery with postoperative RT (50–70 Gy). A complete local and regional response to induction chemotherapy was seen in 54 and 51% of patients respectively. The initial report noted no difference between the two arms with respect to local and regional failures or the rate of second primary tumors. However, there were fewer distant failures in the induction arm (25 vs. 36%) and the median survival was significantly greater (44 vs. 25 months) in the induction arm, despite finding no difference in the 5-year overall survival rate (LEFEBVRE et al. 1996). The updated 10-year overall survival was similar between the two arms, 14% in the surgery arm and 13% in the induction arm, and the 5- and 10-year survival with a functioning larynx in place was 22 and 9% respectively (LEFEBVRE et al. 2004). A summary of the results of this trial is outlined in Table 3.2.

The use of induction chemotherapy gradually fell out of favor in the late 1990s with the maturation of HN cancer meta-analysis data (PIGNON et al. 2000) showing survival benefit with concomitant chemoradiation but little overall impact of induction chemotherapy regimens.

3.6.5
Postoperative Adjuvant Radiation or Chemoradiation Therapy

Many patients treated with primary surgical resection are found to have high-risk pathologic features, triggering a recommendation for postoperative radiation therapy to enhance locoregional control. Classical indications for postoperative radiation include T4 primary tumors, close or positive micro-

Table 3.2. Summary of EORTC 24891 (LEFEBVRE et al. 1996, 2004)

Arms	No. of patients	Local failure (%)	Regional failure (%)	Second primary (%)	Distant failure (%)	5-/10-Year progression-free survival (%)	5/10-Year overall survival (%)
Surgery + RT	94	12	19	16	36	26/8.5	33/14
Induction chemotherapy	100	17	23	13	25	32/11	38/13
p-Value		NS	NS	NS	0.041	NS	NS

scopic margins, cartilage/bony invasion, >1 metastatic lymph node, the presence of extracapsular extension, or perineural/lymphatic/vascular invasion. Recommended doses are 54–63 Gy to all areas at risk with a boost to 60–66 Gy for regions of highest risk. Either a shrinking field conformal technique or IMRT can be used; however, the entire cervical nodal chain from the skull base to the clavicles bilaterally should be included.

Concurrent chemotherapy with postoperative radiation has been evaluated in patients with locally advanced disease and poor pathologic features in two prospective randomized trials by the RTOG and European Organization for the Research and Treatment of Cancer (EORTC) (BERNIER et al. 2004; COOPER et al. 2004, 2006). Ten percent of patients enrolled in the RTOG trial and 20% in the EORTC trial had primary hypopharynx tumors. A joint analysis of these two trials noted that the greatest benefit for postoperative chemoradiation was in patients with positive surgical margins and/or extracapsular nodal extension (BERNIER et al. 2005). Both of these studies show an approximate doubling of the rate of grade 3 or greater toxicity. Therefore, careful clinical judgment regarding the selection of patients most likely to tolerate and thereby benefit from this approach is warranted.

3.6.6
Neck Dissection Following Definitive Radiation or Chemoradiation

Adjuvant neck dissection is generally unnecessary for N0–N1 patients following primary radiation or chemoradiation. However, the role of adjuvant neck dissection is more controversial for patients presenting with advanced N2–N3 neck disease with some proponents of planned, postradiotherapy neck dissection and others of serial observation in light of the advent of improved postradiation imaging with FDG-PET in selecting those at highest risk for failure. Both approaches are readily defendable at present (BOYD et al. 1998; CORRY et al. 2001; MCHAM et al. 2003; MENDENHALL et al. 1988; SEWALL et al. 2007; STENSON et al. 2000; YAO et al. 2005); however, it appears that the global trend is moving towards the incorporation of imaging response at 1–3 months posttreatment to help guide recommendations for adjuvant neck dissection.

3.7
Quality of Life

There have been relatively few prospective assessments of quality of life (QOL) following treatment for HN cancer. Patients with locoregionally advanced hypopharyngeal cancer have historically required radical surgery, such as total laryngectomy and partial pharyngectomy, previously referred to as "mutilating surgery." The functional and psychosocial ramifications of this surgery are substantial. With the support of a knowledgeable health care team, some patients are able to adjust quite well to the functional and cosmetic changes, whereas others cannot despite very best efforts.

With the publication of the Veterans Affairs Larynx Study Group trial and the EORTC 24891 hypopharynx trial in the 1990s, the treatment paradigm shifted towards more frequent consideration of nonoperative approaches in an effort to enable larynx preservation. However, for patients undergoing "organ preservation" with radiation alone or in combination with chemotherapy, it remains important to assess the quality of organ function, and the patient's functional adaptation following therapy. Regardless of the primary treatment approach, these patients often require long-term speech, swallow, and dental rehabilitation.

3.7.1
Quality Of Life in Head and Neck Trials With Regard to Larynx Preservation

Although there has not been a report specifically analyzing the QOL outcomes in patients treated on the EORTC 24891 trial, a reasonable extrapolation can be made from the QOL data from the VA larynx preservation trial. Long-term QOL was assessed in 46 of the 65 surviving patients treated on this trial, including 25 from the surgery arm and 21 from the larynx preservation arm (TERRELL et al. 1998). General health was measured using the Short Form-36 (SF-36) general health measure (eight domains). HN-specific QOL was measured using the HNQOL instrument (four domains), and mental health was measured with the Beck Depression Inventory. Patients who avoided laryngectomy scored significantly higher ($p < 0.5$) on the bodily pain domain and the mental health domain of the SF-36. They also had significantly better scores on the emotional domain ($p = 0.05$) of the HNQOL as well as a better global score for their assessment of their response to treatment ($p = 0.005$). At long-term follow-up, nine of the ten patients with moderate or severe depression had undergone laryngectomy. Of interest, the speech scores on the HNQOL survey were similar between the two groups, which was explained by the fact that 91% of the laryngectomy patients were using some means of artificial voice that allowed them to communicate reasonably well. The authors concluded that the larynx preservation treatment strategy was associated with a better overall QOL. Table 3.3 summarizes the statistically significant differences between patients with laryngeal cancer treated with either laryngectomy and RT vs. those treated with definitive chemoradiation at the University of Arkansas (HANNA et al. 2004).

Not all studies have demonstrated an improved QOL with larynx preservation therapy. Long-term, health-related quality-of-life (HRQOL) outcomes were evaluated in 54 patients (27 matched-pairs) with stage III or IV SCC of the oropharynx, hypopharynx, or larynx treated with either surgery and postoperative radiation therapy (SRT) or concurrent chemoradiation (CRT) at the University of Iowa (EL-DEIRY et al. 2005). They analyzed the domains of speech, eating, aesthetics, social disruption, and depressive symptoms at ≥12 months after diagnosis and did not find any statistically significant differences between the two treatment regimens. However, several of the outcomes demonstrated small clinically important differences (CID), defined as >0.2 but <0.5 standard deviations from the mean score. These included small CID that favored CRT with respect to aesthetics and speech, and a small CID that favored SRT for overall QOL and fewer depressive symptoms. The authors concluded that despite deficits in all domains, the overall QOL was preserved regardless of the treatment method. Indeed, they suggest that the popular assumption that organ preservation approaches routinely provide a higher QOL may be invalid, most likely because nonsurgical strategies have become more aggressive and surgical approaches have become increasingly focused on functional preservation and/or rehabilitation.

Table 3.3. Summary of statistically significant health related quality of life differences, as measured by the EORTC QLQ-C30 and QLQ-H&N 35, comparing laryngectomy + RT vs. chemoradiation; oropharynx vs. hypopharynx primary tumor site; and conventional RT vs. IMRT (GRAFF et al. 2007; HANNA et al. 2004; NORDGREN et al. 2006)

	EORTC QLQ-C30 and EORTC QLQ-H&N 35 domains
S + RT vs. chemoRT	ChemoRT better in senses, coughing, and painkillers domain
	S + RT better in dry mouth domain
Oropharynx vs. hypopharynx primary	Oropharynx better in social, cognitive, diarrhea, coughing, speech, sexuality, and sticky saliva domains
	Hypopharynx not better in any domain
IMRT vs. conformal RT	IMRT better in physical, nausea, dyspnea, pain, dry mouth, sticky saliva, swallowing, social eating, teeth, and opening mouth domains
	Conformal RT not better in any domain

Similar long-term results were found in a group of 24 patients with stage III or IV laryngeal or hypopharyngeal SCC who had survived ≥2 years after treatment with either SRT ($n = 6$) or CRT ($n = 15$). They found no difference between the groups in seven of the eight QOL domains, including physical functioning, bodily pain, energy/fatigue, health perception, social functioning, mental health, or role limitations due to mental health. However, patients treated with CRT were less likely to be limited in their ability to perform activities of daily living (MAJOR et al. 2001).

3.7.2
Altered Fractionation Regimens and Quality Of Life

The impact of altered fractionation on QOL in comparison to conventional fractionation has been analyzed in a prospective fashion in randomized multicenter controlled trials. In patients treated on the CHART trial (DISCHE et al. 1997), two self-reporting questionnaires covering 30 core symptoms in the physical and psychological domains and 14 items regarding anxiety and depression were prospectively administered at ten time-points, from time 0 to 30 months posttreatment. Analysis of short-term symptoms revealed significantly worse pain at 21 days after treatment initiation (63 vs. 39%) in the hyperfractionation arm compared with significantly worse cough (26 vs. 13%) and hoarseness (53 vs. 32%) at 6 weeks in the conventional arm. Since only a limited number of patients reported long-term data, no firm conclusions regarding observed patient reported differences were reported. No differences in anxiety or depression levels were noted in the short- or long term (GRIFFITHS et al. 1999).

Accelerated fractionation can also impact QOL, and patients treated with this regimen on RTOG 9003 were found to have worse diet, eating, and speech at 1 year as evaluated with the Head and Neck Performance Status Scale (HNPSS) (FISHER et al. 2001). Conversely, a prospective study of 21 patients with laryngeal or hypopharyngeal carcinoma treated with accelerated fractionation revealed similar QOL and functional outcome, as assessed by the HNPSS and EORTC QLQ-C30, to those reported for patients treated with conventional or hyperfractionated RT (ALLAL et al. 2000). This series noted that xerostomia had the largest impact on most scales studied, highlighting the importance of the dose to the salivary glands.

3.7.3
Evolution of Quality of Life from Diagnosis to Long-Term Follow-up

The factors affecting QOL in patients with hypopharyngeal cancer can differ between the time of diagnosis, during the treatment course, and in the short- and long-term posttreatment period, mainly because of how the tumor affects HRQOL at diagnosis vs. how the acute and late treatment toxicities impact HRQOL. This evolution of HRQOL from diagnosis through long-term posttreatment follow-up has been studied in the context of prospective clinical trials.

A multicenter prospective Swedish study analyzed changes in HRQOL from completion of radiation therapy until 5 years posttreatment in 89 pharyngeal SCC patients, including 28 with hypopharyngeal carcinoma (NORDGREN et al. 2006). All but five patients received some component of conventional radiation, typically delivered with opposed lateral portals to 62–70 Gy and a separate anterior low-neck field to 50 Gy at 3-cm depth. Forty patients were treated with conventional 2.0 Gy fractions, 44 were treated with hyperfractionated 1.7 Gy b.i.d fractions, 23 were treated with brachytherapy in conjunction with external beam radiation, and 33 received chemotherapy. Emotional functioning, global health, sleep disturbance, and pain improved in a statistically significant manner from diagnosis to 5-year follow-up. Senses, problems with teeth, and problems with dry mouth showed statistically significant deterioration during this time period. A clinically significant, but not statistically significant, deterioration was noted with sexuality, mouth opening, and thick secretions from diagnosis to 5-year follow-up. When comparing HRQOL from the 1-year follow-up to the 5-year follow-up, only pain showed a statistically significant improvement, and only teeth problems and sticky saliva showed a statistically significant deterioration.

A study by MAGNE et al. (2001) similarly analyzed the evolution of HRQOL domains from the end of treatment to 2–7 years posttreatment in 29 patients with stage IV oropharynx or hypopharynx SCC treated with hyperfractionated CRT. They demonstrated corroborative results to the Swedish multicenter study with regards to pain, with 89% experiencing moderate to severe pain at the completion of treatment and only 9% at 2–7 years posttreatment ($p < 0.05$); significant improvements were also seen in moderate to severe psychological problems and swallowing problems. In contrast to the Swedish study, Magne et al. found an improvement in moderate to severe dry mouth and sticky saliva with 97% of patients reporting this at the end of treatment and only 55% at 2–7 years posttreatment ($p < 0.05$). Overall, 76% of patients reported good or very good QOL and 86% said their QOL had improved at long-term follow-up.

3.7.4
Relative Health-Related Quality of Life in Hypopharyngeal Squamous Cell Carcinoma Compared with Other Head and Neck Sites

Despite advances in the diagnosis and treatment of hypopharyngeal cancer, the overall outcome for these patients is relatively poor compared with other HN tumors. Whether or not the QOL for these patients differs from those with other HN cancers has been compared in the context of prospective clinical trials. The Swedish multicenter study compared HRQOL in patients with oropharyngeal SCC to those with hypopharyngeal carcinoma (Nordgren et al. 2006). Patients with oropharyngeal primary tumors had superior scores in 12 scales or single items at diagnosis, including five that achieved statistical significance (cognitive, social, speech, sexuality, and sticky saliva). At 1-year posttreatment, patients with oropharynx SCC demonstrated clinically superior scores in 11 scales or single items, including four that achieved statistical significance (speech, sticky saliva, coughing, and diarrhea). No scale or single item showed any significance in favor of hypopharyngeal SCC. Symptoms typical of those patients with hypopharynx SCC included fatigue, speech, thick secretions, and coughing, whereas patients with oropharyngeal carcinoma reported difficulties with wide mouth opening and dry mouth. Table 3.3 summarizes the statistically significant differences between the patients with oropharynx and hypopharynx primary tumors.

The incidence of pharyngoesophageal stricture and feeding tube dependence may be increased in patients with primary hypopharyngeal tumors compared with other HN primary sites. A report from the Cleveland Clinic revealed a 21% stricture rate in patients treated with concurrent chemoradiation, with hypopharyngeal primary site as a significant predictive factor (Lee et al. 2006). Preliminary results of patients with advanced laryngeal or hypopharyngeal cancer treated with concurrent chemotherapy and IMRT at Memorial Sloan Kettering revealed a 2-year feeding tube dependency rate of 31%, mainly due to pharyngoesophageal stricture, in patients with hypopharyngeal primaries; patients with a laryngeal primary had a 15% 2-year feeding tube dependency rate (Lee et al. 2007).

Functional evaluation using postchemoRT videofluoroscopic swallow function studies in patients with stage III or IV tumors of the hypopharynx ($n = 8$) and oropharynx ($n = 6$) revealed impaired bolus transport in all patients, with more severe anterior pharyngeal dysfunction and a longer duration of laryngeal motion in patients with primary hypopharynx tumors compared with those with oropharynx primaries (Kotz et al. 1999).

3.7.5
The Impact of Intensity-Modulated Radiotherapy on Quality of Life

With the advent of IMRT and its ability to minimize the radiation dose to nearby normal structures, many studies are beginning to report on QOL outcomes with IMRT compared with conventional or 3D-conformal techniques. Studies continue to investigate the role of modifying dose-constraint parameters for various structures, from the commonly constrained salivary glands, to other less commonly delineated structures such as the pharyngeal constrictors and the glottic and supraglottic larynx.

A large French matched-pair comparison of IMRT with conventional RT assessed the benefit of IMRT on QOL on 137 patients with HN cancer (16% with hypopharynx/larynx primary) using the validated EORTC QLQ-30 (cancer specific) and EORTC QLQ-H&N35 (disease specific) (Graff et al. 2007). Patients treated with IMRT had significantly better symptom scores with regard to pain, swallowing, social eating, teeth, opening mouth, dry mouth, and sticky saliva. The mean dose was <30 and <26 Gy for one parotid gland in 63.5 and 34.9% of IMRT patients, respectively. Table 3.3 summarizes the statistically significant differences in QOL scores between patients treated with conventional RT and IMRT.

A smaller prospective, longitudinal matched case–control study reported by Jabbari et al. (2005) compared QOL, measured by the validated xerostomia-specific and HN-cancer-specific QOL questionnaires, in 40 patients with advanced HN cancer (10% with a pyriform sinus primary tumor) treated with either standard RT or IMRT. The trend in both treatment groups was a decline in QOL during the first 3 months posttreatment. However, starting at 6 months posttreatment, patients treated with IMRT showed a trend of improvement, which became statistically significant at 24 months posttherapy. Patients treated with standard RT did not show a trend for improvement. Pretherapy QOL scores were significantly related to posttherapy scores in both groups.

The role of IMRT in reducing dysphagia has been investigated in a prospective, longitudinal study of 36 patients with advanced oropharyngeal or nasopharyngeal cancer treated with chemo-IMRT that spared salivary glands and swallowing structures including the pharyngeal constrictors and the glottic and supraglottic larynx (FENG et al. 2007). Dysphagia endpoints included video fluoroscopy and patient- and observer-reported scores. Significant correlations were observed between aspiration and the mean dose and partial volume doses to the pharyngeal constrictor and glottic and supraglottic larynx, with the highest correlation associated with the dose to the superior pharyngeal constrictor, defined as the portion of the constrictor muscle extending from the caudal tips of the pterygoid plates through the upper edge of the hyoid bone.

3.8
Conclusion

Hypopharynx tumors are a relatively rare subset of HN cancers that tend to present with locoregionally advanced disease. Although early-stage disease can be treated with limited surgery or radiation therapy alone, the majority of these tumors present at an advanced stage requiring multimodality therapy, including surgery with postoperative radiation or chemoradiation, or primary chemoradiation with or without neck dissection. The toxicities of these treatment regimens, compounded by a diminished baseline functional status due to common medical comorbidities in this patient population, make treatment of these tumors quite complex. A multidisciplinary approach with input from surgical, radiation, and medical oncology as well as an experienced HN nursing staff, speech and swallow therapy team, pain and nutritional experts can reduce or minimize unnecessary treatment complications

and delays. The judicious incorporation of new technologies and techniques, such as IMRT, organ sparing surgery, novel chemotherapeutic regimens, molecular targeted therapies, as well as the provision of comprehensive patient support for acute and late treatment toxicities are critical for optimizing overall outcome. Our increasing attention to patient-driven QOL assessments will be important to help evaluate the ultimate impact of these new treatment approaches for hypopharyngeal cancer patients.

References

Adelstein DJ, Li Y, Adams GL et al. (2003) An intergroup phase III comparison of standard radiation therapy and two schedules of concurrent chemoradiotherapy in patients with unresectable squamous cell head and neck cancer. J Clin Oncol 21: 92–98.

Allal AS, Dulguerov P, Bieri S et al. (2000) Assessment of quality of life in patients treated with accelerated radiotherapy for laryngeal and hypopharyngeal carcinomas. Head Neck 22: 288–293.

Barnes L, Johnson JT (1986) Pathologic and clinical considerations in the evaluation of major head and neck specimens resected for cancer. Part I. Pathology Annual 21 Pt 1, 173–250.

Bernier J, Domenge C, Ozsahin M et al. (2004) Postoperative irradiation with or without concomitant chemotherapy for locally advanced head and neck cancer.[see comment]. New England Journal of Medicine 350:1945–1952.

Bernier J, Cooper JS, Pajak TF et al. (2005) Defining risk levels in locally advanced head and neck cancers: a comparative analysis of concurrent postoperative radiation plus chemotherapy trials of the EORTC (#22931) and RTOG (# 9501). Head Neck 27:843–850.

Bonner JA, Harari PM, Giralt J et al. (2006) Radiotherapy plus cetuximab for squamous-cell carcinoma of the head and neck. N Engl J Med 354:567–578.

Bourhis J, Overgaard J, Audry H et al. (2006) Hyperfractionated or accelerated radiotherapy in head and neck cancer: a meta-analysis. Lancet 368:843–854.

Boyd TS, Harari PM, Tannehill SP et al. (1998) Planned postradiotherapy neck dissection in patients with advanced head and neck cancer. Head Neck 20:132–137.

Brizel DM, Albers ME, Fisher SR et al. (1998) Hyperfractionated irradiation with or without concurrent chemotherapy for locally advanced head and neck cancer. N Engl J Med 338: 798–1804.

Brugere J, Guenel P, Leclerc A et al. (1986) Differential effects of tobacco and alcohol in cancer of the larynx, pharynx, and mouth. Cancer 57:391–395.

Carpenter RJ, 3rd DeSanto LW, (1977) Cancer of the hypopharynx. Surg Clin North Am 57, 723–735.

Cooper JS, Pajak TF, Forastiere AA et al. (2004) Postoperative concurrent radiotherapy and chemotherapy for high-risk squamous-cell carcinoma of the head and neck.[see comment]. New England Journal of Medicine 350:1937–1944.

Cooper JS, Pajak TF, Forastiere AA et al. (2006) 25: Long-Term Survival Results of a Phase III Intergroup Trial (RTOG 95-01) of Surgery Followed by Radiotherapy vs. Radiochemotherapy for Resectable High Risk Squamous Cell Carcinoma of the Head And Neck. International journal of radiation oncology, biology, physics 66, S14–S15.

Corry J, Smith JG, Peters LJ (2001) The concept of a planned neck dissection is obsolete. Cancer J 7:472–474.

Davies L, Welch HG (2006) Epidemiology of head and neck cancer in the United States. Otolaryngol Head Neck Surg 135:451–457.

Dische S, Saunders M, Barrett A et al. (1997) A randomised multicentre trial of CHART versus conventional radiotherapy in head and neck cancer. Radiother Oncol 44:123–136.

El-Deiry M, Funk GF, Nalwa S et al. (2005) Long-term quality of life for surgical and nonsurgical treatment of head and neck cancer. Arch Otolaryngol Head Neck Surg 131:879–885.

Feng FY, Kim HM, Lyden TH et al. (2007) Intensity-modulated radiotherapy of head and neck cancer aiming to reduce dysphagia: early dose-effect relationships for the swallowing structures. Int J Radiat Oncol Biol Phys 68:1289–1298.

Fisher J, Scott C, Fu K et al. (2001) Treatment, patient and tumor characteristics impact quality of life (QOL) in patients with locally advanced head and neck cancer: Report of the radiation therapy oncology group (RTOG) trial 90-03. International journal of radiation oncology, biology, physics 51:98.

Frederick Greene L, David Page L, Irvin Fleming D et al. (2002) AJCC Cancer Staging Manual. Springer

Fu KK, Pajak TF, Trotti A et al. (2000) A Radiation Therapy Oncology Group (RTOG) phase III randomized study to compare hyperfractionation and two variants of accelerated fractionation to standard fractionation radiotherapy for head and neck squamous cell carcinomas: first report of RTOG 9003. Int J Radiat Oncol Biol Phys 48:7–16.

Graff P, Lapeyre M, Desandes E et al. (2007) Impact of intensity-modulated radiotherapy on health-related quality of life for head and neck cancer patients: matched-pair comparison with conventional radiotherapy. Int J Radiat Oncol Biol Phys 67:1309–1317.

Griffiths GO, Parmar MK, Bailey AJ (1999) Physical and psychological symptoms of quality of life in the CHART randomized trial in head and neck cancer: short-term and long-term patient reported symptoms. CHART Steering Committee. Continuous hyperfractionated accelerated radiotherapy. Br J Cancer 81, 1196–1205.

Hanna E, Sherman A, Cash D et al. (2004) Quality of life for patients following total laryngectomy vs chemoradiation for laryngeal preservation. Arch Otolaryngol Head Neck Surg 130:875–879.

Ho CM, Lam KH, Wei WI et al. (1993) Squamous cell carcinoma of the hypopharynx--analysis of treatment results. Head & Neck 15:405–412.

Huguenin P, Beer KT, Allal A et al. (2004) Concomitant cisplatin significantly improves locoregional control in advanced head and neck cancers treated with hyperfractionated radiotherapy. J Clin Oncol 22:4665–4673.

Jabbari S, Kim HM, Feng M et al. (2005) Matched case-control study of quality of life and xerostomia after intensity-modulated radiotherapy or standard radiotherapy for head-and-neck cancer: initial report. Int J Radiat Oncol Biol Phys 63:725–731.

Jeremic B, Shibamoto Y, Milicic B et al. (2000) Hyperfractionated radiation therapy with or without concurrent low-dose daily cisplatin in locally advanced squamous cell carcinoma of the head and neck: a prospective randomized trial. J Clin Oncol 18:1458–1464.

Keane TJ, (1982) Carcinoma of the hypopharynx. Journal of Otolaryngology 11:227–231.

Klussmann JP, Weissenborn SJ, Wieland U et al. (2001) Prevalence, distribution, and viral load of human papillomavirus 16 DNA in tonsillar carcinomas. Cancer 92:2875–2884.

Kotz T, Abraham S, Beitler JJ et al. (1999) Pharyngeal transport dysfunction consequent to an organ-sparing protocol. Arch Otolaryngol Head Neck Surg 125:410–413.

Larsson LG, Sandstrom A, Westling P (1975) Relationship of Plummer-Vinson disease to cancer of the upper alimentary tract in Sweden. Cancer Res 35:3308–3316.

Lee NY, O'Meara W, Chan K et al. (2007) Concurrent chemotherapy and intensity-modulated radiotherapy for locoregionally advanced laryngeal and hypopharyngeal cancers. Int J Radiat Oncol Biol Phys 69:459–468.

Lee WT, Akst LM, Adelstein DJ et al. (2006) Risk factors for hypopharyngeal/upper esophageal stricture formation after concurrent chemoradiation. Head Neck 28:808–812.

Lefebvre JL, Chevalier D, Luboinski B et al. (1996) Larynx preservation in pyriform sinus cancer: preliminary results of a European Organization for Research and Treatment of Cancer phase III trial. EORTC Head and Neck Cancer Cooperative Group.[see comment]. Journal of the National Cancer Institute 88:890–899.

Lefebvre JL, Chevalier D, Luboinski B et al. (2004) Is laryngeal preservation (LP) with induction chemotherapy (ICT) safe in the treatment of hypopharyngeal SCC? Final results of the phase III EORTC 24891 trial. J Clin Oncol (Meeting Abstracts) 22:5531–.

Magne N, Marcy PY, Chamorey E et al. (2001) Concomitant twice-a-day radiotherapy and chemotherapy in unresectable head and neck cancer patients: A long-term quality of life analysis. Head Neck 23:678–682.

Major MS, Bumpous JM, Flynn MB et al. (2001) Quality of life after treatment for advanced laryngeal and hypopharyngeal cancer. Laryngoscope 111:1379–1382.

McHam SA, Adelstein DJ, Rybicki LA et al. (2003) Who merits a neck dissection after definitive chemoradiotherapy for N2-N3 squamous cell head and neck cancer? Head Neck 25:791–798.

Mendenhall WM, Parsons JT, Amdur RJ et al. (1988) Squamous cell carcinoma of the head and neck treated with radiotherapy: does planned neck dissection reduce the change for successful surgical management of subsequent local recurrence? Head Neck Surg 10:302–304.

Merino OR, Lindberg RD, Fletcher GH (1977) An analysis of distant metastases from squamous cell carcinoma of the upper respiratory and digestive tracts. Cancer 40:145–151.

Mineta H, Ogino T, Amano HM et al. (1998) Human papilloma virus (HPV) type 16 and 18 detected in head and neck squamous cell carcinoma. Anticancer Res 18:4765–4768.

Mukherji SK, Armao D, Joshi VM (2001) Cervical nodal metastases in squamous cell carcinoma of the head and neck: what to expect. Head & Neck 23:995-1005.

Nakamura K, Shioyama Y, Kawashima M et al. (2006) Multi-institutional analysis of early squamous cell carcinoma of the hypopharynx treated with radical radiotherapy. Int J Radiat Oncol Biol Phys 65:1045–1050.

Nordgren M, Jannert M, Boysen M et al. (2006) Health-related quality of life in patients with pharyngeal carcinoma: a five-year follow-up. Head Neck 28:339–349.

Overgaard J, Hansen HS, SpechtL et al. (2003) Five compared with six fractions per week of conventional radiotherapy of squamous-cell carcinoma of head and neck: DAHANCA 6 and 7 randomised controlled trial. Lancet 362:933–940.

Pignon JP, Bourhis J, Domenge C et al.(2000) Chemotherapy added to locoregional treatment for head and neck squamous-cell carcinoma: three meta-analyses of updated individual data. MACH-NC Collaborative Group. Meta-Analysis of Chemotherapy on Head and Neck Cancer.[see comment]. Lancet 355:949–955.

Pignon JP, le Maitre A, Bourhis J (2007) Meta-Analyses of Chemotherapy in Head and Neck Cancer (MACH-NC): an update. Int J Radiat Oncol Biol Phys 69:S112–114.

Sewall GK, Palazzi-Churas KL, Richards GM et al. (2007) Planned postradiotherapy neck dissection: Rationale and clinical outcomes. Laryngoscope 117:121–128.

Skladowski K, Maciejewski B, Golen M et al. (2006) Continuous accelerated 7-days-a-week radiotherapy for head-and-neck cancer: long-term results of phase III clinical trial. Int J Radiat Oncol Biol Phys 66:706–713.

Spitz MR (1994) Epidemiology and risk factors for head and neck cancer. Semin Oncol 21, 281–288.

Stenson KM, Haraf DJ, Pelzer H et al. (2000) The role of cervical lymphadenectomy after aggressive concomitant chemoradiotherapy: the feasibility of selective neck dissection. Arch Otolaryngol Head Neck Surg 126:950–956.

Terrell JE, Fisher SG, Wolf GT (1998) Long-term quality of life after treatment of laryngeal cancer. The Veterans Affairs Laryngeal Cancer Study Group. Arch Otolaryngol Head Neck Surg 124:964–971.

Yao M, Smith RB, Graham MM et al. (2005) The role of FDG PET in management of neck metastasis from head-and-neck cancer after definitive radiation treatment. International Journal of Radiation Oncology, Biology, Physics 63:991–999.

Laryngeal Cancer:
Epidemiology and Treatment Outcomes

4

WILLIAM M. MENDENHALL, RUSSELL W. HINERMAN, ROBERT J. AMDUR,
MIKHAIL VAYSBERG, and JOHN W. WERNING

CONTENTS

4.1	Anatomy	*43*
4.2	Epidemiology and Risk Factors	*44*
4.3	Diagnostic Evaluation	*44*
4.4	Staging	*44*
4.5	**Selection of Treatment Modality for Glottic Carcinoma**	*44*
4.5.1	Early Vocal Cord Carcinoma	*45*
4.5.2	Moderately Advanced Vocal Cord Cancer	*46*
4.5.3	Advanced Vocal Cord Carcinoma	*46*
4.6	**Selection of Treatment Modality for Supraglottic Carcinoma**	*46*
4.6.1	Early and Moderately Advanced Supraglottic Lesions	*46*
4.6.2	Advanced Supraglottic Lesions	*47*
4.7	**Results of Treatment**	*47*
4.7.1	Vocal Cord Cancer	*47*
4.7.1.1	Supraglottic Results	*49*

References *54*

KEY POINTS

- The 2002 AJCC staging system includes a modification of T2 glottis so that paraglottic space invasion upgrades to T3, resulting in significant stage migration.
- T1–T2 glottic cancers are optimally treated with radiotherapy (RT) or transoral laser. The latter is indicated for limited lesions of the mid-third of the vocal cord. RT is preferred for more extensive tumors. The cure rates are approximately the same. Open partial laryngectomy (OPL) is reserved for salvage of local recurrences.
- Low-volume fixed-cord T3–T4 cancers are treated with RT and concomitant chemotherapy or, in selected cases, OPL.
- High-volume T3–T4 cancers are treated with total laryngectomy, which is usually followed with postoperative RT.
- T1–T2 and low-volume supraglottic (SGL) cancers are treated with either RT or OPL.
- High-volume T3–T4 cancers of the SGL are treated with TL and postoperative RT in most cases.

WILLIAM M. MENDENHALL, MD
Department of Radiation Oncology, University of Florida College
of Medicine, P.O. Box 100385, Gainesville, FL 32610-0385, USA
RUSSELL W. HINERMAN, MD
ROBERT J. AMDUR, MD
Department of Radiation Oncology, University of Florida College
of Medicine, P.O. Box 100385, Gainesville, FL 32610-0385, USA
MIKHAIL VAYSBERG, MD
JOHN W. WERNING, MD
Department of Otolaryngology, University of Florida College of
Medicine, P.O. Box 100264, Gainesville, FL 32610-0264, USA

4.1

Anatomy

The larynx is divided into the supraglottis, glottis, and subglottis. The supraglottis consists of the epiglottis, the false vocal cords, the ventricles, and the aryepiglottic folds, including the arytenoids. The glottis includes the true vocal cords and the anterior commissure. The lateral line of demarcation between the glottis and supraglottis is the apex of the ventricle. The subglottis is located below the vocal cords and is considered to extend from a point 5 mm below the free margin of the vocal cord to the inferior border of the cricoid cartilage.

The supraglottis has a rich capillary lymphatic plexus; the trunks pass through the preepiglottic space and the thyrohyoid membrane and terminate mainly in the level II lymph nodes; a few drain to the level III lymph nodes. There are essentially no capillary lymphatics of the true vocal cords; as a result, lymphatic spread from glottic cancer occurs only if tumor extends to supraglottic or subglottic areas. The subglottis has relatively few capillary lymphatics. The lymphatic trunks pass through the cricothyroid membrane to the pretracheal (Delphian) lymph nodes in the region of the thyroid isthmus. The subglottis also drains posteriorly through the cricotracheal membrane, with some trunks going to the paratracheal lymph nodes and others continuing to the inferior jugular chain.

4.2
Epidemiology and Risk Factors

Cancer of the larynx represents about 2% of the total cancer risk and is the most common head and neck cancer (skin excluded). In 2007 in the United States, there were ~11,300 new cases of cancer of the larynx (8,960 men and 2,340 women) and about 3,660 deaths from laryngeal cancer (JEMAL et al. 2007). Based on 1973–1998 US data, at diagnosis, about 51% of the cases remain localized, 29% have regional spread, and 15% have distant metastases (RIES et al. 2001). The ratio of glottic to supraglottic carcinoma is ~3:1.

Cancer of the larynx is strongly related to cigarette smoking and increases with the number of cigarettes consumed (POLESEL et al. 2008). The risk of tobacco-related cancers of the upper alimentary and respiratory tracts declines among ex-smokers after 5 years and is said to approach the risk of nonsmokers after 10 years of abstention. The role of alcohol in provoking laryngeal cancer is small for moderate consumption, but increases with more than 4 drinks/day and/or with concomitant tobacco use (LA VECCHIA et al. 2008).

4.3
Diagnostic Evaluation

The diagnostic evaluation includes a physical examination (including flexible laryngoscopy), chest radiography, computed tomography (CT) of the larynx and neck, and direct laryngoscopy and biopsy. Nearly all malignant tumors of the larynx arise from the surface epithelium and are squamous cell carcinoma or one of its variants. Position emission tomography and magnetic resonance imaging are obtained only to clarify an equivocal finding on CT or chest radiography.

4.4
Staging

The 2002 American Joint Committee on Cancer (AMERICAN JOINT COMMITTEE ON CANCER 2002) staging system for laryngeal primary cancer is listed in Table 4.1. T2 glottic cancers are stratified into those with normal (T2A) and impaired (T2B) vocal cord mobility. The major difference between the 1998 and 2002 staging systems is that a glottic cancer that invades the paraglottic space is upstaged to T3 in the latter system, even with mobile vocal cords, resulting in significant stage migration. Additionally, T4 has been stratified into T4A and T4B, based on resectability.

4.5
Selection of Treatment Modality for Glottic Carcinoma

The goals of treatment include cure with the best functional result and the least risk of a serious complication. Patients may be considered to be in an early group if the chance of cure with larynx preservation is high, a moderately advanced group if the likelihood of local control is 60–70% but the chance of cure remains good, and an advanced group if the chance of cure is moderate and the likelihood of laryngeal preservation is relatively low. The early group may be treated initially by radiation therapy (RT) or, in selected cases, by partial laryngectomy. The moderately advanced group may be treated with either RT, with laryngectomy reserved for relapse, or by total laryngectomy with or without adjuvant postoperative RT. The obvious advantage

Table 4.1. Staging of laryngeal cancer (Modified from AMERICAN JOINT COMMITTEE ON CANCER 2002)

Supraglottis	
T1	Tumor limited to one subsite of supraglottis with normal vocal cord mobility
T2	Tumor invades mucosa of more than one adjacent subsite of supraglottis or glottis or region outside the supraglottis (e.g., mucosa of base of tongue, vallecula, medial wall of pyriform sinus) without fixation of the larynx
T3	Tumor limited to larynx with vocal cord fixation and/or invades any of the following: postcricoid area, preepiglottic tissues, paraglottic space, and/or minor thyroid cartilage erosion (e.g., inner cortex)
T4a	Tumor invades through the thyroid cartilage and/or invades beyond the larynx (e.g., trachea, soft tissues of neck including deep extrinsic muscle of the tongue, strap muscles, thyroid, or esophagus)
T4b	Tumor invades prevertebral space, encases carotid artery, or invades mediastinal structures
Glottis	
T1	Tumor limited to vocal cord(s) (may involve anterior or posterior commissure) with normal mobility
T1a	Tumor limited to one vocal cord
T1b	Tumor involves both vocal cords
T2	Tumor extends to supraglottis and/or subglottis, and/or with impaired vocal cord mobility
T3	Tumor limited to the larynx with vocal cord fixation and/or invades paraglottic space, and/or minor thyroid cartilage erosion (e.g., inner cortex)
T4a	Tumor invades through the thyroid cartilage and/or invades tissues beyond the larynx (trachea, soft tissues of neck including deep extrinsic muscle of the tongue, strap muscles, thyroid, or esophagus)
T4b	Tumor invades prevertebral space, encases carotid artery, or invades mediastinal structures

of the former strategy, which we use at the University of Florida, is that there is a fairly good chance that the larynx will be preserved. Although some patients may be rehabilitated with a tracheoesophageal puncture after laryngectomy, only about 20% of patients use this device long term and the majority use an electric larynx (MENDENHALL et al. 2002). The advanced group is treated with total laryngectomy and neck dissection with or without adjuvant RT or RT and adjuvant chemotherapy (MENDENHALL et al. 2003). Recent data indicates that induction chemotherapy probably does not improve the likelihood of local-regional control and survival, whereas concomitant chemotherapy and RT results in an improved possibility of cure compared with RT alone (FORASTIERE et al. 2003; MENDENHALL et al. 2003; PIGNON et al. 2000). There is a subset of patients with high volume, unfavorable, advanced cancers who may be cured by chemoradiation but have a useless larynx and permanent tracheostomy and/or gastrostomy (MENDENHALL et al. 2003). These patients are best treated with a total laryngectomy, neck dissection, and postoperative RT.

4.5.1
Early Vocal Cord Carcinoma

In most centers, RT is the initial treatment prescribed for T1 and T2 lesions, with surgery reserved for salvage after RT failure (MENDENHALL et al. 2001, 2004). The likelihood of lymph node metastases is low, so the RT portals include only the primary site with a margin (MILLION et al. 1994). Patients are treated at 2.25 Gy/once daily fraction to 63 Gy for T1–T2A cancers and 65.25 Gy for T2B tumors (MENDENHALL et al. 2001; YAMAZAKI et al. 2006). Although hemilaryngectomy or cordectomy produces comparable cure rates for selected T1 and T2 vocal cord lesions, RT is generally preferred (MENDENHALL et al. 2004; O'SULLIVAN et al. 1994). Supracricoid laryngectomy, as reported by LACCOURREYE et al. (1990), is a procedure designed to remove moderate-sized cancers involving the supraglottic and glottic larynx. The larynx may be removed with preservation of the cricoid and the arytenoid with its neurovascular innervation, and the defect is closed by approximating the base of the tongue to the remaining larynx.

The oncologic and functional results of this procedure in selected patients are reported to be excellent. Transoral laser excision also may provide high cure rates for select patients with small, well-defined lesions limited to the mid-third of one true cord (McGuirt et al. 1994; Steiner 1993). A small subset of transoral laser surgeons successfully uses this technique in moderately advanced cancers (Steiner 1993). The major advantage of RT compared with partial laryngectomy is better voice quality. Partial laryngectomy finds its major use as salvage surgery in suitable cases after RT failure.

4.5.2
Moderately Advanced Vocal Cord Cancer

Fixed-cord lesions (T3) may be subdivided into relatively favorable or unfavorable lesions. Patients with unfavorable lesions usually have extensive bilateral disease with a compromised airway and are considered to be in the advanced group. Patients with favorable T3 lesions have disease confined mostly to one side of the larynx, have a good airway, and are reliable for follow-up. Some degree of supraglottic and subglottic extension usually exists. The extent of disease and tumor volume, in particular, are related to the likelihood of control after RT (Mendenhall et al. 2003).

The patient with a favorable lesion is treated with RT or a partial laryngectomy (Hinni et al. 2007; Lima et al. 2006). Most patients are not candidates for the latter and are irradiated. Recent data suggest that the likelihood of local-regional control is better after some altered fractionation schedules compared with conventional once-daily RT. We currently prefer 74.4 in 62 twice-daily fractions (Fu et al. 2000; Mendenhall et al. 2003). Additionally, concomitant chemotherapy and RT has been shown to improve the likelihood of cure compared with RT alone (Forastiere et al. 2003). The optimal chemotherapy regimen is unclear (Forastiere et al. 2003; Pignon et al. 2000). The risk of subclinical regional disease is 20–30% so that the clinically negative neck is electively irradiated. Follow-up examinations are recommended every 4–6 weeks for the first year, every 6–8 weeks for the second year, every 3 months for the third year, every 6 months for the fourth and fifth years, and annually thereafter.

Patients with unfavorable lesions are usually not cured with chemoradiation and those who are cured less likely to have a functional larynx. Thus, the majority of these patients are best treated with a total laryngectomy.

4.5.3
Advanced Vocal Cord Carcinoma

Advanced lesions usually show extensive subglottic and supraglottic extension, bilateral glottic involvement, and invasion of the thyroid, cricoid, or arytenoid cartilage, or frequently all three (Archer et al. 1984; Mendenhall et al. 1992). The airway is compromised, necessitating a tracheostomy at the time of direct laryngoscopy in ~30% of patients. Clinically positive lymph nodes are found in about 25–30% of patients.

The mainstay of treatment is total laryngectomy and neck dissection, with or without adjuvant RT. The indications for postoperative RT include close or positive margins, subglottic extension (≥1 cm), cartilage invasion, perineural invasion, endothelial-lined space invasion, extension of the primary tumor into the soft tissues of the neck, multiple positive neck nodes, extracapsular extension, and control of subclinical disease in the opposite neck (Amdur et al. 1989; Huang et al. 1992). Concomitant chemotherapy is given with postoperative RT for patients with positive margins and/or extracapsular extension. The postoperative RT dose is as follows: negative margins, 60 Gy in 30 fractions; microscopic positive margins, 66 Gy in 33 fractions; and gross residual, 70 Gy in 35 fractions. The low neck receives 50 Gy in 25 fractions; the stoma is boosted to 60 Gy with electrons if there is subglottic extension. Intensity-modulated RT may be used to avoid a difficult low neck match. Preoperative RT is indicated for patients who have fixed neck nodes, have had an emergency tracheotomy through tumor, or have direct extension of tumor involving the skin.

4.6
Selection of Treatment Modality for Supraglottic Carcinoma

4.6.1
Early and Moderately Advanced Supraglottic Lesions

Treatment of the primary lesion for the early group is by RT or supraglottic laryngectomy, with or without adjuvant RT (Hinerman et al. 2002). Approximately

50% of supraglottic laryngectomies performed at the University of Florida have been followed by postoperative RT because of neck disease and, less often, positive margins. Transoral laser excision is effective in experienced hands for small, selected lesions (STEINER 1993). Total laryngectomy is rarely indicated as the initial treatment for this group of patients and is reserved for treatment failures.

The decision to use RT or supraglottic laryngectomy depends on several factors, including the anatomic extent of the tumor, medical condition of the patient, philosophy of the attending physician(s), and inclination of the patient and family. Extension of the tumor to the true vocal cord, anterior commissure, vocal cord fixation, and/or thyroid or cricoid cartilage invasion precludes supraglottic laryngectomy. The procedure may be extended to include the base of tongue if one lingual artery is preserved. Supracricoid laryngectomy is an option for lesions involving one or both vocal cords; at least one arytenoid must be preserved. Vocal cord fixation and/or cartilage destruction are relative contraindications to this procedure. Overall, about 80% of patients are treated initially by RT. Approximately half of the patients seen in our clinic whose lesions are technically suitable for a supraglottic laryngectomy are not suitable for medical reasons (e.g., inadequate pulmonary status or other major medical problems).

Analysis of local control by anatomic site within the supraglottic larynx shows no obvious differences in local control by RT for similarly staged lesions. Primary tumor volume based on pretreatment CT is inversely related to local tumor control after RT (MENDENHALL et al. 2003). A large, bulky infiltrative lesion is a common reason to select supraglottic laryngectomy, as local control is probably improved compared to treatment with RT alone.

The status of the neck often determines the selection of treatment of the primary lesion. Patients with clinically negative neck nodes have a high risk for occult neck disease and may be treated by RT or supraglottic laryngectomy and bilateral selective neck dissections (levels II–IV).

If a patient has an early-stage primary lesion and N2b or N3 neck disease, combined treatment is frequently necessary to control the neck disease (MENDENHALL et al. 2002). In these cases, the primary lesion is usually treated by RT and concomitant chemotherapy. CT is obtained 4 weeks after RT, and neck dissection is added if the risk of residual cancer in the neck is thought to exceed 5%; otherwise the patient is observed and a CT is repeated in 3 months (MENDENHALL et al. 2002). If the same patient were treated with supraglottic laryngectomy, neck dissection, and postoperative RT, the portals would unnecessarily include the primary site as well as the neck. If the patient has early, resectable neck disease (N1 or N2a) and surgery is elected for the primary site, postoperative RT is added only because of unexpected findings (e.g., positive margins, multiple positive nodes, extensive perineural invasion, or extracapsular extension). The primary site and neck are treated to 55.8 Gy at 1.8 Gy/fraction; the involved neck is boosted to 60–70 Gy depending on the risk of residual disease.

4.6.2 Advanced Supraglottic Lesions

Although a subset of these patients may be suitable for a supraglottic or supracricoid laryngectomy, total laryngectomy is the main surgical option. Selected advanced lesions, especially those that are mainly exophytic, may be treated by RT and concomitant chemotherapy (PIGNON et al. 2000) with total laryngectomy reserved for RT failures.

For patients whose primary lesion is to be treated by a total or partial laryngectomy and who have resectable neck disease, surgery is the initial treatment, and postoperative RT is added if needed. If the neck disease is unresectable, preoperative RT is used. The indications for preoperative and postoperative RT have been previously outlined.

4.7 Results of Treatment

4.7.1 Vocal Cord Cancer

The local control rates after treatment of early-stage glottic carcinoma are depicted in Tables 4.2–4.4 (MENDENHALL et al. 2004). The local control and survival rates are similar for transoral laser excision, open partial laryngectomy, and RT. Larynx preservation and survival rates are also comparable. Voice quality depends on the amount of tissue removed with partial laryngectomy and is probably similar for patients with limited lesions treated with laser to those undergoing RT and poorer for patients undergoing open partial laryngectomy (MENDENHALL et al. 2004).

Table 4.2. Local control after transoral laser excision (MENDENHALL et al. 2004, Table 4.1, p 1787)

Institution	Follow-up[a]	No. of pts.	Stage	Local control (interval) (%)	Local control with larynx preservation (interval) (%)	Ultimate local control (interval) (%)
University of Göttingen (STEINER 1993)	Median, 78 months	159	pTis-pT2	94 (NS)	99 (NS)	–
University of Kiel (RUDERT and WERNER 1995)	Mean, 40 months	8	pTis	100 (NS)	–	–
		88	pT1a	92 (NS)	–	–
		10	pT1b	80 (NS)	–	–
		8	pT2	88 (NS)	–	–
		114	pTis-pT2	–	96 (NS)	–
University of Brescia (PERETTI et al. 2000)	Mean, 76 months	21	pTis	81 (NS)	–	95[b] (5 years)
		96	pT1	82 (NS)	–	87[b] (5 years)
		23	pT2	74 (NS)	–	91[b] (5 years)
		140	pTis-pT2	80 (NS)	97 (NS)	–
Washington University (SPECTOR et al. 1999)	Minimum, 3 years	61	T1	77 (NS)	90 (NS)	98 (NS)
University of Naples (MOTTA et al. 1997)	Minimum, 5 years	321	T1	82[b] (NS)	89[c] (NS)	–
		158	T2	60[b] (NS)	~67[c] (NS)	–
La Sapienza University (GALLO et al. 2003)	Minimum, 3 years	12	Tis	100 (NS)	100 (NS)	–
		120	T1a	94 (NS)	100 (NS)	–
		24	T1b	91 (NS)	100 (NS)	–
Tata Memorial Hospital (PRADHAN et al. 2003)	Minimum, 18 months	52	T1a	90 (NS)	94 (NS)	–
		17	T1b	65 (NS)	88 (NS)	–
		13	T2	77 (NS)	92 (NS)	–

NS not stated
[a]Follow-up period for total number of patients
[b]Ultimate local control with laser treatment alone
[c]Local-regional control rate

FOOTE et al. (1994) reported on 81 patients who underwent laryngectomy for T3 cancers at the Mayo Clinic between 1970 and 1981. Seventy-five patients underwent a total laryngectomy and six underwent a near-total laryngectomy; 53 patients received a neck dissection. No patient underwent adjuvant RT or chemotherapy. The 5-year rates of local-regional control, cause-specific survival, and absolute survival were 74, 74, and 54%, respectively. The results of definitive RT patients with T3 glottic carcinoma are depicted in Table 4.5 (PARSONS et al. 1989) and are similar to the surgical outcomes reported by FOOTE et al. (1994).

The 5-year outcomes after RT (53 patients) vs. surgery with or without RT (65 patients) for patients with T3 fixed-cord lesions treated at the University of Florida were as follows: local-regional control, 62 vs. 75%; ultimate local-regional control, 84 vs. 82%; absolute survival, 55 vs. 45%; and cause-specific survival, 75 vs. 71% (MENDENHALL et al. 1992). There was no relationship between subsequent local control and whether the vocal cord remained fixed or became mobile during irradiation. The incidence of severe complications, including those after the initial treatment and any later salvage procedures, was 15% after RT alone and 15% after surgery alone or combined with adjuvant RT. The vocal quality varied from fair to nearly normal.

The results of treatment of T4 vocal cord carcinoma in four surgical series and three RT series are

Table 4.3. Local control after open partial laryngectomy (MENDENHALL et al. 2004, Table 4.2, p 1788)

Institution	Follow-up	No. of pts.	Stage	Local control (interval) (%)	Local control with larynx preservation (interval) (%)	Ultimate local control (interval) (%)
Universitaire Timone (GIOVANNI et al. 2001)	NS	62	T1	100 (NS)	100 (NS)	–
		65	T2	92 (NS)	92 (NS)	–
Hôpital Saint Charles (CRAMPETTE et al. 1999)	Minimum, 3 years	18	T1a	100 (NS)	–	–
		40	T1b	95 (NS)	–	–
		23	T2a	83 (NS)	–	–
Mayo Clinic (THOMAS et al. 1994)	Median, 6.6 years	159	Tis–T1	93 (5 years)	94 (NS)	100 (NS)
Hôpital Laënnec (LACCOURREYE et al. 1994)	Minimum, 3 years	295	T1	89 (NS)	–	–
		90	T2a	74 (NS)	–	–
		31	T2b	68 (NS)	–	–
		416	T1–T2b	84 (NS)	–	97 (NS)
Washington University (SPECTOR et al. 1999)	Minimum, 3 years	404	T1	92 (NS)	93 (NS)	99 (NS)
Washington University (SPECTOR et al. 1999)	Minimum, 5 years	71	T2	93 (NS)	93 (NS)	99 (NS)

NS not stated

summarized in Table 4.6 (HARWOOD et al. 1981). HINERMAN et al. (2007) reported on 22 highly selected patients with low volume T4 cancers treated with definitive RT; the 5-year local control rate was 81%.

4.7.1.1
Supraglottic Results

The proportion of patients suitable for a supraglottic laryngectomy is variable (HINERMAN et al. 2002). Depending on the referral patterns, a modest subset of patients is suitable for this operation. The extent of neck disease for patients treated with either surgery or radiotherapy is also variable (HINERMAN et al. 2002). In general, patients treated with supraglottic laryngectomy appropriately have earlier stage neck disease and would be anticipated to have a lower risk of distant failure and improved survival.

The local control rates after transoral laser, radiotherapy, and supraglottic laryngectomy are summarized in Tables 4.7–4.9 (HINERMAN et al. 2002). In general, the local control rates after transoral laser excision are fairly good for patients with T1–T2 tumors and tend to deteriorate for those with more advanced disease. The local control rate for patients selected for supraglottic laryngectomy is excellent. However, the incidence of severe complications tends to be higher after supraglottic laryngectomy than after radiotherapy and transoral laser excision (Table 4.10) (HINERMAN et al. 2002).

Acknowledgment

We thank the research support staff of the Department of Radiation Oncology for their help with statistics, editing, and manuscript preparation.

Table 4.4. Local control after radiotherapy (MENDENHALL et al. 2004, Table 4.3, p 1789)

Institution	Follow-up[a]	No. of pts	Stage	Local control (interval) (%)	Local control with larynx preservation (interval) (%)	Ultimate local control (interval) (%)
University of Florida (MENDENHALL et al. 2001)	Minimum, 2 years	230	T1a	94 (5 years)	95 (5 years)	98 (5 years)
	Median, 9.9 years	61	T1b	93 (5 years)	95 (5 years)	98 (5 years)
		146	T2a	80 (5 years)	82 (5 years)	96 (5 years)
		82	T2b	72 (5 years)	76 (5 years)	96 (5 years)
Massachusetts General Hospital (WANG 1997)	NS	665	T1	93 (5 years)	–	–
		145	T2a	77 (5 years)	–	–
				71 (5 years)		
University of California-San Francisco (Le et al., 1997).	Median, 9.7 years	92	T2b		–	–
		315	T1	85 (5 years)	–	96[b] (5 years)
		83	T2	70 (5 years)	–	91[b] (5 years)
Princess Margaret Hospital (WARDE et al. 1998)	Median, 6.8 years	403	T1a	91 (5 years)	–	–
		46	T1b	82 (5 years)	–	–
		286	T2	69 (5 years)	–	–
M. D. Anderson Hospital (GARDEN et al. 2003)	Median, 6.8 years	114	T2a	74 (5 years)	–	–
		116	T2b	70 (5 years)	–	–
		230	T2	72 (5 years)	–	91 (5 years)

NS not stated
[a]Follow-up period for total number of patients
[b]Local-regional control rates

Table 4.5. Stage T3 glottic carcinoma treated with irradiation alone (no chemotherapy) (Modified from PARSONS et al. 1989, Table 4.2, p 127)

Investigator	Institution	No. of pts	Minimum follow-up (years)	Local control (%)	Ultimate control after salvage surgery (%)
HARWOOD et al. (1980)	Princess Margaret (Toronto)	112	3	51	77
WANG (1987)	Mass. General (Boston)	70	4	36	57
FLETCHER et al. (1969)	M.D. Anderson (Houston)	17	2	77	No data
SKOLYSZEWSKI and REINFUSS (1981)	15 European Centers	91	3	50	No data
STEWART et al. (1975)	Manchester (England)	67	10	57	67
MILLS (1979)	Cape Town, South Africa	18	2	44	78
HINERMAN et al. (2007)	U. Florida (Gainesville)	87	2	63	89

Laryngeal Cancer: Epidemiology and Treatment Outcomes 51

Table 4.6. Treatment of stage T4 glottic carcinomas (Modified from HARWOOD et al. 1981, Table 4.4, p 1511)

Investigator	Tumor stage	No. pts.	Method of treatment	Results (NED)
JESSE (1975)	T4N0–N+	48	Laryngectomy	54% at 4 year
OGURA et al. (1975)	T4N0	11	Laryngectomy	45% at 3 year
SKOLNICK et al. (1975)	T4N0	7	Laryngectomy	30% at 5 year
VERMUND (1970)	T4N0	31	Laryngectomy	35% at 5 year
STEWART and JACKSON (1975)	T4N0	13	Radiotherapy with surgery for salvage	38% at 5 year
HARWOOD et al. (1981)	T4N0	56	Radiotherapy with surgery for salvage	49% at 5 year[a]
HINERMAN et al. (2007)	T4N0	22	Radiotherapy with surgery for salvage	81% local control at 5 year[a]

NED no evidence of disease
[a]Life-table method; uncorrected for deaths from intercurrent disease

Table 4.7. Supraglottic Larynx: Local control after transoral laser excision (HINERMAN et al. 2002, Table 4.5, p 463)

Series	Staging	No. pts.	Percent of patients with T1 or T2 tumors	Local control			
				T1 (%)	T2 (%)	T3 (%)	T4 (%)
DAVIS et al. (1991)	P	14 R	57	100	100	50	–
STEINER (1993)[a]	P	81 R	72	–	76	77	100
ZEITELS et al. (1994)	ND	22	100	100	100	–	–
ZEITELS et al. (1994)	ND	23 R	65	100	92	63	–
CSANÁDY et al. (1999)	ND	23	100	70[b]		–	–
RUDERT et al. (1999)	P	34 R	50	100	75	78	38

Some figures were estimated as closely as possible to fit table format if the information was not specifically stated in the cited reference
[a]51 glottic and 30 supraglottic
[b]Overall local control rates for T1 and T2
P pathologic staging; *R* plus or minus radiotherapy; *ND* type of staging not provided

Table 4.8. Supraglottic Larynx: Local control after radiotherapy (HINERMAN et al. 2002, Table 4.6, p 463)

Series	Institution	No. of pts	T1 (%)	T2 (%)	T3 (%)	T4 (%)
FLETCHER and HAMBERGER (1974)	M.D. Anderson Hospital	173	88	79	62	47
GHOSSEIN et al. (1974)	Fondation Curie	203	94	73	46[a]	52
WANG and MONTGOMERY (1991)	Massachusetts General Hospital	229 q.d.	73	60	54	26
		209 b.i.d.	89	89	71	91
NAKFOOR et al. (1998)	Massachusetts General Hospital	164	96	86	76	43
SYKES et al. (2000)	Christie Hospital	331[b]	92[c]	81[c]	67[c]	73[c]
HINERMAN et al. (2002)	University of Florida[d]	274	100	86	62	62

Some figures were estimated as closely as possible to fit table format if the information was not specifically stated in the cited reference
[a]All had cord fixation
[b]All N0
[c]After 17 were salvaged by total laryngectomies
[d]1998 AJCC staging
q.d. once a day; *b.i.d.* twice a day

Table 4.9. Local control after supraglottic laryngectomy (HINERMAN et al. 2002, Table 4.7, p 464)

Series	Institution	No. of pts.	Patients with T1 and T2 tumors (%)	Local control			
				T1 (%)	T2 (%)	T3 (%)	T4 (%)
OGURA et al. (1975)	Washington University	177	78	–	94[a]		–
BOCCA and BAKER (1991)	Milan University						
Stage I		47	100	94	–	–	–
Stage II		252	100	–	82	–	–
Stage III		205	53	–	80[b]	–	–
Stage IV		33	70	–		67[c]	–
LEE et al. (1990)	M.D. Anderson Cancer Center	60	58	100	100	100	100
DeSANTO (1990)	Mayo Clinic	70	100	100	100	–	–
STEINIGER et al. (1997)	Albany Medical College	29	83	–	97[a]		–
SPRIANO et al. (1997)	Varese, Italy	54	100		96[d]	–	–
BURSTEIN and CALCATTERA (1985)	University of California (LA)	40	58	100	85	94	100
ISAACS et al. (1998)	University of Florida	33	76	100	78	71	100
LUTZ et al. (1990)	University of Pittsburgh	72	No data	–	99		–

T stages were not specified

Some figures were estimated as closely as possible to fit table format if the information was not specifically stated in the cited reference

[a] Overall local control rates for T1–T4

[b] Overall local control rates for T1–T3

[c] Overall local control rates for T2–T3

[d] Overall local control rates for T1–T2

Table 4.10. Supraglottic Larynx: Severe complications according to treatment modality (HINERMAN et al. 2002, Table 4.8, p 465)

Series	Institution	No. of severe complications
Radiotherapy		
FLETCHER and HAMBERGER (1974)	M.D. Anderson Cancer Center	10/173 (6%)
GHOSSEIN et al. (1974)	Fondation Curie	8/117 (7%)
NAKFOOR et al. (1998)	Massachusetts General Hospital	12/169 (7%)
SYKES et al. (2000)	Christie Hospital	7/331 (2%)
HINERMAN et al. (2002)	University of Florida	12/274 (4%)
Supraglottic laryngectomy		
LEE et al. (1990)	M.D. Anderson Cancer Center	9/63 (14%)
ISAACS et al. (1998)	University of Florida	14/34 (41%)
BURSTEIN and CALCATERRA (1985)	University of California Los Angeles	14/41 (34%)
STEINIGER et al. (1997)	Albany Medical College	12/29 (41%)
SPRIANO et al. (1997)	Varese, Italy	13/54 (24%)
GALL et al. (1977)	Washington University	20/133 (15%)
WEBER et al. (1993)	University of Pittsburgh	12/69 (17%)
BECKHARDT et al. (1994)	University of Wisconsin	15/50 (30%)
Transoral laser excision		
RUDERT et al. (1999)	University of Kiel, Germany	3/34 (9%)
ZEITELS et al., (1994)	Massachusetts Eye and Ear Infirmary	2/45 (4%)
STEINER (1993)[a]	University of Gottingen, Germany	7/240 (3%)
DAVIS et al. (1991)	University of Utah, Salt Lake City	0/14 (0%)
CSANÁDY et al. (1999)	Albert Szent Gyorgyi Medical University, Szeged, Hungary	0/23 (0%)

Some figures were estimated as closely as possible to fit table format if the information was not specifically stated in the cited reference.

[a]Includes patients with glottic cancer

References

Amdur RJ, Parsons JT, Mendenhall WM et al. (1989) Postoperative irradiation for squamous cell carcinoma of the head and neck: an analysis of treatment results and complications. Int J Radiat Oncol Biol Phys 16:25–36

American Joint Committee on Cancer (2002) Larynx. AJCC cancer staging manual, 6th ed. Springer, New York, pp 47–57

Archer CR, Yeager VL, Herbold DR (1984) Improved diagnostic accuracy in laryngeal cancer using a new classification based on computed tomography. Cancer 53:44–57

Beckhardt RN, Murray JG, Ford CN et al. (1994) Factors influencing functional outcome in supraglottic laryngectomy. Head Neck 16:232–239

Bocca E (1991) Sixteenth Daniel C. Baker, Jr, memorial lecture. surgical management of supraglottic cancer and its lymph node metastases in a conservative perspective. Ann Otol Rhinol Laryngol 100:261–267

Burstein FD, Calcaterra TC (1985) Supraglottic laryngectomy: series report and analysis of results. Laryngoscope 95:833–836

Crampette L, Garrel R, Gardiner Q et al. (1999) Modified subtotal laryngectomy with cricohyoidoepiglottopexy–Long term results in 81 patients. Head Neck 21:95–103

Csanády M, Iván L, Czigner J (1999) Endoscopic CO_2 laser therapy of selected cases of supraglottic marginal tumors. Eur Arch Otorhinolaryngol 256:392–394

Davis RK, Kelly SM, Hayes J (1991) Endoscopic CO_2 laser excisional biopsy of early supraglottic cancer. Laryngoscope 101:680–683

DeSanto LW (1990) Early supraglottic cancer. Ann Otol Rhinol Laryngol 99:593–597

Fletcher GH, Hamberger AD (1974) Causes of failure in irradiation of squamous-cell carcinoma of the supraglottic larynx. Radiology 111:697–700

Fletcher GH, Lindberg RD, Jesse RH (1969) Radiation therapy for cancer of the larynx and pyriform sinus. Eye Ear Nose Throat Digest 31:58–67

Foote RL, Olsen KD, Buskirk SJ et al. (1994) Laryngectomy alone for T3 glottic cancer. Head Neck 16:406–412

Forastiere AA, Goepfert H, Maor M et al. (2003) Concurrent chemotherapy and radiotherapy for organ preservation in advanced laryngeal cancer. N Engl J Med 349:2091–2098

Fu KK, Pajak TF, Trotti A et al. (2000) A Radiation Therapy Oncology Group (RTOG) phase III randomized study to compare hyperfractionation and two variants of accelerated fractionation to standard fractionation radiotherapy for head and neck squamous cell carcinomas: first report of RTOG 9003. Int J Radiat Oncol Biol Phys 48:7–16

Gall AM, Sessions DG, Ogura JH (1977) Complications following surgery for cancer of the larynx and hypopharynx. Cancer 39:624–631

Gallo A, de Vincentiis M, Manciocco V et al. (2003) CO_2 laser cordectomy for early-stage glottic carcinoma: a long-term follow-up of 156 cases. Laryngoscope 112:370–374

Garden AS, Forster K, Wong PF et al. (2003) Results of radiotherapy for T2N0 glottic carcinoma: does the "2" stand for twice-daily treatment? Int J Radiat Oncol Biol Phys 55:322–328

Ghossein NA, Bataini JP, Ennuyer A et al. (1974) Local control and site of failure in radically irradiated supraglottic laryngeal cancer. Radiology 112:187–192

Giovanni A, Guelfucci B, Gras R et al. (2001) Partial frontolateral laryngectomy with epiglottic reconstruction for management of early-stage glottic carcinoma. Laryngoscope 111:663–668

Harwood AR, Beale FA, Cummings BJ et al. (1980) T3 glottic cancer: An analysis of dose-time-volume factors. Int J Radiat Oncol Biol Phys 6:675–680

Harwood AR, Beale FA, Cummings BJ et al. (1981) T4N0M0 glottic cancer: An analysis of dose-time-volume factors. Int J Radiat Oncol Biol Phys 7:1507–1512

Hinerman RW, Mendenhall WM, Amdur RJ et al. (2002) Carcinoma of the supraglottic larynx: treatment results with radiotherapy alone or with planned neck dissection. Head Neck 24:456–467

Hinerman RW, Mendenhall WM, Morris CG et al. (2007) T3 and T4 true vocal cord squamous carcinomas treated with external beam irradiation: a single institution's 35-year experience. Am J Clin Oncol 30:181–185

Hinni ML, Salassa JR, Grant DG et al. (2007) Transoral laser microsurgery for advanced laryngeal cancer. Arch Otolaryngol Head Neck Surg 133:1198–1204

Huang DT, Johnson CR, Schmidt-Ullrich R et al. (1992) Postoperative radiotherapy in head and neck carcinoma with extracapsular lymph node extension and/or positive resection margins: a comparative study. Int J Radiat Oncol Biol Phys 23:737–742

Isaacs JH Jr., Slattery WH, III, Mendenhall WM et al. (1998) Supraglottic laryngectomy. Am J Otolaryngol 19:118–123

Jemal A, Siegel R, Ward E et al. (2007) Cancer statistics 2007. CA Cancer J Clin 57:43–66

Jesse RH (1975) The evaluation of treatment of patients with extensive squamous cancer of the vocal cords. Laryngoscope 85:1424–1429

La Vecchia C, Zhang ZF, Altieri A (2008) Alcohol and laryngeal cancer: an update. Eur J Cancer Prev 17:116–124

Laccourreye H, Laccourreye O, Weinstein G et al. (1990) Supracricoid laryngectomy with cricohyoidoepiglottopexy: a partial laryngeal procedure for glottic carcinoma. Ann Otol Rhinol Laryngol 99:421–426

Laccourreye O, Weinstein G, Brasnu D et al. (1994) A clinical trial of continuous cisplatin-fluorouracil induction chemotherapy and supracricoid partial laryngectomy for glottic carcinoma classified as T2. Cancer 74:2781–2790

Le Q-TX, Fu KK, Kroll S et al. (1997) Influence of fraction size, total dose, and overall time on local control of T1-T2 glottic carcinoma. Int J Radiat Oncol Biol Phys 39:115–126

Lee NK, Goepfert H, Wendt CD (1990) Supraglottic laryngectomy for intermediate-stage cancer: U.T. M.D. Anderson Cancer Center experience with combined therapy. Laryngoscope 100:831–836

Lima RA, Freitas EQ, Dias FL et al. (2006) Supracricoid laryngectomy with cricohyoidoepiglottopexy for advanced glottic cancer. Head Neck 28:481–486

Lutz CK, Johnson JT, Wagner RL et al. (1990) Supraglottic carcinoma: patterns of recurrence. Ann Otol Rhinol Laryngol 99:12–17

McGuirt WF, Blalock D, Koufman JA et al. (1994) Comparative voice results after laser resection or irradiation of T1 vocal cord carcinoma. Arch Otolaryngol Head Neck Surg 120:951–955

Mendenhall WM, Amdur RJ, Morris CG et al. (2001) T1-T2N0 squamous cell carcinoma of the glottic larynx treated with radiation therapy. J Clin Oncol 19:4029–4036

Mendenhall WM, Morris CG, Amdur RJ et al. (2003) Parameters that predict local control following definitive radiotherapy for squamous cell carcinoma of the head and neck. Head Neck 25:535–542

Mendenhall WM, Morris CG, Stringer SP et al. (2002) Voice rehabilitation after total laryngectomy and postoperative radiation therapy. J Clin Oncol 20:2500–2505

Mendenhall WM, Parsons JT, Stringer SP et al. (1992) Stage T3 squamous cell carcinoma of the glottic larynx: a comparison of laryngectomy and irradiation. Int J Radiat Oncol Biol Phys 23:725–732

Mendenhall WM, Riggs CE, Amdur RJ et al. (2003) Altered fractionation and/or adjuvant chemotherapy in definitive irradiation of squamous cell carcinoma of the head and neck. Laryngoscope 113:546–551

Mendenhall WM, Villaret DB, Amdur RJ et al. (2002) Planned neck dissection after definitive radiotherapy for squamous cell carcinoma of the head and neck. Head Neck 24:1012–1018

Mendenhall WM, Werning JW, Hinerman RW et al. (2004) Management of T1-T2 glottic carcinomas. Cancer 100:1786–1792

Million RR, Cassisi NJ, Mancuso AA (1994) Larynx. In: Million RR, Cassisi NJ (eds) Management of head and neck cancer: a multidisciplinary approach, 2nd edn. J. B. Lippincott, Philadelphia, pp 431–497

Mills EE (1979) Early glottic carcinoma: factors affecting radiation failure, results of treatment and sequelae. Int J Radiat Oncol Biol Phys 5:811–817

Motta G, Esposito E, Cassiano B et al. (1997) T1-T2-T3 glottic tumors: Fifteen years experience with CO_2 laser. Acta Otolaryngol Suppl 527:155–159

Nakfoor BM, Spiro IJ, Wang CC et al. (1998) Results of accelerated radiotherapy for supraglottic carcinoma: a Massachusetts General Hospital and Massachusetts Eye and Ear Infirmary experience. Head Neck 20:379–384

Ogura JH, Sessions DG, Ciralsky RH (1975) Supraglottic carcinoma with extension to the arytenoid. Laryngoscope 85:1327–1331

Ogura JH, Sessions DG, Spector GJ (1975) Conservation surgery for epidermoid carcinoma of the supraglottic larynx. Laryngoscope 85:1808–1815

O'Sullivan B, Mackillop W, Gilbert R et al. (1994) Controversies in the management of laryngeal cancer: results of an international survey of patterns of care. Radiother Oncol 31:23–32

Parsons JT, Mendenhall WM, Mancuso AA et al. (1989) Twice-a-day radiotherapy for T3 squamous cell carcinoma of the glottic larynx. Head Neck 11:123–128

Peretti G, Nicolai P, Redaelli De Zinis LO et al. (2000) Endoscopic CO2 laser excision for Tis, T1, and T2 glottic carcinomas: cure rate and prognostic factors. Otolaryngol Head Neck Surg 123:124–131

Pignon JP, Bourhis J, Domenge C et al. (2000) MACH-NC (Meta-Analysis of Chemotherapy on Head and Neck Cancer) Collaborative Group. Chemotherapy added to locoregional treatment for head and neck squamous-cell carcinoma: three meta-analyses of updated individual data. Lancet 355:949–955

Polesel J, Talamini R, La Vecchia C et al. (2008) Tobacco smoking and the risk of upper aero-digestive tract cancers: a reanalysis of case–control studies using spline models. Int J Cancer 122:2398–2402

Pradhan SA, Pai PS, Neeli SI et al. (2003) Transoral laser surgery for early glottic cancers. Arch Otolaryngol Head Neck Surg 129:623–625

Ries LAG, Eisner MP, Kosary CL et al. (2001) SEER cancer statistics review, 1973–1998. National Cancer Institute, Bethesda, MD

Rudert HH, Werner JA (1995) Endoscopic resections of glottic and supraglottic carcinomas with the CO_2 laser. Eur Arch Otorhinolaryngol 252:146–148

Rudert HH, Werner JA, Höft S (1999) Transoral carbon dioxide laser resection of supraglottic carcinoma. Ann Otol Rhinol Laryngol 108:819–827

Skolnik EM, Yee KF, Wheatley MA et al. (1975) Carcinoma of the laryngeal glottis: therapy and end results. Laryngoscope 85:1453–1466

Skolyszewski J, Reinfuss M (1981) The results of radiotherapy of cancer of the larynx in six European countries. Radiobiol Radiother (Berl) 22:32–43

Spector JG, Sessions DG, Chao KS et al. (1999) Stage I (T1 N0 M0) squamous cell carcinoma of the laryngeal glottis: therapeutic results and voice preservation. Head Neck 21:707–717

Spector JG, Sessions DG, Chao KSC et al. (1999) Management of stage II (T2N0M0) glottic carcinoma by radiotherapy and conservation surgery. Head Neck 21:116–123

Spriano G, Antognoni P, Piantanida R et al. (1997) Conservative management of T1-T2N0 supraglottic cancer: a retrospective study. Am J Otolaryngol 18:299–305

Steiner W (1993) Results of curative laser microsurgery of laryngeal carcinomas. Am J Otolaryngol 14:116–121

Steiniger JR, Parnes SM, Gardner GM (1997) Morbidity of combined therapy for the treatment of supraglottic carcinoma: supraglottic laryngectomy and radiotherapy. Ann Otol Rhinol Laryngol 106:151–158

Stewart JG, Brown JR, Palmer MK et al. (1975) The management of glottic carcinoma by primary irradiation with surgery in reserve. Laryngoscope 85:1477–1484

Stewart JG, Jackson AW (1975) The steepness of the dose response curve both for tumor cure and normal tissue injury. Laryngoscope 85:1107–1111

Sykes AJ, Slevin NJ, Gupta NK et al. (2000) 331 cases of clinically node-negative supraglottic carcinoma of the larynx: a study of a modest size fixed field radiotherapy approach. Int J Radiat Oncol Biol Phys 46:1109–1115

Thomas JV, Olsen KD, Neel HB, III et al. (1994) Early glottic carcinoma treated with open laryngeal procedures. Arch Otolaryngol Head Neck Surg 120:264–268

Vermund H (1970) Role of radiotherapy in cancer of the larynx as related to the TNM system of staging. A review. Cancer 25:485–504

Wang CC (1987) Radiation therapy of laryngeal tumors: curative radiation therapy. In: Thawley SE, Panje WR (eds) Comprehensive management of head and neck tumors. WB Saunders, Philadelphia, pp 906–919

Wang CC (1997) Carcinoma of the larynx. In: Wang CC (ed) Radiation therapy for head and neck neoplasms, 3rd ed. Wiley-Liss, New York, pp 221–255

Wang CC, Montgomery WM (1991) Deciding on optimal management of supraglottic carcinoma. Oncology 5: 41–46

Warde P, O'Sullivan B, Bristow RG et al. (1998) T1-T2 glottic cancer managed by external beam radiotherapy: the influence of pretreatment hemoglobin on local control. Int J Radiat Oncol Biol Phys 41:347–353

Weber PC, Johnson JT, Myers EN (1993) Impact of bilateral neck dissection on recovery following supraglottic laryngectomy. Arch Otolaryngol Head Neck Surg 119:61–64

Yamazaki H, Nishiyama K, Tanaka E et al. (2006) Radiotherapy for early glottic carcinoma (T1N0M0): results of prospective randomized study of radiation fraction size and overall treatment time. Int J Radiat Oncol Biol Phys 64:77–82

Zeitels SM, Koufman JA, Davis RK et al. (1994) Endoscopic treatment of supraglottic and hypopharynx cancer. Laryngoscope 104:71–78

Nasopharynx

5

ANNE W. M. LEE, REBECCA M. W. YEUNG, and WAI TONG NG

CONTENTS

5.1	**Epidemiology** *57*	
5.1.1	Distribution Pattern *57*	
5.1.2	Etiology *59*	
5.1.3	Changing Epidemiological Pattern *59*	
5.2	**Current Treatment Recommendations** *59*	
5.2.1	Radiation Therapy *60*	
5.2.2	Chemotherapy *61*	
5.3	**Treatment Outcome** *61*	
5.3.1	Tumor Control and Survival *61*	
5.3.2	Late Toxicity *68*	
5.3.3	Quality of Life *69*	
5.4	**Final Remarks** *70*	
References *70*		

KEY POINTS

- Nasopharyngeal carcinoma (NPC) has a distinct racial and geographic distribution.
- Etiology includes both inherited genetic predisposition and environmental factors. The association of Epstein-Barr virus with nonkeratinizing NPC suggests a probable oncogenic role in pathogenesis.
- Major series (mostly with two-dimensional radiotherapy techniques) during 1990–2000 showed that 5-year overall survival of ~70% could be achieved.
- The current standard recommendation for NPC is radiotherapy alone for early stage and cisplatin-based concurrent chemoradiotherapy for stages III–IVB (± high-risk stage IIB). Intensity-modulated radiotherapy (IMRT) technique is advocated.
- Contemporary series using IMRT report encouraging early results with locoregional control in excess of 90% at 2–4 years. Key remaining problem is distant failure.
- Further enhancement of efficacy by accelerated fractionation and/or altered chemotherapy sequencing is being explored.
- Concurrent chemotherapy significantly increases the risk of late toxicity.
- Although IMRT can reduce xerostomia and improve quality of life, further reduction of other serious late toxicity is needed.

Dr ANNE W. M. LEE, MD
REBECCA M. W. YEUNG, MD
WAI TONG NG, MD
Department of Clinical Oncology, Pamela Youde Nethersole Eastern Hospital, 3 Lok Man Road, Chai Wan, Hong Kong, China

5.1

Epidemiology

5.1.1
Distribution Pattern

Nasopharyngeal carcinoma (NPC) is unique for the distinct racial and geographic distribution (Fig. 5.1). PARKIN et al. (2002) reported that the age-standardized incidence rate (ASR/100,000/year) in 1993–1997 ranged from <1 among Caucasians to >20 among Southern Chinese male populations. There is marked variation in incidence among Chinese residing in different parts of China, with ASR ranging from 1.7

in Tianjin (in the north) to 21.4 in Hong Kong (in the south). There is also marked variation in incidence among different ethnic groups in Singapore, with ASR ranging from 1.3 among Indians to 16.3 among Chinese (Table 5.1).

In low-risk populations, a bimodal age distribution is observed. The first peak incidence occurs at 15–25 and the second peak at 50–59 years of age. In contrast, the incidence in high-risk populations rises after 30 years of age, peaks at 40–60 years, and declines thereafter (FERLAY et al. 2004). The age distribution is similar in both genders. The incidence rates in male are commonly 2–3 fold that of female populations.

Descendants from Chinese who have migrated to western countries show progressively lower risk, but their incidence remains higher than the indigenous populations (BUELL 1973; SUN et al. 2005). The study by DICKSON and FLORES (1985) showed that the incidence rate in Chinese born in the Orient was 20.5, compared with 1.3 for Chinese and 0.2 for white people born in Canada.

Familial aggregation of NPC has been widely reported (FRIBORG et al. 2005; JIA et al. 2004; Ko et al.

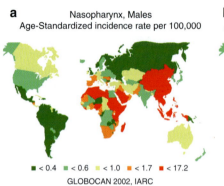
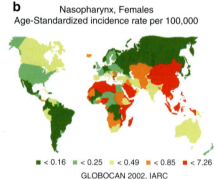

Fig. 5.1. Global incidence of nasopharyngeal cancer: age-standardized rate (world standard population) per 100,000. (a) Males population. (b) Females population (Ferlay 2004, GLOBOCAN 2002; http://www-dep.iarc.fr)

Table 5.1. Age-standardized incidence rate (per 100,000/year) in different communities during different periods

Year	Male				Female			
	1978–1982	1983–1987	1988–1992	1993–1997	1978–1982	1983–1987	1988–1992	1993–1997
China								
Hong Kong	30.0	28.5	24.3	21.4	12.9	11.2	9.5	8.3
Shanghai	4.4	4.0	4.5	4.2	2.0	1.9	1.8	1.5
Singapore								
Chinese	18.1	18.1	18.5	16.3	7.9	7.4	7.3	5.4
Indian	0.3	1.0	0.5	1.3	1.3	0.2	0.5	0.1
United States								
SEER: White	NA	0.5	0.5	0.5	NA	0.2	0.2	0.2
SEER: Black	NA	0.8	0.9	0.9	NA	0.3	0.2	0.3
LA: Chinese	9.9	6.5	9.8	7.6	7.3	3.0	2.8	2.4
England	0.4	0.4	0.4	0.4	0.2	0.2	0.2	0.2
Australia								
NSW	0.8	0.8	0.9	0.9	0.3	0.2	0.3	0.4

SEER surveillance, epidemiology and end-results; *LA* Los Angeles; *NSW* New South Wales

1998; Loh et al. 2006). The excess risk is 4–10 fold among first-degree relatives of patients affected by NPC when compared with cohorts without a family history.

5.1.2
Etiology

The peculiar epidemiological patterns suggest a multifactorial etiology that includes both inherited genetic predisposition and environmental factors. A study in the United States by Burt et al. (1996) showed that the associated haplotypes in human leukocyte antigen (HLA) were different between Chinese and Caucasians; the HLA-A2 allele found specifically in non-Chinese might be associated with a protective effect. Recent linkage analysis of Chinese NPC pedigrees had identified susceptibility loci on chromosomes 4p15.1-q12 (Feng et al. 2002) and 3p21 (Xiong et al. 2004). An extensive review of the genetic changes by Lo et al. (2004b) suggested that involvement of specific haplotypes in HLA, genetic susceptibility factor(s), and loss of heterozygosity at chromosomes 3p and 9p might all play an important part in carcinogenesis. They further postulated that genetic alterations might be induced by chemical carcinogens in the environment that lead to subsequent transformation of normal epithelium to low-grade dysplasia. Latent Epstein-Barr virus (EBV) infection and overexpression of bcl-2 protein (that inhibits apoptosis) might then affect the progression of low-grade precursors to high-grade lesions.

The near constant association of EBV with non-keratinizing NPC, irrespective of ethnic background, indicates a probable oncogenic role in the pathogenesis (Chan et al. 2005a; Pathmanathan et al. 1995; Raab-Traub 2002). Supporting evidence includes presence of EBV-DNA or RNA in practically all tumor cells, presence in a clonal episomal form (indicating that the virus has entered the tumor cell before clonal expansion), and presence in the precursor lesion of NPC (but not in normal nasopharyngeal epithelium). It appears that latent infection of EBV promotes tumorigenicity by enhancing the tumor invading properties (Lo et al. 2004a).

Exposure to carcinogens in traditional southern Chinese diet (Ho 1978), particularly volatile nitrosamines in preserved food (Poirier et al. 1987), has been incriminated. Childhood consumption of salted fish is associated with increased risk of NPC.

The relative risk ranged from 1.4 to 7.5 for cohorts having frequent consumption, compared with those having rare consumption (Armstrong et al. 1998; Yu et al. 1986; Yuan et al. 2000). Cigarette smoking, previous irradiation, occupational exposure to dust, smoke, and chemical fumes has also been implicated, but definitive conclusion is lacking.

5.1.3
Changing Epidemiological Pattern

Table 5.1 shows the changing epidemiology in ethnic groups during different periods. While the incidence remains the same in nonendemic communities, the ASR in Hong Kong shows substantial decrease in the past three decades. The study by Lee et al. (2003) showed steady reduction in the ASR from 28.5 in 1980–1984 to 20.2 in 1995–1999 per 100,000 males, and from 11.2 to 7.8 per 100,000 females, resulting in a total decrease of 30% in both genders over this 20-year period. As there was no substantial change in the proportion of Chinese in the community, this decrease is probably attributed to changing environmental risk factors as the life-style for most Hong Kong citizens changed progressively from traditional southern Chinese to a more western style, particularly in terms of diet.

Furthermore, the magnitude of total decrease in NPC mortality amounted to 43% for males and 50% for females (Fig. 5.2). The age-standardized mortality/incidence ratio decreased from 0.48 to 0.39 for males, and from 0.40 to 0.29 for females in the corresponding periods. This strongly reflects steady improvement in treatment outcome in addition to decreasing incidence.

5.2

Current Treatment Recommendations

Because of the deep-seated location of the nasopharynx and the anatomical proximity to critical structures, radical surgical resection is very difficult. The role of surgery is generally limited to biopsy for histological confirmation and salvage of persistent or recurrent disease.

Megavoltage radiation therapy (RT) has been the primary treatment modality. While excellent control can be achieved for patients with early disease, the results are unsatisfactory for the majority of patients

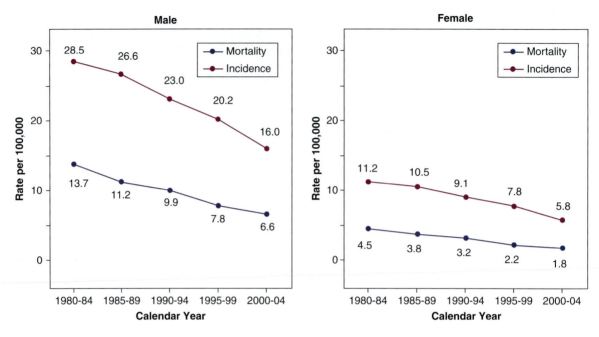

Fig. 5.2. Changing epidemiology of nasopharyngeal carcinoma in Hong Kong from 1980 to 2004

presenting with advanced locoregional diseases. With the notorious predilection for distant metastases, a combination with effective systemic therapy is needed. The meta-analysis by BAUJAT et al. (2006), based on updated patient data of 1,753 patients from eight accepted trials (AL-SARRAF et al. 1998a, b; CHAN et al. 1995, 2005b; CHI et al. 2002; CHUA et al. 1998; CVITKOVIC et al. 1996; HAREYAMA et al. 2002; KWONG et al. 2004b) showed benefit by adding chemotherapy: the absolute gain for 5-year event-free survival (EFS) was 10% (52 vs. 42%) and overall survival (OS) was 6% (62 vs. 56%). The treatment effect was heterogeneous because of significant interaction with the timing of chemotherapy ($p = 0.03$). Concurrent chemotherapy was the most potent combination, and the only sequence that achieved significant benefit in OS: hazard ratio (HR) = 0.71; 95% confidence interval (CI), 0.53–094. Induction chemotherapy per se could significantly reduce the risk of locoregional failures by 24% and distant failures by 35%, though this did not translate into significant benefit in OS, whereas adjuvant chemotherapy failed to achieve significant benefit in any end points.

Hence, the current recommendation is to treat patients with stages I–II disease with RT alone, and those with stages III–IVB (± bulky IIB) disease with concurrent chemoradiotherapy (CRT).

5.2.1
Radiation Therapy

To achieve the best therapeutic ratio, every step in the RT procedure (immobilization, localization of gross tumor and target volumes, optimization of dose fractionation, determination of treatment techniques, and precision in RT delivery) is very important.

Although NPC is a radiosensitive tumor, high dose is needed for complete eradication (PEREZ et al. 1992). The studies by LEE et al. (1995, 1998, 2002a) on patients irradiated by different fractionation schedules showed that total dose was the most important radiation factor ($p = 0.01$): the hazard of local failure decreased by 8% per additional Gray even for T1 tumors. Fractional dose did not affect local control, but it was a significant risk factor for temporal lobe necrosis. KWONG et al. (1997) showed that time factor was significant even for nonkeratinizing tumor, with hazard of local failure increasing by 3% per additional day of prolongation. The general recommendation is to give a total dose of ~70 Gy at conventional fractionation (CF) over 7 weeks to the gross tumor, and 50–60 Gy for elective treatment of potential risk sites. Whether further dose escalation and acceleration can achieve significant benefit is yet to be confirmed.

There is little controversy that intensity-modulated radiotherapy technique (IMRT) is recommended if

A confirmatory trial by WEE et al. (2005) and the NPC-9901 Trial (focusing on patients with N2–3 disease) by LEE et al. (2005a) both supported that the Intergroup-0099 regimen could improve tumor control; the former also showed significant survival benefit. In addition, the NPC-9902 Trial (focusing on patients with T3–4N0–1 disease) by LEE et al. (2006) showed that the concurrent–adjuvant chemotherapy was a significant independent factor for reducing relapse (HR = 0.52; 95% CI, 0.28–0.97; $p = 0.039$).

The other four trials showed less consistent conclusions. LIN et al. (2003) using concurrent cisplatin–fluorouracil reported significant benefit in both EFS and OS. However, subsequent reanalysis by LIN et al. (2004) with retrospective restaging of the accrued patients into different risk groups, showed that the benefit was insignificant for the high-risk group only. The trial by CHAN et al. (2005b) using concurrent weekly cisplatin and that by KWONG et al. (2004b) using concurrent uracil–tegafur with or without adjuvant cisplatin-based combination only showed borderline improvement in OS ($p > 0.06$) and no significant improvement in failure rate ($p > 0.14$). A trial by ZHANG et al. (2005) using concurrent oxaliplatin showed significant improvement in both EFS and OS at 2 years. Longer results are awaited.

Hence, basing on currently available level IA evidence, the Intergroup-0099 regimen remains the standard chemotherapy approach and is commonly recommended outside clinical trials. The outcome of trials with 3-year results are summarized in Table 5.3.

resources permit, as dosimetric studies show clear advantages for improving the conformity of dose distribution for the complex tumor targets, and better protection of the adjacent normal tissues (CHENG et al. 2001; KAM et al. 2003; XIA et al. 2000). Figure 5.3 shows the differences in dose distribution between IMRT and conventional two-dimensional technique.

Skillful specification of dose constraints is important for inverse treatment planning. Current practices in different centers vary in philosophies on defining the clinical target volumes, dose fractionation at different levels, and dose constraint for different organs at risk (Table 5.2). Some centers use simultaneous modulated-accelerated radiation therapy (SMART) as a new way of delivering an accelerated fractionation (AF) schedule, a concept first reported by BUTLER et al. (1999) for the treatment of other head-and-neck cancers with IMRT. One example is the RTOG-0615 study that specifies a total dose of 70 Gy to the planning target volume for gross tumor at 2.12 Gy/fraction for 33 daily fractions. Other centers, for example Pamela Youde Nethersole Eastern Hospital (PYNEH, Hong Kong), prescribe 2 Gy/fraction for 35 daily fractions to avoid potential risk of increase in late toxicities (Fig. 5.4). More long-term data are needed to explore for the best possible optimization.

5.2.2
Chemotherapy

Thus far there have been eight randomized trials to evaluate the therapeutic gain by concurrent with or without adjuvant CRT. The first trial that achieved significant survival benefit was the Intergroup-0099 Study, using cisplatin (100 mg m^{-2}) on days 1, 22, and 43 in concurrence with RT at CF (70 Gy in 35 fractions), followed by a combination of cisplatin (80 mg m^{-2}) and fluorouracil (1,000 mg m^{-2} day^{-1} for 96 h) on days 71, 99, and 127 during the post-RT phase. When compared with RT alone, significant benefit ($p < 0.01$) was noted in both EFS and OS at 3 years in the first report (AL-SARRAF et al. 1998a) and the subsequent update at the fifth year (AL-SARRAF et al. 1998b). However, controversies remain particularly regarding the magnitude of benefit because the results of the RT alone arm were grossly inferior to those achieved by most centers. Chemotherapy in the adjuvant phase was poorly tolerated and therefore the actual contribution is uncertain.

5.3
Treatment Outcome

5.3.1
Tumor Control and Survival

Table 5.4 shows the overall results in major series of patients treated from 1990 onwards. The treatment used in these series was still suboptimal by modern standards, as the RT technique used was mostly conventional two-dimensional technique and only 10% of patients in two of the quoted series had been given concurrent chemotherapy. The average 5-year survival achieved was ~70%, with OS ranging from

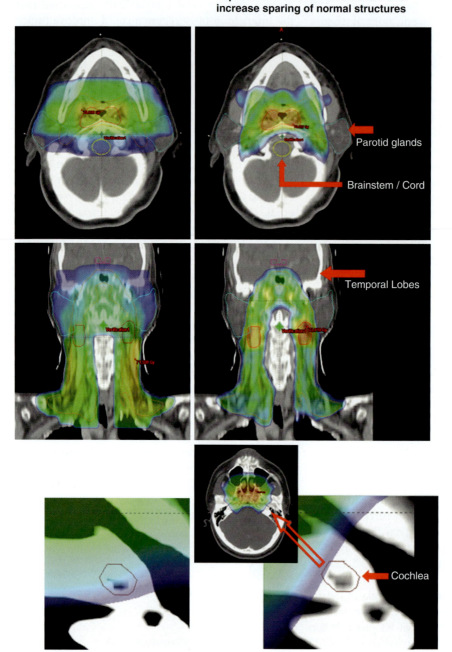

Fig. 5.3. Improvement in dose distribution by intensity-modulated radiation therapy in comparison with conventional two-dimensional technique

Table 5.2. Intensity-modulated radiation therapy for nasopharyngeal carcinoma: methods and results by different centers

References	LEE et al. (2002b)	WOLDEN et al. (2006)	KAM et al. (2004)	KWONG et al. (2004a)	KWONG et al. (2006)
Patient characteristics					
No. of patients	67	74	63	33	50
Treatment period	1995–2000	1998–2004	2000–2002	2000–2002	2000–2004
T4 (%)	21	31	19	0	68
Stage IV (%)	37	47	22	0	72
Intensity-modulated RT					
Total dose (Gy)	65–70	70.2	66	68–70	76
Dose (Gy) per fraction	2.12–2.25	2.34	2	2–2.06	2.17
Additional treatment					
Acceleration (%)	–	80	–	–	–
Boost (%)	39:B	–	32:B, 24:3D	–	–
Chemotherapy (%)	75:C	93:C	25:C, 5:I	0	68°C
Tumor control					
Time point (year)	4	3	3	2	2
Local-FFR (%)	97	91	92	100	96
Regional-FFR (%)	98	93	98	94	98
Distant-FFR (%)	66	78	79	94	94
Overall survival (%)	88	83	90	NR	92
Late toxicity incidence (%)					
Median follow-up (*m*)	31	35	29	14	25
Xerostomia (grade ≥2)	2 (2 year)	32 (1-year)	23 (2-year)	29 (2-year)	–
Deafness (grade >2)	7	>15	15	NR	42
Fibrosis (grade >2)	–	–	11	NR	14
Dysphagia (grade >2)	1	–	5	NR	–
Hypopituitarism	–	0	23	NR	–
Bone/ST necrosis	3	0	2	NR	–
Temporal lobe necrosis		0	3	NR	4
Fatal epistaxis	1	–	–	NR	4[a]

B intracavitary brachytherapy; *3D* 3-dimensional conformal boost; *FFR* failure-free rate; *ST* soft tissue; *I* induction; *C* concurrent ± sequential; *NR* not reported
[a]Bleeding from internal carotid pseudoaneurysm

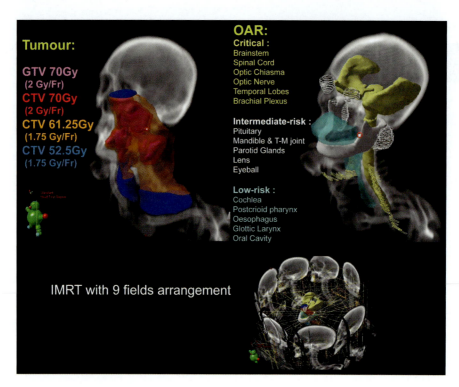

Fig. 5.4. Example of intensity-modulated radiation therapy technique currently used at the Pamela Youde Nethersole Eastern Hospital (Hong Kong), showing the tumor targets and dose prescription, priorities for different organs at risk, and the field arrangement

57 to 76% and disease-specific survival ranging from 67 to 80%. These results are already substantially better than disease-specific survival of around 50% from representative historic series (LEE et al. 1992; GEARA et al. 1997).

Review of these series shows that the average 5-year local failure-free rate (L-FFR) was 80% (range, 75–85%), nodal failure-free rate (R-FFR) was 90% (range, 80–94%), and distant failure-free rate (D-FFR) was 80% (range, 77–83%).

Excellent nodal control can usually be achieved. The average 5-year R-FFR was 97% for N0, 95% N1, 90% N2, and 75% N3 (LEE et al. 2005b; LEUNG et al. 2005). T-category is the most important prognostic factor for local control. The average 5-year L-FFR varied from 90% (range, 88–93%) for T1, 85% (82–87%) for T2, 70% (69–80%) for T3, to 70% (58–77%) for T4 tumors (LEE et al. 2005b; LEUNG et al. 2005; MA et al. 2001).

Distant failure remains a most challenging problem in NPC. The risk correlates significantly with both T and N categories, but N-category is by far the most significant predicting factor. The HR of distant failure in patients with N3b disease was as high as 6.26 (95% CI, 4.42–8.88) when compared with N0 (LEE et al. 2004). The study by LEE et al. (2005b) on 2,070 patients treated by RT alone showed that both the presenting stage and achievement of locoregional control were significant factors affecting distant failure. The 5-year D-FFR for stages I–IIB vs. stages III–IVB were 90 vs. 75% for patients who achieved locoregional control, but 81 vs. 65% for those with locoregional failure.

Presenting stage is one of the most important prognostic factors for survival. The average 5-year OS varied from 90% (range, 88–91%) for stage I, 80% (70–84%) for stage II, 60% (53–76%) for stage III, to 40% (37–52%) for stage IVA–B (HENG et al. 1999; LEE et al. 2005b; LEUNG et al. 2005; MA et al. 2001).

Studies by LEUNG et al. (2003, 2006) show that quantitation of plasma deoxyribonucleic acid (DNA) of EBV could complement staging prognostication particularly for early stages. Among patients with stage I–IIB disease, the 5-year OS for those with pretherapy DNA levels ≥4,000 copies/mL was significantly lower than those with low levels: 64 vs. 91%, $p = 0.0003$. The DNA levels were significantly higher among patients with distant failure than among those without; the actuarial rate of distant failure at 45 months was as high as 37% among patients with IIB diseases having EBV DNA ≥4,000

Table 5.3. Randomized trials comparing concurrent chemoradiotherapy vs. radiotherapy alone for nasopharyngeal carcinoma

	AL-SARRAF et al. (1998a, b)	LIN et al. (2003)	CHAN et al. (2002, 2005a, b)	KWONG et al. (2004b)	WEE et al. (2005)	LEE et al. (2005a)	LEE et al. (2006)	
Patient characteristics								
Number enrolled	193	284	350	222	221	348	189	
Treatment period	1989–1995	1993–1999	1994–1997	1995–2001	1997–2003	1999–2004	1999–2004	
Stage (AJCC/UICC 6th)	II–IVB	II–IVB	II–IVB	II–IVB	III–IVB	III–IVB	III–IVA	
Histology: WHO II (%)	78 vs. 72	98 vs. 96	99 vs. 100	99 vs. 99	All	All	All	
Radiotherapy								
Fractionation	Conventional	Conventional	Conventional	Conventional	Conventional	Conventional	Conventional	Accelerated
Total dose (Gy)	70	70–74	66	62.5–68	70	Mean 68	Mean 69	
Chemotherapy								
Concurrent	P	PF	P	U	P	P	P	P
Adjuvant	PF	–	–	±PF/VBM	PF	PF	PF	PF
Tumor control (%): CRT vs. RT								
Time point (year)	5	5	5	3	3	3	3	
Locoregional control	S	L: 89 vs. 73 $p < 0.01$	NS	80 vs. 72 NS	NR	92 vs. 82 $p = 0.01$	81 vs. 85 NS	94 vs. 85 NS
Distant control	S	79 vs. 70 *MS*	NS	85 vs. 71 $p = 0.03$	87 vs. 70[a] $p < 0.01$	76 vs. 73 NS	89 vs. 81 NS	97 vs. 81 $p = 0.03$
Progression-free survival	58 vs. 29 $p < 0.01$				72 vs. 53 $p = 0.01$	70 vs. 61 NS	73 vs. 68 NS	88 vs. 68 *MS*
Failure-free survival		72 vs. 53 $p = 0.01$	60 vs. 52 NS	69 vs. 58 NS		72 vs. 62 $p = 0.03$	74 vs. 70 NS	94 vs. 70 $p = 0.01$
Overall survival	67 vs. 37 $p < 0.01$	72 vs. 54 $p < 0.01$	70 vs. 59 *MS*	87 vs. 77 *MS*	80 vs. 65 $p = 0.01$	78 vs. 78 NS	87 vs. 83 NS	88 vs. 83 NS

AJCC/UICC 6th American Joint Committee on Cancer/International Union Against Cancer 6th Edition; *WHO II* non-keratinizing/undifferentiated carcinoma; *F* fluorouracil; *U* uracil-tegafur; *V* vincristine; *B* bleomycin; *M* methotrexate; *L* local; *NR* not reported; *S* significant but no detailed data; *MS* marginal significance ($p = 0.06$–0.07); *NS* no statistical significance ($p > 0.1$)

Progression-free survival: defining events included both failures and death; Failure-free survival: defining events included failures only

[a]Two-year incidence of freedom from distant failure as the first site of failure

Table 5.4. Treatment results for different stages by AJCC/UICC Staging System (6th edition)

References	Treatment period	N	RT technique	Chemotherapy	Time (year)	Control rate (%)			Survival (%)					
						Local	Nodal	Distant	End-point	I	IIA–B	III	IVA–B	All
Leung et al. (2005)	1990–1998	1,070	All 2D	19% I, 1% C	5	81	93	77	OS	91	92–78	62	44–43	71
									DSS	85	95–82	67	50–46	67
Palazzi et al. (2004)	1990–1999	171	All 2D	39% I, 23% C	5	84	80	83	OS	–	–	–	–	72
									DSS					74
Yi et al. (2006)	1990–1999	905	All 2D	None	5	58		–	OS	–	–	–	–	76
					10	52			OS					67
Heng et al. (1999)	1992–1994	677	All 2D	None	5	–	–	–	OS	88	75–74	60	35–28	57
Ma et al. (2001)	1993–1994	621	All 2D	None	5	75		77	OS	89	70	53	37	–
Ozyar et al. (1999)	1993–1997	90	All 2D	66% I or C	3	–	–	–	OS	100	72	65	55	65
Lee et al. (2004, 2005b)	1996–2000	2,687	90% 2D, 10% 3D	14% I, 9% C	5	85	94	81	OS	90	84	76	52	75
									DSS	92	87	81	60	80

OS overall survival; *DSS* disease-specific survival; *NR* not reported; *I* induction; *C* concurrent ± sequential; *2D* two-dimensional technique; *3D* conformal technique

copies/mL. Hence, this additional investigation is worth considering for identifying high-risk patients for treatment with CRT.

The treatment outcomes achieved by concurrent with or without adjuvant CRT vs. RT alone in reported randomized trials are summarized in Table 5.3. The RT technique used was mostly conventional two-dimensional technique. The magnitude of improvement in 3-year results achieved by adding the Intergroup-0099 regimen varied. While all three completed trials confirmed statistical significance, the absolute gain in EFS varied from 45% (69 vs. 24% for stage II–IVB) by Al-Sarraf et al. (1998a), to 19% (72 vs. 53% for stage III–IVB) by Wee et al. (2005), and 10% (72 vs. 62% for T1–4N2–3) by Lee et al. (2005a). The absolute gain in OS further varied from 31% (78 vs. 47%) by Al-Sarraf et al. (1998a), to 15% (80 vs. 65%) by Wee et al. (2005) and 0% (78 vs. 78%) by Lee et al. (2005a), though it is possible that the improvement in tumor control might eventually translate into significant survival benefit with longer follow-up.

Early results achieved by contemporary series using IMRT are summarized in Table 5.2. Together with additional treatment by chemotherapy, dose

escalation and/or acceleration, excellent locoregional control at 3 years exceeding 91% could now be achieved. However, distant failure remains a major problem. The report by Lee et al. (2002b) from University of California, San Francisco, showed outstanding 4-year L-FFR of 97%, but the D-FFR was only 66% despite the addition of chemotherapy using the Intergroup-0099 regimen in 75% of the series.

Another report of excellent locoregional control was achieved by Stanford University Medical Center using stereotactic (SRT) boost. The latest update by Hara et al. (2008) on 82 patients (38% T4; 56% stage IV) showed 5-year L-FFR of 98% by adding a single-fraction SRT boost of 7–15 Gy after external RT to 66 Gy. However, the D-FFR was again disappointingly high (68% at 5 years) despite extensive use of the Intergroup-0099 regimen in 85% of the series.

These clinical experience concur with the preliminary results of the NPC-9901 Trial (Lee et al. 2005a), which showed minimal improvement in D-FFR for patients with N2–3 disease (76 vs. 73% at 3 years, $p = 0.47$). Exploration for a more effective strategy is needed.

Table 5.5. New attempts for enhancing efficacy of concurrent chemoradiotherapy for nasopharyngeal carcinoma

Author	No.	Stage IV (%)	Radiotherapy		Chemotherapy			Tumor control (%)			
			Dose (Gy)	Time (weeks)	Induction	Concurrent	Adjuvant	Time-point (year)	LR-FFR	D-FFR	OS
Concurrent-adjuvant chemo-radiotherapy with accelerated fractionation											
Wolden et al. (2001)	50	44	70	6	–	P	PF	3	L:89	79	84
Jian et al. (2002)	48	>77	74	7	–	P	PF	3	L:91	NR	72
Lin et al. (1996)	63	NR	72–74	6	–	PF	±PF	3	L:89	74	74
Induction-concurrent chemo-radiotherapy with conventional fractionation											
Rischin et al. (2002)	35	40	60	6	PEF	P	–	4	L:97	94	90
Oh et al. (2003)	27	NR	70	14[a]	PFI	HF	–	5	93	92	77
Johnson et al. (2005)	44	NR	70	7	PF	PF	–	3	75[c]	89[b]	78
Al-Amro et al. (2005)	110	74	66	6.5	PE	P	–	3	68	74	71
Chan et al. (2004)	31	39	66	6.5	TJ	P	–	2	90[b]	81[b]	92
Hui et al. (2007)	30	NR	66	6.5	DP	P	–	2	NR	NR	93
Induction-concurrent chemo-radiotherapy with accelerated fractionation											
Lee et al. (2005c)	49	100	70	6	PF	P	–	3	77	75	71
Yau et al. (2006)	37	100	70	6	PG	P	–	3	78	76	76

LR-FFR locoregional failure-free rate; *D-FFR* distant failure-free rate; *OS* overall survival; *L* local failure-free rate alone; *NR* not reported; *p* cisplatin; *D* docetaxel; *F* fluorouracil; *E* epirubicin; *I* interferon-α; *H* hydroxyurea, *T* paclitaxel; *J* carboplatin; *G* gemcitabine
[a]Split fractionation (2 Gy/fraction daily × five fraction, q 2 week)
[b]Crude incidence

Table 5.5 summarizes the new strategies explored. One strategy is to enhance the effectiveness of RT by changing from CF to accelerated fractionation (AF). Retrospective studies combining AF with concurrent–adjuvant CRT had shown reasonable tolerability and encouraging preliminary results (Lin et al. 1996; Wolden et al. 2001; Jian et al. 2002). The study by Wolden et al. (2001) showed that 3-year L-FFR of 89% and OS of 84% could be achieved by Intergroup-0099 regimen and AF with concomitant boost. The only randomized trial that attempted to study this combined strategy was the NPC-9902 Trial (Lee et al. 2006) on patients with T3–4N0–1M0 diseases. The fractionation schedule was 2 Gy/fraction, five fractions/week in CF arms and six fractions/week in AF arms. The preliminary results showed that CRT using the Intergroup regimen combined with AF achieved significantly better EFS than CF alone (94 vs. 70% at 3 years, $p = 0.008$). However, further confirmation is needed because the sample size was small and follow-up relatively short.

Another strategy is to enhance the effectiveness of chemotherapy by changing the sequence from concurrent–adjuvant to induction–concurrent. Patient compliance and tolerance is substantially better during the induction phase than the adjuvant phase. Early use of potent combinations of cytotoxic drugs at full dose is likely to be more effective for eradicating micrometastases. Furthermore, this might be particularly advantageous for NPC with extensive locoregional infiltration because shrinking the primary tumor could give wider margin for irradiation. Phase II studies reported encouraging preliminary results (RISCHIN et al. 2002; OH et al. 2003; CHAN et al. 2004; AL-AMRO et al. 2005; JOHNSON et al. 2005; HUI et al. 2007). The first report by RISCHIN et al. (2002) achieved excellent 4-year results in 35 patients (40% stage IV) with OS of 90%, distant control 94% and locoregional control 97%.

For the most difficult stage IV patients with locoregional disease infiltrating or abutting neurological structures, a more aggressive approach combining induction–concurrent CRT with AF has been explored. Two different induction regimens have been tested: cisplatin–fluorouracil was used in the first study by LEE et al. (2005c); a newer combination of cisplatin–gemcitabine was used by YAU et al. (2006). These were then followed by cisplatin in concurrence with RT to 70 Gy using the six fractions/week AF schedule. Given the grave prognosis of this notorious group in the past, 3-year OS of 71 and 76% respectively achieved in the two studies were very encouraging. Further confirmation of efficacy is warranted.

5.3.2
Late Toxicity

With the close proximity of NPC to critical normal tissue structures, the therapeutic margin is notoriously narrow. The importance of best conformity RT technique for maximum protection of normal tissues cannot be overemphasized. Addition of concurrent–adjuvant chemotherapy incurred significant increase in late toxicity, particularly hearing impairment (LEE et al. 2005a). The CRT arm in the NPC-9901 Trial had significantly higher late toxicity rate than the RT alone arm (28 vs. 13% at 3-year, $p = 0.024$).

Recent retrospective study (LEE et al. 2008) of 422 patients treated with three-dimensional conformal technique at 2 Gy/daily fractions to a total of 70 Gy showed that 5-year overall toxicity rate was significantly higher in patients treated with concurrent cisplatin-based chemotherapy compared with those treated by RT alone (37 vs. 27%, $p = 0.009$). The hazard of deafness, adjusted for age, was significantly affected by chemotherapy (HR = 1.89; 95% CI, 1.23–2.88) and the mean dose to the cochlea (HR = 1.03 per Gy increase; 95% CI, 1.01–1.05).

Another observation was that patients given an additional boost (5 Gy in two fractions) had significant increase in temporal lobe necrosis (Fig. 5.5) compared with RT to 70 Gy alone (4.8 vs. 0%, $p = 0.015$). The 5-year necrotic rate amounted to 8.3% among patients boosted by SRT, while none of the patients boosted by brachytherapy were affected. Similar experience of high toxicity rate was reported by other series using SRT boost. The update from Stanford

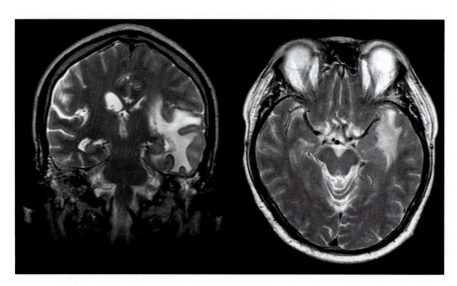

Fig. 5.5. Radiation-induced temporal lobe necrosis

University Medical Center (Hara et al. 2008) with a median follow-up of 41 months reported temporal lobe necrosis in 9.8% (10 of 82) patients. Another serious toxicity reported by Chen et al. (2001) was sudden death due to massive nasal bleeding without any evidence of local recurrence in 4.7% (3 of 64) patients.

With improvement in conformity of physical dose distribution by IMRT, two randomized trials on patients with stage I–II disease confirmed that recovery of stimulated salivary flow was significantly better in patients irradiated with IMRT technique compared with conventional two-dimensional technique. The trial by Pow et al. (2006) showed that the difference in proportion of patients with recovery to above 25% of baseline at 1 year was 83 vs. 10% for parotid flow and 50 vs. 5% for whole salivary flow. The IMRT group showed consistent improvement in xerostomia-related symptoms, and attained significantly higher subscale scores on quality of life. The trial by Kam et al. (2007) further showed significantly lower incidence of xerostomia grade 2–4 at 1 year as scored by physicians (82 vs. 39%, $p = 0.001$), but no difference in xerostomia questionnaire as scored by patients (-24 vs. -33%, $p = 0.32$).

However, it must be cautioned that other serious late toxicities remain substantial (Table 5.2). The study by Kam et al. (2004) at a median follow-up of 2.4 years observed that 2% patients developed osteonecrosis of C1 and C2 vertebrae requiring surgical restoration, 3% temporal lobe necrosis, and 23% endocrine dysfunction. In the study by Lee at al. (2002b), 1.5% (1 of 67) patient died of torrential epistaxis without tumor recurrence. The study by Kwong et al. (2006) that prescribed a total dose of 76 Gy at 2.17 Gy/fraction to the gross tumor showed worrisome toxicities, with 4% (2 of 50) patients suffering from massive epistaxis and another 4% temporal lobe necrosis at a median follow-up of 2.1 years. The bleeding in the two affected patients was found to be due to internal carotid artery pseudo-aneurysm at the skull base (Fig. 5.6); fortunately both survived after emergency treatment by stenting and vascular bypass, respectively.

5.3.3
Quality of Life

Studies in NPC survivors using formal quality of life (QOL) instruments are scanty. Furthermore, prospective longitudinal studies comparing QOL outcomes of different treatment methods are lacking. Thus far, there were two studies that compared the QOL of NPC survivors with the general population (Fang et al. 2002; Wu et al. 2007): both used the SF-36 questionnaire and both showed that NPC survivors had worse QOL.

Swallowing difficulty is a common problem in NPC survivors. Lovell et al. (2005) investigated the impact of dysphagia on QOL using the University of Washington QOL Questionnaire and the Swallow QOL Questionnaire. Eighty-four percent (43 of 51) patients reported swallowing problem, and these patients had worse QOL scores than those without swallowing problems.

Dental and oral health problems are also common. The cross-sectional study on NPC survivors by

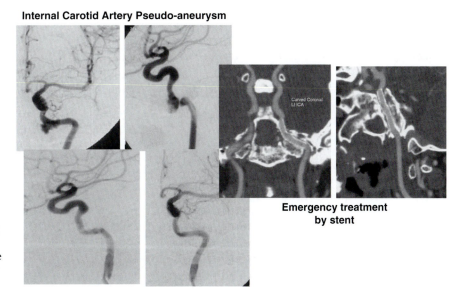

Fig. 5.6. Radiation-induced pseudoaneurysm of the internal carotid artery at the skull base and treatment by insertion of stent

McMILLAN et al. (2004) using the SF-36 questionnaire and the Oral Health Impact Profile showed that NPC survivors had more negative psychosocial and functional impact because of oral problem when compared with controls.

YEUNG et al. (2005) compared the QOL of patients treated with concurrent CRT to those treated by RT alone. Longitudinal assessment using the FACT-H&N questionnaire was done at baseline, at the end of the RT course, and at 3, 12, and 24 months after completion. The results showed that CRT group had worse short-term QOL (related to acute toxicities). However, both groups had good recovery of QOL at 3 months and there was no significant difference in QOL scores at 2 years.

Improvement in RT technique leads to promising improvement in QOL outcomes. Retrospective comparison by FANG et al. (2007) on patients treated at different periods using conventional two-dimensional technique vs. conformal RT (either three-dimensional RT or IMRT) showed that those treated by conformal RT had better QOL scores as assessed by the EORTC questionnaire. FANG et al. (2008) further compared the QOL outcomes for patients treated with IMRT vs. 3D conformal RT by longitudinal assessment with the EORTC questionnaires before RT, during RT, and at 3, 12, and 24 months after completion. The results showed that there was no significant difference in most scales between the two groups at each time point except that IMRT had more improvement at 3 months in items such as global QOL, fatigue, taste/smell, dry mouth, and feeling ill.

As mentioned above, the two randomized trials comparing IMRT vs. conventional two-dimensional (Pow et al. 2006; KAM et al. 2007) showed inconsistent results on QOL despite significant improvement in recovery of salivary function. Further confirmation of the exact benefit remains to be tested.

5.4

Final Remarks

Nasopharyngeal cancer is a fascinating disease with peculiar features in epidemiology, natural history, therapeutic consideration, and treatment response. Medical progress in the battle against NPC is one of the most gratifying successes: a cancer that was invariably lethal before the advent of megavoltage RT can now be effectively treated to achieve 5-year OS of 75% and above. Even better results are expected with further advances in technologies. More accurate prognostication is needed to refine the treatment strategies tailored to individual risk patterns. Furthermore, concerted efforts to minimize toxicities and improve quality of life remain a most challenging mission.

References

Al-Amro A, Al-Rajhi N, Khafaga Y et al. (2005) Neoadjuvant chemotherapy followed by concurrent chemo-radiation therapy in locally advanced nasopharyngeal carcinoma. Int J Radiat Oncol Biol Phys 62:508–513

Al-Sarraf M, LeBlanc M, Giri PG et al. (1998a) Chemoradiotherapy versus radiotherapy in patients with advanced nasopharyngeal cancer: phase III randomized Intergroup study 0099. J Clin Oncol 16(4):1310–1317

Al-Sarraf M, LeBlanc M, Giri PGS et al. (1998b) Chemoradiotherapy (CT-RT) vs radiotherapy (RT) in patients (PTS) with advanced nasopharyngeal cancer (NPC). Intergroup (0099) (SWOG 8892, RTOG 8817, ECOG 2388) Phase III Study: progress report. J Clin Oncol 17:385a [abstract]

Armstrong RW, Imrey PB, Lye MS et al. (1998) Nasopharyngeal carcinoma in Malaysian Chinese: salted fish and other dietary exposures. Int J Cancer 77(2):228–235

Baujat B, Audry H, Bourhis J et al. (2006) Chemotherapy in locally advanced nasopharyngeal carcinoma: An individual patient data meta-analysis of eight randomized trials and 1753 patients. Int J Radiat Oncol Biol Phys 64(1):47–56

Buell P (1973) Race and place in the etiology of nasopharyngeal cancer: a study based on California death certificates. Int J Cancer 11:268–272

Burt RD, Vaughan TL, McKnight B et al. (1996) Associations between human leukocyte antigen type and nasopharyngeal carcinoma in Caucasians in the United States. Cancer Epidemiol Biomarkers Prev 5(11):879–887

Butler EB, Teh BS, Grant WH et al. (1999) SMART (simultaneous modulated accelerated radiation therapy) boost: a new accelerated fractionation schedule for the treatment of head and neck cancer with intensity modulated radiotherapy. Int J Radiat Oncol Biol Phys 45(1):21–32

Chan J, Bray F, McCarron P et al. (2005a) Nasopharyngeal carcinoma. Pathology and genetics of head and neck tumours. World Health Organization Classification of Tumours. IARC, Lyon, pp 85–97

Chan AT, Leung SF, Ngan RK et al. (2005b) Overall survival after concurrent cisplatin-radiotherapy compared with radiotherapy alone in locoregionally advanced nasopharyngeal carcinoma. J Natl Cancer Inst 97(7):536–539

Chan AT, Ma BY, Lo YM et al. (2004) Phase II study of neoadjuvant carboplatin and paclitaxel followed by radiotherapy and concurrent cisplatin in patients with locoregionally advanced nasopharyngeal carcinoma: therapeutic monitoring with plasma Epstein-Barr Virus DNA. J Clin Oncol 22:3053–3060

Chan AT, Teo PM, Leung TW et al. (1995) A prospective randomized study of chemotherapy adjunctive to definitive radiotherapy in advanced nasopharyngeal carcinoma. Int J Radiat Oncol Biol Phys 33(3):569–577

Chan AT, Teo PM, Ngan RK et al. (2002) Concurrent chemotherapy-radiotherapy compared with radiotherapy alone in locoregionally advanced nasopharyngeal carcinoma: Progression-free survival analysis of a phase III randomized trial. J Clin Oncol 20(8):2038–2044

Cheng JC, Chao KS, Low D (2001) Comparison of intensity modulated radiation therapy (IMRT) treatment techniques for nasopharyngeal carcinoma. Int J Cancer 96(2):126–132

Chen HH, Tsai ST, Wang MS et al. (2006) Experience in fractionated stereotactic body radiation therapy boost for newly diagnosed nasopharyngeal carcinoma. Int J Radiat Oncol Biol Phys 66(5):1408–1414

Chen HJ, Leung SW, Su CY (2001) Linear accelerator based radiosurgery as a salvage treatment for skull base and intracranial invasion of recurrent nasopharyngeal carcinomas. Am J Clin Oncol 24(3):255–258

Chi KH, Chang YC, Guo WY et al. (2002) A phase III study of adjuvant chemotherapy in advanced nasopharyngeal carcinoma patients. Int J Radiat Oncol Biol Phys 52(5):1238–1244

Chua DT, Sham JS, Choy D et al. (1998) Preliminary report of the Asian-Oceanian Clinical Oncology Association randomized trial comparing cisplatin and epirubicin followed by radiotherapy versus radiotherapy alone in the treatment of patients with locoregionally advanced nasopharyngeal carcinoma. Asian-Oceanian Clinical Oncology Association Nasopharynx Cancer Study Group. Cancer 83(11):2270–2283

Cvitkovic E, Eschwege F, Rahal M et al. (1996) Preliminary results of trial comparing neoadjuvant chemotherapy (cisplatin, epirubicin, bleomycin) plus radiotherapy vs radiotherapy alone in stage IV ($\geq$N2, M0) undifferentiated nasopharyngeal carcinoma: a positive effect on progression free survival. I Int J Radiat Oncol Biol Phys 35:463–469

Dickson RI, Flores AD (1985) Nasopharyngeal carcinoma: an evaluation of 134 patients treated between 1971–1980. Laryngoscope 95(3):276–283

Fang FM, Chien CY, Tsai WL et al. (2008) Quality of life and survival outcome for patients with nasopharyngeal carcinoma receiving three-dimensional conformal radiotherapy vs. intensity-modulated radiotherapy-a longitudinal study. Int J Radiat Oncol Biol Phys 72:356–364

Fang FM, Chiu HC, Kuo WR et al. (2002) Health-related quality of life for nasopharyngeal carcinoma patients with cancer-free survival after treatment. Int J Radiat Oncol Biol Phys 53(4):959–968

Fang FM, Tsai WL, Chen HC et al. (2007) Intensity-modulated or conformal radiotherapy improves the quality of life of patients with nasopharyngeal carcinoma: comparisons of four radiotherapy techniques. Cancer 109(2):313–321

Ferlay J, Bray F, Pisani P et al. (2004) GLOBOCAN 2002. Cancer incidence, mortality, and prevalence worldwide. IARC Cancer Base No. 5, version 2.0. IARC, Lyon

Feng BJ, Huang W, Shugart YY et al. (2002) Genome-wide scan for familial nasopharyngeal carcinoma reveals evidence of linkage to chromosome 4. Nat Genet 31:395–399

Friborg J, Wohlfahrt J, Koch A et al. (2005) Cancer susceptibility in nasopharyngeal carcinoma families–a population-based cohort study. Cancer Res 65:8567–8572

Geara FB, Sanguineti G, Tucker SL et al. (1997) Carcinoma of the nasopharynx treated by radiotherapy alone: determinants of distant metastasis and survival. Radiother Oncol 43(1):53–61

Hara W, Loo BW, Goffinet DR et al. (2008) Excellent local control with stereotactic radiotherapy boost after external beam radiotherapy in patients with nasopharyngeal carcinoma. Int J Radiat Oncol Biol Phys 71(2):393–400

Hareyama M, Sakata K, Shirato H et al. (2002) A prospective, randomized trial comparing neoadjuvant chemotherapy with radiotherapy alone in patients with advanced nasopharyngeal carcinoma. Cancer 94(8):2217–2223

Heng DM, Wee J, Fong KW et al. (1999) Prognostic factors in 677 patients in Singapore with nondisseminated nasopharyngeal carcinoma. Cancer 86(10):1912–1920

Ho JH (1978) An epidemiologic and clinical study of nasopharyngeal carcinoma. Int J Radiat Oncol Biol Phys 4(4):182–198

Hui EP, Ma BB, Leung SF et al. (2007) Efficacy of neoadjuvant docetaxel and cisplatin followed by concurrent cisplatin-radiotherapy in locally advanced nasopharyngeal carcinoma (NPC): a randomized phase II study. J Clin Oncol 25(18S):6037

Jia WH et al. (2004) Familial risk and clustering of nasopharyngeal carcinoma in Guangdong, China. Cancer 101(2):363–369

Jian JJ, Cheng SH, Tsai SY et al. (2002) Improvement of local control of T3 and T4 nasopharyngeal carcinoma by hyperfractionated radiotherapy and concomitant chemotherapy. Int J Radiat Oncol Biol Phys 53:344–352

Johnson FM, Garden AS, Palmer JL et al. (2005) A phase I/II study of neoadjuvant chemotherapy followed by radiation with boost chemotherapy for advanced T-stage nasopharyngeal carcinoma. Int J Radiat Oncol Biol Phys 63:717–724

Kam MK, Chau RM, Suen J et al. (2003) Intensity-modulated radiotherapy in nasopharyngeal carcinoma: dosimetric advantage over conventional plans and feasibility of dose escalation. Int J Radiat Oncol Biol Phys 56(1):145–157

Kam MK, Leung SF, Zee B et al. (2007) Prospective randomized study of intensity-modulated radiotherapy on salivary gland function in early-stage nasopharyngeal carcinoma patients. J Clin Oncol 25:4873–4879

Kam MK, Teo PM, Chau RM, et al. (2004) Treatment of nasopharyngeal carcinoma with intensity-modulated radiotherapy: the Hong Kong experience. Int J Radiat Oncol Biol Phys 60(5):1440–1450

Ko JY, Sheen TS, Hsu MM et al. (1998) Familial clustering of nasopharyngeal carcinoma. Otolaryngol Head Neck Surg 118:736–737

Kwong DL, Pow EH, Sham JS et al. (2004a) Intensity-modulated radiotherapy for early-stage nasopharyngeal carcinoma: a prospective study on disease control and preservation of salivary function. Cancer 101(7):1584–1593

Kwong DL, Sham JS, Au GK et al. (2004b) Concurrent and adjuvant chemotherapy for nasopharyngeal carcinoma: a factorial study. J Clin Oncol 22(13):2643–2653

Kwong DL, Sham JS, Chua DT et al. (1997) The effect of interruptions and prolonged treatment time in radiotherapy for nasopharyngeal carcinoma. Int J Radiat Oncol Biol Phys 39(3):703–710

Kwong DL, Sham JS, Leung LH et al. (2006) Preliminary results of radiation dose escalation for locally advanced nasopharyngeal carcinoma. Int J Radiat Oncol Biol Phys 64(2):374–381

Lee AW, Au JS, Teo PM et al. (2004) Staging of nasopharyngeal carcinoma: suggestions for improving the current UICC/AJCC staging system. Clin Oncol 16(4):269–276

Lee AW, Chan DK, Fowler JF et al. (1995) Effect of time, dose and fractionation on local control of nasopharyngeal carcinoma. Radiother Oncol 36(1):24–31

Lee AW, Foo W, Chappell R et al. (1998) Effect of time, dose, and fractionation on temporal lobe necrosis following radiotherapy for nasopharyngeal carcinoma. Int J Radiat Oncol Biol Phys 40(1):35–42

Lee AW, Foo W, Mang O et al. (2003) Changing epidemiology of nasopharyngeal carcinoma in Hong Kong over a 20-year period (1980–99): an encouraging reduction in both incidence and mortality. Int J Cancer 103(5):680–685

Lee AW, Kwong DL, Leung SF et al. (2002a) Factors affecting risk of symptomatic temporal lobe necrosis: significance of fractional dose and treatment time. Int J Radiat Oncol Biol Phys 53(1):75–85

Lee AW, Lau WH, Tung SY et al. (2005a) Preliminary results of a randomized study on therapeutic gain by concurrent chemotherapy for regionally-advanced nasopharyngeal carcinoma: NPC-9901 Trial by the Hong Kong Nasopharyngeal Cancer Study Group. J Clin Oncol 23:6966–6975

Lee AWM, Ng WT, Hung WM et al. (2009) Major Late Toxicities Following Conformal Radiotherapy for Nasopharyngeal Carcinoma – Patient and Treatment Related Risk Factors. Int J Radiat Oncol Biol Phys 73(4):1121–1128

Lee AW, Poon YF, Foo W et al. (1992) Retrospective analysis of 5037 patients with nasopharyngeal carcinoma treated during 1976–1985: overall survival and patterns of failure. Int J Radiat Oncol Biol Phys 23(2):261–270

Lee AW, Sze WM, Au SK et al. (2005b) Treatment results for nasopharyngeal carcinoma in the modern era: the Hong Kong experience. Int J Radiat Oncol Biol Phys 61:1107–1116

Lee AW, Tung SY, Chan AT et al. (2006) Preliminary results of a randomized study (NPC-9902 Trial) on therapeutic gain by concurrent chemotherapy and/or accelerated fractionation for locally-advanced nasopharyngeal carcinoma. Int J Radiat Oncol Biol Phys 66:142–151

Lee AW, Yau TK, Wong HM et al. (2005c) Treatment of stage IV(A-B) nasopharyngeal carcinoma by induction-concurrent chemoradiotherapy and accelerated fractionation. Int J Radiat Oncol Biol Phys 63:1331–1338

Lee N, Xia P, Quivey JM et al. (2002b) Intensity-modulated radiotherapy in the treatment of nasopharyngeal carcinoma: an update of the UCSF experience. Int J Radiat Oncol Biol Phys 53(1):12–22

Leung SF, Chan AT, Zee B et al. (2003) Pretherapy quantitative measurement of circulating Epstein-Barr virus DNA is predictive of posttherapy distant failure in patients with early-stage nasopharyngeal carcinoma of undifferentiated type. Cancer 98(2):288–291

Leung TW, Tung SY, Sze WK et al. (2005) Treatment results of 1070 patients with nasopharyngeal carcinoma: an analysis of survival and failure patterns. Head Neck 27(7):555–565

Leung SF, Zee B, Ma B et al. (2006) Plasma Epstein-Barr viral deoxyribonucleic acid quantitation complements tumor node-metastasis staging prognostication in nasopharyngeal carcinoma. J Clin Oncol 24:5414–5418

Lin JC, Chen KY, Jan JS et al. (1996) Partially hyperfractionated accelerated radiotherapy and concurrent chemotherapy for advanced nasopharyngeal carcinoma. Int J Radiat Oncol Biol Phys 36:1127–1136

Lin JC, Jan JS, Hsu CY et al. (2003) Concurrent chemoradiotherapy versus radiotherapy alone for advanced nasopharyngeal carcinoma: positive effect on overall and progression-free survival. J Clin Oncol 21:631–637

Lin JC, Liang WM, Jan JS et al. (2004) Another way to estimate outcome of advanced nasopharyngeal carcinoma–is concurrent chemoradiotherapy adequate. Int J Radiat Oncol Biol Phys 60:156–164

Lo AK, Huang P, Lo KW et al. (2004a) Phenotypic alterations induced by the Hong Kong-prevalent Epstein-Barr virus-encoded LMP1 variant (2117-LMP1) in nasopharyngeal epithelial cells. Int J Cancer 109(6):919–925

Lo KW, To KF, Huang DP (2004b) Focus on nasopharyngeal carcinoma. Cancer Cell 5(5):423–428

Loh KS, Goh BC, Lu J et al. (2006) Familial nasopharyngeal carcinoma in a cohort of 200 patients. Arch Otolaryngol Head Neck Surg 132(1):82–85

Lovell SJ, Wong HB, Loh KS et al. (2005) Impact of dysphagia on quality-of-life in nasopharyngeal carcinoma. Head Neck 27(10):864–872

Ma J, Mai HQ, Hong MH et al. (2001) Is the 1997 AJCC staging system for nasopharyngeal carcinoma prognostically useful for Chinese patient populations? Int J Radiat Oncol Biol Phys 50(5):1181–1189

McMillan AS, Pow EH, Leung WK et al. (2004) Oral health-related quality of life in southern Chinese following radiotherapy for nasopharyngeal carcinoma. J Oral Rehabil 31(6):600–608

Oh JL, Vokes EE, Kies MS et al. (2003) Induction chemotherapy followed by concomitant chemoradiotherapy in the treatment of locoregionally advanced nasopharyngeal cancer. Ann Oncol 14:564–569

Ozyar E, Yildiz F, Akyol FH et al. (1999) Comparison of AJCC 1988 and 1997 classifications for nasopharyngeal carcinoma. American Joint Committee on Cancer. Int J Radiat Oncol Biol Phys 44(5):1079–1087

Palazzi M, Guzzo M, Tomatis S et al. (2004) Improved outcome of nasopharyngeal carcinoma treated with conventional radiotherapy. Int J Radiat Oncol Biol Phys 60(5):1451–1458

Parkin DM, Whelan SL, Ferlay J et al. (2002) Cancer incidence in five continents, vol VIII. IARC, Lyon

Pathmanathan R, Prasad U, Sadler R et al. (1995) Clonal proliferations of cells infected with Epstein-Barr virus in preinvasive lesions related to nasopharyngeal carcinoma. N Engl J Med 333:693–698

Perez CA, Devineni VR, Marcial-Vega V et al. (1992) Carcinoma of the nasopharynx: factors affecting prognosis. Int J Radiat Oncol Biol Phys 23(2):271–280

Poirier S, Ohshima H, de-The G et al. (1987) Volatile nitrosamine levels in common foods from Tunisia, south China and Greenland, high-risk areas for nasopharyngeal carcinoma (NPC). Int J Cancer 39(3):293–296

Pow HN, Kwong LW, McMillan S et al. (2006) Xerostomia and quality of life after intensity-modulated radiotherapy vs conventional radiotherapy for early-stage nasopharyngeal carcinoma: initial report on a randomized controlled clinical trial. Int J Radiat Oncol Biol Phys 66(4):981–991

Raab-Traub N (2002) Epstein-Barr virus in the pathogenesis of NPC. Semin Cance Biol 12(6):431–441

Rischin D, Corry J, Smith J et al. (2002) Excellent disease control and survival in patients with advanced nasopharyngeal cancer treated with chemoradiation. J Clin Oncol 20:1845–1852

Sun LM, Epplein M, Li CI et al. (2005) Trends in the incidence rates of nasopharyngeal carcinoma among Chinese Americans living in Los Angeles County and the San Francisco metropolitan area, 1992–2002. Am J Epidemiol 162(12):1174–1178

Wee J, Tan EH, Tai BC et al. (2005) Randomized trial of radiotherapy versus concurrent chemoradiotherapy followed by adjuvant chemotherapy in patients with American Joint Committee on Cancer/International Union Against Cancer Stage III and IV nasopharyngeal cancer of the endemic variety. J Clin Oncol 23:6730–6738

Wolden SL, Chen WC, Pfister DG et al. (2006) Intensity-modulated radiation therapy (IMRT) for nasopharynx cancer: update of the Memorial Sloan-Kettering experience. Int J Radiat Oncol Biol Phys 64(1):57–62

Wolden SL, Zelefsky MJ, Kraus DH et al. (2001) Accelerated concomitant boost radiotherapy and chemotherapy for advanced nasopharyngeal carcinoma. J Clin Oncol 19:1105–1110

Wu Y, Hu WH, Xia YF et al. (2007) Quality of life of nasopharyngeal carcinoma survivors in Mainland China. Qual Life Res 16(1):65–74

Xia P, Fu KK, Wong GW et al. (2000) Comparison of treatment plans involving intensity-modulated radiotherapy for nasopharyngeal carcinoma. Int J Radiat Oncol Biol Phys 48(2):329–337

Xiong W, Zeng ZY, Xia JH et al. (2004) A susceptibility locus at chromosome 3p21 linked to familial nasopharyngeal carcinoma. Cancer Res 64(6):1972–1974

Yau TK, Lee AW, Wong HM et al. (2006) Induction chemotherapy with Cisplatin and Gemcitabine followed by accelerated radiotherapy and concurrent Cisplatin in patients with stage IV(A-B) Nasopharyngeal Carcinoma. Head Neck 28:880–887

Yeung RM, Wong D, Au KH et al. (2005) To compare the quality of life of patients with advanced nasopharyngeal carcinoma treated with radical radiotherapy alone versus concurrent chemoradiotherapy. East-West Symposium on Nasopharyngeal Cancer, Toronto, (15):19–20 [abstract]

Yi JL, Gao L, Huang XD et al. (2006) Nasopharyngeal carcinoma treated by radical radiotherapy alone: ten-year experience of a singly institution. Int J Radiat Oncol Biol Phys 65(1):161–168

Yu MC, Ho JH, Lai SH et al. (1986) Cantonese-style salted fish as a cause of nasopharyngeal carcinoma: report of a case–control study in Hong Kong. Cancer Res 46(2):956–961

Yuan J, Wang XL, Xiang YB et al. (2000) Preserved foods in relation to risk of nasopharyngeal carcinoma in Shanghai, China. Int J Cancer 85(3):358–363

Zhang L, Zhao C, Peng PJ et al. (2005) Phase III study comparing standard radiotherapy with or without weekly oxaliplatin in treatment of locoregionally advanced nasopha-ryngeal carcinoma: preliminary results. J Clin Oncol 23:8461–8468

Paranasal Sinus and Nasal Cavity

6

CLAUS ANDRUP KRISTENSEN

CONTENTS

6.1   Epidemiology   76

6.2   Diagnosis and Staging   76

6.3   Treatment   76
6.3.1   Surgery   79
6.3.2   Radiotherapy   80
6.3.2.1 Radiotherapy Technique   80
6.3.2.2 Radiation Dose and Fractionation   81
6.3.2.3 Doses to Organs at Risk   82
6.3.2.4 Target Definition   82
6.3.2.5 Particle Therapy   82
6.3.2.6 Brachytherapy   83
6.3.3   Systemic Therapy   83
6.3.3.1 Sinonasal Neuroendocrine
        Carcinomas   83
6.3.3.2 Sinonasal Undifferentiated
        Carcinoma   83
6.3.3.3 Intra-Arterial Infusion   83
6.3.4   Treatment Results   83

6.4   Follow-Up   84

6.5   Treatment of Recurrence   84

6.6   Cancer of the Nasal Vestibule   84

Abbreviations   84

References   85

CLAUS ANDRUP KRISTENSEN, MD, PhD
Department of Oncology 5073, The Finsen Centre,
Rigshospitalet, Blegdamsvej 9, 2100 Copenhagen, Denmark

KEY POINTS

- Sinonasal carcinoma occurs more frequently in wood dust-exposed individuals and occupational history is particularly important for this patient group.
- CT scans and MRI are complementary and both are necessary for diagnosis, staging, and planning of surgery and radiotherapy. ^{18}F-FDG-PET/CT can be used as a supplement to other diagnostic and treatment planning procedures.
- Multidisciplinary conferences are essential for optimal diagnosis and treatment planning.
- Surgery is the primary treatment of sinonasal cancer. Postoperative radiotherapy is recommended in cases of incomplete surgery, advanced stage disease, or adenoid cystic carcinoma. Most studies report 5-year overall survival rates on the order of 50–60%.
- In selected cases, radical surgery is feasible with endoscopic techniques with excellent cosmetic result.
- Increasing radiation dose conformality leads to increased functional preservation of organs at risk (OARs). IMRT and proton therapy reduce mean dose to OARs significantly. Doses of 60–70 Gy should be applied.
- Induction and concomitant chemotherapy should be considered in sinonasal undifferentiated carcinoma. For other histologies, the indication is not clear-cut and should be decided in each individual case.
- Follow-up with MRI and/or PET/CT at regular intervals is recommended.
- Local recurrences should be evaluated for reirradiation and surgery before palliative chemotherapy is offered.

6.1

Epidemiology

Carcinoma of the paranasal sinuses and nasal cavity is relatively rare with an incidence of ~1/100.000 inhabitants; 60–80% of patients are males. The most common histologic subtype is squamous cell carcinoma (40–80%) followed by adenocarcinoma (10–20%) (Barnes et al. 2005). Less frequently occurring are salivary gland tumors (mainly adenoid cystic carcinoma), sinonasal undifferentiated carcinoma (SNUC), and neuroendocrine carcinomas (small cell carcinoma and esthesioneuroblastoma).

Smoking increases the risk of squamous cell carcinoma with a factor of 1.7–3.1 (t'Mannetje et al. 1999; Hayes et al. 1987), whereas the main etiological factor for development of adenocarcinoma is occupational wood dust exposure. There is a clear correlation between cancer risk and prolonged exposure to high concentrations of wood dust (t'Mannetje et al. 1999). The role of inhalation of formaldehyde and dust from the preparation of leather and textiles is more controversial, but these agents may increase the risk of sinonasal adenocarcinoma (Luce et al. 2002; Coggon et al. 2003).

6.2

Diagnosis and Staging

Due to the anatomy of the area with large mucosa-lined cavities, the tumor may grow for a very long time without causing any symptoms. Patients often ignore the initial unspecific symptoms, e.g., anosmia, nasal obstruction, discharge, and epistaxis; but eventually the tumor will invade the osseous walls of the cavities leading to local pain, headache, facial swelling, and orbital symptoms (proptosis, vision loss, diplopia) after invasion of the orbit and/or the skull base (Jiang et al. 1998; Dias et al. 2003). Consequently, most patients are diagnosed in advanced stages (Myers and Oxford 2004).

Carcinomas should be staged according to the UICC/AJCC classification (Table 6.1). The first clinical staging system for esthesioneuroblastomas was developed by Kadish et al. (1976) (Table 6.2) and later modified by Morita et al. (1993). The Kadish classification was criticized for distributing a population of patients unevenly in stages A–C with very few patients in stage A and a large inhomogeneous group of patients in stage C. In a recent comparison of different classification systems, the Kadish classification was the only staging system able to show a statistically significant discrimination between stages regarding relapse-free survival (Dias et al. 2003).

The diagnosis and staging is based on physical examination, imaging, and biopsy. Fiberoptic nasal endoscopy may provide important information about local tumor extension. Since large areas of the nose and paranasal sinuses are inaccessible for visualization even by nasal endoscopy, the use of imaging modalities is particularly important for staging and assessment of exact tumor extension. Combined CT scanning and MRI is recommended for determination of tumor stage and tumor extension before surgery and/or radiotherapy (Raghavan and Phillips 2007). Most comparative studies of imaging modalities are of patients with nasopharyngeal carcinoma; but due to the close proximity of nasopharyngeal and sinonasal tumors and the propensity for both tumor types to invade the skull base and intracranial space, extrapolations from one tumor type to the other seem acceptable. CT is excellent for assessment of cortical bone destruction, whereas MR provides more information than CT regarding soft tissue involvement, skull base erosion/invasion along cranial nerve foramina, dural and orbital invasion (Fig. 6.1) (Ng et al. 1997; Raghavan and Phillips 2007). The exact role of PET and PET/CT in diagnosis, treatment planning, and evaluation has not been determined, but uptake of ^{18}F-FDG seems to be particularly high in squamous cell carcinomas and undifferentiated carcinomas (Ninomiya et al. 2004; Wild et al. 2006).

Lymph node metastases are generally not frequent; they are present in 2–10% of patients at the time of diagnosis and lymph node recurrences occur in 7–12% (Cantù et al. 2008; Dulguerov et al. 2001; Grau et al. 2001; Le et al. 2000; Logue and Slevin 1991; Myers et al. 2002), approximately half of these recurrences occur in lymph nodes only (Dulguerov et al. 2001). Elective lymph node irradiation was not given consistently in these studies, but in a study of 49 $T_{3-4}N_0M_0$ tumors, two patients (4.5%) had lymph node recurrences after elective radiotherapy (Jeremic et al. 2000).

6.3

Treatment

The location of sinonasal tumors in close proximity to high-priority organs at risk (OAR) such as the eye(s), the optic nerve(s), the optic chiasm, and the

Table 6.1. UICC/AJCC 2002 system for staging of cancer in the nasal cavity and paranasal sinuses

Primary tumor (T)	
Tx: Primary tumor cannot be assessed	
T0: No evidence of primary tumor	
Tis: Carcinoma in situ	

Maxillary sinus	Nasal cavity and ethmoid sinus
T1: Tumor limited to maxillary sinus mucosa with no erosion or destruction of bone	T1: Tumor restricted to any one subsite, with or without bony invasion
T2: Tumor causing bone erosion or destruction including extension into the hard palate and/or middle nasal meatus, except extension to posterior wall of maxillary sinus and pterygoid plates	T2: Tumor invading two subsites in a single region or extending to involve an adjacent region within the nasoethmoidal complex, with or without bony invasion
T3: Tumor invades any of the following – bone of the posterior wall of maxillary sinus, subcutaneous tissues, floor or medial wall of orbit, pterygoid fossa, ethmoid sinuses	T3: Tumor extends to invade the medial wall or floor of the orbit, maxillary sinus, palate, or cribriform plate
T4a: Tumor invades anterior orbital contents, skin of cheek, pterygoid plates, infratemporal fossa, cribriform plate, sphenoid or frontal sinuses	T4a: Tumor invades any of the following – anterior orbital contents, skin of nose or cheek, minimal extension to anterior cranial fossa, pterygoid plates, sphenoid or frontal sinuses
T4b: Tumor invades any of the following–orbital apex, dura, brain, middle cranial fossa, cranial nerves other than maxillary division of trigeminal nerve (V_2), nasopharynx or clivus	T4b: Tumor invades any of the following – orbital apex, dura, brain, middle cranial fossa, cranial nerves other than maxillary division of trigeminal nerve (V_2), nasopharynx or clivus

Regional lymph nodes (N)	Stage grouping
Nx: Regional lymph nodes cannot be assessed	
N0: No regional lymph node metastasis	
N1: Metastasis in a single ipsilateral lymph node, 3 cm or less in greatest dimension	
N2a: Metastasis in a single ipsilateral lymph node, more than 3 cm but not more than 6 cm in greatest dimension	
N2b: Metastases in multiple ipsilateral lymph nodes, not more than 6 cm in greatest dimension	
N2c: Metastasis in bilateral or contralateral lymph nodes, not more than 6 cm in greatest dimension	
N3: Metastasis in a lymph node, more than 6 cm in greatest dimension	

Stage grouping:

	T1	T2	T3	T4a	T4b
N0	I	II			
N1			III		
N2				IVA	
N3					IVB

Distant metastasis (M)	
Mx: Distant metastasis cannot be assessed	IVC: Any T, Any N, M1
M0: No distant metastasis	
M1: Distant metastasis	

Table 6.2. The Kadish staging system for esthesioneuroblastoma

Stage	Tumor extension
A	Tumor limited to the nasal cavity
B	Tumor involving nasal cavity and paranasal sinuse(s)
C	Tumor extending beyond the nasal cavity and paranasal sinuses

brainstem makes these tumors a particular challenge to the surgeon and the radiation oncologist. Surgery and radiotherapy represent the two available curative treatment modalities, but randomized studies of surgery vs. radiotherapy and the sequence of these modalities in combination treatment have not been published.

Most authors recommend surgery followed by radiotherapy for all stages (WALDRON et al. 1998; TRAN et al. 1989; TIWARI et al. 2000; PAULINO et al.

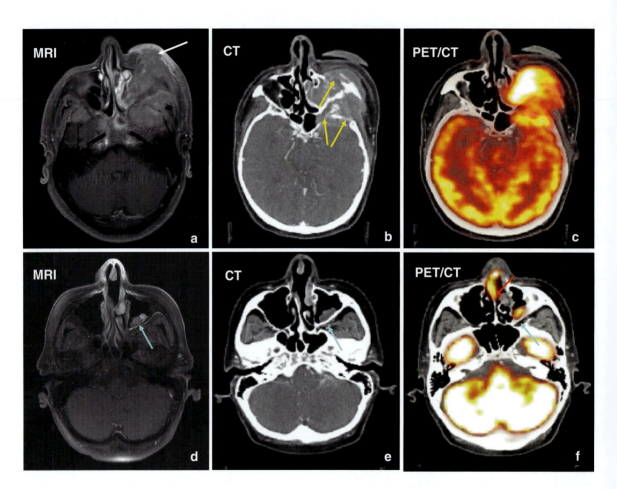

Fig. 6.1. MRI, CT, and PET/CT scans of a patient with a maxillary tumor (**a–c**) and a patient with a tumor of the nasal septum (**d–f**). The imaging modalities complement each other and all contributes to the staging and target volume delineation. MRI (**a**) is excellent for visualization of tumor extension in soft tissue; in this case, the tumor is invading the subcutis (*white arrow*). The bone destruction (*yellow arrows*) is clearly visible by CT (**b**), and FDG-PET/CT shows the overall tumor extension (**c**). The tumor in the mucosa of the nasal septum is not clearly visible by neither MRI nor CT, but obvious on PET/CT (*red arrow*). In contrast, the tumor in the left maxillary sinus (*blue arrows*) is clearly visible by all three imaging modalities. In both patients, the MR and PET/CT scans have been performed in different patient positions; hence the anatomical differences between MR and PET/CT scans. For fusion of scans for target volume delineation, these differences in patient positioning are adjusted by software correction (with kind assistance from A. K. Berthelsen, Rigshospitalet, Denmark)

1998) except small nasal or maxillary tumors, where surgery can be the only treatment (LE et al. 2000). If primary surgery is not possible due to tumor extension, initial radiotherapy may be followed by surgery (GIRI et al. 1992). Superiority of the combined-therapy approach seems to be supported by a study of nasal and paranasal salivary gland tumors by TRAN et al. (1989), in which patients treated with postoperative radiotherapy had an improved local control compared with patients treated with either surgery or radiotherapy, despite having a higher fraction of patients with advanced stage and residual disease in the combination therapy group. Thus, radiotherapy alone is considered to be inferior to combination therapy, but survival data comparable to survival after combination treatment have been reported (LOGUE and SLEVIN 1991).

6.3.1
Surgery

Anterior craniofacial resection (ACFR) is the gold standard of sinonasal surgery techniques (LUND et al. 2007). An extended lateral rhinotomy incision or a combined bicoronal (or rarely spectacle) incision with midfacial degloving is used (HOWARD et al. 2006). Intracranial access is achieved by a frontal osteotomy (LUND et al. 1998). This open surgery technique allows for radical en bloc tumor removal and for bioptic evaluation of treatment response, but tumor involvement of critical structures as eyes, nerves, arteries, or brain may jeopardize resection with clear margins, which seems to be an independent predictor of survival (GANLY et al. 2005). The margin to intraorbital structures is particularly important for decisions regarding surgical extent, since orbital exenteration or clearance (where the eyelids and palpebral conjunctiva is preserved) leads to a major decrease in the patients' quality of life. An aggressive surgical approach including orbital clearance is only justified if the decrease in quality of life is balanced by an improved survival rate. The criteria for orbital clearance are still highly controversial, and different surgical strategies have been outlined. Some authors recommend orbital clearance if the periorbital fascia is invaded (TIWARI et al. 2000) or transgressed (LUND et al. 1998) by tumor tissue, others only if orbital fat, muscle, or apex is invaded

(MAGHAMI and KRAUS 2004). In one study, there was no difference in locoregional control between patients treated with orbital preservation ($n = 54$) and those undergoing exenteration ($n = 12$), and among the 54 patients treated with periorbital resection only, acceptable vision without diplopia was retained in 91% of patients, 54% had no visual impairment (IMOLA and SCHRAMM 2002). It seems acceptable to conclude that selective orbital preservation is safe and allows for functional preservation of the eye (SUÁREZ et al. 2008).

The combination of functional endoscopic sinus surgery (FESS) and computer-aided surgery (CAS) enables the surgeon to navigate the surgical instruments in a three-dimensional CT image acquired preoperatively. Thus, it is possible to relate the position of the instruments in the surgical field to tumor tissue and critical structures visualized on the CT scanning. The use of FESS in treatment of malignant tumors in the sinonasal cavities has been controversial, mainly because of concerns that surgical radicality may be compromised in the attempt to decrease morbidity. In endoscopic sinus surgery, the tumor is removed by piecemeal technique followed by a step-by-step dissection with constant evaluation of tumor boundaries and surgical margins by frozen-section analysis as opposed to the en bloc removal of tumor by ACFR (NICOLAI et al. 2007).

Piecemeal removal may predispose to local contamination with cancer cells or cancer cell spread through blood or lymph vessels, but a retrospective study compared the outcome of nonendoscopic piecemeal vs. en bloc resection of 30 malignant paranasal sinus tumors and found no apparent difference in survival between the two groups (WELLMAN et al. 1999). The complication rate seemed lower after piecemeal procedures. Similar results have been published in a retrospective comparison of endoscopic ($n = 9$) and craniofacial ($n = 16$) resection of anterior skull base tumors; no difference in complication rates, recurrence rates, or survival was found between the two groups (BATRA et al. 2005). Most specialists agree that endoscopic resection of sinonasal tumors located in the anterior skull base is safe and feasible in carefully selected patients (BOGAERTS et al. 2008). Surgeons with experience in endoscopic as well as external approaches and a close collaboration between ENT surgeons and neurosurgeons in multidisciplinary teams are absolute necessities (BATRA et al. 2005; NICOLAI et al. 2007).

6.3.2
Radiotherapy

The precise role of radiotherapy in the treatment of sinonasal carcinomas has never been assessed in randomized trials. There seems to be no doubt that radiotherapy alone can induce complete and lasting responses with locoregional control rates of 40–50%; the corresponding figure for surgery alone is 70% (Dulguerov et al. 2001; Katz et al. 2002). Obviously, these figures are not comparable; patients with low disease stages were selected for surgery alone, whereas radiotherapy as the only treatment modality usually is given in situations where surgery is not possible due to tumor extension or comorbidity. Thus, radiotherapy may be an excellent single-modality treatment, but high doses ($\geq$66 Gy) are necessary for complete tumor control. It is complicated to achieve this dose with conventional techniques without a major risk of severe toxicity to OARs, and in a study where radical radiotherapy has been employed in the majority of cases, a high frequency of unilateral (35%) and bilateral (7%) radiation-induced blindness has been reported (Katz et al. 2002). With modern conformal radiotherapy techniques with CT (and MRI)-based planning and intensity-modulated radiation therapy (IMRT), significant sparing of OARs and further dose intensification is possible; this may justify radiotherapy as the primary treatment for sinonasal cancers. Based on the published reports, however, there seems to be a general agreement that the major part of patients with tumor stages > T1 should be treated with a combination of surgery and radiotherapy (Dulguerov et al. 2001; Jansen et al. 2000; Claus et al. 2002b; Ozsaran et al. 2003; Padovani et al. 2003; Porceddu et al. 2004; Hicsonmez et al. 2005; Duthoy et al. 2005; Daly et al. 2007; Dirix et al. 2007; Hoppe et al. 2007). Surgery as the only treatment modality can be used for T1 tumors (Blanch et al. 2004; Dulguerov et al. 2001).

Having reached consensus on combined surgery and radiotherapy for advanced stage sinonasal cancers, further unresolved issues are whether to irradiate before or after surgery, doses to target volumes, and whether or not to treat the neck lymph nodes electively.

Usually, combined modality treatment leads to increased morbidity because of contributions to toxicity from both/all modalities. Consequently, it would be an obvious advantage if one of the treatment modalities could minimize the toxicity of the other: preoperative radiotherapy may decrease the tumor volume and allow for less radical surgery, and surgery with clear (or close) margins allows for a radiotherapy dose reduction from $\geq$66 to 60 Gy. In situations where the tumor has been growing in a sinus without invading the opposite mucous membrane, it may be safe to include only the mucosa at the origin of the tumor in the clinical target volume (CTV) after debulking surgery, enabling a significant reduction of the irradiated volume (Jansen et al. 2000). However, it is often very complicated to localize areas with involved margins precisely, and in most cases the postsurgical CTV includes the entire presurgical tumor volume with a margin. In general, compromises regarding surgical radicality should be made with caution – avoiding orbital clearance when indicated will force the radiation oncologist to treat the orbital content to very high radiation doses, which inevitably will lead to loss of vision or other severe morbidity. Again, multidisciplinary conferences between ENT surgeons, neurosurgeons, maxillary-facial surgeons, neuroradiologists, anesthetists, pathologists, medical oncologists, and radiation oncologists are of great importance.

The optimal sequence of surgery and radiotherapy in head and neck cancer has been investigated in a randomized study from 1980 (Snow et al. 1980). Unfortunately, only very few sinonasal cancers were included in this study, and there was no difference in local control rate or survival between patients treated with pre- and postoperative radiotherapy. In a review from 1995, it is concluded that postoperative radiotherapy seems to improve locoregional control compared with preoperative irradiation (Wennerberg 1995), but the reviewed studies included only patients with squamous cell head and neck carcinoma, and the conclusions may not be valid for sinonasal cancer patients.

6.3.2.1
Radiotherapy Technique

Positioned between the orbits in front of the optic chiasm and the brainstem, the nasal cavity (with the intimately related paranasal sinuses) is the most complicated target to irradiate without exceeding the maximal tolerated doses to the surrounding and very radiosensitive OARs. Conventional two-dimensional photon treatment consisted of one anterior and two wedged lateral fields. The fields were shaped to shield the orbit, brain and brainstem, but full doses were often given to the optic nerve(s) and chiasm because of their close proximity to the tumor. Introduction of CT-planning and three-dimensional conformal radiotherapy made it possible to

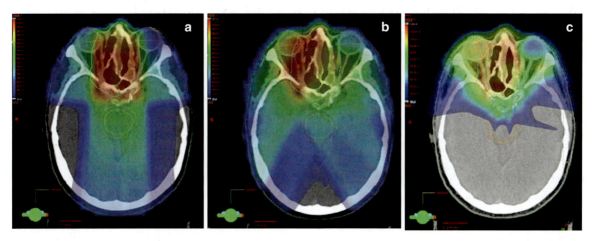

Fig. 6.2. Dose distribution (6.8 Gy–maximum dose) in a single CT slice shown as color-wash images of (**a**) a three-field conventional photon dose plan, (**b**) a seven-field IMRT plan, and (**c**) a five-field intensity-modulated proton therapy (IMPT) plan from the same patient. Selective sparing of the left eye and the left optic nerve/chiasm is possible with IMRT (**b**) and IMPT (**c**), whereas more than 68 Gy is given to the optic chiasm and parts of both optic nerves by conventional radiotherapy (**a**). Proton therapy (**c**) reduces doses to OARs and low-dose irradiation to normal tissue compared with photon therapy (**a** and **b**) (with kind assistance from W. Sapru and J. Medin, Rigshospitalet, Denmark)

transfer tumor volumes and OARs to dose plans and shape the fields not only to cover target volumes but also to attempt to spare vital organs. Multileaf collimators and IMRT is a further step in optimizing conformity and improving the therapeutic ratio particularly in sinonasal tumors. IMRT has been demonstrated to decrease morbidity from curative radiotherapy for sinonasal tumors, particularly regarding dry-eye syndrome and optic neuropathy (VELDEMAN et al. 2008). An increase in local control by IMRT has not been demonstrated, but there is no doubt that IMRT enables a dose increment while decreasing the doses to OARs (PACHOLKE et al. 2005; DALY et al. 2007) (Fig. 6.2).

However, the increased conformity introduces new problems in radiotherapy planning. Local control is essential for the prognosis of patients with cancer of the paranasal sinuses and nasal cavity. An exact definition of target volumes has become increasingly important, but the target is often very difficult to delineate and it may not be visible on CT at all. Furthermore, there is substantial interobserver variation in target contouring (RASCH et al. 2002). Accounting for this variation by increasing margins around target volumes decreases conformity and may lead to loss of a part of what has been gained by introducing IMRT. Instead, the observer variation should be minimized by fusion of pre- and postoperative MRI and CT images, PET/CT-based treatment planning, and delineation consensus between oncologists, surgeons, pathologists, and radiologists on multidisciplinary target definition conferences.

Still, it may not be possible to cover the target volume without overdosing OARs. Particularly in the sinonasal area, the tumor tissue or the surgical field is often involving or directly bordering vital structures and it is not possible to cover the target volume and spare, e.g., the optic apparatus in cases where these structures overlap. Whether to sacrifice the vision on one (or both) eye(s) or to deliberately underdose the target volume depends on several factors: Most importantly, the patient should be informed in detail about these dilemmas and about the risks regarding functional preservation of the eye(s). If chemotherapy is given concomitantly, it may be acceptable in certain situations to underdose small volumes of the CTV close to OARs. Regarding postoperative radiotherapy, lower doses than prescribed may also be acceptable in small areas of the surgical field where margins are found or presumed to be clear.

6.3.2.2
Radiation Dose and Fractionation

In most studies, the GTV has been treated to 66–70 Gy and areas with clear or close margins to ~60 Gy, usually 1.8–2 Gy/fraction, five fractions/week. The effect of accelerated and/or hyperfractionated radiotherapy has never been assessed for sinonasal cancer, but a survival benefit has been demonstrated for squamous cell carcinomas of other head and neck localizations (BOURHIS et al. 2006). In the sinonasal area, accelerated radiotherapy regimens are used at some centers (WEBER et al. 2006). The patient should be immobilized with a mask extending to the shoulders if the treatment of the neck is planned. A bite block should be positioned in the mouth to hold the tongue and most of the oral mucosa out of the irradiation field.

6.3.2.3
Doses to Organs at Risk

Recommended maximum doses to OARs and planning risk volumes (PRVs) are given in Table 6.3. Particularly at risk are the visual pathways surrounding the target volume. With IMRT, it is possible to keep doses to risk organs below the maximally allowed, but in certain situations, dose constraints must be exceeded at least on one side to cover critical areas of the target volume.

Radiation-induced fibrosis of the nasolacrimal duct can be treated with dilatation. Keratitis, keratoconjunctivitis sicca, and ultimately the dry-eye syndrome may lead to enucleation to alleviate pain (PARSONS et al. 1994), but severe dry-eye syndrome seems to be avoidable if doses to the lacrimal glands are kept below 30 Gy (CLAUS et al. 2002a). Cataracts are difficult to avoid since they occur after very low radiation doses, but fortunately they are treatable by surgery and do not constitute a major problem. Retinopathy and glaucoma are serious late-occurring complications probably avoidable if doses to the posterior part of the eye are kept below 45 Gy (TAKEDA et al. 1999). Doses to the

optic nerves, and chiasm should be kept below 54 Gy. The brainstem tolerance is particularly important since progressing neurologic loss is a devastating complication. Even though the dose tolerance of the brainstem seems to be volume dependent, only a very small volume (<0.9 cc) of the brainstem tolerates doses above 60 Gy (DEBUS et al. 1997).

6.3.2.4
Target Definition

The gross tumor volume (GTV) should be delineated from (PET/)CT scans and MRI, with specific attention to the description of tumor extension from the clinical and endoscopic examination, since tumor extension to the superior alveololabial sulcus and/or palate is often not visualized with conventional imaging modalities. In the postoperative setting, information from surgical and pathological reports should be considered in the GTV delineation.

It is not possible to outline exact recommendations regarding the margin from the GTV to the CTV. In general, 10 mm seems appropriate but the margin can be much narrower in areas bordering intact bone. Regional lymph nodes (facial nodes and levels Ib, II, and III) should be included in the CTV in cases with lymph node involvement (N+) and in cases where the primary tumor involves the oral cavity, the pharynx, or the skin. If the nasopharynx is involved, levels I–V should be included. Unilateral lymph node irradiation can be used for maxillary tumors not involving the midline.

Margins to the planning target volume (PTV) may vary depending on the immobilization procedure and the daily setup control procedure and cannot be generalized.

6.3.2.5
Particle Therapy

Table 6.3. Recommended maximum doses to critical normal tissues (OARs and PRVs) (from http://www.dahanca.dk)

	OAR (Gy)	PRV (Gy)
Spinal cord	45	50
Brainstem	54	60
Optic chiasm	54	60
Optic nerve	54	60
Posterior eye	45	50
Anterior eye	30	35
Inner ear	54	60

Parotid gland: mean dose ≤ 26 Gy; Larynx: 2/3 of total volume should be kept below 50 Gy

The role of proton or carbon ion therapy has not yet been fully elucidated but there is no doubt that a further increase in conformity is obtainable with particle therapy and will result in further sparing of OARs, particularly in this anatomical area (Fig. 6.2). The use of proton therapy has been demonstrated to reduce the mean doses to OARs compared with conventional, 3D conformal, and IMRT photon techniques (MOCK et al. 2004; LOMAX et al. 2003; MIRALBELL et al. 1992) and improvement in target coverage as well as dose reduction to OARs seems to be obtainable by photon IMRT with carbon ion boost compared with photon IMRT alone for adenoid cystic carcinomas involving the skull base (SCHULZ-ERTNER et al. 2003). Twenty-one patients were treated with this technique, resulting in 3-year locoregional control and disease-specific survival of 62 and 40%, respectively (SCHULZ-ERTNER et al. 2004).

6.3.2.6
Brachytherapy

Brachytherapy in combination with external beam radiotherapy makes it possible to increase the dose to surgical areas with involved margins. The technique can be applied after external beam radiotherapy (TIWARI et al. 1999) or as intraoperative high-dose rate brachytherapy (IOHDR) with placement of gold marker seeds at the resection margins. IOHDR can be used in combination with external beam radiotherapy with 5-year local control and overall survival rates of 65 and 44%, respectively (NAG et al. 2004).

6.3.3
Systemic Therapy

Chemotherapy has been used for all subgroups of sinonasal cancer, mainly as induction treatment before surgery with the purpose of shrinking the tumor and thereby increasing the possibility of radical surgery. Most studies of chemotherapy are retrospective, and no randomized studies have been performed.

Sinonasal tumors are generally chemosensitive with response rates for induction therapy with cisplatin and 5-FU of up to 70% (BJÖRK-ERIKSSON et al. 1992) and 5-year survival rates of 72–76% (FUJII et al. 1998; LEE et al. 1999). These survival data seem impressive but may not be significantly different from survival data from study populations, in which only a small fraction of patients have been given chemotherapy (DULGUEROV et al. 2001). Again, the studies should be compared with caution and the inevitable selection of patients with a fair prognosis for aggressive multimodality regimens resulting in high survival rates should be kept in mind.

6.3.3.1
Sinonasal Neuroendocrine Carcinomas

These tumors (esthesioneuroblastomas and small cell carcinomas) seem to be particularly chemosensitive with response rates of 60–82% to cisplatin and etoposide combined with other cytostatic agents, e.g., ifosfamide, cyclophosphamide, doxorubicin, or vin-cristine (FITZEK et al. 2002; KIM et al. 2004; MISHIMA et al. 2004; ROSENTHAL et al. 2004). In patients with esthesioneuroblastoma, distant metastases occur rarely and local therapy with combined surgery and radiotherapy results in excellent survival rates of up to 93%; consequently, it may be reasonable to reserve chemotherapy for histological subtypes with higher rates of systemic failure and a poorer prognosis (ROSENTHAL et al. 2004). The prognosis of patients with small cell carcinoma is very poor; in spite of aggressive therapy including chemotherapy, all of 16 tumors seemed to recur (ROSENTHAL et al. 2004).

6.3.3.2
Sinonasal Undifferentiated Carcinoma

Aggressive behavior, high frequency of distant metastases, and a poor prognosis characterize SNUCs, and it seems reasonable to include systemic chemotherapy in the multimodality treatment of these histologic subgroups (ROSENTHAL et al. 2004). Even with aggressive multimodality treatment, the prognosis of patients with SNUC remains poor (CHEN et al. 2008).

6.3.3.3
Intra-Arterial Infusion

Intra-arterial infusion of cisplatin (MADISON MICHAEL et al. 2005) or 5-FU (YOSHIMURA et al. 2002) has been investigated and seems to lead to high rates of local control and survival in retrospective studies, but randomized studies have not been conducted.

In conclusion, chemotherapy (particularly cisplatin and 5-FU) induces relatively high response rates in sinonasal cancers, but the effect of chemotherapy on locoregional control, distant metastases, and survival is still unresolved. Systemic therapy in the primary treatment of sinonasal cancer should be used with caution – unexpected toxicity and complications may occur when intensive multimodality regimens are used in this anatomical area. Studies on the effect of other systemic therapies as antibodies, tyrosine kinase inhibitors, and radiosensitizers in sinonasal cancer have not been published.

6.3.4
Treatment Results

Several reports on the effect of combined modality treatment have been published. In general, the studies are retrospective and the populations of patients included are very heterogeneous regarding tumor localization, stage, histology, and treatment; this complicates the interpretation and comparison of data significantly. The majority of patients were treated with a combination of surgery and radiotherapy. The 5-year locoregional control rate in recently published studies is 54–62% and the 5-year overall survival rate is 45–62%. The prognosis for patients with cancer of the paranasal sinus or nasal cavity seems to have improved during the last four decades (DULGUEROV et al. 2001).

6.4

Follow-Up

Follow-up after treatment has the purpose of diagnosing recurrences and late-occurring adverse effects as early as possible. The program should include clinical examination, endoscopy, and MRI and/or PET/CT scanning. MRI and CT are complementary in the diagnosis of recurrent head and neck tumors (LELL et al. 2000). FDG-PET was found superior to MR and CT in the diagnosis of local residual and recurrent nasopharyngeal carcinoma in a review of 21 articles including 1,813 patients (LIU et al. 2007), and may also be the method of choice for detection of residual or recurrent sinonasal cancers. Increased FDG uptake early after irradiation may be caused by a post-treatment inflammatory reaction, and PET should not be performed earlier than 3 months after radiotherapy (LIU et al. 2007).

Late-occurring side effects of radiotherapy are mainly ophthalmologic or related to mucous membranes or salivary glands (CHEN et al. 2008; HOPPE et al. 2007; BRISTOL et al. 2007).

Control of visual function should be performed with regular intervals after radiotherapy.

Surgical and dental rehabilitation is of major importance; defects after removal of tumors should be closed by surgical reconstruction if possible and dental implants should be considered. Involvement of anaplastologists already in the planning phase of surgery is a great advantage in situations where an external prosthesis (orbital and/or nasal) is necessary.

6.5

Treatment of Recurrence

Studies addressing the treatment of recurrent or metastasizing sinonasal cancer are very rare, and no randomized trials have been conducted. At diagnosis of a local recurrence, radical surgery and/or reirradiation should be considered since salvage therapy may result in lasting local control (KIM et al. 2008). If none of these options are possible, systemic chemotherapy should be offered according to histology. Patients with squamous cell carcinoma have been included in the published randomized studies on the effect of different combination chemotherapy regimens in patients with recurrent or metastasizing head and neck cancer reviewed by COHEN et al. (2004).

6.6

Cancer of the Nasal Vestibule

Nasal vestibule carcinomas are mainly squamous cell carcinomas of the skin. For small tumors, excellent local control rates (>90%) and cosmetic results have been obtained by radiotherapy (external beam or brachytherapy) alone (LANGENDIJK et al. 2004), but surgery may be the treatment of choice for selected small superficial tumors. In a recently published study of 36 T4 tumors, the 5-year local control rate after radiotherapy ± surgery was 71%. Larger tumors (>4 cm) or tumors invading the bone should be treated with combined surgery and radiotherapy (WALLACE et al. 2007).

Abbreviations

5-FU	5-Fluorouracil
ACFR	Anterior craniofacial resection
AJCC	American Joint Commission on Cancer
CAS	Computer-aided surgery
CGE	Cobalt Gray equivalent
CTV	Clinical target volume
ENT	Ear, nose, and throat
FDG	2-Fluoro-2-deoxy-D-glucose
FESS	Functional endoscopic sinus surgery
GTV	Gross tumor volume
IMRT	Intensity-modulated radiotherapy
IOHDR	Intraoperative high-dose-rate brachytherapy
MRI	Magnetic resonance imaging
OAR	Organ at risk
PRV	Planning organ at risk volume
SNUC	Sinonasal undifferentiated carcinoma
UICC	Union Internationale Contre le Cancer

References

Barnes L, Eveson JW, Reichart P et al. (eds) (2005) World Health Organisation classification of tumours. Pathology and genetics of head and neck tumours. IARC Press, Lyon

Batra PS, Citardi MJ, Worley S et al. (2005) Resection of anterior skull base tumors: Comparison of combined traditional and endoscopic techniques. Am J Rhinol 19:521–528

Björk-Eriksson T, Mercke C, Petruson B et al. (1992) Potential impact on tumor control and organ preservation with cisplatin and 5-fluorouracil for patients with advanced tumors of the paranasal sinuses and nasal fossa. A prospective pilot study. Cancer 70:2615–2620

Blanch JL, Ruiz AM, Alos L et al. (2004) Treatment of 125 sinonasal tumors: Prognostic factors, outcome, and follow-up. Otolaryngol Head Neck Surg 131:973–976

Bogaerts S, Vander Poorten V, Nuyts S et al. (2008) Results of endoscopic resection followed by radiotherapy for primarily diagnosed adenocarcinomas of the paranasal sinuses. Head Neck 30:728–736

Bourhis J, Overgaard J, Audry H et al. (2006) Hyperfractionated or accelerated radiotherapy in head and neck cancer. Lancet 368:843–854

Bristol IJ, Ahamad A, Garden AS et al. (2007) Postoperative radiotherapy for maxillary sinus cancer: Long-term outcomes and toxicities of treatment. Int J Radiat Oncol Biol Phys 68:719–730

Cantù G, Bimbi G, Miceli R et al. (2008) Lymph node metastases in malignant tumors of the paranasal sinuses. Arch Otolaryngol Head Neck Surg 134:170–177

Chen AM, Daly ME, El-Sayed I et al. (2008) Patterns of failure after combined-modality approaches incorporating radiotherapy for sinonasal undifferentiated carcinoma of the head and neck. Int J Radiat Oncol Biol Phys 70:338–343

Claus F, Boterberg T, Ost P et al. (2002a) Short term toxicity profile for 32 sinonasal cancer patients treated with IMRT. Can we avoid dry eye syndrome? Radiother Oncol 64:205–208

Claus F, Boterberg T, Ost P et al. (2002b) Postoperative radiotherapy for adenocarcinoma of the ethmoid sinuses: Treatment results for 47 patients. Int J Radiat Oncol Biol Phys 54:1089–1094

Coggon D, Harris EC, Poole J et al. (2003) Extended follow-up of a cohort of British chemical workers exposed to formaldehyde. J Natl Cancer Inst 95:1608–1615

Cohen EEW, Lingen MW, Vokes EE (2004) The expanding role of systemic therapy in head and neck cancer. J Clin Oncol 22:1743–1752

Daly ME, Chen AM, Bucci MK et al. (2007) Intensity-modulated radiation therapy for malignancies of the nasal cavity and paranasal sinuses. Int J Radiat Oncol Biol Phys 67:151–157

Debus J, Hug EB, Liebsch NJ et al. (1997) Brainstem tolerance to conformal radiotherapy of skull base tumors. Int J Radiat Oncol Biol Phys 39:967–975

Dias FL, Sa GM, Lima RA et al. (2003) Patterns of failure and outcome in esthesioneuroblastoma. Arch Otolaryngol Head Neck Surg 129:1186–1192

Dirix P, Nuyts S, Geussens Y et al. (2007) Malignancies of the nasal cavity and paranasal sinuses: Long-term outcome with conventional or three-dimensional conformal radiotherapy. Int J Radiat Oncol Biol Phys 69:1042–1050

Dulguerov P, Jacobsen MS, Allal AS et al. (2001) Nasal and paranasal sinus carcinoma. Are we making any progress? Cancer 92:3012–3029

Duthoy W, Boterberg T, Claus F et al. (2005) Postoperative intensity-modulated radiotherapy in sinonasal carcinoma: Clinical results in 39 patients. Cancer 104:71–82

Fitzek MM, Thornton AF, Varvares M et al. (2002) Neuroendocrine tumors of the sinonasal tract. Results of a prospective study incorporating chemotherapy, surgery, and combined proton-photon radiotherapy. Cancer 94: 2623–2634

Fujii M, Ohno Y, Tokumaru Y et al. (1998) Adjuvant chemotherapy with oral tegaful and uracil for maxillary sinus carcinoma. Oncology 55:109–115

Ganly I, Patel SG, Singh B et al. (2005) Craniofacial resection for malignant paranasal sinus tumors: Report of an international collaborative study. Head Neck 27:575–584

Giri SP, Reddy EK, Gemer LS et al. (1992) Management of advanced squamous cell carcinomas of the maxillary sinus. Cancer 69:657–661

Grau C, Jakobsen MH, Harbo G et al. (2001) Sino-nasal cancer in Denmark 1982–1991. A nationwide survey. Acta Oncol 40:19–23

Hayes RB, Kardaun JW, de Bruyn A (1987) Tobacco use and sinonasal cancer: A case–control study. Br J Cancer 56: 843–846

Hicsonmez A, Andrieu MN, Karaca M et al. (2005) Treatment outcome of nasal and paranasal sinus carcinoma. J Otolaryngol 34:379–383

Hoppe BS, Stegman LD, Zelefsky MJ et al. (2007) Treatment of nasal cavity and paranasal sinus cancer with modern radiotherapy techniques in the postoperative setting – The MSKCC experience. Int J Radiat Oncol Biol Phys 67:691–702

Howard DJ, Lund VJ, Wei WI (2006) Craniofacial resection for tumors of the nasal cavity and paranasal sinuses: A 25-year experience. Head Neck 28:867–873

Imola MJ, Schramm VL Jr (2002) Orbital preservation in surgical management of sinonasal malignancy. Laryngoscope 112:1357–1365

Jansen EPM, Keus RB, Hilgers FJM et al. (2000) Does the combination of radiotherapy and debulking surgery favor survival in paranasal sinus carcinoma? Int J Radiat Oncol Biol Phys 48:27–35

Jeremic B, Shibamoto Y, Milicic B et al. (2000) Elective ipsilateral neck irradiation of patients with locally advanced maxillary sinus carcinoma. Cancer 88:2246–2251

Jiang GL, Morrison WH, Garden AS et al. (1998) Ethmoid sinus carcinomas. Natural history and treatment results. Radiother Oncol 49:21–27

Kadish S, Goodman M, Wang CC (1976) Olfactory neuroblastoma. A clinical analysis of 17 cases. Cancer 37:1571–1576

Katz TS, Mendenhall WM, Morris CG et al. (2002) Malignant tumors of the nasal cavity and paranasal sinuses. Head Neck 24:821–829

Kim DW, Jo YH, Kim JH et al. (2004) Neoadjuvant etoposide, ifosfamide, and cisplatin for the treatment of olfactory neuroblastoma. Cancer 101:2257–2260

Kim HJ, Cho HJ, Kim KS et al. (2008) Results of salvage therapy after failure of initial treatment for advanced olfactory neuroblastoma. J Craniomaxillofac Surg 36:47–52

Langendijk JA, Poorter R, Leemans CR et al. (2004) Radiotherapy of squamous cell carcinoma of the nasal vestibule. Int J Radiat Oncol Biol Phys 59:1319–1325

Le QT, Fu KK, Kaplan MJ et al. (2000) Lymph node metastasis in maxillary sinus carcinoma. Int J Radiat Oncol Biol Phys 46:541–549

Lee MM, Vokes EE, Rosen A et al. (1999) Multimodality therapy in advanced paranasal sinus carcinoma: Superior long-term results. Cancer J Sci Am 5:219–223

Lell M, Baum U, Greess H et al. (2000) Head and neck tumors: Imaging recurrent tumor and post-therapeutic changes with CT and MRI. Eur J Radiol 33:239–247

Liu T, Xu W, Yan W-L et al. (2007) FDG-PET, CT, MRI for diagnosis of local residual or recurrent nasopharyngeal carcinoma, which one is the best? A systematic review. Radiother Oncol 85:327–335

Logue JP, Slevin NJ (1991) Carcinoma of the nasal cavity and paranasal sinuses: An analysis of radical radiotherapy. Clin Oncol (R Coll Radiol) 3:84–89

Lomax AJ, Goitein M, Adams J (2003) Intensity modulation in radiotherapy: Photons versus protons in the paranasal sinus. Radiother Oncol 66:11–18

Luce D, Leclerc A, Begin D et al. (2002) Sinonasal cancer and occupational exposures: A pooled analysis of 12 case–control studies. Cancer Causes Control 13:147–157

Lund V, Howard DJ, Wei WI (2007) Endoscopic resection of malignant tumors of the nose and sinuses. Am J Rhinol 21:89–94

Lund V, Howard DJ, Wei WI et al. (1998) Craniofacial resection for tumors of the nasal cavity and paranasal sinuses – A 17-year experience. Head Neck 20:97–105

Madison Michael L II, Sorenson JM, Samant S et al. (2005) The treatment of advanced sinonasal malignancies with pre-operative intra-arterial cisplatin and concurrent radiation. J Neurooncol 72:67–75

Maghami E, Kraus DH (2004) Cancer of the nasal cavity and paranasal sinuses. Expert Rev Anticancer Ther 4:411–424

Miralbell R, Crowell C, Suit HD (1992) Potential improvement of three dimension treatment planning and proton therapy in the outcome of maxillary sinus cancer. Int J Radiat Oncol Biol Phys 22:305–310

Mishima Y, Nagasaki E, Terui Y et al. (2004) Combination chemotherapy (cyclophosphamide, doxorubicin, and vincristine with continuous-infusion cisplatin and etoposide) and radiotherapy with stem cell support can be beneficial for adolescents and adults with esthesioneuroblastoma. Cancer 101:1437–1444

Mock U, Georg D, Bogner J et al. (2004) Treatment planning comparison of conventional, 3D conformal, and intensity-modulated photon (IMRT) and proton therapy for paranasal sinus carcinoma. Int J Radiat Oncol Biol Phys 58:147–154

Morita A, Ebersold MJ, Olsen KD et al. (1993) Esthesioneuroblastoma: Prognosis and management. Neurosurgery 32:706–715

Myers LL, Nussenbaum B, Bradford CR et al. (2002) Paranasal sinus malignancies: An 18-year single institution experience. Laryngoscope 112:1964–1969

Myers LL, Oxford LE (2004) Differential diagnosis and treatment options in paranasal sinus cancers. Surg Oncol Clin N Am 13:167–186

Nag S, Tippin D, Grecula J et al. (2004) Intraoperative high-dose-rate brachytherapy for paranasal sinus tumors. Int J Radiat Oncol Biol Phys 58:155–160

Ng SH, Chang TC, Ko SF et al. (1997) Nasopharyngeal carcinoma: MRI and CT assessment. Neuroradiology 39:741–746

Nicolai P, Castelnuovo P, Lombardi D et al. (2007) Role of endoscopic surgery in the management of selected malignant epithelial neoplasms of the naso-ethmoidal complex. Head Neck 29:1075–1082

Ninomiya H, Oriuchi N, Kahn N et al. (2004) Diagnosis of tumor in the nasal cavity and paranasal sinuses with [11C] choline PET: Comparative study with 2-[18F]fluoro-2-deoxy-D-glucose (FDG) PET. Ann Nucl Med 18:29–34

Ozsaran Z, Yalman D, Baltalarli B et al. (2003) Radiotherapy in maxillary sinus carcinomas: Evaluation of 79 cases. Rhinology 41:44–48

Pacholke HD, Amdur RJ, Louis DA et al. (2005) The role of intensity modulated radiation therapy for favorable stage tumor of the nasal cavity or ethmoid sinus. Am J Clin Oncol 28:474–478

Padovani L, Pommier P, Clippe S et al. (2003) Three-dimensional conformal radiotherapy for paranasal sinus carcinoma: Clinical results for 25 patients. Int J Radiat Oncol Biol Phys 56:169–176

Parsons JT, Bova FJ, Fitzgerald CR et al. (1994) Severe dry-eye syndrome following external beam irradiation. Int J Radiat Oncol Biol Phys 30:775–780

Paulino AC, Marks JE, Bricker P et al. (1998) Results of treatment of patients with maxillary sinus carcinoma. Cancer 83:457–465

Porceddu S, Martin J, Shanker G et al. (2004) Paranasal sinus tumors: Peter Maccallum Cancer Institute experience. Head Neck 26:322–330

Raghavan P, Phillips CD (2007) Magnetic resonance imaging of sinonasal malignancies. Top Magn Reson Imaging 18:259–267

Rasch C, Eisbruch A, Remeijer P et al. (2002) Irradiation of paranasal sinus tumors, a delineation and dose comparison study. Int J Radiat Oncol Biol Phys 52:120–127

Rosenthal DI, Barker JL, El-Naggar AK et al. (2004) Sinonasal malignancies with neuroendocrine differentiation. Patterns of failure according to histologic phenotype. Cancer 101:2567–2573

Schulz-Ertner D, Didinger B, Nikoghosyan A et al. (2003) Optimization of radiation therapy for locally advanced adenoid cystic carcinomas with infiltration of the skull base using photon intensity-modulated radiation therapy (IMRT) and a carbon ion boost. Strahlenther Onkol 179:345–351

Schulz-Ertner D, Nikoghosyan A, Thilmann C et al. (2004) Results of carbon ion radiotherapy in 152 patients. Int J Radiat Oncol Biol Phys 58:631–640

Snow JB Jr, Gelber RD, Kramer S et al. (1980) Randomized preoperative and postoperative radiation therapy for patients with carcinoma of the head and neck: Preliminary report. Laryngoscope 90:930–945

Suárez C, Ferlito A, Lund VJ et al. (2008) Management of the orbit in malignant sinonasal tumors. Head Neck 30:242–250

t'Mannetje A, Kogevinas M, Luce D et al. (1999) Sinonasal cancer, occupation, and tobacco smoking in European women and men. Am J Ind Med 36:101–107

Takeda A, Shigematsu N, Suzuki S et al. (1999) Late retinal complications of radiation therapy for nasal and paranasal malignancies: Relationship between irradiated-dose area and severity. Int J Radiat Oncol Biol Phys 44:599–605

Tiwari R, Hardillo JA, Mehta D et al. (2000) Squamous cell carcinoma of the maxillary sinus. Head Neck 22:164–169

Tiwari R, Hardillo JA, Tobi H et al. (1999) Carcinoma of the ethmoid: Results of treatment with conventional surgery and post-operative radiotherapy. Eur J Surg Oncol 25:401–405

Tran L, Sidrys J, Horton D et al. (1989) Malignant salivary gland tumors of the paranasal sinuses and nasal cavity. The UCLA experience. Am J Clin Oncol 12:587–592

Veldeman L, Madani I, Hulstaert F et al. (2008) Evidence behind use of intensity-modulated radiotherapy: A systematic review of comparative clinical studies. Lancet Oncol 9:367–375

Waldron JN, O'Sullivan B, Warde P et al. (1998) Ethmoid sinus cancer: Twenty-nine cases managed with primary radiation therapy. Int J Radiat Oncol Biol Phys 41:361–369

Wallace A, Morris CG, Kirwan J et al. (2007) Radiotherapy for squamous cell carcinoma of the nasal vestibule. Am J Clin Oncol 30:612–616

Weber DC, Chan AW, Lessell S et al. (2006) Visual outcome of accelerated fractionated radiation for advanced sinonasal malignancies employing photons/protons. Radiother Oncol 81:243–249

Wellman BJ, Traynelis VC, McCulloch TM et al. (1999) Midline anterior craniofacial approach for malignancy: Results of en bloc versus piecemeal resections. Skull Base Surg 9:41–46

Wennerberg J (1995) Pre versus post-operative radiotherapy of resectable squamous cell carcinoma of the head and neck. Acta Otolaryngol 115:465–474

Wild D, Eyrich GK, Ciernik IF et al. (2006) In-line (18) F-fluorodeoxyglucose positron emission tomography with computed tomography (PET/CT) in patients with carcinoma of the sinus/nasal area and orbit. J Craniomaxillofac Surg 34:9–16

Yoshimura R-I, Shibuya H, Ogura I et al. (2002) Trimodal combination therapy for maxillary sinus carcinoma. Int J Radiat Oncol Biol Phys 53:656–663

Salivary Glands and Quality of Life

7

CHRIS TERHAARD

CONTENTS

7.1   Introduction   *89*

7.2   Epidemiology and Treatment Outcome   *90*

7.3   The Role of Radiotherapy   *92*

7.4   Factors Influencing QOL in Salivary Gland Tumors   *92*
7.4.1   Comorbidity   *92*
7.4.2   Facial Nerve Function   *93*
7.4.3   Hearing Loss   *94*
7.4.4   Xerostomia   *95*
7.4.5   Mastoiditis/Temporal Bone Osteoradionecrosis   *95*

7.5   Radiation Techniques to Reduce the Complication Risks   *96*

7.6   Conclusion   *98*

References   *99*

KEY POINTS

- Only 2% of the head and neck (HN) malignancies originate in the salivary glands.
- The parotid gland is most frequently involved.
- Unlike other HN cancer sites, smoking and alcohol are no etiological factors, and so comorbidity is less predominant compared with other HN sites.
- Postoperative radiotherapy improves locoregional control for cases with poor prognostic factors.
- Pre- and posttreatment facial nerve dysfunction has an impact on quality of life (QOL).
- Side effects after radiotherapy for salivary gland tumors, including hearing loss, mastoiditis, and

xerostomia, may influence QOL, although no specific prospective studies on QOL and radiotherapy for salivary gland tumors are available.
- New radiotherapy techniques, such as intensity-modulated radiotherapy may reduce the risk on side effects, and so, probably improve QOL.

7.1
Introduction

A review of quality of life (QOL) concerning the salivary glands may focus on treatment of a salivary gland tumor, or xerostomia as a side effect of radiotherapy.

Quality of life studies about treatment of salivary gland tumors mainly focus on facial nerve function after surgery with or without postoperative radiotherapy. Prospective longitudinal studies on QOL issues concerning radiotherapy for salivary gland tumors cannot be found in the literature. As an indirect indicator of QOL, treatment resulting in improvement of locoregional control, and risk factors such as comorbidity and treatment-related side effects may be studied. For parotid gland tumors, the main side effects are facial nerve dysfunction, hearing loss, xerostomia, and temporal bone necrosis. Side effects of treatment of the submandibular gland and the minor salivary gland tumors strongly relate to the location of the tumor, and the possible need for elective or curative treatment of the neck nodes.

Data about the loss of the function of the salivary glands after radiotherapy, especially the parotid glands, are published increasingly in the literature. Results of objective salivary flow measurements, the subjective judgment of the salivary function by the patient, and results of QOL questionnaires may not always correlate.

CHRIS TERHAARD, MD, PhD
Department of Radiotherapy, UMC Utrecht, Huispost D01.213, Postbus 85500, 3508 GA Utrecht, The Netherlands

7.2
Epidemiology and Treatment Outcome

Two percent of all head and neck tumors are localized in the salivary glands. In the USA the incidence of salivary gland cancer did not change between 1973 and 1992, with an average per 100,000 persons of 1.2 in males and 0.8 in females (SUN et al. 1999). Etiologic factors are not clearly defined. Particularly mucoepidermoid cancer may be related to previous radiation, although this is the cause in less than 1% of salivary gland cancer (BEAL et al. 2003). Relationship between salivary gland cancer and hairdressers and people working in beauty shops has been found (SWANSON and BURNS 1997).

Of all salivary glands the parotid gland is most frequently (70%) involved. The tumor is located in the submandibular glands and minor salivary glands in 8 and 22%, respectively (SPIRO 1986). The risk of lymph node involvement depends on tumor localization, T-stage, and histology (TERHAARD et al. 2005). Lymph node involvement is around 25% for a parotid localization, and for submandibular and minor salivary gland tumor of the oral cavity up to 42 and 10%, respectively (TERHAARD et al. 2004, 2005; BHATTACHARYYA and FRIED 2005; RÉGIS DE BRITO SANTOS et al. 2001; VANDER POORTEN et al. 1999; THERKILDSEN et al. 1998; JONES et al. 1998; LOPES et al. 1998; PARSONS et al. 1996). The risk of a positive node for a salivary tumor of the nasopharynx is around 50% (SCHRAMM and IMOLA 2001).

Results, with a long follow-up, derived from a large retrospective study of the Dutch Head and Neck Oncology Group (NWHHT), concerning locoregional control, distant metastasis, and overall survival are shown in Fig. 7.1 (TERHAARD et al. 2004). Overall survival depends on histological subtype (Fig. 7.2). Acinic cell subtype is associated with the best prognosis; however, 10 years of survival for undifferentiated and squamous cell subtype is only 30% (TERHAARD et al. 2004). Prognosis of patients with distant metastases from adenoid cystic or acinic cell carcinoma is significantly better than from all other subtypes (TERHAARD et al. 2004).

Data derived from studies using multivariate analyses on prognostic factors for locoregional control, and disease-free and overall survival have been summarized in Table 7.1 (BHATTACHARYYA and FRIED 2005; THERKILDSEN et al. 1998; TERHAARD et al. 2004, 2006; JONES et al. 1998; LOPES et al. 1998; PARSONS et al. 1996; MENDENHALL et al. 2005; CHEN

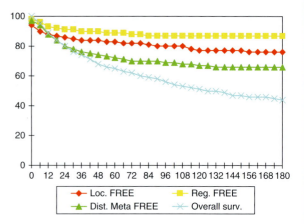

Fig. 7.1. Regional (Reg.) recurrence-free survival, Local (Loc.) recurrence-free survival, Distant (Dist.) metastasis-free survival and overall survival vs. months after diagnosis, in 666 patients with salivary gland cancer. Data derived from the Dutch NWHHT study

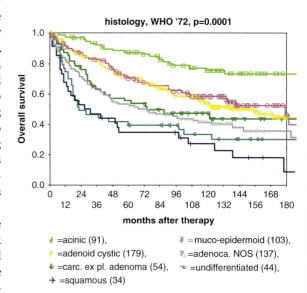

Fig. 7.2. Overall survival of salivary gland cancer, depending on histology. Data derived from the Dutch NWHHT study

et al. 2007; SPIRO et al. 1989; POULSEN et al. 1992; GARDEN et al. 1995; KOUL et al. 2007; CARRILLO et al. 2007; BHATTACHARYYA 2004; STOREY et al. 2001; BECKHARDT et al. 1995). Minor salivary gland tumors of the oral cavity are associated with the best local control and overall survival rates. As expected, more advanced age results in lower overall survival rates (BHATTACHARYYA and FRIED 2005; VANDER POORTEN et al. 1999; TERHAARD et al. 2004; SPIRO et al. 1989; POULSEN et al. 1992; KOUL et al. 2007; CARRILLO et al. 2007; BHATTACHARYYA 2004; KIRKBRIDE et al. 2001;

Table 7.1. Prognostic factors for salivary gland cancer; selection of studies with multivariate analyses

	All sites combined	Parotid	Submandibular	Minor
Loco-regional control	T-stage (Terhaard et al. 2004; Mendenhall et al. 2005) Site (Therkildsen et al. 1998; Terhaard et al. 2004) N-stage (N) (Therkildsen et al. 1998; Terhaard et al. 2004) Surgical margin (Therkildsen et al. 1998; Terhaard et al. 2004) Bone invasion (Terha ard et al. 2004) Histology (N) (Therkildsen et al. 1998; Chen et al. 2007) Therapy: S + RT > S (Therkildsen et al. 1998; Terhaard et al. 2004)	Age (Poulsen et al. 1992; Terhaard et al. 2006) N-stage (Garden et al. 1995; Terhaard et al. 2006) T-stage (Poulsen et al. 1992; Terhaard et al. 2006) Surgical margin (Poulsen et al. 1992; Terhaard et al. 2006) Grade (Poulsen et al. 1992) N VII-dysf. (N) (Garden et al. 1995; Terhaard et al. 2006) Bone invasion (Terhaard et al. 2006) Therapy: S + RT > S (Terhaard et al. 2006)	Grade (Storey et al. 2001) Histology (Storey et al. 2001) Surgical margin (Storey et al. 2001) Early years (Storey et al. 2001)	T-stage (Jones et al. 1998; Parsons et al. 1996) N-stage (Jones et al. 1998; Lopes et al. 1998; Parsons et al. 1996) Histology (Lopes et al. 1998; Beckhardt et al. 1995) Bone invasion (Lopes et al. 1998) Therapy: S + RT > S (Parsons et al. 1996)
Disease free survival	Histology (Therkildsen et al. 1998) Stage (Therkildsen et al. 1998; Mendenhall et al. 2005) Surgical margin (Therkildsen et al. 1998)	Age (Koul et al. 2007; Carrillo et al. 2007) Sex (Garden et al. 1995) $N > 4$ nodes (Garden et al. 1995) T-stage (Koul et al. 2007; Carrillo et al. 2007; Terhaard et al. 2006) Grade (Koul et al. 2007; Carrillo et al. 2007) N VII-dysf. (Garden et al. 1995; Carrillo et al. 2007; Terhaard et al. 2006) Surgical margin (Carrillo et al. 2007) Extragl. ext. (Garden et al. 1995) Bone invasion (Terhaard et al. 2006) Skin invasion (Terhaard et al. 2006) Therapy: S + RT > S (Koul et al. 2007)	Early years (Storey et al. 2001)	Grade (Lopes et al. 1998; Beckhardt et al. 1995) Stage (Parsons et al. 1996; Beckhardt et al. 1995) Surgical margin (Beckhardt et al. 1995) Therapy: S + RT > S (Lopes et al. 1998; Parsons et al. 1996)
Overall survival	Age (Terhaard et al. 2004) Sex (Terhaard et al. 2004) T-stage (Terhaard et al. 2004) Skin invasion (Terhaard et al. 2004) Bon-invasion (Terhaard et al. 2004)	Age (Bhattacharyya and Fried 2005; Spiro et al. 1989) T-stage (Bhattacharyya and Fried 2005; Spiro et al. 1989) N-stage (Bhattacharyya and Fried 2005; Spiro et al. 1989) Site (Spiro et al. 1989) Histology (Spiro et al. 1989) Extragl. ext. (Bhattacharyya and Fried 2005)	Age (Bhattacharyya 2004) Grade (Bhattacharyya 2004)	T-stage (Jones et al. 1998) General condition (Jones et al. 1998)

S surgery; *RT* postoperative radiotherapy; *N VII dysf.* facial nerve dysfunction; *Extragl. ext.* extraglandular extension

POHAR et al. 2005). However, more advanced age was in some studies also related to locoregional control (RÉGIS DE BRITO SANTOS et al. 2001; KIRKBRIDE et al. 2001; POHAR et al. 2005). As found in most head and neck cancers, T- and N-stage are prognostic factors for both locoregional control and survival (TERHAARD et al. 2004; MENDENHALL et al. 2005; GARDEN et al. 1995). Based on a weighted combination of prognostic factors, a prognostic score may be developed. T-stage, age, facial nerve dysfunction, surgical margins, and grade were identified as significant prognostic factors for parotid gland cancer by Carrillo et al. Three prognostic score categories for disease-free survival could be separated (CARRILLO et al. 2007). In the study of VANDER POORTEN et al. (1999), besides the above-mentioned factors, pain, N-stage, skin invasion, and perineural growth were also included. They could identify four categories, and could validate their results using another data set (VANDER POORTEN et al. 2003).

In search for additional prognostic factors, immunohistochemical staining of salivary gland cancers has been performed. Elevated levels of matrix metalloproteinases (MMP) have been associated with invasion capacity of cancer, and high MMP-9 intensity predicted poor overall survival in adenoid cystic and salivary duct carcinoma in a study by LUUKKAA et al. (2008). Maspin is a serine protease inhibitor with an inhibitory effect on tumor-induced angiogenesis, tumor cell motility, invasion, and metastases. Loss of nuclear and cytoplasmic maspin was an independent prognostic factor for survival of intermediate malignancy grade salivary gland cancer, as shown by SCHWARZ et al. (2008). High expression of p53, and overexpression of HER-2neu may be found in salivary gland cancer, and is related to poor survival (GALLO et al. 1995; PRESS et al. 1994; LIM et al. 2003; JAEHNE et al. 2005). Based on the expression, in future molecularly targeted therapy may become an option for poor prognostic salivary gland tumors.

7.3
The Role of Radiotherapy

Preventing locoregional recurrence is the major goal of postoperative radiotherapy for salivary gland cancer. Since radiotherapy may be associated with complications, possibly resulting in impaired QOL, the positive effect has to be proven, preferably in prospective studies. However, only results of retrospective studies are available. In some detailed studies the prognostic importance of a large number of patients has been studied extensively. In these studies, postoperative radiotherapy is a strong prognostic factor for locoregional control (THERKILDSEN et al. 1998; TERHAARD et al. 2004; PARSONS et al. 1996) and disease-specific survival in some studies (PARSONS et al. 1996; KOUL et al. 2007; CARRILLO et al. 2007). Based on these studies, postoperative radiotherapy to enhance locoregional control is recommended for T3–4 tumors, close or incomplete resection margins, bone involvement, perineural invasion, lymph node metastasis, and high-grade and recurrent cancer (TERHAARD et al. 2005; THERKILDSEN et al. 1998; PARSONS et al. 1996; STOREY et al. 2001; KIRKBRIDE et al. 2001, GARDEN et al. 1997; EADH NORTH et al. 1990; CHEN et al. 2006). In the nationwide Dutch study the relative risk (RR) for surgery alone, compared with combined treatment, was 9.7 for local recurrence and 2.3 for regional recurrence (TERHAARD et al. 2005). The advised dose is 60 Gy in case of close (<5 mm) resection margin and 66 Gy for incomplete resection margin (<1 mm) (TERHAARD et al. 2005). Radiation doses higher than 66 Gy as definitive management for salivary gland cancer may result in >50% local control (TERHAARD et al. 2005; CHEN et al. 2006).

On the one hand radiotherapy may enhance QOL by improving locoregional control, and on the other hand radiation side effects may decrease the QOL. Most series of radiotherapy for salivary gland cancer report results of patients treated during a long time period. In a series of MD Anderson Houston studies the percentage hearing loss and bone necrosis were respectively 7 and 18%, and 9 and 8% after radiotherapy for respectively minor and parotid glands (GARDEN et al. 1994, 1997). However, most complications were seen in patients treated in the early years, and the risk was substantially reduced by more modern techniques (GARDEN et al. 1994). In what follows, some factors influencing QOL will be discussed.

7.4
Factors Influencing QOL in Salivary Gland Tumors

7.4.1
Comorbidity

Salivary gland tumors are generally not included in QOL studies for head and neck cancer. One of the main reasons for this exclusion may be the difference in etiology. In contrast to most other sites of head and neck cancer, chronic tobacco and alcohol consumption play no role in the cancer of the salivary gland. Longstanding exposure to tobacco and alcohol is also associated with cardiovascular, pulmonary, hepatic, and metabolic diseases. In a prospective study in Utrecht, patients with head and neck cancer and a low Karnofsky performance status were at risk for physical and psychological morbidity after treatment (GRAEFF et al. 2000). Besides, these comorbidities may influence the choice and the outcome of treatment (DERKS et al. 2005). In elderly patients (>70 years) with head and neck carcinoma, comorbidities were present in 75%, and appeared to be a prognostic factor for overall survival in a study by SANABRIA et al. (2007). However, in this study the cancer-specific survival was not related with comorbidity. This is in contrast with a study of PICIRRILLO and COSTAS (2004), who showed a significant correlation between developing recurrence and increasing levels of comorbidity. In both studies the Adult Comorbidity Evaluation-27 (ACE)-27 index, which is a modification of the Kaplan–Feinstein index, was measured (KAPLAN and FEINSTEIN 1974). In recent years the ACE-27 has become a common method of scoring comorbidity. The ACE-27 adds several important comorbid conditions such as AIDS and diabetes mellitus (PICCIRILLO and COSTAS 2004). The ACE-27 is a validated 27-item comorbidity item, and grades specific comorbid conditions into one of four levels of comorbidity: none (0), mild (1), moderate (2), or severe (3). Besides, for overall survival and possibly disease-free survival, comorbidity is an important predictor of major complications in head and neck surgery (FERRIER et al. 2005), especially for grade 2 and 3. TERELL et al. (2004) studied the impact of comobidity on QOL for head and neck cancer. The presence of a feeding tube had the most negative impact on QOL, followed by comorbidity. Grade 2 and 3 comorbidities were associated with impaired general health, physical, emotional, and social functioning, vitality and pain, conform results of a prospective study of BORGGREVEN et al. (2007), in patients with cancer of the oral cavity and oropharynx. The NWHHT studied the role of comorbity in salivary (major and minor) gland cancer, since comorbidity will influence QOL (TERHAARD et al. 2008). The prevalence and the prognostic importance of comorbidity (ACE-27) were evaluated in a group of 613 patients. The number of cases with ACE-27 grade 0, 1, 2, and 3, was 64, 19, 12, and 5%, respectively. The type of treatment performed was influenced by ACE-27

comorbidity in case of grade 3 only. Comorbidity was associated with overall survival, but not with disease-free survival. For all histological subtypes distribution of ACE-27 was equal, except for squamous cell carcinoma. Two thirds of patients with squamous cell carcinoma of the major salivary gland (5% of the cases) had an ACE-27 grade 1–3, compared with one-third in all other cases. It seems that patients with salivary gland cancer have significantly less comorbidity, compared with that of other head and neck cancer patients (see Table 7.2), except for squamous cell cancer of the major salivary glands. Quality of life data were not available in this study. However, owing to its low incidence it seems likely that comorbidity plays a less important role in salivary gland cancer compared with other head and neck cancer cases.

7.4.2
Facial Nerve Function

Impairment of the facial nerve function at diagnosis of a parotid gland cancer may vary between 12 and 35%. In the Dutch study partially impaired function was found in 14%, and complete paralysis was noted in 7% (TERHAARD et al. 2006). Independent high-risk factors of facial nerve dysfunction are tumors originating from the medial lobe, N-stage, pain, age, and perineural invasion (VANDER POORTEN et al. 1999; TERHAARD et al. 2006; BRON and O'BRIEN 1997). The RR on facial nerve dysfunction for medial tumors was 8.4, compared with lateral tumors (TERHAARD et al. 2006). Pretreatment facial nerve dysfunction was an independent prognostic factor for neck node recurrence and disease-free survival, with an RR of 4.8 for complete paralysis compared with normal function (TERHAARD et al. 2006). As is shown in this study, for patients with pretreatment intact or partially impaired facial nerve function, conservation of the facial nerve, if combined with postoperative radiotherapy, did not result in increased local recurrence rates when compared with sacrifice of the facial nerve (Table 7.3) (TERHAARD et al. 2006). In other words, aggressive surgery does not improve disease-free survival, as shown by others (CARINCI et al. 2001; MAGNANO et al. 1999). Nerve grafting is used in a minority of cases (KERREBIJN and FREEMAN 1988). Recovery after facial nerve reconstruction may be disappointing (BRON and O'BRIEN 1997). Radiotherapy does not negatively influence facial nerve function after reconstruction (BROWN et al. 2000; REDDY et al. 1999). Therefore,

Table 7.2. Comparison between comorbidity (*ACE* adult comorbidity evaluation) in salivary gland carcinoma and head- and neck cancer (From TERHAARD et al. 2008)

Study	Types of tumors	n	ACE = 0 (%)	ACE = 1 (%)	ACE = 2 (%)	ACE $\geq$ 2 (%)	ACE = 3 (%)	χ^{2a}
FERRIER et al. (2005)	HNSCC; sinus, lip, oral cavity, nasopharynx, oropharynx, hypopharynx, and larynx.	117	48 (Sanabria et al. 2007)	35 (29.9)	–	34 (29.1)	–	22.6[b]
BORGGREVEN et al. (2007)	HNSCC; oral cavity, oropharynx	100	17 (17)	36 (36)	34 (34)	–	13 (13)	83.4[b]
ROGERS	HNSCC; hypopharynx, larynx, oropharynx	157	74 (47)	57 (36)	–	26 (17)	–	21.6[b]
SANABRIA et al. (2007)	HNSCC; nasopharynx, nose/paranasal, hypo- and oropharynx, larynx and oral cavity	309	77 (25)	141 (46)	48 (15)	–	43 (14)	136.9[b]
PICCIRILLO and COSTAS (2004)	HNSCC; lip, oral cavity, nasopharynx, oropharynx, hypopharynx, larynx and thyroid gland	341	188 (55)	82 (24)	53 (16)	–	18 (5)	8.0[b]
CHRIS TERHAARD (2009)	Salivary glands	613	394 (64)	119 (19)	71 (12)	–	29 (5)	

[a]Test statistic using the Kruskal-Wallis test (comparing the study given with this paper).
[b]p-value < 0.05

nerve-sparing surgery with postoperative radiotherapy is the preferable treatment (SPIRO and SPIRO 2003). Facial nerve palsy, and as a consequence disfigurement, may have important impact on QOL. However, only few papers have been published on this subject. Objective facial nerve dysfunction and disfigurement did not reliably reflect the patients' own perceptions in a study ($n = 23$) by KWOK et al. (2002). However, this retrospective study may have been biased by availability. In another retrospective study, in 49 patients QOL was evaluated after facial nerve repair (39% of the patients were treated for parotid cancer), and compared with a cohort of the normal population (GUNTINAS-LICHIUS et al. 2007). Despite surgical nerve repair, significant lower scores were noted for social functioning, emotional role, general mental health, and vitality. Avoidance of soiling their clothes while drinking and eye problems were both experienced by the patients in 69%. The patient-perceived facial function correlated significantly with the QOL scores (GUNTINAS-LICHIUS et al. 2007). A significant reduction in social functioning in patients with facial nerve paralysis was also shown in a cross-sectional study by COULSON et al. (2002). On the basis of these studies, albeit retrospective, sparing the facial nerve in parotid gland cancer is of utmost importance for the QOL of the patient.

Table 7.3. Correlation between facial nerve function *before* treatment, conservation or sacrificing the facial nerve during operation and percentage local recurrence (From TERHAARD et al. (2006))

Surgery alone	N VII conservation	N VII sacrificed
Pretreatment intact N VII	6/28 = 21%	1/2
partially impaired	3/3	2/3
complete paralysis	–	–
Surgery + postoperative RT		
Pre-treatment intact N VII	11/180 = 6%	3/22 = 14%
partially impaired	1/12 = 8%	3/21 = 14%
complete paralysis	0/1	1/11 = 9%

7.4.3
Hearing Loss

In the acute phase of radiotherapy, secretory otitis media, caused by edema around the Eustachian tube, is the main, although mostly reversible, cause of hearing loss. As a late consequence of radiotherapy, conductive (external auditory canal stenosis, chronic otitis media, and/ or Eustachian tube pathology), sensorineural, or mixed hearing loss may be seen (BHIDE et al. 2006). Sensorineural hearing loss (SNHL) may be caused by changes in the cochlea and/or retrocochlear damage (auditory nerve/auditory brain stem). The etiology may be vascular, leading to degeneration and atrophy of the cochlea structures, cartilage necrosis, and mastoiditis, and/or focal brain necrosis (JERECZEK-FOSSA et al. 2003). Hearing loss is mainly seen after (chemo) radiotherapy for nasopharyngeal or parotid carcinoma. The definition of relevant hearing loss may differ between 10 and 15 dB or ≥20 dB between the irradiated and nonirradiated ear for minimal two frequencies (JERECZEK-FOSSA et al. 2003; ANTEUNIS et al. 1994; CHEN et al. 2006). Hearing loss is mostly seen in the higher frequencies (4 kHz) (ANTEUNIS et al. 1994; Low et al. 2006; RAAIJMAKERS and ENGELEN 2002). In a prospective study in patients receiving postoperative radiotherapy for parotid tumors, clinically relevant hearing loss was seen in 8 of 18 patients, affecting QOL in 6 of 18 (ANTEUNIS et al. 1994). The incidence of SNHL depends not only on the dose to the cochlea, but also on (increasing) age and (decreasing) pretherapeutic hearing level (HONORÉ et al. 2002). In a randomized study the possible synergistic ototoxicity of cisplatin and radiotherapy in nasopharyngeal cancer was studied. Especially for the threshold at 4 kHz, cisplatin and radiotherapy resulted in significant higher SNHL compared with radiation alone (Low et al. 2006). Several (possible) thresholds in cochlear dose–response have been published, with a dose range between 40 and 60 Gy (CHEN et al. 2006; HONORÉ et al. 2002; CHEN et al. 1999; PAN et al. 2005). HONORÉ et al. (2002) presented a nomogram for the estimation of a 15% risk of SNHL based on age, pretherapeutic hearing loss, and dose to the cochlea. This nomogram may be used for dose constraints in treatment planning.

7.4.4
Xerostomia

Partial xerostomia may be seen after radiotherapy for parotid or submandibular cancer. Complete dryness may result from radiotherapy of the minor salivary gland tumors of the pharynx, and less frequently the oral cavity. Xerostomia results in impaired QOL and oral discomfort (DIRIX et al. 2006). Objective methods, such as salivary flow measurements, and/or subjective observer-based or patient self-reported toxicity scoring questionnaires are used to quantify xerostomia. Based on salivary flow measurements, a parotid flow of 25% or less after radiotherapy relative to preradiotherapy is defined as a complication. Using flow measurements, a steep parotid complication dose–response curve was found by EISBRUCH et al. (1999), with a threshold of 26 Gy. However, less steep dose–response curves have been published, with a 50% complications risk 1 year after radiotherapy for a mean parotid dose of 39 Gy, and ±10% for a dose of 26 Gy (ROESINK et al. 2001). A mean parotid dose of 26 Gy has been used in several studies, using intensity-modulated radiotherapy IMRT to reduce mean parotid dose. Parotid flow measurements and subjective patient scores were analyzed in a prospective randomized study for patients with nasopharyngeal cancer. IMRT was compared with conventional radiotherapy (KAM et al. 2007). Parotid flow was significantly higher after IMRT. However, subjective xerostomia patient scores did not improve significantly. Similar findings were found in a study in Utrecht, comparing IMRT with conventional radiotherapy in oropharyngeal cancer (BRAAM et al. 2006). In both studies, the dose to both submandibular glands was >50 Gy. At daytime most saliva is produced by the parotid glands, at night by the submandibular glands. The EORTC questionnaire does not distinguish xerostomia at night or daytime. In 66 patients treated with IMRT in Utrecht for oropharyngeal cancer, a more detailed xerostomia questionnaire was used. Sparing both parotid glands resulted in significant lower scores for dry mouth at daytime, but not at night (Fig. 7.3). So, for prevention of xerostomia at night sparing of at least one submandibular gland is advisable. A threshold of 40 Gy has been published for a complication of submandibular flow (MURDOCH-KINCH et al. 2008). Therefore, for radiotherapy of salivary gland tumors, dose constraints for the noninvolved major salivary glands should be 26 Gy for the parotid gland, and 40 Gy for the submandibular gland. Primary and postoperative radiotherapy for parotid gland tumors is generally unilateral; sparing the ipsilateral submandibular gland in N0 cases should be aimed for. To prevent xerostomia at night, in submandibular cancer the contralateral submandibular gland should be spared.

7.4.5
Mastoiditis/Temporal Bone Osteoradionecrosis

This is an unusual complication after radiotherapy; however, it may occur many years after radiotherapy. As a late complication, meningitis, temporal lobe or

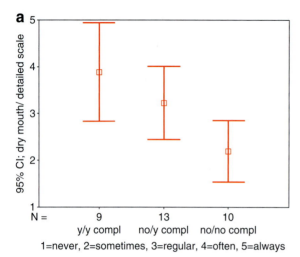

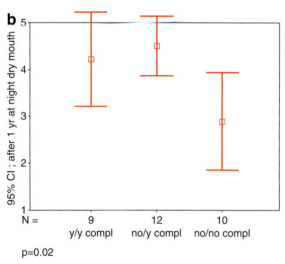

Fig. 7.3. IMRT for oropharyngeal cancer (*n* = 66). Data from Utrecht. Submandibular dose ≥50/2 Gy/fraction; mean xerostomia score (1 = none, 5 = always); *compl.* complication; parotid gland: <25% flow 1 year after RT; y/y: two parotid glands complication; y/n: one parotid gland complication; n/n: both parotid glands no complication; (**a**) dry mouth at daytime; (**b**) dry mouth at night

cerebellar abscess, and cranial neuropathies may occur (GUIDA et al. 1990). Localized necrosis may be treated conservatively; however, more severe temporal bone necrosis requires surgical intervention (PATHAK and BRYCE 2000). Radiation otomastoiditis may be demonstrated on T2-weighted MR examination as a high-signal intensity area. The incidence of radiation otomastoiditis is increased after 50 Gy (NISHIMURA et al. 1997). So, the part of the temporal bone receiving 50 Gy or more should be as small as possible (NISHIMURA et al. 1997).

7.5
Radiation Techniques to Reduce the Complication Risks

Besides photon and/or electron therapy, neutron therapy is used for primary treatment of salivary gland cancer. Although in a prospective study neutron therapy compared with photon resulted in superior locoregional control rates, overall survival was equal (LARAMORE et al. 1993). In a study of Heidelberg, combination of neutrons with photons resulted in decreased severe late toxicity compared with neutrons only. However, for advanced, inoperable, recurrent and incompletely resected adenoid cystic carcinoma, 5-year local control was 30%, comparable to photons only, and lower than with neutrons only (75%); overall survival was equal (HUBER et al. 2001). In a study of Douglas et al., the use of a gamma knife stereotactic radiosurgical boost after primary neutron therapy for salivary gland tumors invading the base of skull resulted in a local control of 7 of 8. However, follow-up was short (DOUGLAS et al. 2004). Owing to its increased severe late toxicity and sparse availability, neutrons are not commonly used in salivary gland cancer. Other options, besides photons only, are the use of a combination of carbon ions or protons with photons. These techniques have been tested to improve the poor results (0–30% local control) with photons only in advanced adenoid cystic tumors invading the base of skull. Three-year local control was 65% after a combination of carbon ions with photons in a series of 16 patients (SCHULZ-ERTNER et al. 2003). In a comparable selection of 23 patients, combined photon/proton treatment resulted in 93% 5-year local control, with acceptable toxicity (POMMIER et al. 2006). However, larger and multi-institutional studies with a long follow-up are necessary to rate these expensive techniques at their true value.

In the vast majority of patients treated with radiotherapy for salivary gland tumors photon beam therapy will be used. For tumors of the parotid gland the clinical target volume includes the entire parotid gland, including the parapharyngeal space and infratemporal fossa (GARDEN et al. 1997; NUTTING et al. 2001). A bolus on the scar is only advised in case of a very superficial tumor or skin invasion (KIRKBRIDE et al. 2001). In case of named perineural invasion, the nerve should be treated up to the base of skull (GARDEN et al. 1995). In case of a clinical N0 neck, the indication for elective treatment of the neck nodes may be based on site, histology, and T-stage (Spiro 1986). For example, in submandibular cancer, except for T1 acinic and adenoid cystic carcinoma, elective treatment is recommended in all cases (Spiro 1986).

Planning studies have been performed to compare conventional, three-dimensional conformal (3DCRT), and intensity-modulated techniques (IMRT) for the treatment of parotid cancer (Nutting et al. 2001; Bragg et al. 2002; Lamers-Kuijper et al. 2007). Based on a study on dose distributions and dose–volume histograms, optimal conventional techniques for unilateral treatment of parotid tumors are an ipsilateral wedge-pair technique, a three-field wedged AP/PA and lateral portal technique, or a mixed electron-photon beam (Yaparpalvi et al. 1998). However, with 3DCRT a reduction in dose to the critical normal tissues was demonstrated in a planning study by Nutting et al. (2001). A four-field class solution IMRT technique produced a further reduction in the dose to the cochlea and oral cavity (Nutting et al. 2001). Bragg et al. (2002) proposed a five-field IMRT. In this planning study, IMRT resulted in higher uncomplicated tumor control probability compared with 3DCRT (Bragg et al. 2002). A four-beam IMRT technique was superior to a wedge pair technique for sparing the auditory system and the oral cavity in a retrospective planning study of 20 patients with parotid gland tumors, shown by Lamers-Kuijper et al. (2007). However, IMRT resulted in a small increase in dose inhomogeneity compared with the conventional technique (Lamers-Kuijper et al. 2007). Helical tomotherapy treatment for parotid gland tumors leads to comparable sparing of normal structures, with slightly better target dose homogeneity, compared with IMRT (Lee et al. 2008).

Three patients treated in Utrecht for salivary gland tumors are discussed to demonstrate the value of IMRT. All have been treated with 6 MV photons on a cone beam accelerator with micro-leaves, with a 3-mm margin between the clinical target volume and PTV. The first patient is an 11-year-old boy, who had an enucleation of a pleomorphic adenoma of 2.5 × 2 cm^2, incomplete resection, 2 years before referral. A wait and see policy was followed. Two years later a recurrence was seen, and a parotidectomy was performed. This surgery was incomplete, and postoperative radiotherapy was advised. A conventional four-field wedge technique was compared with a unilateral IMRT technique with five fields and 76 segments. The dose applied to the PTV was 50 Gy in 25 fractions. The number of monitor units per fraction, important for the risk of radiation-induced tumors, was 468 for IMRT, compared with 682 for the wedge technique. The mean dose to the cochlea, the jaw, the mastoid, and right submandibular gland was 43, 32, 31, and 47% lower for IMRT compared with conventional, respectively (see Fig. 7.4a, b). The dose homogeneity improved with IMRT.

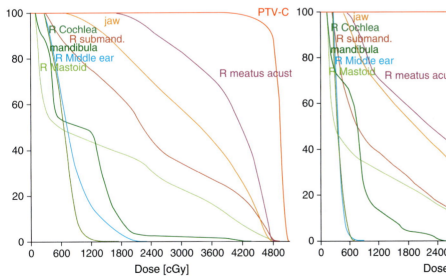

Fig. 7.4. Case 1: Recurrent pleomorphic adenoma; dose–volume histogram (DVH): (**a**) four-field conventional radiotherapy, (**b**) five-field inverse IMRT; *PTV-C* PTV-CTV; *submand* submandibular gland; *R* right = ipsilateral; *meatus acust. ext.* meatus acusticus externus

The second patient is a 57-year-old man with a poorly differentiated acinic cell carcinoma, $pT_{4a} pN_1$ (no extranodal spread), incompletely resected parotid carcinoma. In the postoperative setting a five-field IMRT technique was used, with 65 segments. The dose applied to the PTV was 66 Gy in 33 fractions; the dose for level Ib-V was 50 Gy in 25 fractions. In Fig. 7.5 the beam configurations are shown for a conventional and the used IMRT technique.

In Table 7.4, a comparison between the doses for different structures using a conventional or IMRT technique is given.

The third patient is a 23-year-old woman with a low-grade myoepithelial carcinoma of the left tonsil and anterior pillar. A tonsillectomy was performed. The tumor was re-excised with a close margin. Postoperative radiotherapy was administered with a dose of 60 Gy in 30 fractions; the neck nodes were not treated. A five-field IMRT-technique with 71 segments was used. The dose distribution for a three-dimensional conformal and IMRT technique is shown in Fig. 7.6 doses to the ipsilateral parotid gland, the contralateral submandibular gland, and the maximum dose to the brain were 42.4, 30.6, and 41.8 vs. 27.6, 21.9, and 31.1 for conventional vs. IMRT, respectively.

7.6
Conclusion

Side effects after radiotherapy for salivary gland tumors, including hearing loss, mastoiditis, and xerostomia, may influence QOL. New radiotherapy techniques, such as intensity-modulated radiotherapy, may reduce the risk on side effects, and so, probably improve QOL.

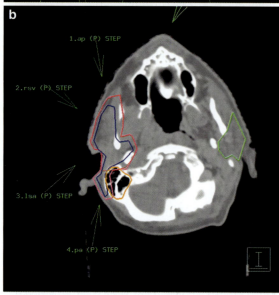

Fig. 7.5. Beam, set-up, Patient 2, (a) three-field wedge pair technique, (b) five-field IMRT

Table 7.4. Patient 2: comparison between mean and maximum dose for postoperative radiotherapy, 66 Gy, for a $pT_{4a} pN_1$ parotid cancer, comparing three-field conventional with five-field IMRT

	3D conventional	IMRT
PTV: mean/max (Gy)	65.6/68.2	66.9/69.9
Ipsilat. cochlea: mean/max (Gy)	23.4/44.6	18.9/35.2
Ipsilat. mastoid: mean/max (Gy)	53.7/66.5	48.8/68.7
Contralat. subm: mean/max (Gy)	9.2/10.4	4.0/6.8
Contralat. parotid: mean/max (Gy)	7.6/8.9	2.8/7.5
Ipsilat. eye: mean/max (Gy)	6.3/19.0	3.9/11.6

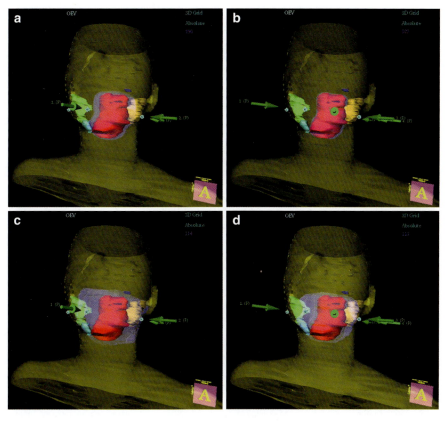

Fig. 7.6. Patient 3: Low grade myoepithelial carcinoma of the oropharynx, close resection margin, postoperative radiotherapy (60 Gy); (**a** and **c**) Conventional technique; (**b** and **d**) IMRT; (**a** and **b**) 95% of 60 Gy isodose; (**c** and **d**) *blue*: 40 Gy isodose; *pink* = PTV of CTV; *light blue* = submandibular gland; *green* = contralateral parotid gland; *yellow* = ipsilateral parotid gland

References

Anteunis LJC, Wanders SL, Hendriks JJT et al. (1994) A prospective longitudinal study on radiation-induced hearing loss. Am J Surg 168:408–411

Beal KP, Singh B, Kraus D et al. (2003) Radiation-induced salivary gland tumors: a report of 18 cases and a review of the literature. Cancer J 9:467–471

Beckhardt RN, Weber RS, Zane R et al. (1995) Minor salivary gland tumors of the palate: clinical and pathologic correlates of outcome. Laryngoscope 105:1155–1160

Bhattacharyya N (2004) Survival and prognosis for cancer of the submandibular gland. J Oral Maxillofac Surg 62:427–430

Bhattacharyya N, Fried MP (2005) Determinants of survival in parotid gland carcinoma: a population-based study. Am J Otolaryngol-Head Neck Med Surg 26:39–44

Bhide SA, Harrington KJ, Nutting CM (2006) Otological toxicity after postoperative radiotherapy for parotid tumours. Clinical Oncol 19:77–82

Borggreven PA, Verdonck-de Leeuw IM, Muller MJ et al. (2007) Quality of life and functional status in patients with cancer of the oral cavity and oropharynx: pre-treatment values of a prospective study. Eur Arch Otorhinolaryngol 264:651–657

Braam PM, Terhaard CH, Roesink JM et al. (2006) Intensity-modulated radiotherapy significantly reduces xerostomia compared with conventional radiotherapy. Int J Radiat Oncol Biol Phys 66:975–980

Bragg CM, Conway J, Robinson MH (2002) The role of intensity-modulated radiotherapy in the treatment of parotid tumors. Int J Radiat Oncol Biol Phys 52:729–738

Bron LP, O'Brien CJ (1997) Facial nerve function after parotidectomy. Arch Otolaryngol Head Neck Surg 123(10):1091–1096

Brown PD, Eshleman JS, Foote RL et al. (2000) An analysis of facial nerve function in irradiated and unirradiated facial nerve grafts. Int J Radiat Oncol Biol Phys 48(3):737–743

Carinci F, Farina A, Pelucchi S et al. (2001) Parotid gland carcinoma: 1987–1997 UICC T classifications compared for prognostic accuracy at 5 years. Eur Arch Otorhinolaryngol 258:150–154

Carrillo JF, Vazquez R, Ramirez-Ortega M et al. (2007) Multivariate prediction of the probability of recurrence in patients with carcinoma of the parotid gland. Cancer 109:2043–2051

Chen AM, Bucci MK, Quivey JM et al. (2006) Long-term outcome of patients treated by radiation therapy alone for salivary gland carcinomas. Int J Radiation Oncology Biol Phys 67:1044–1050

Chen AM, Granchi PJ, Garcia J et al. (2007) Local-regional recurrence after surgery without postoperative irradiation for carcinomas of the major salivary glands: implications for adjuvant therapy. Int J Radiat Oncol Biol Phys 67:982–987

Chen WC, Jackson A, Budnick AS et al. (2006) Sensorineural hearing loss in combined modality treatment of nasopharyngeal carcinoma. Cancer 106:820–829

Chen W-C, Liao C-T, Tsai H-C et al. (1999) Radiation-induced hearing impairment in patients treated for malignant parotid tumor. Ann Rhinol Laryngol 108:1159–1164

Coulson S, O'Dwyer NJ, Adams RG et al. (2002) Expression of emotion and quality of life after facial nerve paralysis. Otol Neurotol 25:1014–1019 de Graeff A, Leeuw JRJ de, Ros, WJG et al. (2000) Pretreatment factors predicting quality of life after treatment for head and neck cancer. Head Neck 22:398–407

Derks W, de Leeuw JR, Hordijk GJ et al. (2005) Reasons for non-standard treatment in elderly patients with advanced head and neck cancer. Eur Arch Otorhinolaryngol 262(1):21–26

Dirix P, Nuyts S, Van den Bogaert W (2006) Radiation-induced xerostomia in patients with head and neck cancer. Cancer 107:2525–2534

Douglas JG, Silbergeld DL, Laramore GE (2004) Gamma Knife stereotactic radiosurgical boost for patients treated primarily with neutron radiotherapy for salivary gland neoplasms. Stereotact Funct Neurosurg 82:84–89

Eisbruch A, Ten Haken RK, Kim HM et al. (1999) Dose, volume, and function relationships in parotid salivary glands following conformal and intensity-modulated irradiation of head and neck cancer. Int J Radiat Oncol Biol Phys 45:577–587

Ferrier MB, Spuesens EB, Le Cessie S et al. (2005) Comorbidity as a major risk factor for mortality and complications in head and neck surgery. Arch Otolaryngol Head Neck Surg 131:27–32

Gallo O, Franchi A, Bianchi S et al. (1995) P53 oncoprotein expression in parotid gland carcinoma is associated with clinical outcome. Cancer 75:2037–2044

Garden AS, el-Naggar AK, Morrison WH et al. (1997) Postoperative radiotherapy for malignant tumors of the parotid gland. Int J Radiat Oncol Biol Phys 37:79–85

Garden AS, Weber RS, Ang KK et al. (1994) Postoperative radiation therapy for malignant tumors of minor salivary glands. Outcome and patterns of failure. Cancer 73:2563–2569

Garden AS, Weber RS, Morrison WH et al. (1995) The influence of positive margins and nerve invasion in adenoid cystic carcinoma of the head and neck treated with surgery and radiation. Int J Radiat Oncol Biol Phys 32:619–626

Guida RA, Finn DG, Buchalter IH et al. (1990) Radiation injury to the temporal bone. Am J Otol 11:6–11

Guntinas-Lichius O, Straesser A, Streppel M (2007) Quality of life after facial nerve repair. Laryngoscope 117:421–426

Honoré HB, Bentzen SM, Moller K et al. (2002) Sensori-neural hearing loss after radiotherapy for nasopharyngeal carcinoma: individualized risk estimation. Radioth Oncol 65:9–16

Huber PE, Debus J, Latz D et al. (2001) Radiotherapy for advanced adenoid cystic carcinoma: neutrons, photons or mixed beam? Radiother Oncol 59:161–167

Jaehne M, Roeser K, Jaekel T et al. (2005) Clinical and immuno-histologic typing of salivary duct carcinoma. A report of 50 cases. Cancer 103:2526–2533

Jereczek-Fossa BA, Zarowski A, Milani F et al. (2003) Radiotherapy-induced ear toxicity. Cancer Treat Rev 29:417–430

Jones AS, Beasley NJP, Houghton DJ et al. (1998) Tumours of the minor salivary glands. Clin Otolaryngol 23:27–33

Kam MK, Leung SF, Zee B et al. (2007) Prospective randomized study of intensity-modulated radiotherapy on salivary gland function in early-stage nasopharyngeal carcinoma patients. J Clin Oncol 25:4873–4879

Kaplan MH, Feinstein AR (1974) The importance of classifying initial co-morbidity in evaluating the outcome of diabetes mellitus. J Chronic Dis 27(7–8):387–404

Kerrebijn JD, Freeman JL (1988) Facial nerve reconstruction: outcome and failures. J Otolaryngol 27(4):183–186

Kirkbride P, Liu FF, O'Sullivan B et al. (2001) Outcome of curative management of malignant tumors of the parotid gland. J Otolaryngol 30:271–279

Koul R, Dubey A, Butler J et al. (2007) Prognostic factors depicting disease-specific survival in parotid-gland tumors. Int J Radiat Oncol Biol Phys 68:714–718

Kwok HCK, Morton R, Chaplin JM et al. (2002) Quality of life after parotid and temporal bone surgery for cancer. Laryngoscope 112:820–833

Lamers-Kuijper E, Schwarz M, Rasch C et al. (2007) Intensity-modulated vs. conventional radiotherapy of parotid gland tumors: potential impact on hearing loss. Med Dosim 32:237–245

Laramore GE, Krall JM, Griffin TW et al. (1993) Neutron versus photon irradiation for unresectable salivary gland tumors: final report of an RTOG-MRC randomized clinical trial. Int J Radiat Oncol Biol Phys 235–240

Lee TK, Rosen II, Gibbons JP et al. (2008) Helical tomotherapy for parotid gland tumors. Int J Radiat Oncol Biol Phys 70:883–891

Lim JJ, Kang S, Lee MR et al. (2003) Expression of vascular endothelial growth factor in salivary gland carcinomas and its relation to p53, Ki-67 and prognosis. J Oral Pathol Med 32:552–561

Lopes MA, Santos GC, Kowalski LP (1998) Multivariate survival analysis of 128 cases of oral cavity minor salivary gland carcinomas. Head Neck 20:699–706

Low WK, Toh ST, Wee J et al. (2006) Sensorineural hearing loss after radiotherapy and chemoradiotherapy: a single, blinded, randomized study. J Clin Oncol 24:1904–1909

Luukkaa H, Klemi P, Hirsimali P et al. (2008) Matrix metalloproteinase (MMP)-1, -9, and -13 as prognostic factors in salivary gland cancer. Acta Oto-Laryngologica 128: 482–490

Magnano M, Gervasio CF, Cravero L et al. (1999) Treatment of malignant neoplasms of the parotid gland. Otolaryngol Head Neck Surg 121(5):627–632

Mendenhall WM, Morris CG, Amdur RJ et al. (2005) Radiotherapy alone or combined with surgery for salivary gland carcinoma. Cancer 103:2544–2550

Murdoch-Kinch CA, Kim HM, Vineberg KA et al. (2008) Dose-effect relationships for the submandibular salivary glands and implications for their sparing by intensity modulated radiotherapy. Int J Radiat Oncol Biol Phys 72(2):373–82

Nishimura R, Baba Y, Murakimi R et al. (1997) MR evaluation of radiation otomastoiditis. Int J Radiat Oncol Biol Phys 39:155–160

North CA, Lee DJ, Piantadosi S et al. (1990) Carcinoma of the major salivary glands treated by surgery or surgery plus postoperative radiotherapy. Int J Radiat Oncol Biol Phys 18:1319–1326

Nutting CM, Rowbottom CG, Cosgrove VP et al. (2001) Optimisation of radiotherapy for carcinoma of the parotid gland: a comparison of conventional, three-dimensional conformal, and intensity-modulated techniques. Radiother Oncol 60:163–172

Pan CC, Eisbruch A, Lee SJ et al. (2005) Prospective study of inner ear radiation dose and hearing loss in head-and-neck cancer patients. Int J Radiat Oncol Biol Phys 61:1393–1402

Parsons JT, Mendenhall WM, Stringer SP et al. (1996) Management of minor salivary gland carcinomas. Int J Radiat Oncol Biol Phys 35:443–454

Pathak I, Bryce G (2000) Temporal bone necrosis: diagnosis, classification, and management. Otolaryngol Head Neck Surg 123:252–257

Piccirillo JF, Costas I (2004) The impact of comorbidity on outcomes. ORL 66:180–185

Pohar S, Gay H, Rosenbaum P et al. (2005) Malignant parotid tumors: presentation, clinical/pathologic prognostic factors, and treatment outcomes. Int J Radiat Oncol Biol Phys 61:112–118

Pommier P, Liebsch NJ, Deschler DG et al. (2006) Proton beam radiation therapy for skull base adenoid cystic carcinoma. Arch Otolaryngol Head Neck Surg 132:1242–1249

Poulsen MG, Pratt GR, Kynaston B et al. (1992) Prognostic variables in malignant epithelial tumors of the parotid. Int J Radiat Oncol Biol Phys 23:327–330

Press MF, Pike MC, Hung G et al. (1994) Amplification and overexpression of HER-2/neu in carcinomas of the salivary gland: correlation with poor prognosis. Cancer Res 54:5675–5682

Raaijmakers E, Engelen AM (2002) Is sensorineural hearing loss a possible side effect of nasopharyngeal and parotid irradiation? A systematic review of the literature. Radioth Oncol 65:1–7

Reddy PG, Arden RL, Mathog RH (1999) Facial nerve rehabilitation after radical parotidectomy. Laryngoscope 109(6):894–899

Régis de Brito Santos I, Kowalski LP, Cavalcante de Araujo V et al. (2001) Multivariate analysis of risk factors for neck metastases in surgically treated parotid carcinoma. Arch Otolaryngol Head Neck Surg 127:46–60

Roesink J, Moerland M, Battermann J et al. (2001) Quantative dose-volume response analysis of changes in parotid gland function after radiotherapy in the head-and-neck region. Int J Radiat Oncol Biol Phys 51:938–946

Rogers SN, Aziz A, Lowe D et al. (2006) Feasibility study of the retrospective use of the Adult Comorbidity Evaluation index (ACE-27) in patients with cancer of the head and neck who had radiotherapy. Br J Oral Maxillofac Surg 44(4):283–8

Sanabria A, Carvalho AL, Vartanian JG et al. (2007) Comorbidity is a prognostic factor in elderly patients with head and neck cancer. Ann Surg Oncol 14(4):1449–1457

Schramm VL, Imola MJ (2001) Management of nasopharyngeal salivary gland malignancy. Laryngoscope 111: 1533–1544

Schulz-Ertner D, Nikoghosyan A, Jäkel et al. (2003) Feasibility and toxicity of combined photon and carbon ion radiotherapy for locally advanced adenoid cystic carcinomas. Int J Radiat Oncol Biol Phys 56:391–398

Schwarz S, Ettl T, Kleinsasser N et al. (2008) Loss of Maspin expression is a negative prognostic factor in common salivary gland tumors. Oral Oncol 44:563–570

Spiro RH (1986) Salivary neoplasms: overview of a 35-year experience with 2,807 patients. Head Neck Surg 8:177–184

Spiro RH, Armstrong J, Harrison L et al. (1989) Carcinoma of major salivary glands. Arch Otolaryngol Head Neck Surg 115:316–321

Spiro JD, Spiro RH (2003) Cancer of the parotid gland: role of the 7th nerve preservation. World J Surg 27(7):863–867

Storey MR, Garden AS, Morrison WH et al. (2001) Postoperative radiotherapy for malignant tumors of the submandibular gland. Int J Radiat Oncol Biol Phys 51:952–958

Sun EC, Curtis R, Melbye M et al. (1999) Salivary gland cancer in the United States. Cancer Epidemiol Biomark Prev 8:1095–1100

Swanson GM, Burns PB (1997) Cancers of the salivary gland: workplace risk among women and men. Ann Epidemiol 7:639–374

Terell JE, Ronis DL, Fowler KE et al. (2004) Clinical predictors of quality of life in patients with head and neck cancer. Arch Otolaryngol Head Neck Surg 130:401–408

Terhaard C, Lubsen H, Tan B et al. (2006) Facial nerve function in carcinoma of the parotid gland. Eur J Cancer 42(16): 2744–2750

Terhaard CHJ, Lubsen H, Rasch CRN et al. (2005) The role of radiotherapy in the treatment of malignant salivary gland tumours. Int J Radiat Oncol Biol Phys 61(1):103–111

Terhaard CHJ, Lubsen H, Van der Tweel et al. (2004) Salivary gland carcinoma: independent prognostic factors for locoregional control, distant metastases, and overall survival: results of the Dutch Head and Neck Oncology Cooperative Group. Head Neck 26:681–693

Terhaard CHJ, van der Schroeff MP, Schie K van et al. (2008) Prognostic role of comorbidity in salivary gland carcinoma. Cancer 113:1572–1576

Therkildsen MH, Christensen M, Andersen LJ et al. (1998) Salivary gland carcinomas–prognostic factors. Acta Oncol 37:701–713

Vander Poorten V, Balm AJ, Hilgers FJ et al. (1999) The development of a prognostic score for patients with parotid carcinoma. Cancer 85(9):2057–2067

Vander Poorten VLM, Hart AAM, Van der Laan BFAM et al. (2003) Prognostic index for patients with parotid carcinoma. External validation using the nationwide 1985–1994 Dutch Head and Neck Oncology Cooperative Group Database. Cancer 97:1453–1463

Yaparpalvi R, Fontenla DP, Tyerech SK et al. (1998) Parotid gland tumors: a comparison of postoperative radiotherapy techniques using three dimensional (3D) dose distributions and dose-volume histograms (DVHS). Int J Radiat Oncol Biol Phys 40:43–49

Head and Neck Sarcomas and Lymphomas

8

Brian O'Sullivan, Jonathan Irish, and Richard Tsang

CONTENTS

8.1	**Introduction**	*104*
8.2	**Evaluation and Diagnosis**	*104*
8.2.1	Sarcoma	*104*
8.2.2	Lymphoma	*105*

8.3 **Treatment of Sarcoma** *106*
8.3.1 Surgery of Sarcoma *106*
8.3.1.1 Soft Tissue Sarcoma *106*
8.3.1.2 Osteosarcoma and Chondrosarcoma *107*
8.3.2 Radiotherapy of Sarcoma *108*
8.3.2.1 Soft Tissue Sarcoma *108*
8.3.2.2 Bone Sarcomas *108*
8.3.2.3 Scheduling of Radiotherapy
(Preoperative vs. Postoperative
Radiotherapy) *109*
8.3.2.4 Radiation Target Volumes
and Dose-Fractionation *109*
8.3.2.5 High Precision Radiotherapy
(Particle Beam and IMRT) *110*
8.3.2.6 Radiotherapy Alone *111*
8.3.3 Adjuvant Chemotherapy *111*
8.3.3.1 Soft Tissue Sarcoma *111*
8.3.3.2 Bone Sarcoma *112*
8.3.4 Targeted Approaches *112*

8.4 **Treatment of Lymphomas
of the Head and Neck** *112*
8.4.1 Indolent Lymphoma *112*
8.4.2 Aggressive Histology Lymphoma *113*

References *113*

Brian O'Sullivan, MD, FRCPC
Department of Radiation Oncology, Princess Margaret Hospital, University of Toronto, 610 University Avenue, Toronto, ON M5G 2M9, Canada
Jonathan Irish, MD, FRCSC
Department of Surgical Oncology, Princess Margaret Hospital, University of Toronto, 610 University Avenue, Toronto, Ontario M5G 2M9, Canada
Richard Tsang, MD, FRCPC
Department of Radiation Oncology, Princess Margaret Hospital, University of Toronto, 610 University Avenue, Toronto, Ontario M5G 2M9, Canada

KEY POINTS

- Head and neck (HN) sarcoma and lymphoma share similarities in being uncommon mesenchymal tumors where the goal of treatment should emphasize methods of achieving disease control while maximizing preservation of cosmesis and function.
- Cross-sectional imaging is best undertaken in sarcomas before any biopsy or intervention to avoid compromising the planning of appropriate management; in lymphomas this is also needed for local radiotherapy (RT) but should be especially remembered if systemic treatment is undertaken initially to facilitate subsequent RT planning.
- Pathological grading provides an important prognostic measure and has been incorporated into the staging system of sarcomas.
- Clear surgical margin resection with or without RT is almost exclusively the mainstay of management of HN sarcoma. The indication for adjuvant systemic treatments is generally based on the experience of sarcomas in more common anatomic sites elsewhere.
- HN bone sarcomas differ from soft tissue lesions in that RT is much less established as a component of treatment, but chemotherapy is usually indicated in osteosarcoma and the very rarely seen HN Ewing's tumor.
- In the combined RT and surgery approach to HN sarcoma, preoperative RT seems particularly suited, because of the smaller RT volumes and lower doses to critical anatomy where wide margins cannot be obtained.
- The management of non-Hodgkin's lymphoma (NHL) in the HN is primarily influenced by histology and the Ann Arbor stage.

- Optimal pathology interpretation of NHL involves immunophenotypic and sometimes molecular studies. Although surgical treatment for lymphoma is rarely required, open surgical approaches for tissue acquisition may be necessary.
- Stages I and II indolent lymphomas are treated with low to moderate dose involved-field RT with the expectation of a local control rate exceeding 95%, and long-term disease-free survival of 50–70%.
- Aggressive histology lymphomas presenting in early stage (I–II) is still associated with high risk for occult systemic disease and the use of anthracycline-based chemotherapy is required.

8.1

Introduction

Sarcoma and lymphoma are tumors of mesenchymal origin that comprise a contrasting subset of uncommon head and neck (HN) neoplasms. Lymphomas enjoy excellent response to chemotherapy and radiotherapy (RT) and almost never require surgery. In contrast, sarcomas almost always require surgery to achieve local control, and rarely develop regional metastases other than for some uncommon histological subtypes so that elective neck management is generally unnecessary.

Sarcomas comprise less than 1% of all HN cancers and their management follows principles extrapolated from other anatomic sites where the disease is more common (O'SULLIVAN et al. 2007). Surgery with or without RT is almost exclusively the mainstay of management. The indication for adjuvant systemic treatments relies for the most part on published meta-analyses for soft tissue sarcoma (STS) and some overviews for HN osteosarcoma.

HN lymphomas can present in lymph nodes or in extranodal organs. In virtually all cases a philosophy of functional preservation without resorting to ablative surgery should be followed. The need for chemotherapy and/or radiation therapy is not diminished following surgical excision of lymphoma. Advanced stages (stages III–IV) of lymphoma are treated primarily with chemotherapy and will not be further discussed. For stage I–II presentations in the HN area, the treatment approach involves radiation alone, or combined modality therapy (CMT) with chemotherapy followed by consolidation radiation, with curative intent. The description of management that follows later will address two broad categories, specifically indolent lesions and the contrasting group with aggressive histology lymphoma.

While dramatically contrasting in terms of management approaches, both HN sarcoma and lymphoma share similarities in that the goal of treatment should emphasize methods of achieving disease control while maximizing preservation of cosmesis and function. This philosophy will be maintained in the discussion that follows, although no formal quality of life or functional assessment studies specific to these HN tumors are available. Some illustrative cases will complement the discussion to demonstrate anatomic challenges that can be met with individualized approaches to the choice of RT and surgical techniques.

8.2

Evaluation and Diagnosis

8.2.1
Sarcoma

Local management of STS and bone sarcoma starts with imaging and physical examination to determine whether soft tissue lesions originate superficial or deep to the muscle investing fascia and whether bone tumors are intramedullary or have invaded into the extra-osseous compartment. Cross-sectional imaging is best undertaken before any biopsy or intervention to avoid compromising the planning of appropriate management since even needle tracts are potential sites of tumor contamination. Ideally the surgeon and radiation oncologist should be involved in planning the optimal biopsy route and be aware of potential contamination. Computerized tomography of the chest is required, excepting very low grade lesions where a plain chest radiograph may be sufficient because of the low risk of distant metastases.

The prototypical STS has been malignant fibrous histiocytoma but additional unique predispositions in the HN include angiosarcoma of the scalp and facial regions, hemangiopericytoma of the sinonasal region, dermatofibrosarcoma protruberans of the dermal regions of the low neck and supraclavicular area and rhabomyosarcoma which preferentially afflicts younger adults and children. Primary malignant tumors of bone are predominantly confined to two histological types: osteosarcoma and chondrosarcoma. Other histologies, including primitive neuroectodermal tumor/Ewing's sarcoma, are much less frequent in the HN and will not be discussed.

The HN accounts for about 5–10% of all osteosarcomas, with the mandible (40%) and maxilla the most frequent bones involved (SMITH et al. 2003). In general it is perceived that they have a lower potential for metastatic spread compared with other sites. However local relapse is disappointingly high, resulting in survival rates in the 30–60% range (HA et al. 1999; MARK et al. 1991; KASSIR et al. 1997; SMEELE et al. 1997). The recent National Cancer Data Base (NCDB) report showed a year disease-specific survival rate of 60% (SMITH et al. 2003). After osteosarcoma, chondrosarcoma is the second most common malignancy of bone and constitutes ~10% of bone malignancy. In an NCDB report, HN lesions were grade 1 (50%) or grade 2 (37%) and only a minority have unfavorable higher grade pathology (KOCH et al. 2000). Chondrosarcoma of the petrous temporal and clival bones and of the cricoid lamina of the larynx are intriguing rare presentations and typically low-grade tumors. Metastases are rare and dedifferentiation to high-grade sarcoma is exceptional.

In both STS and bone sarcoma, pathological grading provides an important prognostic measure and has been incorporated in the TNM staging system (GREENE et al. 2002; SOBIN and Wittekind 2002). The system is optimally designed to stage extremity tumors and while patients with HN sarcoma present with earlier T-category size and favorable pathology grade the patient survival may be offset by the more complicated anatomical sites of origin.

8.2.2
Lymphoma

The management of non-Hodgkin's lymphoma (NHL) in the HN is primarily influenced by histology and the Ann Arbor stage (represented in the TNM system (GREENE et al. 2002; SOBIN and Wittekind 2002). Optimal pathology interpretation involves immunophenotypic and sometimes molecular studies. Although surgical treatment for lymphoma is rarely required, open surgical approaches for tissue acquisition may be necessary. Attention to ensure fresh tissue is appropriately handled is essential for accurate pathological diagnosis. The surgeon should excise the largest node in a group of nodes whenever possible. The node should be removed intact with minimal crushing or handling. It should be wrapped in gauze soaked in normal saline and transported to the pathology laboratory for touch prep processing and for fixation in B5 and formalin media; a small portion should be snap frozen in liquid nitrogen. Standard staging investigations involve cross-sectional and functional imaging, assessment of blood indices and bone marrow biopsy and should be undertaken before initiation of chemotherapy so that RT target design can be implemented later.

The most common indolent lymphomas are of follicular histology followed in incidence by mucosa-associated lymphoid tissue (MALT) lymphoma. Follicular lymphoma often involves lymph nodes and the bone marrow, and is widely regarded as a systemic disease. However, up to one third of patients at the time of presentation have localized (stages I–II) disease after standard staging investigations (ARMITAGE and WEISENBURGER 1998), although the addition of FDG-PET may reduce this to 15–20% (WIRTH et al. 2008). In contrast, MALT lymphomas present with localized (stage IE–IIE) disease in 70–90% of cases (ZUCCA et al. 2003; TSANG et al. 2003), involving a variety of extranodal sites, and many will present in the HN area. The most common sites are orbital adnexa, major salivary glands, and the thyroid gland. Lymphocytic infiltration of the tissues associated with infection (Chlamydia psittaci in orbital site), or autoimmune diseases (Sjögren's disease in salivary gland site, Hashimoto's thyroiditis in thyroid site) are predisposing factors to MALT lymphomas.

Aggressive lymphomas also arise in the HN and also have the potential for systemic disease. The HN region is one of the most common sites of extranodal NHL accounting for 10–20% of cases of NHL (SHIMA et al. 1990). Most cases occur in Waldeyer's ring (LOPEZ-GUILLERMO et al. 2005; EZZAT et al. 2001) and the majority of patients are elderly males, except for thyroid lymphomas, where there is a female predominance. The most common histology is diffuse large B-cell lymphoma, for which standard therapy has been well established based on phase III clinical trials. Other uncommon aggressive lymphomas (e.g., T-cell lymphomas) are based on a similar philosophy of therapy with CMT and functional preservation.

8.3
Treatment of Sarcoma

HN sarcomas usually do not enjoy the high local control rates seen in similar histologies in the extremity and this may be the reason for poorer survival in these lesions. This has been attributed to the traditional inability to deliver aggressive treatments because of their location in the critical anatomy of the HN.

In a systematic literature review of HN STS MENDENHALL et al. (2005) showed that the local control rate after surgery alone or combined with RT is ~60–70%. The probability of local control is influenced by histological grade, tumor size, and surgical margins and appears to be improved by adjuvant RT.

HN bone sarcomas differ from STS in that RT is much less established as a component of treatment, but chemotherapy is usually indicated in osteosarcoma and the very rarely seen HN Ewing's tumors.

Elective neck management with surgery or RT is rarely indicated in HN sarcomas because of the rarity of lymph node involvement particularly for those histologies that require surgery. Some rare histological subtypes (i.e., rhabdomyosarcoma, clear cell, epithelioid and potentially synovial sarcoma and angiosarcoma) have a greater risk of regional lymph node involvement.

8.3.1
Surgery of Sarcoma

8.3.1.1
Soft Tissue Sarcoma

The natural history of sarcomas requires a surgical margin approximating 2 cm in dimension unless an intact barrier to tumor spread exists within a region with a closer surgical margin. Generally this will be provided by intact fascia in the radial distribution of the lesion, though bone or other skeletal anatomy may also provide the protection needed. In the HN, these margin recommendations are rarely achievable because of constraints posed by the desire to preserve functional anatomy and minimize cosmetic changes. Lesions judged not to be resectable with secure margins on the basis of their presentation and proximity to critical anatomy, or due to the wish to preserve functional anatomy or cosmetic outcome, should be considered for adjuvant RT to achieve optimal local

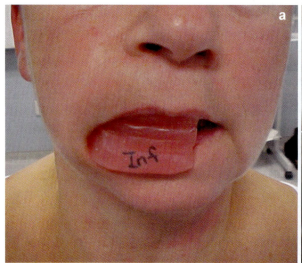 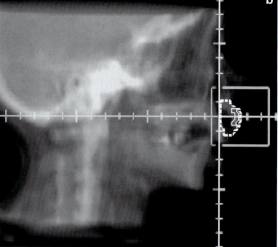

Fig. 8.1. A 50-year-old woman presented with a recently excised STS on the oral aspect of her right upper lip. The surgical margins were positive. An obvious re-excision was needed. This could readily have been performed with a full thickness excision through the lip and without RT. The patient insisted on the avoidance of a cosmetically obvious scar in this location. Instead preoperative RT (50 Gy in 25 fractions using 6 MV photon) was administered with opposed lateral beams using a custom "spacer" to maximally deviate the lip from other oral anatomy and spare these tissues from the RT volume (**a**). The digitally reconstructed radiograph (DRR) for one beam is shown with the clinical target volume (CTV) outlined in *dashed line* and radio-opaque marking for the site of the original tumor are apparent within the CTV volume (**b**). Very conservative surgery was subsequently applied to protect the external lip entirely and re-excise the risk area on the inner lip incorporating ~5-mm margins around the previous surgical incision. Advancement flaps were utilized to provide for a primary closure. The deep margins were carried down to the level of the muscle, but preserving the muscle. The patient remains disease-free 5 years later with no external cosmetic changes of any type

control when surgical margins are closer than is optimum. Therefore the extent of the surgery needed may be modified when RT is applied strategically in situations where surgery alone would have been sufficient but would have needed a wider excision (Fig. 8.1). In other circumstances, a conservative function sparing operation may again be accomplished using RT, though RT is frequently needed irrespective of the form of operation (conservative or ablative) if there has been prior contamination of tissues from prior ill-advised and unsuccessful excision attempts or by previous aberrant biopsy procedures. Such problems apply to both STS and bone tumors, as illustrated for a patient with a grade 2 chondrosarcoma of the larynx (see Fig. 8.2). These tailored approaches should be discussed and planned in advance in a multidisciplinary setting especially involving surgical and radiation oncologists.

Rare exceptions to the use of surgery in STS include many rhabdomyosarcomas where exquisite RT and chemotherapy sensitivity makes this unnecessary and the overwhelming risk is distant metastasis to bone marrow, meninges, and lung typically. Scalp and facial angiosarcomas often pose an overwhelming challenge to surgery because of the improbable ability to achieve useful margins in advanced lesions and such tumors are frequently managed with RT or chemotherapy on a palliative basis.

8.3.1.2
Osteosarcoma and Chondrosarcoma

Surgery accomplished with clear resection margins is the foundation of local treatment of osteosarcoma and chondrosarcoma. Neoadjuvant chemotherapy is indicated in the case of osteosarcoma but not in

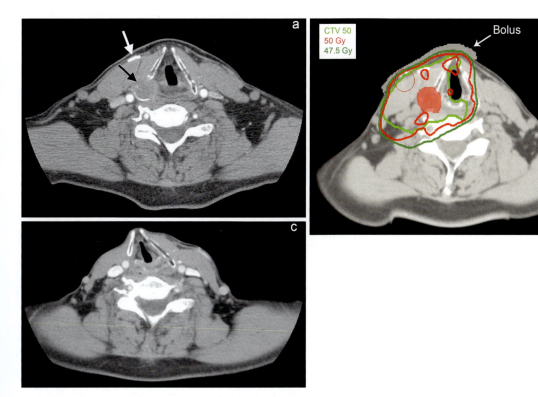

Fig. 8.2. Axial view of a computerized tomography (CT) of a 60-year-old man who presented with an expansile lesion (*black arrow*) of the posterior right thyroid cartilage (**a**). Biopsy had been performed through the right neck by the referring surgeon revealing a grade 2 chondrosarcoma. The *white arrow* identifies a surgical clip in the superficial tissues indicating the entry route of the biopsy and the consequent region of contamination from skin to the tumor area. Although such lesions may be recommended for total laryngectomy, our preference was for laryngeal preserving surgery combined with adjuvant RT since the tissues at risk did not require total laryngeal ablation. In this patient the initial soft tissue contamination mandated the use of RT irrespective of the surgical approach chosen at this time. A course of moderate dose preoperative RT (50 Gy in 25 fractions with 6 MV photons delivered with IMRT) was used (**b**). Coverage of the necessary CTV by the 50 Gy isodose required bolus to be placed over the superficially contaminated tissues for this moderate dose treatment course. The gross tumor volume (GTV) is shown in *red* color wash. The patient underwent resection of the tumor that included partial resection of the laryngeal framework and remains disease-free with excellent voice and swallowing function with 4 years of follow-up (**c**)

chondrosarcoma. RT as a local adjuvant to surgery has a role in high-risk chondrosarcoma but data justifying this approach are far less prevalent for osteosarcoma. The local resection should be planned with a very clear definition of tumor extent, particularly the intramedullary component. Any biopsy scars or other access routes for disease to "track" from the primary site should also be excised especially if the contaminated area is not intended for inclusion in the RT target volume (see Fig. 8.2). It is important to emphasize that wide excision beyond the pseudo-capsule is especially required for chondrosarcomas which tend to have microscopic fingerlike extensions and a notorious propensity to seed the wound with later nodular recurrence if the tumor is violated.

Chondrosarcoma is the most common sarcoma of the larynx and usually presents with a long history from a mass originating on the posterior cricoid lamina eventually resulting in airway compromise and voice dysfunction. These patients are generally older males (>50 years), and usually have low-grade lesions. Complete laryngectomy is virtually always curable but more conservative and single modality surgery when possible may be more appropriate in such low-grade tumors given the excellent survival rates (LEWIS et al. 1997; KOZELSKY et al. 1997). These lesions differ from the rarer higher grade tumor of the thyroid cartilage depicted in Fig. 8.2 that requires a more aggressive approach that may include RT. As noted earlier, chondrosarcoma of the skull, especially those arising in the petrous temporal bone or clivus, is typically also low grade in type. Surgery is indicated but proximity to critical anatomy, including the internal carotid artery, brain stem, and the optic nerves makes surgery problematic and RT is commonly performed on an adjuvant basis or alone as outlined below (see Sect. 8.3.2.5).

8.3.2
Radiotherapy of Sarcoma

8.3.2.1
Soft Tissue Sarcoma

Adjuvant RT was widely adopted for the management of STS following the observation that RT, in combination with conservative excision, could achieve equivalent results to more ablative surgery. The landmark observation was a trial that randomized

high-grade sarcoma of the extremities to receive amputation vs. a limb-sparing operation followed by adjuvant RT (ROSENBERG et al. 1982). Conservative surgical resection with or without adjuvant RT was compared in two further randomized clinical trials that showed superior local control with combined RT and surgery (PISTERS et al. 1996; YANG et al. 1998). Of interest, no improvement in local control was evident from the use of brachytherapy (BRT) in low-grade tumors in one of the trials, but this effect was not present in the second trial where external beam RT was used. These data are important for the general treatment of STS, though no specific trials have been undertaken for the HN.

The advantage of a combined RT and surgery approach is also evident in one series where local control was 52% in those treated with surgery alone vs. 90% in those treated with the combination (TRAN et al. 1992). Another report showed that HN STS patients with either clear surgical margins or microscopic residuum had similar local control rates (26 and 30% failure, respectively) provided RT was administered (LE VAY et al. 1994). Finally, we also reported a prospective series of high-risk cases that has been treated on a consistent protocol by a limited number of radiation oncologists using preoperative RT (O'SULLIVAN et al. 2003). The results are comparable to extremity sarcoma of similar histology and are superior to historical series with less consistent approaches at our institution (LE VAY et al. 1994; O'SULLIVAN et al. 2003).

8.3.2.2
Bone Sarcomas

After surgery with involved resection margins in HN osteosarcoma, revision surgery is advisable when feasible because the outlook for these patients is bleak and adjuvant RT does not appear to confer the high rates of local control seen in STS and in most other tumors. The literature is scant in this area and concludes that outcome with RT is unrewarding because of a preponderance of unresectable lesions or the presence of residual disease after surgery. Reports have suggested that RT either confers no significant value (SMEELE et al. 1997), or is associated with worse outcome (KASSIR et al. 1997; ODA et al. 1997).

Despite the general pessimistic views expressed in the literature, DELANEY et al. (2005a) described an overall local control rate at 5 years of 68% (±8.3%) in 41 osteosarcoma patients in whom surgical resection

Head and Neck Sarcomas and Lymphomas

with widely negative margins was not possible. Seventeen of these patients also had their tumor arising in the HN and eight were of spinal origin. They concluded that RT can enhance local control of osteosarcoma and appears most effective in situations in which only microscopic or minimal residual disease is being treated (DeLaney et al. 2005a).

RT can be a very effective adjunct for chondrosarcoma when there is concern about the adequacy of resection (Harwood et al. 1980; McNaney et al. 1982), although it is acknowledged that opinions vary as to its value but was used as a component of management in more than 20% of cases in a large NCDB study (Koch et al. 2000). At our center we have always regarded positive resection margins as an indication for adjuvant RT especially in lesions that are at least grade 2 in type (Harwood et al. 1980; Krochak et al. 1983). Both adjuvant RT and RT as a sole modality should follow similar principles as for STS regarding planning, dose-fractionation parameters, and target volumes (Fig. 8.2).

8.3.2.3
Scheduling of Radiotherapy (Preoperative vs. Postoperative Radiotherapy)

The scheduling of RT (pre- vs. postoperative) remains controversial and has been discussed extensively (Pisters et al. 2007). Our randomized trial comparing preoperative and postoperative RT in extremity STS showed that local control was equivalent in both groups (93%) (O'Sullivan et al. 2002). We also showed that there is concern about preoperative RT due to the increased risk of wound complications in some anatomic extremity sites, but not in others (O'Sullivan et al. 2002). Similarly, we found this was very uncommon in the separate prospective assessment of HN STS (O'Sullivan et al. 2003). In the combined RT and surgery approach to HN STS and chondrosarcoma, preoperative RT seems particularly suited, because of the smaller RT volumes and lower doses to critical anatomy where wide margins cannot be obtained. This is especially notable in proximity to ocular structures. At present, our guidelines for using preoperative RT are (1) the need to maximally restrict RT volumes in some anatomic sites, (2) the desire to minimize RT dose in some situations (e.g., where critical neurological tissues are in close proximity), and (3) a desire to not irradiate new tissues, especially complex reconstructions that may be vulnerable to the effects of high dose postoperative RT.

8.3.2.4
Radiation Target Volumes and Dose-Fractionation

Soft tissue sarcomas tend to invade locally in a longitudinal fashion while respecting barriers to spread that especially include fascial planes in the axial planes. While our preferred philosophy is to consider surgery alone for these relatively modest sized lesions (in comparison to other anatomic sites), the surgical margins required are rarely achievable in the HN and either pre or postoperative RT is usually needed to secure control. For preoperative RT our policy has been to strive for a longitudinal RT target volume that encompasses a 3.5-cm clinical target volume (CTV) margin surrounding gross tumor, including peritumoral edema where possible (equivalent to field margins of ~5 cm in traditional planning), irrespective of grade or size of the tumor to a dose of 50 Gy in 25 fractions over 5 weeks to be followed by surgery 4–6 weeks later. Radial margins can generally be restricted to 1.5-cm CTV coverage from the closest region of the gross tumor or surgically disrupted tissues (including biopsies).

For postoperative RT planning the high-risk target area includes the surgical field containing all tissues handled during the surgical procedure, including scars and drain sites with a CTV margin of 3.5 cm to address the potential presence of microscopic disease (O'Sullivan et al. 2002). This is often not feasible in the complex anatomy of the HN and compromise is frequently necessary. The "subsequent" phase to deliver a dose of 66 Gy in the postoperative setting is administered with a CTV margin approximating 1 cm surrounding the original tumor site. Some centers may use an "in-field boost" technique with intensity-modulated radiotherapy (IMRT) from the outset to avoid the need for a subsequent additional IMRT "boost" plan. While published results with this approach are unavailable for STS at this time, prescriptions generally use the approach used for more common HN cancers. The wider microscopic volume is treated to 56 Gy in 33 fractions, or equivalent regimens, while simultaneously delivering 66 Gy to the "boost" region (also in 33 fractions) (Fig. 8.3).

In contrast, BRT protocols generally use margins of only 2 cm around the surgical bed (Pisters et al. 1996), although cases may not always be selected similarly for external beam and BRT protocols. In practice these volumes resemble the longitudinal coverage used in preoperative RT. Most experience has been with monotherapy low dose rate treatments to 45–50 Gy at 0.45 Gy h^{-1} with the skin dose restricted

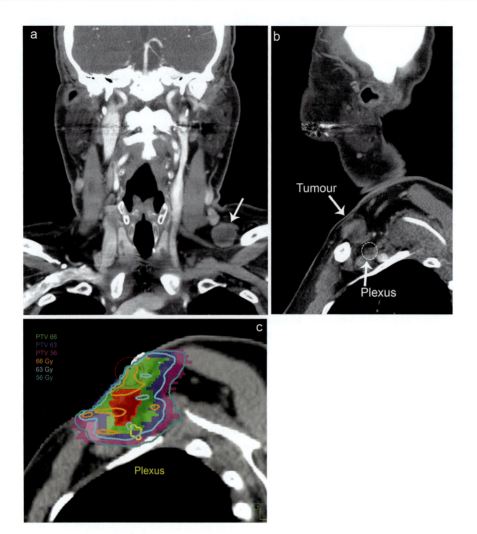

Fig. 8.3. Computerized tomography (CT) coronal view shows a STS (*white arrow*) in proximity to the brachial plexus above the left clavicle in a 65-year-old man (**a**). The brachial plexus is identifiable within the *dotted circle* in the sagittal CT view that also shows the tumor (*white arrow*) (**b**). The lesion was resected with very close margins (<1 mm) and required postoperative RT to a dose of 66 Gy in 33 fractions to the main risk area with a wider area treated to 56 Gy in 33 fractions using IMRT with optimization to reduce dose to vulnerable anatomy (**c**). The original tumor site prior to resection with immediate risk zone for tumor contamination is shown in *red* color wash with surrounding PTV66, PTV63, and PTV56 in different colors. On the sagittal IMRT distribution shown, a heterogeneous pattern is apparent attempting to treat the highest risk area to 66 Gy but maintaining the dose to the brachial plexus to 63 Gy to minimize the risk of functional limiting brachial plexopathy. The surgical scar is evident by the radio-opaque skin marker placed on the skin. This case illustrates the way dose distributions can be tailored to protect vulnerable anatomy using precision RT techniques

to doses of 20–25 Gy. BRT doses of 15–20 Gy are used if combined external beam to a dose of 45–50 Gy. BRT requires specific technical expertise with surgical support and should ordinarily not be used as a sole RT method in the presence of the following: involved resection margins, low-grade histology, proximity of tumor to skin, and complex anatomic locations where the zone of risk is difficult to access (NAG et al. 2001).

8.3.2.5
High Precision Radiotherapy (Particle Beam and IMRT)

The combination of surgical debulking and high-dose precision RT results in durable local control in a large proportion of skull base chondrosarcomas (more than 80%) with modest late toxicity (DELANEY et al. 2005b). The outcome of lesions <25 mL in volume is especially good if adequate doses are administered with a combination of photons and protons (e.g., to ~70 cobalt Gray equivalent) (HUG et al. 1999). Others have reported similar impressive results in smaller series with either protons or fractionated stereotactic RT (NOEL et al. 2001; DEBUS et al. 2000).

Schulz-Ertner et al. recently reported the outcome of 54 patients with gross residual low- and intermediate-grade chondrosarcomas of the skull base using carbon ion RT. The actuarial local control rates were 96.2 and 89.8% at 3 and 4 years; overall survival was 98.2% at 5 years. Only one patient had grade 3 toxicity (SCHULZ-ERTNER et al. 2007).

Until recently particle beam approaches were the only method of treating complex tumors at the skull base with high-dose RT. Presently stereotactic fractionated RT or IMRT may provide similar outcomes. IMRT has provided a 3-year actuarial local control of 95%, and regional node control rate of 90%, in 28 younger patients aged 1–29 years (median age, 8 years) with rhabdomyosarcoma despite the use of relatively close RT margins (1.5-cm margin) (WOLDEN et al. 2005). COMBS et al. (2007) have also reported excellent outcomes using IMRT and fractionated stereotactic RT in children with head-and-neck rhabdomyosarcoma with a low incidence of treatment-related side effects. Confirmatory reports are awaited.

The ability of IMRT to selectively target areas of the volume to avoid delivering doses to vulnerable regions while maintaining high dose gradients between target and normal tissue interphases can be especially useful in the treatment of sarcoma where adjuvant doses are relatively high to complex volumes and normal tissue protection is desirable (Fig. 8.3).

8.3.2.6
Radiotherapy Alone

RT alone may be the only option of management in selected adverse presentations in the HN where surgical management is not feasible and 5-year local control rates are reported as 51% for small lesion. Doses of at least 63 Gy are recommended (KEPKA et al. 2005) and 70 Gy in 35 fractions should be administered if technically feasible.

An exception to the almost universal need for combined surgery and RT in STS is in the treatmentof rhabdomyosarcoma, where control with RT alone with chemotherapy is an expected result

because of the unusual radioresponsive nature of these lesions.

Angiosarcoma is unfortunately well represented in the HN (approximately half of all angiosarcomas), especially in the scalp or facial skin (GLICKSTEIN et al. 2006). Local control is an overwhelming problem because of the difficulty determining the optimal extent of surgical and RT margins in these apparently multifocal tumors, and local recurrence beyond the treatment areas seems to be almost invariable. It remains uncertain whether wide surgical excision is benefiting many of these typically elderly patients, and palliative RT alone may be the optimal approach.

RT as sole modality for chondrosarcomas in difficult locations, such as the clival regions, can be accomplished with proton beam RT or IMRT. Ten-year control rates of 70–80% have been reported from experienced centers using proton beam RT. Indication include the need to sacrifice critical vascular supply in clival lesions and especially where the lesion is of small volume.

At present the literature does not provide convincing evidence that RT as a sole modality is useful for the local management of osteosarcoma and is typically reserved for palliation. Even in this setting it is often not helpful.

8.3.3
Adjuvant Chemotherapy

8.3.3.1
Soft Tissue Sarcoma

Chemotherapy is controversial in STS other than for specific histologies such as rhabdomyosarcoma, and potentially for larger synovial sarcoma where a good response is expected though the true value is uncertain. An individual patient data meta-analysis from the 1,568 patients randomized in 14 trials addressed the role of doxorubicin-based adjuvant chemotherapy in STS (Sarcoma Meta-analysis COLLABORATION 1997). The results were in favor of the use of adjuvant chemotherapy for recurrence-free survival and distant metastases, but not for overall survival ($p = 0.12$). HN STS were included to varying degrees in half of the studies (WILSON et al. 1986; ALVEGARD et al. 1989; ANTMAN et al. 1990; BAKER 1988; GLENN et al. 1985; RAVAUD et al. 1990; BRAMWELL et al. 1994). In the largest trial ($n = 468$) (that of the EORTC), relapse-free survival was significantly better (56 vs. 43% for controls; $p = 0.007$) and local recurrence significantly reduced by chemotherapy (17 vs. 31%; $p = 0.01$) (BRAMWELL et al. 1994). This favorable finding appeared to be confined to HN and trunk tumors and may provide an opportunity to improve local control in a situation where local control has traditionally not been as satisfactory as extremity STS.

In childhood rhadomyosarcoma, chemotherapy has facilitated the local management due to the excellent response in addition to local effect from RT. Current research efforts are even exploring the potential of relying on chemotherapy as the sole therapy given the devastating local sequelae of RT that may arise in young children (STEVENS 2002).

8.3.3.2
Bone Sarcoma

Chemotherapy is not ordinarily a component of management of chondrosarcoma, in contrast with osteosarcoma. The exception is in the mesenchymal subtype where chemotherapy was used in the majority of mesenchymal chondrosarcoma cases (57.5%) in the NCDB series (KOCH et al. 2000) and has been our policy at Princess Margaret Hospital (HARWOOD et al. 1981).

Intense chemotherapy approaches are often recommended for HN osteosarcoma because of the pivotal role they had in the introduction of limb preservation for osteosarcoma of limb bones. Trials exist in extremity osteosarcoma but prospective studies in the HN are lacking and approaches are inconsistent. As a result, there is disagreement about the role of chemotherapy in seemingly more favorable osteosarcomas of the mandible and maxilla compared with extremity lesions. Two independent overviews of the retrospective data regarding the role of adjuvant chemotherapy were reported simultaneously (KASSIR et al. 1997; SMEELE et al. 1997). As discussed earlier, both studies suggested that RT was unhelpful. However, KASSIR et al. (1997) concluded that the role of chemotherapy in HN osteosarcoma remains unproven, while SMEELES et al. (1997) maintained that chemotherapy does improve survival. The two studies differed in that the former accepted all nonmetastatic patients while the latter restricted entry to those studies that reported on the status of surgical margins. In the NCDB report, no substantial difference in the 5-year survival rate was noted between treatment with surgery alone (74.7%) and surgery with adjuvant chemotherapy (71.3%) (SMITH et al. 2003).

8.3.4
Targeted Approaches

Proven therapeutic molecular targets have remained elusive in sarcoma (WUNDER et al. 2007). Several situations are emerging that may offer opportunities in this regard.

The recent observations of response to imatinib (STI 571, Gleevec®) in DFSP predicted by the presence of the t(17;22) translocation (MCARTHUR et al. 2005) provide possibilities for molecular target therapies in the future. Bevacizumab, a humanized monoclonal antibody to vascular endothelial growth factor, is an attractive agent to consider in angiosarcoma given its ability to inhibit tumor growth. KOONTZ et al. (2008) recently reported promising results in two patients using neoadjuvant bevacizumab combined with radiation therapy. Follicular dendritic cell sarcoma is a rare, malignant, non-lymphoid-cell-derived tumor that originates from B-lymphoid follicles of nodal and extranodal sites. Surgery and RT are the mainstay of treatment for localized disease. Classic lymphoma and sarcoma regimens have shown dismal responses in the metastatic setting. An imatinib-based combination has been reported recently to provide a potential therapeutic strategy (AZIM et al. 2007).

8.4
Treatment of Lymphomas of the Head and Neck

8.4.1
Indolent Lymphoma

Both follicular lymphoma and MALT lymphoma are known to be radiation-sensitive diseases. Stages I and II of the disease are treated with involved-field radiation therapy (RT), expecting a local control rate exceeding 95%, and long-term disease-free survival of 50–70% (ZUCCA et al. 2003; TSANG et al. 2003; TSANG and GOSPODAROWICZ 2005, 2007). Because of exquisite radiation sensitivity, low to moderate doses (25–35 Gy, fractionated over 2–3 weeks) have been the standard approach. Short-term toxicity is mild and serious long-term toxicity is rare in virtually all HN tissues or organs that commonly harbor lymphoma. Perhaps the only exception is in patients with MALT lymphoma of the parotid gland(s), where existing xerostomia due to Sjögren's syndrome will be exacerbated by RT and due to the underlying autoimmune disease, the patient will continue to have progressive xerostomia even with control and cure of the lymphoma. In the orbital site, provided that the disease is not in the retroorbital location, it is often possible to shield the anterior chamber of the eye and the lens and if done successfully the risk of cataracts is low (<20%).

8.4.2
Aggressive Histology Lymphoma

Despite a presentation in early stage (I–II), the recognition of the high risk for occult systemic disease mandates the use of anthracycline-based chemotherapy to achieve the best cure rates. Patients are treated with CMT, with chemotherapy first for 3–6 cycles, followed by moderate dose radiation (30–40 Gy) 3–6 weeks later. A combined chemotherapy–RT approach has been shown in a phase III trial of stage I Waldeyer's ring lymphoma to be superior to radiation therapy alone, or chemotherapy alone (AVILES et al. 1996). In general, a cure rate ranging from 60 to 80% is achieved, depending on age, tumor burden, and other prognostic factors such as performance status and LDH level (LOPEZ-GUILLERMO et al. 2005; EZZAT et al. 2001). Clinical outcomes appear to be best with lymphomas located in the tonsil, compared with other HN sites such as paranasal sinus or major salivary glands (LOPEZ-GUILLERMO et al. 2005; EZZAT et al. 2001). For B-cell lymphomas, the addition of immunotherapy with anti-CD20 antibody (rituximab) in combination with chemotherapy improves the clinical outcome (PFREUNDSCHUH et al. 2006, 2008; COIFFIER et al. 2002). Where disease is infiltrating or located in proximity to the meninges (e.g., base of skull and paranasal sinuses), or for rare very aggressive histologies (e.g., lymphoblastic lymphoma, Burkitt lymphoma) with a predilection for spread to the central nervous system, the addition of central nervous system prophylaxis is indicated. This consists of intrathecal chemotherapy, with or without low-dose cranial irradiation depending on the institutional protocol followed. Because of the moderate radiation doses required (30–40 Gy), short-term toxicity is mild and serious long-term toxicity is rare, particularly with current precision RT techniques such as IMRT with improved ability to further reduce the dose to uninvolved normal tissues such as the salivary glands, pharynx, and oral cavity.

References

Alvegard TA, Sigurdsson H, Mouridsen H et al. (1989) Adjuvant chemotherapy with doxorubicin in high-grade soft tissue sarcoma: a randomized trial of the Scandinavian Sarcoma Group. J Clin Oncol 7:1504–1513

Antman K, Ryan L, Borden E (1990) Pooled results from three randomized adjuvant studies of doxorubicin versus observation in soft tissue sarcoma: 10 year results and review of literature. In: Salmon SE (ed) Adjuvant therapy of cancer, vol VI. WB Saunders, Philadelphia, pp 529–543

Armitage JO, Weisenburger DD (1998) New approach to classifying non-Hodgkin's lymphomas: clinical features of the major histologic subtypes. Non-Hodgkin's lymphoma classification project. J Clin Oncol 16:2780–2795

Aviles A, Delgado S, Ruiz H et al. (1996) Treatment of non-Hodgkin's lymphoma of Waldeyer's ring: radiotherapy versus chemotherapy versus combined therapy. Eur J Cancer Oral Oncol 32B:19–23

Azim HA, Elsedewy E, Azim HA, Jr. (2007) Imatinib in the treatment of follicular dendritic sarcoma: a case report and review of literature. Onkologie 30:381–384

Baker LH (1988) Adjuvant therapy for soft tissue sarcomas. In: Ryan JR, Baker L (eds) Recent concepts in sarcoma treatment. Kluwer, Dordecht, pp 131–136

Bramwell V, Rouesse J, Steward W et al. (1994) Adjuvant CYVADIC chemotherapy for adult soft tissue sarcoma – reduced local recurrence but no improvement in survival: a study of the European Organization for Research and Treatment of Cancer Soft Tissue and Bone Sarcoma Group. J Clin Oncol 12:1137–1149

Coiffier B, Lepage E, Briere J et al. (2002) CHOP chemotherapy plus rituximab compared with CHOP alone in elderly patients with diffuse large-B-cell lymphoma. N Engl J Med 346:235–242

Combs SE, Behnisch W, Kulozik AE et al. (2007) Intensity modulated radiotherapy (IMRT) and fractionated stereotactic radiotherapy (FSRT) for children with head-and-neck-rhabdomyosarcoma. BMC Cancer 7:177

Debus J, Schulz-Ertner D, Schad L et al. (2000) Stereotactic fractionated radiotherapy for chordomas and chondrosarcomas of the skull base. Int J Radiat Oncol Biol Phys 47:591–596

DeLaney TF, Park L, Goldberg SI et al. (2005a) Radiotherapy for local control of osteosarcoma. Int J Radiat Oncol Biol Phys 61:492–498

DeLaney TF, Trofimov AV, Engelsman M et al. (2005b) Advanced-technology radiation therapy in the management of bone and soft tissue sarcomas. Cancer Control 12:27–35

Ezzat AA, Ibrahim EM, El Weshi AN et al. (2001) Localized non-Hodgkin's lymphoma of Waldeyer's ring: clinical features, management, and prognosis of 130 adult patients. Head Neck 23:547–558

Glenn J, Kinsella T, Glatstein E et al. (1985) A randomized, prospective trial of adjuvant chemotherapy in adults with soft tissue sarcomas of the head and neck, breast, and trunk. Cancer 55:1206–1214

Glickstein J, Sebelik ME, Lu Q (2006) Cutaneous angiosarcoma of the head and neck: a case presentation and review of the literature. Ear Nose Throat J 85:672–674

Greene FL, Page D, Norrow M et al. (2002) AJCC cancer staging manual, 6 edn. Springer, New York

Ha PK, Eisele DW, Frassica FJ et al. (1999) Osteosarcoma of the head and neck: a review of the Johns Hopkins experience. Laryngoscope 109:964–969

Harwood AR, Krajbich JI, Fornasier VL (1980) Radiotherapy of chondrosarcoma of bone. Cancer 45:2769–2777

Harwood AR, Krajbich JI, Fornasier VL (1981) Mesenchymal chondrosarcoma: a report of 17 cases. Clin Orthop (158): 144–148

Hug EB, Loredo LN, Slater JD et al. (1999) Proton radiation therapy for chordomas and chondrosarcomas of the skull base. J Neurosurg 91:432–439

Kassir RR, Rassekh CH, Kinsella JB et al. (1997) Osteosarcoma of the head and neck: meta-analysis of nonrandomized studies. Laryngoscope 107:56–61

Kepka L, Delaney TF, Suit HD et al. (2005) Results of radiation therapy for unresected soft-tissue sarcomas. Int J Radiat Oncol Biol Phys 63:852–859

Koch BB, Karnell LH, Hoffman HT et al. (2000) National cancer database report on chondrosarcoma of the head and neck. Head Neck 22:408–425

Koontz BF, Miles EF, Rubio MA et al. (2008) Preoperative radiotherapy and bevacizumab for angiosarcoma of the head and neck: two case studies. Head Neck 30:262–266

Kozelsky TF, Bonner JA, Foote RL et al. (1997) Laryngeal chondrosarcomas: the Mayo Clinic experience. J Surg Oncol 65:269–273

Krochak R, Harwood AR, Cummings BJ et al. (1983) Results of radical radiation for chondrosarcoma of bone. Radiother Oncol 1:109–115

Le Vay J, O'Sullivan B, Catton C et al. (1994) An assessment of prognostic factors in soft-tissue sarcoma of the head and neck. Arch Otolaryngol Head Neck Surg 120:981–986

Lewis JE, Olsen KD, Inwards CY (1997) Cartilaginous tumors of the larynx: clinicopathologic review of 47 cases. Ann Otol Rhinol Laryngol 106:94–100

Lopez-Guillermo A, Colomo L, Jimenez M et al. (2005) Diffuse large B-cell lymphoma: clinicobiological characterization and outcome according to the nodal or extranodal primary origin. J Clin Oncol 23:2797–2804

Mark RJ, Sercarz JA, Tran L et al. (1991) Osteogenic sarcoma of the head and neck. The UCLA experience. Arch Otolaryngol Head Neck Surg 117:761–766

McArthur GA, Demetri GD, van Oosterom A et al. (2005) Molecular and clinical analysis of locally advanced dermatofibrosarcoma protuberans treated with imatinib: Imatinib Target Exploration Consortium Study B2225. J Clin Oncol 23:866–873

McNaney D, Lindberg RD, Ayala AG et al. (1982) Fifteen year radiotherapy experience with chondrosarcoma of bone. Int J Radiat Oncol Biol Phys 8:187–190

Mendenhall WM, Mendenhall CM, Werning JW et al. (2005) Adult head and neck soft tissue sarcomas. Head Neck 27:916–922

Nag S, Shasha D, Janjan N et al. (2001) The American Brachytherapy Society recommendations for brachytherapy of soft tissue sarcomas. Int J Radiat Oncol Biol Phys 49:1033–1043

Noel G, Habrand JL, Mammar H et al. (2001) Combination of photon and proton radiation therapy for chordomas and chondrosarcomas of the skull base: the Centre de Protontherapie D'Orsay experience. Int J Radiat Oncol Biol Phys 51:392–398

O'Sullivan B, Chung P, Euler C et al. (2007) Soft tissue sarcoma. In: Gunderson LL, Tepper JE (eds) Clinical radiation oncology, 2nd edn. Churchill Livingston, Philadelphia, pp 1519–1549

O'Sullivan B, Davis A, Turcotte R et al. (2002) Pre-operative versus post-operative radiotherapy in soft issue sarcoma of the limbs: a randomized trial. Lancet 359:2235–2241

O'Sullivan B, Gullane P, Irish J et al. (2003) Preoperative radiotherapy for adult head and neck soft tissue sarcoma: assessment of wound complication rates and cancer outcome in a prospective series. World J Surg 27:875–883

Oda D, Bavisotto LM, Schmidt RA et al. (1997) Head and neck osteosarcoma at the University of Washington. Head Neck 19:513–523

Pfreundschuh M, Schubert J, Ziepert M et al. (2008) Six versus eight cycles of bi-weekly CHOP-14 with or without rituximab in elderly patients with aggressive CD20+ B-cell lymphomas: a randomised controlled trial (RICOVER-60). Lancet Oncol 9:105–116

Pfreundschuh M, Trumper L, Osterborg A et al. (2006) CHOP-like chemotherapy plus rituximab versus CHOP-like chemotherapy alone in young patients with good-prognosis diffuse large-B-cell lymphoma: a randomised controlled trial by the MabThera International Trial (MInT) Group. Lancet Oncol 7:379–391

Pisters PW, Harrison LB, Leung DH et al. (1996) Long-term results of a prospective randomized trial of adjuvant brachytherapy in soft tissue sarcoma. J Clin Oncol 14:859–868

Pisters PW, O'Sullivan B, Maki RG (2007) Evidence-based recommendations for local therapy for soft tissue sarcomas. J Clin Oncol 25:1003–1008

Ravaud A, Bui NB, Coindre JM (1990) Adjuvant chemotherapy with Cyvadic in high risk soft tissue sarcoma: a randomized prospective trial. In: Salmon SE (ed) Adjuvant therapy of cancer, vol VI. WB Saunders, Philadelphia, pp 556–566

Rosenberg SA, Tepper J, Glatstein E et al. (1982) The treatment of soft-tissue sarcomas of the extremities: prospective randomized evaluations of (1) limb-sparing surgery plus radiation therapy compared with amputation and (2) the role of adjuvant chemotherapy. Ann Surg 196:305–315

Sarcoma Meta-analysis Collaboration (1997) Adjuvant chemotherapy for localised resectable soft-tissue sarcoma of adults: meta-analysis of individual data. Lancet 350: 1647–1654

Schulz-Ertner D, Nikoghosyan A, Hof H et al. (2007) Carbon ion radiotherapy of skull base chondrosarcomas. Int J Radiat Oncol Biol Phys 67:171–177

Shima N, Kobashi Y, Tsutsui K et al. (1990) Extranodal non-Hodgkin's lymphoma of the head and neck. A clinicopathologic study in the Kyoto-Nara area of Japan. Cancer 66:1190–1197

Smeele LE, Kostense PJ, van der Waal I et al. (1997) Effect of chemotherapy on survival of craniofacial osteosarcoma: a systematic review of 201 patients. J Clin Oncol 15: 363–367

Smith RB, Apostolakis LW, Karnell LH et al. (2003) National Cancer Data Base report on osteosarcoma of the head and neck. Cancer 98:1670–1680

Sobin L, Wittekind CH (2002) TNM classification of malignant tumours, 6 edn. Wiley-Liss, New York

Stevens MCG (2002) Malignant mesenchymal tumours of childhood. In: Souhami RL, Tannock I, Hohenberger P, Horiot J-C (eds) Oxford textbook of oncology, 2nd edn. Oxford University Press, Oxford, pp 2525–2538

Tran LM, Mark R, Meier R et al. (1992) Sarcomas of the head and neck. Cancer 70:169–177

Tsang RW, Gospodarowicz MK (2007) Low-grade non-Hodgkin lymphomas. Semin Radiat Oncol 17:198–205

Tsang RW, Gospodarowicz MK, Pintilie M et al. (2003) Localized mucosa-associated lymphoid tissue lymphoma treated with radiation therapy has excellent clinical outcome. J Clin Oncol 21:4157–4164

Tsang RW, Gospodarowicz MK (2005) Radiation therapy for localized low-grade non-Hodgkin's lymphomas. Hematol Oncol 23:10–17

Wilson RE, Wood WC, Lerner HL et al. (1986) Doxorubicin chemotherapy in the treatment of soft-tissue sarcoma. Combined results of two randomized trials. Arch Surg 121:1354–1359

Wirth A, Foo M, Seymour JF et al. (2008) Impact of [18f] fluorodeoxyglucose positron emission tomography on staging and management of early-stage follicular non-Hodgkin lymphoma. Int J Radiat Oncol Biol Phys 71:213–219

Wolden SL, Wexler LH, Kraus DH, Laquaglia MP, Lis E, Meyers PA. Intensity-modulated radiotherapy for head-and-neck rhabdomyosarcoma. Int JRadiat Oncol Biol Phys 2005; 61:1432–1438

Wunder JS, Nielsen TO, Maki RG et al. (2007) Opportunities for improving the therapeutic ratio for patients with sarcoma. Lancet Oncol 8:513–524

Yang JC, Chang AE, Baker AR et al. (1998) Randomized prospective study of the benefit of adjuvant radiation therapy in the treatment of soft tissue sarcomas of the extremity. J Clin Oncol 16:197–203

Zucca E, Conconi A, Pedrinis E et al. (2003) Nongastric marginal zone B-cell lymphoma of mucosa-associated lymphoid tissue. Blood 101:2489–2495

Thyroid Cancer

9

Li Ning, Herbert Chen, and Rebecca S. Sippel

CONTENTS

9.1   Incidence   *117*

9.2   Types of Thyroid Cancer   *118*

9.3   Diagnosis   *118*

9.4   Management   *120*
9.4.1   Well-Differentiated Thyroid Cancer   *120*
9.4.1.1   Surgery   *120*
9.4.1.2   Radioiodine Ablation   *121*
9.4.1.3   External Beam
          Radiotherapy   *122*
9.4.1.4   Chemotherapy   *122*
9.4.2   Poorly Differentiated and
          Anaplastic Thyroid Cancer   *122*
9.4.2.1   Surgery   *122*
9.4.2.2   Radiotherapy   *122*
9.4.2.3   Chemotherapy   *123*
9.4.3   Medullary Thyroid
          Cancer   *123*
9.4.3.1   Surgery   *123*
9.4.3.2   Radiotherapy   *123*
9.4.3.3   Chemotherapy   *123*

Abbreviations   *123*

References   *124*

KEY POINTS

- Thyroid cancer accounts for 1% of all cancers diagnosed in the United States per year.
- Surgery, consisting of a total thyroidectomy, is the primary treatment modality for patients with thyroid cancer.
- Postoperatively patients with well-differentiated thyroid cancer are usually treated with radioactive iodine
- External beam radiation is rarely indicated in the treatment of well-differentiated thyroid cancer, but can play an important role in the treatment of poorly differentiated or anaplastic thyroid cancers.
- The prognosis of most patients with thyroid cancer is excellent.
- Traditional chemotherapy is of little utility in treatment of metastatic thyroid cancer that is not responsive to radioactive iodine; therefore enrollment in clinical trials should be encouraged.

Li Ning, MD
Department of Surgery, H4750 CSC, University of Wisconsin, 600 Highland Avenue, Madison, WI 53792, USA
Herbert Chen, MD
Department of Surgery, University of Wisconsin, H4/750 CSC, 600 Highland Avenue, Madison, WI 53792, USA
Rebecca S. Sippel, MD
Department of Surgery, H4/755 CSC, University of Wisconsin, 600 Highland Ave., Madison, WI 53792, USA

9.1

Incidence

Although thyroid nodules are extremely common, malignant lesions of the thyroid are relatively uncommon. In the United States, thyroid cancer accounts for only 1% of all human malignant tumors and 0.5% of cancer-related deaths (Landis et al. 1998). The American Cancer Society estimates that 37,340 new cases of thyroid cancer are diagnosed annually in the United States and that 1,590 thyroid-cancer-related deaths occur annually (JEMAL et al. 2008). Despite its infrequent occurrence, thyroid cancer is the most common malignant endocrine lesion (90% of all endocrine cancers) and is responsible for more deaths than all other endocrine cancers combined (LANDIS et al. 1998).

9.2 Types of Thyroid Cancer

Thyroid cancers are classified by their predominant histologic cell types. (1) Follicular cell origin: papillary, follicular, Hürthle cell, and anaplastic cancer; (2) parafollicular or C cell origin: medullary cancer; and (3) other tumors, including lymphomas and metastatic tumors.

Most thyroid cancers are of follicular cell origin. Four distinct histologic types of follicular cell-derived cancers are recognized: papillary, follicular, Hürthle cell, and anaplastic (Fig. 9.1). Malignant tumors of thyroid follicular cell origin have traditionally been classified as either well-differentiated thyroid cancer, which is composed of papillary, follicular, and Hürthle cell thyroid cancer, or undifferentiated/anaplastic thyroid cancer. The majority of patients with well-differentiated thyroid cancer have an excellent prognosis, whereas patients with anaplastic thyroid cancer uniformly have a poor prognosis. In 1983, Sakamoto et al. introduced a group of tumors that fall between well-differentiated and anaplastic thyroid cancer in terms of both morphologic appearance and biologic behavior. Patients with these tumors, which they termed poorly-differentiated thyroid cancer, often have rapid progression and a poor outcome despite appropriate treatment. However, controversy surrounding poorly differentiated persists because there is no consensus regarding the diagnostic criteria or definition.

9.3 Diagnosis

The majority of patients with thyroid cancer present with a neck mass originating from the thyroid gland. Therefore, a thorough history and neck examination should be the first evaluation of a thyroid mass. Symptoms such as hoarseness, dysphagia, dyspnea, hemoptysis, difficulty swallowing, and rapid enlargement of the mass may occur with thyroid carcinomas but are not diagnostic of malignancy. A history of head and neck irradiation, especially in childhood, is an important risk factor for thyroid cancer. Previous thyroid diseases such as goiter, Hashimoto's disease and Grave's disease can also be risk factors for thyroid cancer. A family history of thyroid cancer is also an important risk factor. Well-differentiated thyroid cancer is believed to have a familial origin in 5% of cases. Medullary thyroid cancer, which constitutes ~7% of all thyroid malignancies, occurs within a familial setting in 20% of cases, usually as part of the multiple endocrine neoplasia type 2A or 2B syndrome. Systemic disorder such as Gardner's syndrome, Cowden's disease, lymphoma, or other malignant diseases can also be associated with thyroid nodules. Physical examination includes a thorough neck examination. A malignant tumor is usually firmer and may be fixed to the surrounding and underlying tissues. Neck examination may also reveal palpable metastatic cervical lymph nodes, especially in the anterior compartment (levels III, IV, VI) and less commonly in the posterior compartment (level V).

Fine-needle aspiration (FNA) is the gold standard for the evaluation of a new thyroid nodule. This technique can be performed by palpation or under ultrasound guidance (Fig. 9.2). FNA is an accurate diagnostic procedure in papillary, medullary, metastatic, and anaplastic thyroid cancers, as well as in malignant lymphomas. In our experience, FNA is a

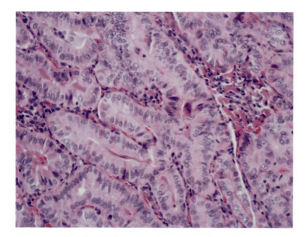

Fig. 9.1. Histology of a tall-cell variant of papillary thyroid cancer. Note that the cells are twice as tall as they are wide. This subtype of thyroid cancer is associated with a more aggressive course

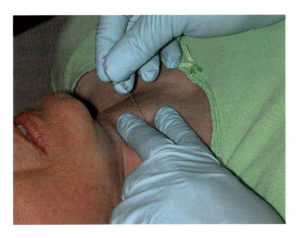 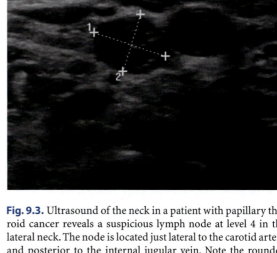

Fig. 9.2. Palpation-guided fine-needle aspiration of a large thyroid nodule can easily be performed at the bedside using a 25-gauge needle. A syringe can be used to apply gentle aspiration pressure, or the sample can be obtained through simple capillary filling of the needle obtained with 3–4 passes of the needle

Fig. 9.3. Ultrasound of the neck in a patient with papillary thyroid cancer reveals a suspicious lymph node at level 4 in the lateral neck. The node is located just lateral to the carotid artery and posterior to the internal jugular vein. Note the rounded appearance of the node with the prominent anterior/posterior diameter as well as the contained microcalcifications

valuable tool in determining the optimal operative approach for a patient with a thyroid nodule, and can help to avoid unplanned reoperations. Therefore, we recommend routine use of preoperative thyroid FNA, even in those patients in whom a resection is already planned (Greenbelt et al. 2006). One of the limitations of FNA is its inability to differentiate between benign/malignant follicular and Hürthle cell neoplasms of the thyroid. This distinction is based on the presence or absence of a capsular or vascular invasion, which can usually only be seen on the permanent pathologic evaluation after the nodule has been removed. Ashcraft and Van Herle (1981), in a comprehensive review comparing the accuracy of FNA and core biopsy, concluded that neither biopsy technique is superior, but FNA was almost free of complications. In recent reports, the sensitivity of the procedure is 89–94% and the specificity is 92–98.5% (Greenbelt et al. 2006; Yang et al. 2007). Therefore, a malignant specimen on FNA is a strong indication for surgery; however, a negative result cannot rule out cancer entirely. FNA may be less accurate in some clinical diseases, including predominantly cystic lesions, large nodules, multinodular goiters, and in the presence of underlying thyroiditis.

For most patients a thyroid stimulating hormone (TSH) level is the only blood test that is needed. If the TSH is abnormal, then additional thyroid function testing is indicated. TSH is a known thyroid growth factor, which may be involved in thyroid cancer growth and development. Haymart et al. (2008) reported that the likelihood of thyroid cancer increases with higher serum TSH concentration. Even within normal TSH ranges, a TSH level above the population mean is associated with significantly greater likelihood of thyroid cancer than a TSH below the mean. Thyroglobulin is usually measured as a baseline following surgery for well-differentiated thyroid cancer because it correlates well with tumor volume. Recurrent tumors are usually associated with an elevation in the thyroglobulin level. Calcitonin is a useful test to confirm a diagnosis of medullary thyroid cancer; however, it is not a cost-effective screening tool.

Thyroid cancers can require multimodal imaging evaluations. Ultrasound is the main modality for the initial assessment of a new thyroid nodule (Wong and Ahuja 2005). It provides an accurate tridimensional location, gives the nodule size, and indicates the nodule location for FNA. Ultrasound can also identify features of the nodule which are associated with a higher risk of malignancy (microcalcifications, intranodular hypervascularity, irregular borders). Ultrasound can detect nodules as small as 2–3 mm and can differentiate between solitary and multinodular disease. Ultrasound is also a highly sensitive technique for detecting lymph node disease (Fig. 9.3).

Chest X-ray is helpful in detecting tracheal deviation or airway narrowing due to large lesions. Chest X-ray can also help to identify lung and bone metastasis. Thyroid cancers, especially when located posteriorly can invade the recurrent laryngeal nerve, causing vocal cord paralysis. Therefore, preoperative laryngoscopy to evaluate for vocal cord paralysis should be performed in suspected carcinomas, especially if there have been any voice changes.

Radioactive iodine scanning has little value in the routine evaluation of solitary thyroid nodules because the majority of both benign and malignant thyroid nodules are hyporeactive compared with adjacent tissues. However, radioactive iodine scanning is useful in the subgroups of patients with hyperthyroidism (suppressed TSH) to identify autonomously functioning thyroid nodules. Radioactive iodine scanning is also used postoperatively to detect and treat remaining thyroid tissue after surgical resection as well as metastatic disease (BUSCOMBE 2007).

Magnetic resonance imaging (MRI) and computed tomography (CT) are useful tools for the evaluation of extrathyroidal invasion to the surrounding organs such as larynx and trachea. CT and MRI are also better than ultrasound for evaluating the deep cervical lymph nodes, including retropharyngeal, deep cervical, and substernal regions (MIYAKOSHI et al. 2007). The advantages of MRI over CT include multiplane evaluation, better tissue contrast, and no radiation to the thyroid gland (MIYAKOSHI et al. 2007). MRI is also very useful to detect residual, recurrent, and metastatic cancers. T2 imaging can be used to differentiate between tumor and fibrosis in the previously operated neck, and can detect muscle invasion.

Increasingly thyroid nodules are detected as incidental findings on an 18F-FDG PET scan for another indication. When thyroid nodules have high FDG uptake, they have a risk of malignancy up to 50% and need further assessment (AL-NAHHAS et al. 2008). An emerging role for 18F-FDG PET is in the investigation of cases of established well-differentiated thyroid cancer presenting with high serum

thyroglobulin levels and negative radioiodine imaging (DEBATIN and BRANDAU 2004; AL-NAHHAS et al. 2008). FREUDENBERG et al. (2007) compared the positron emission tomography (PET)/CT results with ^{131}I whole-body scintigraphy in patients with differentiated thyroid cancer, and they concluded that PET imaging is valuable in patients suffering from advanced differentiated thyroid cancer prior to radioiodine therapy and in patients with suspected recurrence and potential metastatic disease.

9.4
Management

9.4.1
Well-Differentiated Thyroid Cancer

9.4.1.1
Surgery

The mainstay of treatment of well-differentiated thyroid cancer is surgery. The surgical procedures include total thyroidectomy or thyroid lobectomy. Total thyroidectomy is usually performed for well-differentiated thyroid cancer. For most patients with papillary thyroid cancer, especially those with tumors greater than 1 cm in diameter, multifocal disease, extrathyroidal spread, familial disease, and those with clinically involved nodes, total thyroidectomy is indicated (MAZZAFERRI 1994) (Table 9.1 and 9.2). Patients with follicular thyroid cancer showing evidence of vascular invasion or tumor more than 4 cm in diameter should also be treated with total thyroidectomy or near-total thyroidectomy (removal of all grossly visible thyroid tissue, leaving only a small amount of tissue near the recurrent laryngeal nerve as it enters into the cricothyroid muscle) (WATKINSON et al. 2006). Tumor size correlates directly with malignant potential in patients with Hürthle cell neoplasms of the thyroid. Since the

Table 9.1. Comparison of thyroid cancer staging systems

	Age	Metastases	Extent/invasion	Tumor size	Tumor grade	Complete resection	Nodal disease
AMES	•	•	•	•			
AGES	•	•	•	•	•		
MACIS	•	•	•			•	
TNM	•	•	•				•

Table 9.2. TNM staging classification system for differentiated thyroid cancer

Stages	Patient age < 45 years	Patient aged 45 years or older
Stage I	Any T, any N, MO	T1, NO, MO
Stage II	Any T, any N, M1	T2, NO, MO
Stage III		T3, NO, MO or T1–T3, N1a, MO
Stage IVA		T4a, NO-N1a, MO or T1–T4a, N1b, MO
Stage IVB		T4b, any N, MO
Stage IVC		Any T, any N, M1

T1 tumor diameter 2 cm or smaller; T2 primary tumor diameter: 2–4 cm; T3 primary tumor diameter: 4 cm limited to the thyroid or with minimal extrathyroidal extension; T4a tumor of any size extending beyond the thyroid capsule to invade subcutaneous soft tissues, larynx, trachea, esophagus, or recurrent laryngeal nerve; T4b tumor invades prevertebral fascia or encases carotid artery or mediastinal vessels; TX primary tumor size unknown, but without extrathyroidal invasion; NO no metastatic nodes; N1a metastases to level VI (pretracheal, paratracheal, and prelaryngeal/Delphian lymph nodes); N1b metastasis to unilateral, bilateral, contralateral cervical or superior mediastinal mode metastases; NX nodes not assessed at surgery; MO no distant metastases; M1 distant metastases; MX distant metastases not assessed
The original source for this material is the AJCC Cancer Staging Manual, Sixth Edition (2002). Springer, New York

risk of malignancy is about 55–65% in patients with a tumor larger than 4 cm in diameter, consideration should be given for an initial total thyroidectomy in these patients (CHEN et al. 1998; SIPPEL et al. 2008a, b). Patients with bilateral nodular disease or those who prefer to undergo bilateral thyroidectomy to avoid the possibility of requiring a future surgery on the contralateral lobe should also undergo total thyroidectomy. Thyroid lobectomy is probably adequate in patients with well-differentiated thyroid cancer of 1 cm diameter or less or those with only minimal capsular invasion (MAZZAFERRI 1999).

The role of neck dissection in conjunction with thyroidectomy for well-differentiated thyroid cancer is a controversial topic. Several studies have shown that elective neck dissection does not improve the survival rate in papillary thyroid cancer. However, bilateral central (compartment VI) node dissection may reduce the risk for recurrence and in some patients may improve survival, especially in patients who are considered high risk (male sex, age > 45 years, tumor greater than 4 cm in diameter, extracapsular or extrathyroidal disease) (Cooper et al. 2006). For these reasons, central-compartment (level VI) neck dissection should be considered at the primary operation for patients with papillary thyroid cancer and in those with suspected Hürthle cell cancer. Lateral neck compartment lymph node dissection should be performed for patients with biopsy-proven metastatic cervical lymphadenopathy detected either clinically or by preoperative imaging.

9.4.1.2
Radioiodine Ablation

Following a total or near-total thyroidectomy, some radioiodine uptake is usually demonstrable in the thyroid bed. ^{131}I-induced destruction of this residual thyroid tissue is known as radioiodine remnant ablation. ^{131}I ablation can eradicate all remaining thyroid cells, including possible residual microscopic disease and thus possibly reduces the risk of local and distant tumor recurrence. On the basis of a number of large, retrospective studies, most patients with well-differentiated tumors greater than 1–1.5 cm in diameter receive ^{131}I ablation (HAY et al. 2002; MAZZAFERRI 1997). However, other similar studies show no such benefit, at least among the majority of patients with papillary thyroid cancer, who are at the lowest risk for mortality. However, no prospective studies have been performed to address this question (SAWKA et al. 2004). Moreover, recent data indicate that the incidence of a secondary malignancy after radioiodine might be higher than previously thought (SANDEEP et al. 2006). For these reasons, the decision about ^{131}I ablation should be individualized. Several factors other than size of tumor, such as the presence of metastases, completeness of excision, age, degree of invasion, and associated comorbidities should be taken into account. ^{131}I ablation may not be helpful in patients with Hürthle cell cancer because this tumor often takes up ^{131}I poorly.

To undergo successful treatment with radioactive iodine, patients must have an elevated TSH level ($>30 \text{ uIU mL}^{-1}$), which is usually obtained by withdrawing thyroid hormone for a period of 4 weeks. Recombinant human TSH (rhTSH) has recently been approved by the US Food and Drug Administration for use in radioiodine scanning of patients with follicular cell-derived cancers. Some patients, unable to tolerate hypothyroidism or unable to generate an elevated TSH, have undergone successful remnant ablation with rhTSH (PACINI et al. 2002; ROBBINS et al. 2002). An international, randomized, controlled study demonstrates comparable remnant ablation rates in patients prepared for ^{131}I remnant ablation with 3.7 GBq by either administering rhTSH or with-holding thyroid hormone. rhTSH-prepared patients maintained a higher quality of life and received less radiation exposure to the blood (PACINI et al. 2006). On the basis of clinical trials, adverse reactions include nausea, headaches, asthenia, vomiting, dizziness or paresthesias, chills, fever, and other nonspecific symptoms. These side effects were transient and never serious.

9.4.1.3
External Beam Radiotherapy

Postoperative adjuvant external beam radiotherapy (EBRT) is infrequently indicated for well-differentiated thyroid cancer. The main indications for adjuvant radiotherapy are (1) gross evidence of local tumor invasion at surgery, presumed to have significant macro- or microscopic residual disease, particularly if the residual tumor fails to concentrate sufficient amounts of radioiodine; and (2) extensive T_4 disease in patients older than 60 years of age with extensive extranodal spread after optimal surgery, even in the absence of evidence residual disease. There are reports of responses among patients with locally advanced disease, with improved relapse-free and cause-specific survival (MEADOWS et al. 2006; BIERMANN et al. 2005). It remains unknown whether EBRT might reduce the risk for recurrence in the neck after adequate primary surgery and/or radioiodine treatment. Owing to the scarring that is caused by EBRT, most surgeons only resort EBRT when surgery is no longer feasible or when there is known untreated residual disease.

9.4.1.4
Chemotherapy

There are no data to support the use of adjunctive chemotherapy in the management of well-differentiated thyroid cancer. Doxorubicin (adriamycin) may act as a radiation sensitizer in some tumors of thyroid origin, and could be considered for patients with locally advanced disease undergoing external beam radiation.

9.4.2
Poorly Differentiated and Anaplastic Thyroid Cancer

9.4.2.1
Surgery

Surgical management is the principal treatment approach for poorly differentiated thyroid cancer (PAREL and SHAHA 2006). Owing to the aggressive nature of this tumor, a total thyroidectomy is necessary. The role of surgery in anaplastic thyroid cancer, with removal of all gross disease, remains controversial. Complete surgical resection is rarely feasible because patients often present at an advanced stage. A recent consensus on the treatment of anaplastic thyroid cancer suggests that total thyroidectomy is justified if cervical and mediastinal disease can be resected with limited morbidity (AACE/ACE 2001). Resection of vital structures, such as the larynx, pharynx, and esophagus, should be avoided. Palliative management is meant to prevent death from asphyxiation. Tracheostomy is considered when the airway is compressed by local disease.

9.4.2.2
Radiotherapy

The use of radioiodine ablation and EBRT in poorly differentiated thyroid cancer is still controversial. Although prospective evidence for its use and efficacy is not available, most surgeons advocate the use of radioiodine ablation and L-thyroxine because these tumors display differentiated epithelial function with aggressive behavior, with high rates of regional and distant metastases. No studies have specially evaluated the use of EBRT in poorly differentiated thyroid cancer. On the basis of the characteristics of the tumor and the patient, EBRT may represent an added treatment modality. Patients with unresectable disease, incompletely excised tumors, and locoregional recurrences might benefit from EBRT.

Anaplastic thyroid cancer does not concentrate ^{131}I. Therefore, the only radiation option is EBRT. The effect of EBRT is limited, and most patients progress and ultimately die of their disease. In select cases, EBRT, in combination with surgery and/or chemotherapy, can improve short-term survival and provide some palliation (Lo et al. 1999). However, the timing, dose, and mode of delivery of EBRT remain controversial.

9.4.2.3
Chemotherapy

Most data for the use of chemotherapy in thyroid cancer are based on studies performed for anaplastic thyroid cancer. The most effective agent is adriamycin (doxorubicin). The approved combination by the FDA includes adriamycin and cisplatin with hyperfractionated radiotherapy with or without debulking surgery.

Currently many new agents that inhibit a variety of signaling pathways are under investigation for their use in anaplastic and poorly-differentiated thyroid cancers. These agents have shown some promise in early clinical studies. Given the poor efficacy of traditional chemotherapy, these patients should be encouraged to participate in clinical trials.

9.4.3
Medullary Thyroid Cancer

9.4.3.1
Surgery

Because of the frequent multicentricity of sporadic medullary thyroid cancer (about 20%), total thyroidectomy is appropriate for all cases, irrespective of primary tumor size (CLARK 1997). Controversy exists, however, regarding the indications for and the extent of lymph node surgery. All patients with established medullary thyroid cancer should undergo a bilateral central compartment node dissection, because recent results have demonstrated that the central neck lymph node compartment is involved in 33% of cases with tumors 10 mm or less (pT1) in diameter (UKKAT et al. 2004). Patients with pT2–4 tumors, or palpable lymph nodes in the central or lateral compartment without distant metastases, should in addition undergo bilateral selective neck dissection of levels IIa–Vb (UKKAT et al. 2004). Patients with distant metastases at presentation usually have an unfavorable course that does not warrant extended surgery apart from total thyroidectomy and selective removal of symptomatic lymph nodes or tumor infiltrates to prevent local complications (BTA/RCP 2007). Even with widespread disease, patients often have a prolonged survival despite debilitating symptoms from tumor persistence or progression.

Prophylactic surgery should be offered to patients identified through genetic screening to be carriers of germ line RET mutations (DE GROOT et al. 2006). Germ line RET mutations are associated with nearly a 100% lifetime risk of developing medullary thyroid cancer

(DE GROOT et al. 2006). Children with multiple endocrine neoplasia (MEN) 2B should undergo prophylactic thyroidectomy within the first year of life (OGILVIE and KEBEBEW 2006). Children with MEN 2A should undergo prophylactic thyroidectomy before the age of 5 years. In children with MEN 2A under the age of 10, it may be unnecessary to perform a lymph node dissection (BTA/RCP 2007). However, in older children and those with MEN 2B, central compartment lymphadenectomy should probably be performed at the time of thyroidectomy (BTA/RCP 2007).

9.4.3.2
Radiotherapy

MTC is not very sensitive to EBRT. Routine EBRT has not been shown to improve survival but may improve the relapse-free rate if there is gross microscopic residual disease or extensive nodal disease (PINCHERA and ELISEI 2006). In the event of local-regional recurrence, reoperation is the preferred treatment. Radiation therapy should be avoided unless local disease is symptomatic or rapidly progressing and is not amenable to resection. Conversely, irradiation may be beneficial in treating symptomatic distant metastases, especially bone metastases (PINCHERA and ELISEI 2006).

9.4.3.3
Chemotherapy

Experience with chemotherapy is limited in advanced or metastatic medullary thyroid cancer. Drugs investigated include cisplatin, cyclophosphamide, dacarbazine, doxorubicin, 5-fluorouracil, streptozocin, vincristine, and vindesine. Unfortunately, traditional chemotherapy is generally ineffective in this disease. Several new agents that inhibit a variety of signaling pathways, including RET, VEGF, EGFR, and PDGF, are currently undergoing evaluation for their use in metastatic medullary thyroid cancer (SIPPEL et al. 2008a, b).

Abbreviations

CT	Computed tomography
EBRT	External-beam radiation therapy
FNA	Fine needle aspiration
MRI	Magnetic resonance imaging
MEN	Multiple endocrine neoplasia
PET	Positron emission tomography
RAI	Radioactive iodine
TSH	Thyroid stimulating hormone

References

AJCC Cancer Staging Manual, Sixth Edition (2002). Greene, Frederick. Springer Publications. Part 2, Chapter 8 Thyroid. Pgs 89–98.

Al-Nahhas A, Khan S, Gogbashian A et al. (2008) 18F-FDG PET in the diagnosis and follow-up of thyroid malignancy. In Vivo 22:109–114

American Association of Clinical Endocrinologists (AACE). American College of Endocrinology (ACE). Thyroid Carcinoma Task Force (2001) AACE/AAES medical/surgical guidelines for clinical practice: management of thyroid carcinoma. Endocr Pract 7:202–220

Ashcraft MW, Van Herle AJ (1981) Management of thyroid nodules. II: scanning techniques, thyroid suppressive therapy, and fine needle aspiration. Head Neck Surg 3:297–322

BTA (British Thyroid Association)/Royal College of Physicians (RCP) (2007) Guidelines for the management of thyroid cancer, 2nd edn. BTA/RCP, London

Biermann M, Pixberg M, Schuck A et al. (2005) External beam radiotherapy. In: Biersack H-J, Grünwald F (eds). Thyroid cancer. Springer, Heidelberg, pp 139–161

Buscombe JR (2007) Radionuclides in the management of thyroid cancer. Cancer Imaging 7:202–209

Chen H, Nicol TL, Zeiger MA et al. (1998) Ann Surg 277:542–546

Clark OH (1997) Fine-needle aspiration biopsy and management of thyroid tumors. Am J Clin Pathol. Oct;108 (4 Suppl 1): S22–5.

Cooper DS, Doherty GM, Haugen BR et al. (2006) The American Thyroid Association Guidelines Taskforce. Management guidelines for patients with thyroid nodules and differentiated thyroid cancer. Thyroid 16:109–142

de Groot JW, Links TP, Plukker JT et al. (2006) RET as a diagnostic and therapeutic target in sporadic and hereditary endocrine tumors. Endocr Rev 27:535–560

Debatin JF, Brandau W (2004) Value of (124) I-PET/CT in staging of patients with differentiated thyroid cancer. Eur Radiol 14:2092–2098

Freudenberg LS, Antoch G, Jentzen W et al. (2007) Magnetic resonance imaging of thyroid cancer. Top Magn Reson Imaging 18:293–302

Greenbelt DY, Woltman T, Harter J et al. (2006) Fine-needle aspiration optimizes surgical management in patients with thyroid cancer. Ann Surg Oncol 13:859–863

Hay ID, Thompson GB, Grant CS et al. (2002) Papillary thyroid carcinoma managed at the Mayo Clinic during six decades (1940–1999): temporal trends in initial therapy and long-term outcome in 2444 consecutively treated patients. World J Surg 26:879–885

Haymart MR, Repplinger DJ, Leverson GE et al. (2008) Higher serum thyroid stimulating hormone level in thyroid nodule patients is associated with greater risks of differentiated thyroid cancer and advanced tumor stage. J Clin Endocrinol Metab 93:809–814

Jemal A, Siegel R, Ward E et al. (2008) Cancer statistics, 2008. CA Cancer J Clin 58:71–96

Parel KN, Shaha AR (2006) Poorly differentiated and anaplastic thyroid cancer. Cancer control 13:119–128

Landis SH, Murray T, Bolden S et al. (1998) Cancer statistics CA. Cancer J Clin 48:6–29

Lo CY, Lam KY, Wan KY et al. (1999) Anaplastic carcinoma of the thyroid. Am J Surg 177:337–339

Mazzaferri EL, Jhiang SM (1994) Long-term impact of initial surgical and medical therapy on papillary and follicular thyroid cancer. Am J Med 97:418–428

Meadows KM, Amdur RJ, Morris CG et al. (2006) External beam radiotherapy for differentiated thyroid cancer. Am J Otolaryngol 27:24–28

Mazzaferri EL (1997) Thyroid remnant 131I ablation for papillary and follicular thyroid carcinoma. Thyroid 7:265–271

Mazzaferri EL (1999) An overview of the management of papillary and follicular thyroid carcinoma. Thyroid 9:421–417

Ogilvie JB, Kebebew E (2006) Indication and timing of thyroid surgery for patients with hereditary medullary thyroid cancer syndromes. J Natl Compr Canc Netw 4:139–147

Pacini F, Molinaro E, Castagna MG et al. (2002) Ablation of thyroid residues with 30 mCi 131I: a comparison in thyroid cancer patients prepared with recombinant human TSH or thyroid hormone withdrawal. J Clin Endocrinol Metab 87:4063–4068

Pacini F, Ladenson PW, Schlumberger M et al. (2006) Radioiodine ablation of thyroid remnants after preparation with recombinant human thyrotropin in differentiated thyroid carcinoma: results of an international, randomized, controlled study. J Clin Endocrinol Metab 91:926–932

Pinchera A, Elisei R (2006) Medullary thyroid caner: diagnosis and management. In: Mazzaferri EL, Harmer C, Mallick UK, Kendall-Taylor P (eds) Practical management of thyroid cancer: a multidisciplinary approach. Springer, London, pp 255–280

Robbins RJ, Larson SM, Sinha N et al. (2002) A retrospective review of the effectiveness of recombinant human TSH as a preparation for radioiodine thyroid remnant ablation. J Nucl Med 43:1482–1488

Sawka AM, Thephamongkhol K, Brouwers M et al. (2004) Clinical review 170: a systematic review and metaanalysis of the effectiveness of radioactive iodine remnant ablation for well-differentiated thyroid cancer. J Clin Endocrinol Metab 89:3668–3676

Sandeep TC, Strachan MW, Reynolds RM et al. (2006) Second primary cancers in thyroid cancer patients: a multinational record linkage study. J Clin Endocrinol Metab 91: 1819–1825

Sakamoto A, Kasai N, Sugano H. (1983) Poorly differentiated carcinoma of the thyroid. A clinicopathologic entity for a high-risk group of papillary and follicular carcinomas. Cancer 52:1849–1855

Sippel RS, Elaraj DM, Khanafshar E et al. (2008a) Tumor size predicts malignant potential in hürthle cell neoplasms of the thyroid. World J Surg 32:702–707

Sippel RS, Kunnimalaiyaan M, Chen H (2008b) Current management of medullary thyroid cancer. Oncologist 13:539–547

Ukkat J, Gimm O, Brauckhoff M et al. (2004) Single center experience in primary surgery for medullary thyroid carcinoma. World J Surg 28:1271–1274

Watkinson JC, Franklyn JA, Olliff JF (2006) Detection and surgical treatment of cervical lymph nodes in differentiated thyroid cancer. Thyroid 16:187–194

Wong KT, Ahuja AT (2005) Ultrasound of thyroid cancer. Cancer Imaging 5:157–166

Yang J, Schnadig V, Logrono R et al. (2007) Fine-needle aspiration of thyroid nodules: a study of 4703 patients with histologic and clinical correlations. Cancer 111(5):306–15.

Cervical Lymph Node Metastases from Unknown Primary Tumors

10

Cai Grau

CONTENTS

10.1 **Introduction** *125*

10.2 **Incidence** *126*

10.3 **Diagnostic Workup** *126*

10.4 **Treatment** *127*
10.4.1 Surgery *127*
10.4.2 Radiotherapy *127*
10.4.3 Chemotherapy *129*

10.5 **Follow-Up** *129*

10.6 **Prognostic Factors** *129*

10.7 **Patterns of Failure** *130*

10.8 **Morbidity** *131*

10.9 **Conclusions and Future Directions** *131*

References *131*

KEY POINTS

- Patients with neck node metastases from occult squamous cell or undifferentiated head and neck cancer (CUP) constitute 2–3% of all head and neck malignancies.
- Diagnostic imaging with computer tomography or magnetic resonance and FDG-PET followed by panendoscopy with biopsies from potential primary sites are recommended for patients presenting with CUP.

CAI GRAU, MD, DMSC
Department of Oncology, Aarhus University Hospital, Noerrebrogade 44, DK-8000 Aarhus C, Denmark

- Treatment options include neck dissection alone, neck dissection with postoperative radiotherapy, or definite radiotherapy. Prospective or randomized studies are not available.
- Early stages (N1 and selected N2a disease) can be managed with neck dissection alone or radiotherapy alone.
- Advanced disease (N2 and N3 patients) can be managed with neck dissection and postoperative radiotherapy or radiotherapy alone.
- Extensive irradiation of both sides of the neck and the mucosa results in fewer emerging primaries and regional failures, compared with patients treated with ipsilateral techniques or surgery, but the effect on survival is less clear. Prospective studies on this topic are warranted.
- The value of chemotherapy in CUP is unknown, but concomitant chemoradiotherapy may be justified based on the documented value in patients with nodal metastasis from a known primary tumor.

10.1
Introduction

Cervical lymph node metastases from squamous cell or undifferentiated unknown primary tumors (CUP) are rare, constituting 2–3% of all new head and neck cancers. The management of these patients remains a major challenge in oncology. The diagnosis of CUP relies on the absence of a primary tumor after the completion of an extensive workup. Recent developments in imaging and pathology have increased our diagnostic spectrum considerably, but the impact of these techniques on decision-making has not been well documented. The selection and timing of the diagnostic measures in the workup process are still under debate, and the choice of treatment is controversial. Treatment options and recommendations vary from surgery alone in selected cases, limited field radiotherapy, where only the ipsilateral neck is treated, or extensive prophylactic irradiation of all potential mucosal sites as well as both sides of the neck. While these strategies may differ in the rate of emerging primary tumors and morbidity, no randomized or prospective studies are available to support either of these approaches in particular. These issues are summarized and discussed in this chapter. More detailed reviews are given in Jereczek-Fossa et al. (2004) and Nieder et al. (2001).

10.2
Incidence

The reported incidence of CUP is about 2–3% of all head and neck cancers (Grau et al. 2000; Jereczek-Fossa et al. 2004). In the Danish national study, the annual incidence of CUP was 0.34 cases/100,000/year, and was stable over a 20-year period (Grau et al. 2000). CUP is one of the most frequent causes of isolated mass in the neck. Enlarged lymph nodes are most frequently observed in level II, followed by level III. Lymph nodes in levels I, IV, and V are much less frequent (Fig. 10.1). Unilateral lymph node involvement is more common; bilateral involvement is present in about 10% of patients. Median nodal size is 5 cm (Grau et al. 2000).

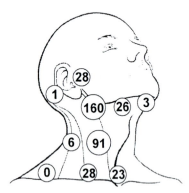

Fig. 10.1. The distribution of enlarged lymph nodes according to anatomical levels in a retrospective series of 277 CUP patients. Adapted from Grau et al. (2000)

Metastases in the upper and middle neck are generally related to cancers of the head and neck region, whereas metastases limited to the lower neck (supraclavicular area) are often associated with primaries below the clavicles.

As for other head and neck cancers, the age at diagnosis is generally between 55 and 65 years. Younger median age in some series may partially be explained by the inclusion of more undifferentiated tumors. The majority of patients are males.

10.3
Diagnostic Workup

Classification of a patient as having CUP is done if adequate investigations fail to detect a possible primary tumor when a final treatment decision is made (Grau et al. 2000). Typically, the diagnosis of a CUP requires a proper examination of the head and neck mucosa with a fiber-optic and a rigid endoscopy under general anesthesia in addition to state-of-the-art imaging. Biopsies are taken from any suspicious site and blindly from sites of possible origin of the primary, e.g., base of tongue, piriform sinus, or nasopharynx. A systematic tonsillectomy has been recommended since up to 25% of invasive squamous cell carcinomas are detected here (Jereczek-Fossa et al. 2004; Issing et al. 2003). Some authors recommend bilateral tonsillectomy, since about 10% of all tonsillary carcinomas are bilateral (Issing et al. 2003; Haas et al. 2002).

A search for a thoracic primary tumor is justified in patients presenting with pathologic lymph nodes in the lower neck. Whether-laser induced fluorescence imaging will be useful to guide biopsy sampling requires further assessment.

Imaging includes computer tomography (CT) scan and/or magnetic resonance (MRI), as well as positron-emission tomography using 18-flourine-labeled deoxyglucose (FDG-PET) (Rades et al. 2001; Stoeckli et al. 2003; Issing et al. 2003; Fogarty et al. 2003; Lassen et al. 1999; Regelink et al. 2002). The detection rate with the use of CT or MR scan is about 20%. FDG-PET has an overall staging accuracy of 75%, a positive predictive value of 70%, a negative predictive value of 80%, a sensitivity of 63–100%, and a specificity of 90% (Stoeckli et al. 2003; Regelink et al. 2002). A Danish multicenter study with 60 patients showed that FDG-PET found a primary tumor or further (distant) metastatic disease in 30 patients (JOHANSEN et al. 2008). When FDG-PET was performed before panendoscopy fewer false-positive pathological foci were found, compared with when FDG-PET was done after biopsy. Another study showed that a therapeutic change of treatment was made in 20 or 69%, respectively, as a consequence of FDG-PET (REGELINK et al. 2002; RADES et al. 2001). On the basis of such studies FDG-PET is now recommended as an early diagnostic modality in the workup of CUP. Biopsies should preferably be performed after PET scan has been done, since such a sequence allows for sampling of the areas suspected in PET and avoids false-positive PET scans at biopsy site. PET may play a role to exclude other metastases, in selection of patients with residual disease after radiotherapy and subsequent monitoring.

The presence of Epstein-Barr virus detected with in situ hybridization in metastatic lymph nodes from CUP may be suggestive for nasopharyngeal tumor (LEE et al. 2000). Human papillomavirus detected by polymerase chain reaction may indicate oropharyngeal cancer. More studies are needed to evaluate the role of molecular investigations and to understand the biology of CUP.

10.4
Treatment

Various curative treatment options have been proposed for patients with CUP: neck dissection alone, neck dissection with postoperative radiotherapy, node excision (for small single node) with postoperative radiotherapy, or radiotherapy followed by some form of salvage surgery (ASLANI et al. 2007; GRAU et al. 2000; WEIR et al. 1995; GLYNNE-JONES et al. 1990; JERECZEK-FOSSA et al. 2004; NIEDER et al. 2001; COLLETIER et al. 1998). There are no prospective or randomized studies to guide us to the best treatment, so treatment decisions must rely on data from retrospective series and individual considerations. A review of the literature suggests that early stages (N1 and selected N2a disease) can be managed with neck dissection alone or radiotherapy alone with equally satisfactory nodal control, whereas combined modalities are recommended for N2b, N2c, and N3 patients. For the latter group, nodal resection and radiotherapy to bilateral neck nodes and potential mucosal sites seem to result in better locoregional control and survival, compared with patients receiving either

nodal resection and ipsilateral irradiation, or radiation alone. More details are given in JERECZEK-FOSSA et al. (2004).

10.4.1
Surgery

The extent of surgery, in addition to the diagnostic excisional biopsy, and the combination of surgical procedures with radiotherapy are still controversial. A review showed that the emergence rate of the primary tumor after surgery alone was about 25%, the median nodal recurrence rate 34%, and the 5-year overall survival rate 66% (NIEDER et al. 2001). Surgery alone was therefore recommended in selected patients with N1 disease without extracapsular extension and with no history of incisional or excisional biopsy (ERKAL et al. 2001b; NIEDER et al. 2001; GLYNNE-JONES et al. 1990). In the case of a history of incisional or excisional biopsy for N1 disease, postoperative irradiation is indicated (HARPER et al. 1990). Planned neck dissection after radiotherapy has shown persistence of nodal disease in up to 44% of patients (NIEDER et al. 2001). Such a sequence was associated with poorer survival and with higher postoperative morbidity when compared with surgery followed by radiotherapy. However, selection bias may be involved, since the use of radiotherapy is typically attempted in patients with advanced, inoperable neck disease. In the absence of randomized studies this issue will remain unresolved.

10.4.2
Radiotherapy

Radiotherapy may be given in combination with surgery or as definitive treatment, reserving surgery for salvage. Most patients managed with surgery receive adjuvant postoperative irradiation. Various radiotherapy techniques have been used, but they can be divided into two groups, one treating ipsilateral neck only, the other treating bilateral neck, including head and neck mucosa sites in the pharyngeal axis as a potential site of primary.

Target volume for *ipsilateral* irradiation includes the ipsilateral neck only or both ipsilateral neck and ipsilateral oral cavity, oropharynx, and larynx. The target volume for *extensive* irradiation depends on the nodal involvement. For patients with level II and V nodal involvement, the target volume should include naso- and oropharynx mucosa. In patients with level III involvement, oropharynx should always be included, as it is the most common site of emerging primary. Naso- and hypopharynx, as well as larynx, are generally also included, but subsites may be individually avoided based on the probability of occult squamous cell carcinoma and the potential complications of large-volume radiotherapy. A small study has suggested that limited larynx blocking may be safe in CUP (Barker et al. 2005).

The choice of including mucosal sites or not remains one of the most controversial topics in the management of occult head and neck primaries. In many countries mucosal irradiation to prevent emerging primaries has been the rule over the last two decades (Grau et al. 2000; Nieder et al. 2001). Irradiation of the entire pharyngeal axis and the larynx causes significant acute and late morbidity. Although not demonstrated in retrospective analyses, it is well known from other head and neck series that radiation morbidity is highly related to the irradiated volume. The arguments for ipsilateral treatment have been that by sparing most of the mucosa and the entire contralateral neck, patients will tolerate treatment much better and have the same survival rate (Weir et al. 1995). On the other hand, the arguments for large mucosal fields have been to prevent potentially incurable locoregional relapses. This dilemma between safety and morbidity is evident from the data in the large Danish study (Grau et al. 2000). Patients treated with ipsilateral technique had a relative risk of recurrence in the head and neck region of 1.9 ($p = 0.05$), compared with patients treated to both neck and mucosa (Fig. 10.2). At 5 years, the estimated control rates were 27 and 51%, respectively. For disease-specific survival, N-stage, gender, and overall treatment time were independent factors. The irradiated volume did not significantly influence survival; when adjusted for cofactors the 5-year disease-specific survival estimates were 28 and 45%, respectively ($p = 0.10$). In contrast, two recent analyses of patient series from Italy found significantly better survival in the group treated with extensive radiotherapy (Beldi et al. 2007; Boscolo-Rizzo et al. 2006). Unfortunately, there will probably not be data available from randomized trials on this subject. A worldwide intergroup comparative study, including quality of life measures, was stopped prematurely because of poor accrual.

Radiotherapy significantly reduces the risk of having an emerging mucosal primary when compared with patients treated with surgery alone. In fact, the incidence of emerging primary after radiotherapy seems to be similar to the incidence of metachronous cancers in other head and neck cancer series, where a constant rate of 3%/year has been reported (see Sect. 10.7).

Patients presenting with poor performance status, very extensive nodal involvement, distant metastases, or bilateral low neck involvement can be offered palliative irradiation. A study has shown that palliative radiotherapy is associated with an objective response rate of 65%, the symptomatic response rate of 57% at 1 year, and 25% 1-year survival (Erkal et al. 2001a).

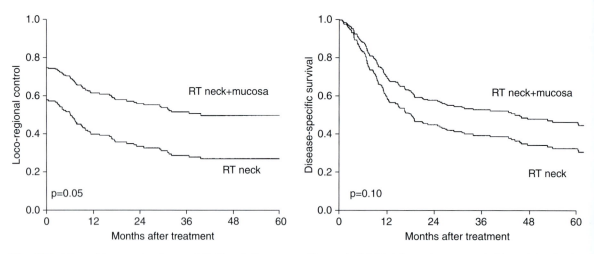

Fig. 10.2. Adjusted loco-regional control (*left*) and disease-specific survival (*right*) for patients treated either with selective ipsilateral radiotherapy or extensive radiotherapy to both sides of the neck and mucosal surfaces. The two groups are plotted at means of covariates. Reprinted with permission from Grau et al. (2000)

10.4.3
Chemotherapy

There is no clear evidence supporting the systematic use of chemotherapy in patients with CUP. Platinum-based chemotherapy preceding radiotherapy for CUP is recommended for N3 disease by the European Society of Medical Oncology, whereas irradiation alone is suggested for N1 and N2 patients (JERECZEK-FOSSA et al. 2004). The role of chemotherapy in patients with CUP could however be inferred from what is known of the value of chemotherapy for treating other head and neck cancers. For patients with stage III or IV squamous cell carcinoma with a known primary site, a large meta-analysis concluded that chemotherapy were advantageous only when chemotherapy was given concomitantly to radiation (PIGNON et al. 2000). Level I evidence has also been established for the postoperative adjuvant treatment of patients with selected high-risk locally advanced head and neck cancers, with the publication of the results of two trials conducted by the European Organization Research and Treatment of Cancer (BERNIER et al. 2004) and in the United States by the Radiation Therapy Oncology Group (COOPER et al. 2004).

10.5
Follow-Up

Clinical follow-up with a complete clinical examination of the oral cavity, pharynx, larynx, and the neck, and routine use of endoscopic evaluation and post-treatment imaging for response evaluation are generally recommended after treatment for CUP. Suspicious recurrence in the neck and/or emergence of a primary tumor should be confirmed by appropriate imaging modalities (CT, MRI, PET) and by histopathological examination of biopsy specimen or fine-needle aspiration from lymph node. In patients subjected to neck irradiation, thyroid function testing should be considered prior to therapy and as a follow-up procedure, since up to 30% of patients may develop hypothyroidism (JERECZEK-FOSSA et al. 2004).

10.6
Prognostic Factors

Depending on patient and tumor characteristics, reported 5-year actuarial survival rates of patients with cervical nodal metastasis from an unknown primary carcinoma range from 18 to 63% (NIEDER and ANG 2002). Prognostic factors for survival include N-stage, number of nodes, grading, extracapsular extension, and performance status. Retrospective studies suggest that neck relapse is more common than are distant metastases or emergence of mucosal primary tumors. For the 277 patients in the large Danish series, the 5-year estimates of neck control, disease-specific and overall survival for radically treated patients were 51, 48, and 36%, respectively (GRAU et al. 2000). The most important factor for treatment outcome and survival was the nodal stage. Figure 10.3 shows the locoregional tumor control in the three N-stages. Patients with N1 and N2 disease had a significantly better prognosis, compared with N3 patients. These figures are comparable to those observed in patients with known primary sites and similar extent of disease in the neck. Other important factors for treatment outcome were gender (females did better), hemoglobin (high hemoglobin was better), and differentiation. Differentiation was especially important for the risk of emerging primary, as significantly fewer patients with undifferentiated/poorly differentiated lymph node metastases experienced an emerging primary in the head and neck mucosa. This group also had a marginally better 5-year disease-specific survival (51 vs. 43%; $p = 0.05$) and overall survival (40 vs. 30%; NS).

For patients treated with neck dissection, other prognostic factors for survival included the number of positive nodes, the histopathological grading, and the extracapsular extension. Again, these prognostic

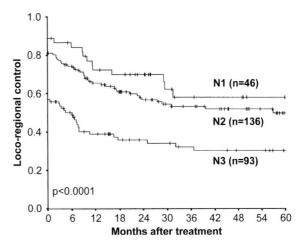

Fig. 10.3. The most important factor for treatment outcome and survival in CUP is the nodal stage. The figure shows the locoregional tumor control in the three N-stages in a series of 277 CUP patients. Reprinted with permission from GRAU et al. (2000)

factors are similar to those that have been reported in patients with a known primary site.

The Danish series showed that for patients receiving radiotherapy, there was a significant negative influence of prolonged overall treatment (50+ days) compared with shorter schedules (GRAU et al. 2000). This effect was evident for neck control and locoregional tumor control, but it was not significant for survival.

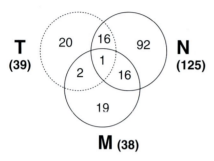

Fig. 10.4. The failure pattern observed in 166 recurrences from a series of 277 patients treated with radical intent. Data from GRAU et al. (2000)

10.7
Patterns of Failure

The pattern of failure depends on the treatment. After extensive radiotherapy, the most common site of failure is the neck nodes. Figure 10.4 shows the failure pattern observed in the Danish series.

The rate of emerging primaries is around 15% after 5 years, ranging from 0 to 57%. In the Danish series, half of the emerging primaries occurred in the head and neck region (GRAU et al. 2000). Oropharynx, especially base of tongue, was the most common site of emerging primary, whereas other occult sites in the head and neck region were rare. Emerging primaries outside the head and neck region were primarily located in the lung and esophagus. Figure 10.5 shows the actuarial probability of being free of emerging primary in the head and neck region for radically treated patients treated with neck dissection only ($n=23$), unilateral radiotherapy with or without neck surgery ($n = 26$), or radiation treatment to both sides of the neck and the mucosal sites

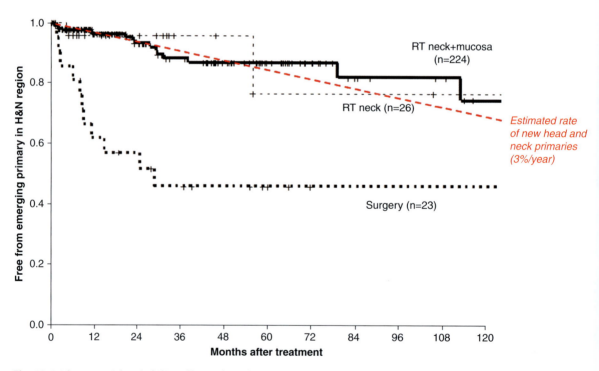

Fig. 10.5. The actuarial probability of being free of emerging primary in the head and neck region for 277 radically treated patients assigned to neck dissection only, unilateral radiotherapy with or without neck surgery, or radiation treatment to both sides of the neck and the mucosal sites in the pharynx and larynx. Adapted from GRAU et al. (2000)

in the pharynx and larynx ($n = 224$). The actuarial values at 10 years were 46, 77, and 75%, respectively. Both radiotherapy groups were significantly better than surgery to control occult mucosal primaries ($p < 0.05$), and there was no difference between the two radiotherapy groups.

The annual rate of 3% for emerging head and neck primaries after radiotherapy is similar to the rate of subsequent primary tumors reported after treatment of squamous cell primary tumors of the head and neck. One explanation for the "mucosal effectiveness" of ipsilateral treatment may be that it unintentionally involves some mucosal irradiation. This effect may be especially important in sterilizing potential lateral tumors in the oropharynx, because this region lies just medially to the commonly involved subdigastric nodes. From such indirect evidence it seems logic to include the ipsilateral tonsillar fossa and base of tongue if decision is made to use unilateral fields.

10.8
Morbidity

Apart from small studies with larynx blocking (BARKER et al. 2005) or intensity-modulated radiotherapy (IMRT) (MADANI et al. 2008), data are lacking on treatment-related morbidity or quality of life for patients with CUP. Such data would be particularly useful for comparing extended and selective irradiation. There are however data supporting the use of parotid-sparing irradiation technique for patients with squamous cell carcinoma in the head and neck, either ipsilateral conformal radiotherapy (JENSEN et al. 2007) or using IMRT (LIN et al. 2003; LEE et al. 2002). More aggressive multimodality approaches may be advantageous, but will be so at the cost of increased morbidity.

10.9
Conclusions and Future Directions

Management of CUP continues to represent a major challenge in head and neck oncology. Conventional diagnostic workup with CT or MRI, FDG-PET, and panendoscopy with random biopsies is recommended. The optimal extent and combination of surgery and radiotherapy are not well defined. Although patients

with minimal nodal disease and no extracapsular spread can be managed with neck dissection without radiotherapy, the majority of patients will need radiotherapy, either postoperatively after neck dissection, or as radiotherapy alone. Retrospective studies suggest that neck relapse is more common than emergence of mucosal primary tumors. Selective radiation to the ipsilateral neck may result in survival and locoregional control rates not significantly worse than irradiation of mucosal sites and bilateral neck nodes, but prospective studies on this topic are warranted. Also the value of adjuvant chemotherapy and molecular targeted therapy should be further investigated.

References

Aslani M, Sultanem K, Voung T et al. (2007) Metastatic carcinoma to the cervical nodes from an unknown head and neck primary site: is there a need for neck dissection? Head Neck 29:585–590

Barker CA, Morris CG, Mendenhall WM (2005) Larynx-sparing radiotherapy for squamous cell carcinoma from an unknown head and neck primary site. Am J Clin Oncol 28:445–448

Beldi D, Jereczek-Fossa BA, D'Onofrio A et al. (2007) Role of radiotherapy in the treatment of cervical lymph node metastases from an unknown primary site: retrospective analysis of 113 patients. Int J Radiat Oncol Biol Phys 69:1051–1058

Bernier J, Domenge C, Ozsahin M et al. (2004) Postoperative irradiation with or without concomitant chemotherapy for locally advanced head and neck cancer. N Engl J Med 350:1945–1952

Boscolo-Rizzo P, Da Mosto MC, Gava A et al. (2006) Cervical lymph node metastases from occult squamous cell carcinoma: analysis of 82 cases. ORL J Otorhinolaryngol Relat Spec 68:189–194

Colletier PJ, Garden AS, Morrison WH et al. (1998) Postoperative radiation for squamous cell carcinoma metastatic to cervical lymph nodes from an unknown primary site: outcomes and patterns of failure. Head Neck 20(8):674–681

Cooper JS, Pajak TF, Forastiere AA et al. (2004) Postoperative concurrent radiotherapy and chemotherapy for high-risk squamous-cell carcinoma of the head and neck. N Engl J Med 350:1937–1944

Erkal HS, Mendenhall WM, Amdur RJ et al. (2001a) Squamous cell carcinomas metastatic to cervical lymph nodes from an unknown head and neck mucosal site treated with radiation therapy with palliative intent. Radiother Oncol 59: 319–321

Erkal HS, Mendenhall WM, Amdur RJ et al. (2001b) Squamous cell carcinomas metastatic to cervical lymph nodes from an unknown head-and-neck mucosal site treated with radiation therapy alone or in combination with neck dissection. Int J Radiat Oncol Biol Phys 50:55–63

Fogarty GB, Peters LJ, Stewart J et al. (2003) The usefulness of fluorine 18-labelled deoxyglucose positron emission tomography in the investigation of patients with cervical lymphadenopathy from an unknown primary tumor. Head Neck 25:138–145

Glynne-Jones RG, Anand AK, Young TE et al. (1990) Metastatic carcinoma in the cervical lymph nodes from an occult primary: a conservative approach to the role of radiotherapy. Int J Radiat Oncol Biol Phys 18:289–294

Grau C, Johansen LV, Jakobsen J et al. (2000) Cervical lymph node metastases from unknown primary tumours. Results from a national survey by the Danish Society for Head and Neck Oncology. Radiother Oncol 55:121–129

Haas I, Hoffmann TK, Engers R et al. (2002) Diagnostic strategies in cervical carcinoma of an unknown primary (CUP). Eur Arch Otorhinolaryngol 259:325–333

Harper CS, Mendenhall WM, Parsons JT et al. (1990) Cancer in neck nodes with unknown primary site: role of mucosal radiotherapy. Head Neck 12:463–469

Issing WJ, Taleban B, Tauber S (2003) Diagnosis and management of carcinoma of unknown primary in the head and neck. Eur Arch Otorhinolaryngol 260:436–443

Jensen K, Overgaard M, Grau C (2007) Morbidity after ipsilateral radiotherapy for oropharyngeal cancer. Radiother Oncol 85:90–97

Jereczek-Fossa BA, Jassem J, Orecchia R (2004) Cervical lymph node metastases of squamous cell carcinoma from an unknown primary. Cancer Treat Rev 30:153–164

Johansen J, Buus S, Loft A et al. (2008) Prospective study of 18FDG-PET in the detection and management of patients with lymph node metastases to the neck from an unknown primary tumor. Results from the DAHANCA-13 study. Head Neck 30:471–478

Lassen U, Daugaard G, Eigtved A et al. (1999) 18F-FDG whole body positron emission tomography (PET) in patients with unknown primary tumours (UPT). Eur J Cancer 35:1076–1082

Lee N, Xia P, Quivey JM et al. (2002) Intensity-modulated radiotherapy in the treatment of nasopharyngeal carcinoma: an update of the UCSF experience. Int J Radiat Oncol Biol Phys 53:12–22

Lee WY, Hsiao JR, Jin YT et al. (2000) Epstein-Barr virus detection in neck metastases by in-situ hybridization in fine-needle aspiration cytologic studies: an aid for differentiating the primary site. Head Neck 22:336–340

Lin A, Kim HM, Terrell JE et al. (2003) Quality of life after parotid-sparing IMRT for head-and-neck cancer: a prospective longitudinal study. Int J Radiat Oncol Biol Phys 57:61–70

Madani I, Vakaet L, Bonte K et al. (2008) Intensity-modulated radiotherapy for cervical lymph node metastases from unknown primary cancer. Int J Radiat Oncol Biol Phys 71:1158–1166

Nieder C, Ang KK (2002) Cervical lymph node metastases from occult squamous cell carcinoma. Curr Treat Options Oncol 3:33–40

Nieder C, Gregoire V, Ang KK (2001) Cervical lymph node metastases from occult squamous cell carcinoma: cut down a tree to get an apple? Int J Radiat Oncol Biol Phys 50:727–733

Pignon JP, Bourhis J, Domenge C et al. (2000) Chemotherapy added to locoregional treatment for head and neck squamous-cell carcinoma: three meta-analyses of updated individual data. MACH-NC Collaborative Group. Meta-analysis of chemotherapy on head and neck cancer. Lancet 355:949–955

Rades D, Kuhnel G, Wildfang I et al. (2001) Localised disease in cancer of unknown primary (CUP): the value of positron emission tomography (PET) for individual therapeutic management. Ann Oncol 12:1605–1609

Regelink G, Brouwer J, de BR et al. (2002) Detection of unknown primary tumours and distant metastases in patients with cervical metastases: value of FDG-PET versus conventional modalities. Eur J Nucl Med Mol Imaging 29:1024–1030

Stoeckli SJ, Mosna-Firlejczyk K, Goerres GW (2003) Lymph node metastasis of squamous cell carcinoma from an unknown primary: impact of positron emission tomography. Eur J Nucl Med Mol Imaging 30:411–416

Weir L, Keane T, Cummings B et al. (1995) Radiation treatment of cervical lymph node metastases from an unknown primary: an analysis of outcome by treatment volume and other prognostic factors. Radiother Oncol 35:206–211

Treatment Techniques with Potential Impact on QOL

Dysphagia-Related Quality of Life of Patients with Cancer in the Oropharynx: An Advantage for Brachytherapy?

PETER C. LEVENDAG, PETER VAN ROOIJ, DAVID N. TEGUH, INGE NOEVER, PETER VOET, HENRIE VAN DER EST, and PAUL I. M. SCHMITZ

CONTENTS

11.1   Introduction   *136*

11.2   Patients and Methods   *136*
11.2.1 Dysphagia   *138*
11.2.2 Xerostomia   *138*
11.2.3 Univariate Dose–Response
        Relationship   *139*

11.3   Results   *139*

11.4   Discussion   *139*

11.5   Conclusions   *142*

References   *143*

PETER C. LEVENDAG, MD, PhD
PETER VAN ROOIJ, MSc
DAVID N. TEGUH, MD
INGE NOEVER, RTT
PETER VOET, RTT
HENRIE VAN DER EST, RTT
Department of Radiation Oncology, Erasmus MC, Daniel den
Hoed Cancer Center, Groene Hilledijk 301, 3075 EA Rotterdam,
The Netherlands
PAUL I. M. SCHMITZ, PhD
Departments of Biostatistics, Erasmus MC, Daniel den Hoed
Cancer Center, Groene Hilledijk 301, 3075 EA Rotterdam,
The Netherlands

KEY POINTS

- Results of conventional head and neck radiotherapy by external beam radiotherapy, including a boost of external beam radiation, with or without concurrent chemotherapy, include a number of side effects among which are dysphagia and xerostomia.
- In addition to side effects, the quality of life is also negatively affected.
- In brachytherapy (BT), high doses are used in a short overall treatment time in relatively small volume disease (accelerated conformal treatment), with excellent tumor control rates.
- The current chapter describes the outcome in 155 patients with tonsillar fossa and/or soft palate tumors ($n = 108$) or cancers of the base of tongue ($n = 47$). Overall, according to chart review, a severe degree of dysphagia (RTOG grades III and IV) was experienced in 31% of the patients. Similarly, according to responses to the EORTC H&N35 QOL questionnaires, severe dysphagia was observed in about 20% of the BT group and about 38% in the non-BT group.
- Univariate analysis demonstrated less dysphagia for the following conditions: lower mean doses applied to swallowing muscles, BT treatment, single neck irradiation, and in case a neck dissection is performed. The multivariate analysis shows a significant effect for BT (~ implicating less swallowing complaints due to the lower doses of radiation received by the swallowing muscles).
- For improvement of the dysphagia-related QOL, it is suggested to try and further optimize the dose distribution.

11.1
Introduction

In organ preservation therapy, for cancer in the head and neck, over the years a number of investigators have noted a significant increase in dysphagia, defined as swallowing problems that most likely relate to more aggressive treatment regimes used in order to obtain better tumor control rates. The aggressive nature of the treatment modalities is exemplified by high doses of radiation and/or (accelerated) fractionation regimens, with or without (concomitant) chemotherapy (LEVENDAG et al. 2004). Xerostomia has been well documented in patients treated with chemotherapy (CHT) and/or radiation. It has been argued that the degree of xerostomia corresponds with the amount of dysphagia experienced by the patient (LOGEMANN et al. 2001, 2003). To define potential rehabilitation strategies, it is important to investigate first the anatomical structures and functionality of the swallowing apparatus. Examples of preventative measures are the pre- and posttreatment exercises and/or the introduction of Therabite (BURKHEAD et al. 2006; KULBERSH et al. 2006). Few studies have examined the association of dysphagia with the location of the primary tumor site (PAULOSKI et al. 2000, 2002).

This chapter analyses the response to validated QOL questionnaires in search of (severe) late side effects, such as swallowing disorders and xerostomia, in patients with oropharyngeal cancers treated between 1991 and 2005 in a single institution (Erasmus MC). The patient retrieval for the current analysis consisted of patients with tonsillar fossa and/or soft palate (TF and/or SP) or base-of-tongue (BOT) tumors treated by radiation therapy (RT). Over time the primary tumor was boosted by various RT techniques, that is, by either a parallel-opposed (P-O) field configuration, or by 3D conformal radiotherapy (3DCRT), intensity-modulated radiotherapy (IMRT), or brachytherapy (BT). A treatment regime using conventional 2 Gy/day fractionation, combined with a BT boost, has been applied in our institute by far the most over a great number of years (1991–2008) for various reasons: With regard to tumor control, HDR/PDR fractionation is given in an accelerated fashion with intrinsic dose escalation. A high conformality is obtained because of an accurate CTV delineation, no PTV margin (because catheters move with movement of target area), and rapid dose fall-off. The invasiveness of the procedure, the need for albeit some dexterity, the logistics in the OR, and patients being medically unfit for any type of surgical procedure are some of the disadvantages of BT. This chapter reports in particular those patients treated with BT.

11.2
Patients and Methods

All patients with squamous cell carcinoma of the oropharynx were treated by RT in the Erasmus MC. Patients were seen in joint consultation by the radiation-oncologist and HN surgeon. Diagnosis was established by clinical examination, and preferentially by panendoscopy, CT, and/or MRI of the head and neck. Biopsy of the primary tumor and, in the majority of cases, ultrasound-guided fine-needle aspiration of the suspicious regional lymph nodes were performed. Staging was done according to the TNM classification, 2002 edition (GREENE et al. 2006).

The actuarial loco-regional control rate, disease-free survival, and overall survival of the 336 patients, stratified for type of booster technique (BT vs. non-BT), are depicted in Fig. 11.1 (LRC; 5 years 84 vs. 60%), Fig. 11.2 (DFS; 5 years 59 vs. 43%), and Fig. 11.3, (OS; 5 years 64 vs. 39%).

Of the 336 patients treated, 155 were disease free with a minimum follow-up of 1 year and were selected for the purpose of the present QOL analysis.

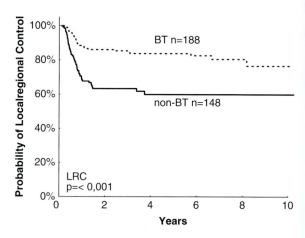

Fig. 11.1. Loco-regional control of tumors in the oropharynx, treated between 1991 and 2005 in the Erasmus Medical Center – Daniel den Hoed Cancer Center. (BT, non-BT): primary tumors (tonsillar fossa and soft palate, base of tongue) were boosted by BT or by non-BT techniques

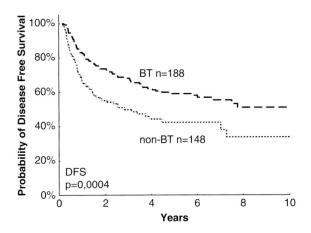

Fig. 11.2. Disease-free survival of patients with tumors in the oropharynx, treated between 1991 and 2005 in the Erasmus Medical Center – Daniel den Hoed Cancer Center.

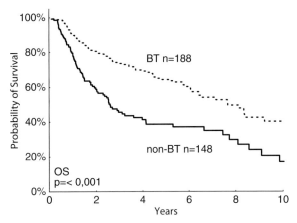

Fig. 11.3. Overall survival of patients with tumors in the oropharynx, treated between 1991 and 2005 in the Erasmus Medical Center – Daniel den Hoed Cancer Center

Ninety-one patients were male, and 64 female; mean age was 56 years (range, 35–78). Primary tumor sites were TF or SP ($n = 108$), or BOT ($n = 47$); 119/155 (77%) of patients were stages III and IV; for stage grouping, see also Tables 11.1 and 11.2.

Over the years, the treatment of preference for T1–T3 TF and/or SP tumors and T1–T4 cancer of the BOT consisted of a first series of 46 Gy (2 Gy/fraction, five fractions/week; as of 2000, six fractions/week) by a P-O technique, 3DCRT, or IMRT to the neck and primary tumor, followed by a boost of fractionated high dose rate/or pulsed dose rate BT to the primary tumor. The doses of the external beam radiotherapy techniques are prescribed according to the International Commission on Radiation Units and Measurement 50 and 62 recommendations. In case of BT, the dose was prescribed to 0.5–0.75 cm of the catheter plane (TF and/or SP tumors; single plane implant), or to 85% of the mean central dose (BOT volume implant). The total dose of fractionated HDR was 20 Gy (4 Gy, 4 × 3 Gy, 4 Gy; two fractions/day 8-h interval minimum); in case of PDR, 22 Gy (2 Gy, 18 × 1 Gy, 2 Gy; interval 3 h) was given. In case of neck nodes, a neck dissection (ND) was executed in the same surgical session as BT was applied. All patients were treated preferably by a BT boost (BT group; $n = 107$; 83 TF/SP, 24 BOT); in case BT was not feasible, non-BT boost techniques were used (non-BT group; $n = 48$; 25 TF/SP, 23 BOT). The non-BT techniques used consisted of P-O techniques (P-O; $n = 24$), 3DCRT ($n = 9$), or IMRT ($n = 15$). For more details regarding the protocol, see LEVENDAG et al. (2004) and TEGUH et al. (2008b).

All 155 patients without evidence of disease for a minimum of 1 year received three types of questionnaires: (1) The EORTC H&N35 swallowing scale, including four items (problems with swallowing of liquid, pureed food, or solid food, and aspiration when swallowing) (BJORDAL et al. 2000), (2) The performance status scale (PSS) of LIST et al. (1996) with item normalcy of diet, and (3) The MD Anderson Dysphagia Inventory (MDADI), (CHEN et al. 2001) consisting of 20 questions with global, emotional, functional, and physical subscales.

Treatment plans of previously irradiated patients were retrieved, with the previously defined five muscular structures of the swallowing apparatus delineated on the axial CT slices (LEVENDAG et al. 2007). Thus the mean dose contribution by the 3DCRT or IMRT technique to the muscular structures could be computed using the original treatment plan. From the patients treated by P-O fields and if a CT scan for treatment planning purposes was available, also the dose contribution to the swallowing muscles was calculated (HOOGEMAN et al. 2006). From the available CT-based 3D dose distributions of patients boosted by means of BT, the mean BT dose was calculated. For the patients boosted by BT, the 3DCRT, IMRT, or P-O dose and the boost doses were physically summated. Finally, the relationship of the mean total dose received by the five swallowing muscles to the responses of the three–dysphagia-related–QOL questionnaires (mean QOL scores; H&N35, PSS, and MDADI) is reported per tumor site (i.e., the TF and/or SP or BOT) and per treatment technique (BT vs. non-BT).

Table 11.1. UICC/AJCC 2002 edition TNM stage distribution for TF/SP tumors boosted by BT or non-BT techniques

| | Tonsillar fossa/soft palate (n = 108) | | | | | | | | | | | | | |
| | Brachytherapy (n = 83) | | | | | | | Non-brachytherapy (n = 25) | | | | | | |
	N0	N1	N2a	N2b	N2c	N3	Total	N0	N1	N2a	N2b	N2c	N3	Total
T1	2	4	3	5	0	2	16	0	0	0	1	0	0	1
T2	28	9	6	4	4	0	51	3	1	1	1	1	3	10
T3	9	1	3	2	0	0	15	3	5	0	0	2	0	10
T4a	0	0	0	0	0	0	0	2	1	0	0	0	0	3
T4b	1	0	0	0	0	0	1	1	0	0	0	0	0	1
Total	40	14	12	11	4	2	83	9	7	1	2	3	3	25

Table 11.2. UICC/AJCC 2002 edition TNM stage distribution for BOT tumors boosted by BT or non-BT techniques

| | Base of tongue (n = 47) | | | | | | | | | | | | | |
| | Brachytherapy (n = 24) | | | | | | | Non-brachytherapy (n = 23) | | | | | | |
	N0	N1	N2a	N2b	N2c	N3	Total	N0	N1	N2a	N2b	N2c	N3	Total
T1	1	0	3	3	2	0	9	0	0	0	0	0	1	1
T2	1	0	1	2	1	0	5	1	2	0	0	2	1	6
T3	1	1	3	1	0	1	7	2	0	0	2	1	0	5
T4a	3	0	0	0	0	0	3	4	1	0	4	1	0	10
T4b	0	0	0	0	0	0	0	0	0	0	0	1	0	1
Total	6	1	7	6	3	1	24	7	3	0	6	5	2	23

11.2.1
Dysphagia

From responses to the H&N35 (swallowing scale), PSS (normalcy diet), and to the MDADI questionnaires, prevalence of dysphagia was computed. Also, a moderate and severe degree of dysphagia is established by clustering, that is, e.g., regarding the charts, the RTOG grade 3 and 4 scores were combined. Similarly, for H&N35 (swallowing) "quite a bit" and "very much" dysphagia (score $\leq$ 50) was scored as grade 3 and 4, respectively, and clustered as "severe." The PSS (normalcy diet) score $\leq$ 50 and total MDADI score $\leq$ 50 were taken as the prevalence of a significant degree (equivalent to RTOG grade 3 or 4) of dysphagia.

11.2.2
Xerostomia

Patients were also asked to respond to the dry mouth scale in the QOL questionnaire H&N35. The outcome was correlated to the dysphagia-related scale of the EORTC H&N35.

A univariate and a multivariate analysis were performed for the parameters T-stage, N-stage, sex, age, dose in superior constrictor muscle (scm), dose in medial constrictor muscle (mcm), dose in inferior constrictor muscle (icm), dose in cricopharyngeal muscle (cphm), dose in first centimeter of esophageal inlet (eim), site, neck irradiation unilateral, neck irradiation bilateral, neck irradiation plus ND, treatment before or after 2000 in relation to the QOL questionnaires.

11.2.3
Univariate Dose–Response Relationship

For the scm, mcm, icm, cphm and eim, the correlations of dose in these muscular structures and the absence or presence of dysphagia grade 3 and 4 combined (dataset dichotomized) were calculated using logistic regressions. For example:

$$\Pr\{H\&N35 \text{ swallowing} \geq 50|\text{Dose in scm}\}$$
$$=1/(1 + \exp{(- (\alpha + \beta * \text{Dose scm})))}$$

We calculated coefficients for α and β and p-values for testing if $\beta = 0$.

11.3
Results

Between 1991 and 2005, 155 oropharyngeal cancer patients were treated by RT; 107 were boosted by BT, and 48 boosted by non-BT techniques. At the censor date 1 January 2006, every patient without evidence of disease after a follow-up period of at least 1 year was asked to respond to three validated questionnaires, that is, the EORTC H&N35, PSS, and MDADI. Out of the patients alive NED, 93% responded. We have focused the data analysis in this chapter on calculating the mean number of patients with late side effects "dysphagia" (and "xerostomia"). Table 11.3 presents an overview of the boost techniques with the respective follow-up times. Tables 11.4 and 11.5 summarize the QOL scores of the EORTC H&N35 for the BT group and the non-BT group with regard to the scales "swallowing" and "dry mouth," respectively. Table 11.6 presents QOL data with respect to the PSS scores, item "normalcy of diet." Table 11.7 shows the QOL mean scores of the MDADI. From the Tables 11.4–11.7 one can appreciate differences in QOL outcome per validated questionnaire, per boost technique, and per tumor site. In short, the mean QOL scores for swallowing and dry mouth were better for BT patients as opposed to non-BT patients, for TF and/or SP tumors as opposed to BOT tumors and for those patients treated with BT and CHT vs. patients treated with CHT in combination with non-BT boost techniques. Better QOL scores were also observed in patients radiated to a single neck as opposed to bilateral neck. The outcome data are consistent for all three QOL questionnaires and summarized in Table 11.8. From the univariate and multivariate analyses one can conclude that BT and boost treatment are significant parameters ($p < 0.001$) (Table 11.9). Also from Fig. 11.4 one can appreciate a significant dose–effect relationship regarding swallowing; i.e., 20% increase points per 10 Gy was found (Fig. 11.4).

11.4
Discussion

This chapter analyzes the dose–volume relationships for swallowing problems (dysphagia) in oropharyngeal cancer. It particularly focuses on the relationship of swallowing disorders caused by BT as opposed to other treatment techniques that have been used over the years to boost the primary tumor. Swallowing is a complex action requiring coordination between sensory input and motor function of the swallowing apparatus (ROSENTHAL et al. 2006). Intensification of therapy for head and neck cancer in general, either by altered fractionation RT schemes and/or by the addition of concomitant chemotherapy, results in improved loco-regional tumor control (FRANZMANN et al. 2006; LEE et al. 2006; ROSENTHAL and ANG 2004), and increase of late sequelae, such as dysphagia

Table 11.3. Mean follow-up times for patients treated with different boost techniques: BT, IMRT, 3DCRT, P-O

Boost technique	Number of patients	Mean FU years	Range FU years
Brachytherapy	107	6.7	1.3–14.7
Non-brachytherapy	48	3.7	1.0–10.5
IMRT	15	1.8	1.0–2.4
3DCRT	9	4.2	1.1–5.7
Parallel-opposed	24	4.7	1.5–10.5

IMRT intensity-modulated radiotherapy; *3DCRT* 3D conformal radiotherapy; *P-O* parallel-opposed

Table 11.4. Outcome QOL for oropharyngeal cancer patients treated between 1991 and 2005 in the Erasmus Medical Center-Daniel den Hoed Cancer Center (*): H&N35 swallowing scale: high scores, more problems

EORTC H&N35 swallowing scale (mean scores)*						
Quality of life categories	BT			Non-BT		
	TF/SP[a]	BOT[b]	Total	TF/SP	BOT	Total
All patients	19	22	19	30	47	38
Ipsilateral neck RT	9	No data	9	17	No data	17
Bilateral neck RT	24	22	23	31	47	39
Ipsilateral RT + ND	10	No data	10	0	No data	0
Bilateral neck RT + ND	21	23	22	28	40	32
Chemotherapy	12	14	13	33	42	38

ND neck dissection; *RT* radiation therapy
[a]Tonsillar fossa and/or soft palate
[b]Base of tongue

Table 11.5. Outcome QOL for oropharyngeal cancer patients treated between 1991 and 2005 (*) in the Erasmus Medical Center-Daniel den Hoed Cancer Center: H&N35 dry mouth scale

EORTC H&N35 dry mouth scale (mean scores)*						
Quality of Life categories	BT			Non-BT		
	TF/SP[a]	BOT[b]	Total	TF/SP	BOT	Total
All patients	49	54	50	71	71	71
Ipsilateral neck RT	35	33	35	78	No data	78
Bilateral neck RT	56	55	56	70	71	71
Ipsilateral RT + ND	35	No data	35	33	No data	33
Bilateral neck RT + ND	49	50	49	56	58	57
Chemotherapy	40	41	40	72	70	71

ND neck dissection; *RT* radiation therapy; *BT* brachytherapy; *Non-BT* non-brachytherapy
[a]Tonsillar fossa and/or soft palate
[b]Base of tongue

(PIGNON et al. 2000). In general, the prevalence of dysphagia is probably being underreported because of its (sometimes) clinically silent nature, but can be as high as 50% according to some papers on head and neck cancer survivors (EISBRUCH et al. 2002; MITTAL et al. 2003; NGUYEN et al. 2006; TROTTI 2006). Swallowing disorders are most likely caused by radiation-induced edema and neuromuscular fibrosis (MITTAL et al. 2003). Consequentially, a reduced pharyngeal contraction results in an impaired bolus transport through the pharynx (KOTZ et al. 2004). Some controversy exists whether the various primary disease sites have a different impact on the severity and/or frequency of dysphagia. Pretreatment swallowing therapy may improve dysphagia and reduce the need for tube feedings (LAZARUS 1993; LOGEMANN et al. 1997).

The majority of our patients had stage III and IV disease (77%). After 2000, stage III and IV patients were offered more routinely concomitant CHT. In fact, before 2000 concomitant CHT was given to 11% of the advanced-staged patients, as opposed to 48% in advanced cases after 2000. Also, as of 2000, according to protocol, RT allowed for six fractions/

Table 11.6. Outcome QOL for oropharyngeal cancer patients treated between 1991 and 2005 (*) in the Erasmus Medical Center-Daniel den Hoed Cancer Center: PSS (performance status scale), item "normalcy of diet"

PSS normalcy of diet (mean scores)*						
Quality of life categories	BT			Non-BT		
	TF/SP[a]	BOT[b]	Total	TF/SP	BOT	Total
All patients	75	78	75	64	51	58
Ipsilateral neck RT	84	No data	84	75	No data	75
Bilateral neck RT	70	78	73	63	51	57
Ipsilateral RT + ND	81	No data	81	100	No data	100
Bilateral neck RT + ND	72	78	74	75	67	72
Chemotherapy	85	98	92	58	52	54

High scores better functions; *ND* neck dissection; *RT* radiation therapy
[a]Tonsillar fossa and/or soft palate
[b]Base of tongue

Table 11.7. Outcome QOL for Oropharyngeal cancer patients treated between 1991 and 2005 (*) in the Erasmus Medical Center: MDADI (MD Anderson Dysphagia Inventory), function scale

MDADI (mean scores)*						
Quality of life categories	BT			Non-BT		
	TF/SP[a]	BOT[b]	Total	TF/SP	BOT	Total
All patients	75	74	75	59	52	55
Ipsilateral neck RT	80	No data	80	55	No data	55
Bilateral neck RT	71	74	72	60	52	55
Ipsilateral RT + ND	82	No data	82	81	No data	81
Bilateral neck RT + ND	66	78	69	63	52	58
Chemotherapy	78	80	79	61	50	54

High scores better functions; *ND* neck dissection; *RT* radiation therapy
[a]Tonsillar fossa and/or soft palate
[b]Base of tongue

week as opposed to (conventionally) five fractions. Between 1991 and 2005, 336 oropharyngeal cancers were treated. The LRC, DFS, and OS of the TF and/or SP and BOT tumors, boosted by BT or by non-BT techniques, are shown in Figs. 11.1–11.3. From this series of patients, chart review revealed that roughly 31% of patients experienced moderate to severe dysphagia (RTOG grade 3 and 4). Moreover, dysphagia was more of a problem in patients with BOT (40%) cancer as opposed to patients with cancer of the TF and/or SP (26%). When grouped by the boost technique BT vs. non-BT, severe dysphagia (problem score of QOL H&N35 with swallowing item ≥50) was observed in patients with TF and/or SP tumors in 19% and for BOT tumors in 22%. For the non-BT group, severe dysphagia was found in 30% of the TF/SP tumors and in 47% for the BOT tumors (see also Tables 11.4 and 11.5). A further breakdown of the non-BT group with respect to the booster technique used showed severe dysphagia in 42% for P-O, 25% for 3DCRT, and 25% for IMRT (data not shown in Tables 11.4 and 11.5). Also, more complaints were reported with higher doses, in particular with regard to the superior-and medial

Table 11.8. For some of the relevant patient/tumor characteristics, comparison between the outcome of three QOL questionnaires used in the present chapter (i.e., EORTC H&N35, PSS, MDADI)

Quality of life categories	H&N35 swallowing	PSS normalcy of diet	MDADI dysphagia
BT all patients vs. non-BT all patients	BT > 0	BT > 0	No data
Ipsilateral neck RT vs. bilateral neck RT	Ipsilateral > 0	Ipsilateral > 0	No data
Ipsilateral neck RT + ND vs. bilateral neck RT	Ipsilateral > 0	Ipsilateral > 0	No data
Chemotherapy BT vs. chemotherapy non-BT	CHT BT > 0	CHT BT > 0	No data
TF/SP BT vs. BOT BT	TF = BOT	TF = BOT	TF = BOT
TF/SP non-BT vs. BOT non-BT	TF > BOT	TF > BOT	TF > BOT

The compared outcome data were taken from Tables 11.4–11.7. That is, the differences in sparing capacity (e.g., less problems with swallowing, better functioning in general) is based on responses to the validated QOL questionnaires EORTC H&N35 (see Table 11.4 item "swallowing" and see Table 11.5 item "dry mouth"), PSS (see Table 11.6 item "normalcy of diet"), and MDADI (see Table 11.7 item "dysphagia")
> better; = equivalent; *ND* neck dissection; *RT* radiation therapy

Table 11.9. Univariate analysis: parameters found to be significant in relation to outcome of QOL questionnaires H&N35 (swallowing, dry mouth), MDADI (dysphagia) and PSS (normalcy of diet)

	Univariate/multivariate analysis						
	T-stage	Brachy therapy	Boost treatment	Surgery neck	Neck irradiation	Dose scm	Dose mcm
H&N35 swallowing	0.005	*0.006*	0.012	0.012	–	*<0.001*	<0.001
H&N35 Dry mouth	–	–	0.003	*0.01*	0.006	*<0.001*	*<0.001*
MDADI	0.018	*0.002*	0.026	–	–	*<0.001*	0.001
PSS normalcy of diet	–	–	*<0.001*	–	0.02	*<0.001*	<0.001

Multivariate analysis: the parameters of the univariate analysis found to be significant for H&N35 (swallowing), H&N35 (dry mouth), MDADI (swallowing) and PSS (normalcy of diet). The significant *p*-values are given in italic. *scm* superior constrictor muscle; *mcm* medial constrictor muscle

constrictor muscles. Figure 11.4 shows an example of the dose–effect relationship computed by logistic regression. The steepness of the curve from 60 Gy, can be expressed by 20% increase/10 Gy. Furthermore, next to dose being a significant factor, other variables of importance with respect to dysphagia are treatment of the unilateral (vs. bilateral neck), and ND (see also Table 11.8). We speculate that this increase in dysphagia (high dose, no BT, bilateral neck irradiation, no ND) has to do with the increase in irradiated volume and radiation dose. Finally, for the same reason, xerostomia and dysphagia are also strongly correlated; that is, $p \leq 0.001$

for the parameter dose in the scm/mcm vs. the parameter dry mouth (TEGUH et al. 2008a).

11.5
Conclusions

Overall, according to chart review, a severe degree of dysphagia (RTOG grade III and IV) was experienced in 31% of the patients. Similarly, according to responses to the EORTC H&N35 QOL questionnaires, severe dysphagia was observed in about 20%

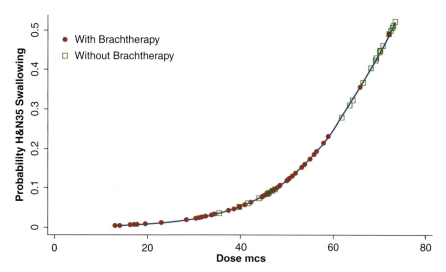

Fig. 11.4. Univariate dose–response relationship: for the scm, mcm, icm, cphm, and eim. The correlations of dose in these muscular structures and the absence or presence of dysphagia grade 3 and 4 combined (data set dichotomized) were calculated using logistic regressions. For example: Pr{H&N35 swallowing ≥ 50|Dose in scm} $= 1/(1+\exp(-(\alpha+\beta^*\text{Dose scm})))$. We calculated coefficients for α and β and p-values for testing if $\beta = 0$. This graph exemplifies the D–E curve for the superior constrictor muscle (scm).

of the BT group and about 38% in the non-BT group. Univariate analysis demonstrated less dysphagia for the following conditions: lower mean doses applied to swallowing muscles, BT treatment, single neck irradiation, and in case a ND is performed. The multivariate analysis shows a significant effect for BT (~implicating less swallowing complaints due to the lower doses of radiation received by the swallowing muscles).

For improvement of the dysphagia-related QOL, it is suggested to try and further optimize the dose distribution.

References

Bjordal K, de Graeff A, Fayers PM et al.; for EORTC Quality of Life Group (2000) A 12 country field study of the EORTC QLQ-C30 (version 3.0) and the head and neck cancer specific module (EORTC QLQ-H&N35) in head and neck patients. Eur J Cancer 36:1796–1807

Burkhead LM, Rosenbek J, Sapienza C et al. (2006) The effect of jaw and tongue position on suprahyoid muscle function during swallowing. Dysphagia 21:298

Chen AY, Frankowski R, Bishop-Leone J et al. (2001) The development and validation of a dysphagia-specific quality-of-life questionnaire for patients with head and neck cancer: the M. D. Anderson dysphagia inventory. Arch Otolaryngol Head Neck Surg 127:870–876

Eisbruch A, Lyden T, Bradford CR et al. (2002) Objective assessment of swallowing dysfunction and aspiration after radiation concurrent with chemotherapy for head-and-neck cancer. Int J Radiat Oncol Biol Phys 53:23–28

Franzmann EJ, Lundy DS, Abitbol AA et al. (2006) Complete hypopharyngeal obstruction by mucosal adhesions: a complication of intensive chemoradiation for advanced head and neck cancer. Head Neck 28:663–670

Greene FL, Page DL, Fleming ID et al. (2006) AJCC cancer staging manual, 6th edn. Springer, New York

Hoogeman MS, Herk van M, Zijp L (2006) The design and implementation of a multicenter volumetric and dosimetric database. Springer, Berlin, pp 82–84

Kotz T, Costello R, Li Y et al. (2004) Swallowing dysfunction after chemoradiation for advanced squamous cell carcinoma of the head and neck. Head Neck 26:365–372

Kulbersh BD, Rosenthal EL, McGrew BM et al. (2006) Pretreatment, preoperative swallowing exercises may improve dysphagia quality of life. Laryngoscope 116:883–886

Lazarus CL (1993) Effects of radiation therapy and voluntary maneuvers on swallow functioning in head and neck cancer patients. Clin Commun Disord 3:11–20

Lee WT, Akst LM, Adelstein DJ et al. (2006) Risk factors for hypopharyngeal/upper esophageal stricture formation after concurrent chemoradiation. Head Neck 28:808–812

Levendag P, Nijdam W, Noever I et al. (2004) Brachytherapy versus surgery in carcinoma of tonsillar fossa and/or soft palate: late adverse sequelae and performance status: can we be more selective and obtain better tissue sparing? Int J Radiat Oncol Biol Phys 59:713–724

Levendag PC, Teguh DN, Voet P et al. (2007) Dysphagia disorders in patients with cancer of the oropharynx are significantly affected by the radiation therapy dose to the superior and middle constrictor muscle: a dose–effect relationship. Radiother Oncol 85:64–73

List MA, D'Antonio LL, Cella DF et al. (1996) The performance status scale for head and neck cancer patients and the functional assessment of cancer therapy head and neck scale – A study of utility and validity. Cancer 77:2294–2301

Logemann JA, Pauloski BR, Rademaker AW et al. (1997) Super-supraglottic swallow in irradiated head and neck cancer patients. Head Neck 19:535–540

Logemann JA, Pauloski BR, Rademaker AW et al. (2003) Xerostomia: 12-month changes in saliva production and its relationship to perception and performance of swallow function, oral intake, and diet after chemoradiation. Head Neck 25:432–437

Logemann JA, Smith CH, Pauloski BR et al. (2001) Effects of xerostomia on perception and performance of swallow function. Head Neck 23:317–321

Mittal BB, Pauloski BR, Haraf DJ et al. (2003) Swallowing dys-function–preventative and rehabilitation strategies in patients with head-and-neck cancers treated with surgery, radiotherapy, and chemotherapy: a critical review. Int J Radiat Oncol Biol Phys 57:1219–1230

Nguyen NP, Frank C, Moltz CC et al. (2006) Aspiration rate following chemoradiation for head and neck cancer: an underreported occurrence. Radiother Oncol 80:302–306

Pauloski BR, Rademaker AW, Logemann JA et al. (2000) Pretreatment swallowing function in patients with head and neck cancer. Head Neck 22:474–482

Pauloski BR, Rademaker AW, Logemann JA et al. (2002) Swallow function and perception of dysphagia in patients with head and neck cancer. Head Neck 24:555–565

Pignon JP, Bourhis J, Domenge C et al.; for MACH-NC Collaborative Group (2000) Chemotherapy added to locoregional treatment for head and neck squamous-cell carcinoma: three meta-analyses of updated individual data. Lancet 355:949–955

Rosenthal DI, Ang KK (2004) Altered radiation therapy frac-tionation, chemoradiation, and patient selection for the treatment of head and neck squamous carcinoma. Semin Radiat Oncol 14:153–166

Rosenthal DI, Lewin JS, Eisbruch A (2006) Prevention and treatment of dysphagia and aspiration after chemoradiation for head and neck cancer. J Clin Oncol 24:2636–2643

Teguh DN, Levendag PC, Noever I et al. (2008a) Treatment tech-niques and site considerations regarding dysphagia-related quality of life in cancer of the oropharynx and nasophar-ynx. Int J Radiat Oncol Biol Phys 72(4):1119–1127

Teguh DN, Levendag PC, Voet P et al. (2008b) Trismus in patients with oropharyngeal cancer: relationship with dose in struc-tures of mastication apparatus. Head Neck 30:622–630

Trotti A (2006) Toxicity in head and neck cancer: a review of trends and issues. Int J Radiat Oncol Biol Phys 47(1):1–12

Improving the Quality of Life of Patients with Head and Neck Cancer by Highly Conformal Radiotherapy

12

AVRAHAM EISBRUCH

CONTENTS

12.1 Introduction *145*

12.2 Evolution of Highly Conformal RT: From 2D to 3D and to Intensity-Modulated Radiotherapy and Tomotherapy *146*

12.3 IMRT: General Aspects *146*

12.4 IMRT for Head and Neck Cancer *146*

12.5 Reducing Xerostomia by Highly Conformal Radiotherapy *147*

12.6 Efforts to Reduce Dysphagia Related to Chemo-RT of Head and Neck Cancer *149*

12.7 Using IMRT to Reduce the Doses to the Swallowing Structures *150*

12.8 Effects of Highly Conformal RT on Broad Aspects of QOL *151*

References *152*

> ## KEY POINTS
>
> - Xerostomia has been the most common late sequel of radiotherapy for head and neck cancer.
> - Highly conformal radiotherapy has concentrated on the sparing of the parotid glands to reduce xerostomia, achieving moderate improvements.

AVRAHAM EISBRUCH, MD
Department of Radiation Oncology, University of Michigan Health System, UH B2C490, 1500 East Medical Center Drive, SPC 5010, Ann Arbor, MI 48109, USA

- It is likely that sparing minor salivary glands dispersed in the oral cavity, and the submandibular glands will further improve these gains.
- Dose–response relationships for the major salivary glands demonstrate significant relationships with the mean doses.
- The effects of the spatial dose distributions within the glands may be important and requires further research.
- Weak correlations have been observed between the amount of the spared saliva and patient-reported xerostomia, requiring further research.

12.1
Introduction

Efforts to improve quality of life (QOL) by highly conformal radiotherapy (RT) rely on its ability to conform the high radiation dose to the targets and partly spare organs whose damage causes long-term symptoms, which affect the QOL of survivors. The symptom that highly conformal RT sought to reduce has been xerostomia, where efforts to spare the salivary glands have been a main goal of this technology in head and neck (HN) cancer. In recent years, dysphagia has emerged as a major late sequel following treatment intensification for HN cancer. Efforts to define the anatomical structures whose damage by intensive chemo-RT causes dysphagia, and to assess the ability of highly conformal RT to spare these structures, have been made very recently. This chapter will describe the evolution of highly conformal RT and its utilization in studies aiming to reduce xerostomia and dysphagia, and their effect on broad aspects of QOL.

12.2
Evolution of Highly Conformal RT: From 2D to 3D and to Intensity-Modulated Radiotherapy and Tomotherapy

In traditional irradiation of HN cancer, the placement of the radiation fields and their shapes are based on the bony anatomy acquired by the simulator diagnostic-quality films. During the late 1980s, advancements in computer technology and imaging introduced methods to identify the targets on computed tomography (CT) scans, and display the radiation beams in three dimensions (3D) relative to the anatomy. In addition, calculation and display of the radiation dose distributions and methods to evaluate and compare rival plans using dose–volume histograms became available. The introduction of multileaf collimators facilitated an increase in the number of beams that could be delivered without a large extension of treatment time. Treatment could then be delivered from multiple angles, including noncoplanar directions, when required. The result was the emergence of 3D conformal radiotherapy (3DCRT), which allowed better precision of irradiation delivery to image-based targets, and some improvements in the sparing of noninvolved critical tissue. Early studies of the utility of 3DCRT in HN demonstrated a significant benefit from 3DCRT: better coverage of the tumors and reduced doses to critical tissue, compared with standard techniques. A step forward was gained in the mid-1990s by intensity-modulated radiotherapy (IMRT), which facilitated a higher degree of dose conformality and offered opportunities for additional clinical gains. More recently, imaging-guided radiotherapy has emerged, providing opportunities for better precision of patient setup and for tracking tumor regression and anatomical changes in the noninvolved tissue during the course of radiation. Tracking these anatomical changes may facilitate future replanning during the course of therapy to address them. Other emerging technologies include new imaging modalities that provide opportunities to study the customization of the radiation dose depending on the expected tumor biology, and the use of heavy particles such as protons or carbon ions, which offer additional advantages in dose conformality.

12.3
IMRT: General Aspects

IMRT implies the use of radiation fields whose intensity varies across the field, depending on the thickness of the target and the existence of critical organs or critical noninvolved tissue in their path. Treating the targets with multiple beams of varying intensity allows a relatively uniform dose in an irregularly shaped target while avoiding a high dose to the surrounding structures. Two technological developments made IMRT possible: the introduction of computer-controlled multileaf collimators, and the development of computerized optimization, or "inverse planning," that determines the intensity of the beams that is required to satisfy a specified set of dose distributions.

Currently, most IMRT delivery systems use conventional multileaf collimators. Delivering IMRT using a conventional multileaf collimator can be made in a "dynamic" or "static" form. In the dynamic form, the leaves at each gantry position are swept across the target while the beam is on and their speed determines the radiation fluency. In static or segmental multileaf IMRT, each field consists of multiple segments with different intensities. These forms of IMRT are currently offered by most manufacturers of linear accelerators. A helical tomotherapy design has been developed at the University of Wisconsin and is similar in its operation to the helical CT, delivering essentially an infinite number of beams while the gantry rotates around the patient. This design has been available commercially in recent years.

12.4
IMRT for Head and Neck Cancer

The anatomy of the neck is complex, with many critical and radiation-sensitive organs in close proximity to the targets. Tight dose gradients around the targets that limit the doses to the noninvolved tissue, features characteristic of IMRT, are desirable and offer the potential for therapeutic gains. Noninvolved tissue whose sparing may offer tangible gains include the major salivary glands, minor salivary glands dispersed within the oral cavity, the mandible, and the pharyngeal musculature. In the cases of nasopharyngeal and paranasal sinus cancer, critical normal tissue that may be partly spared using IMRT include the inner and middle ears, the temporomandibular joints, temporal brain lobes, and the optic pathways. While the sparing of any of these structures may improve the QOL of patients who would have received high doses using previous, conventional RT, the following discussion will concentrate on efforts to reduce xersostomia and dysphagia, which are thought to be the main QOL-related issues in head and neck RT.

12.5

Reducing Xerostomia by Highly Conformal Radiotherapy

Limiting the volume of the major salivary glands receiving a high radiation dose has long been recognized as a major factor in reducing the severity of xerostomia. Relatively simple RT planning and delivery tools can be used to treat only the unilateral neck in patients with small, lateral tumors of the oral cavity and the oropharynx. This would exclude the contralateral parotid and submandibular glands and result in mild xerostomia (Hazuka et al. 1993; O'Sullivan et al. 2001). Partial sparing of the parotid glands in patients requiring bilateral neck RT became feasible following the introduction to the clinic of 3DCRT (Eisbruch et al. 1996; Maes et al. 2002) and IMRT tools (Eisbruch et al. 1998; Butler et al. 1999; Wu et al. 2000; Chao et al. 2000; Hunt et al. 2001; De Neve et al. 1999; Lee et al. 2002; Vineberg et al. 2002) to the clinic. These studies have demonstrated significant sparing of the parotid glands, reducing their mean doses such that significant retention of the salivary output is possible. Reducing the mean doses to the parotid glands to levels below 26–39 Gy has enabled the retention of more than 25% of the pre-RT salivary flow rates, in various studies (Maes et al. 2002; Eisbruch et al. 2001a). This range of mean doses is readily achievable by IMRT in the contralateral parotid glands and in cases where the tumor is centrally located, also in the ipsilateral glands. The sparing of the parotid glands, in conjunction with the relative sparing of the oral cavity achieved by the conformal dose distributions of IMRT, contributes to reduced observer-rated and patient-reported xerostomia, compared with that expected following standard RT.

Studies of dose–volume–response relationships in the major salivary glands are essential to effectively plan their sparing. These studies have primarily focused on the parotid glands because they typically lie outside or at the periphery of the targets in HN cancer. In contrast, the submandibular glands often lie within nodal targets (submandibular lymph nodes, or nodal level IB), or, if they lie outside the targets, they are immediately anterior to upper neck jugular nodes (level II) which are almost always included in the targets. Recent advances in RT treatment planning include the ability to construct dose–volume histograms, facilitating an accurate assessment of the dose distributions in the glands. Several recent studies have been published assessing dose–response relationships based on dose–volume histograms (Maes et al. 2002; Eisbruch et al. 1998, 1999, 2001a, b; Butler et al. 1999; Wu et al. 2000; Chao et al. 2000, 2001a, b; Hunt et al. 2001; De Neve et al. 1999; Lee et al. 2002; Vineberg et al. 2002; Roesink et al. 2001; Schilstra and Meertens 2001). The common finding in all these studies is the correlation of the post-RT gland function with the mean gland dose. This is expected in an organ with a "parallel" organization of its functional subunits (Withers et al. 1988). The studies differ in the methods of salivary collection: selective parotid flows (Eisbruch et al. 1999; Roesink et al. 2001; Schilstra and Meertens 2001) or whole mouth saliva (Chao et al. 2001a, b); and in the RT technique: standard 3-field RT (Roesink et al. 2001; Schilstra and Meertens 2001) or various methods of IMRT (Maes et al. 2002; Eisbruch et al. 1999; Chao et al. 2001a, b), causing different spatial dose distributions within the glands.

Different models have been fitted in these studies to the resulting data. As would be expected from this variability, these studies have reported different relationships between the mean doses and residual gland function. Defining as an end point a reduction of the salivary output to ≤25% of the pre-RT flow rate (RTOG/EORTC xerostomia grade IV); the mean parotid gland doses reported in these studies were in the range of 26–39 Gy. Similar dose range (Marks et al. 1981; Leslie and Dische 1994) or higher (Franzen et al. 1992) were reported to cause long-term dysfunction in previous studies, which used crude estimates of the gland doses. Studies are currently being conducted using salivary gland single photon emission computed tomography, assessing the relationships between the 3D scintigraphy results and the mean parotid gland dose (Van Acker et al. 2001).

What is the extent of improvement in xerostomia following IMRT, compared with the improvement observed following the administration of radiation protectors or salivary stimulants to patients treated with standard RT? Lacking a randomized study of IMRT vs. standard RT, this question can only be addressed indirectly (a randomized study is planned in Britain; Nutting, personal communication). In a study of 66 patients receiving IMRT for nasopharyngeal cancer, grade 2 xerostomia according to the RTOG scale was noted in ~30% of the patients 1 year after therapy, and no grade 3 was observed (Lee et al. 2002). Two years after therapy, the rate of grade 2 xerostomia decreased to 3%. In comparison, the rate of xerostomia grade ≥2 1 year after RT in the randomized study of amifostine was 34% in the treated patients, and 57% in the controls (Brizel et al. 2000). It is likely that in the amifostine study, in which most patients had nonnasopharyngeal cancers and many received postoperative RT, the doses and the extent of salivary gland RT were lower than in the nasopharyngeal IMRT study. Chao et al. (2001a, b) compared patients with oropharyngeal cancer receiving IMRT to similar patients who had received standard RT. RTOG-graded xerostomia scores were determined prospectively in the IMRT patients and retrospectively in the standard RT patients and it was concluded that significant improvement in late xerostomia was demonstrated in those receiving IMRT. A validated patient-reported xerostomia questionnaire (XQ) was used in a nonrandomized study at the University of Michigan to compare patients receiving bilateral neck RT by multisegmental IMRT or by standard RT (Malouf et al. 2003). One year after therapy, the mean xerostomia scores were 3.1 and 5.1, respectively, on a 0–10-point scale (higher scores denote worse xerostomia). Thus, patients receiving IMRT showed on average a 2-point advantage over patients receiving standard RT. A difference of that magnitude is considered clinically relevant in QOL studies (Osoba et al. 1998). Notwithstanding the lack of randomization, this was a larger relative difference than that noted in the randomized amifostine study (Brizel et al. 2000). Two years after therapy, the salivary flow rates from the spared parotid glands have recovered to their pre-RT levels (Eisbruch et al. 2001a, b). At the same time, the xerostomia scores reported by the patients who received bilateral neck IMRT were close to those reported by patients receiving unilateral neck RT. These results, as well as the 2-year results of the nasopharyngeal IMRT study (Lee et al. 2002), suggest that following IMRT, both the preservation of the measured salivary output and the long-term reduction in symptoms are

favorable compared with other methods aiming to reduce xerostomia.

As parotid salivary output is partly preserved and increases over time, it has been predicted that parallel improvements in the symptoms of xerostomia would follow. However, this issue was found to be much more complex and uncertain. The uncertainties relate to the poor correlation between the parotid flow rates and xerostomia, and questions about which is the best way to measure xerostomia. Two recent randomized studies comparing IMRT to conventional RT for early nasopharyngeal cancer have demonstrated a dichotomy between the preserved parotid saliva and xerostomia symptoms: Kam et al. (2007) found that the salivary flows, but not patient-reported xerostomia scores, were significantly better following IMRT than following conventional RT, and Pow et al. (2006) reported substantially higher salivary flow rates in the IMRT group; however, the improvement in symptoms, while statistically significant, was quite modest. The primary end point in the study of Kam et al. (2007) was RTOG/EORTC late xerostomia scores, demonstrating significant difference favoring the IMRT arm compared with the 2D RT arm. This is consistent with observations in previous single-arm series of IMRT for nasopharyngeal cancer, which reported no, or very low, xerostomia measured by RTOG/EORTC scores (Lee et al. 2002). On the other hand, the differences between the arms in patient-reported xerostomia were not statistically significant. What was the reason for this difference in outcome, which seems to relate to the method of assessment?

The RTOG/EORTC is an observer-based grading system that has been widely used, and has recently been replaced by the similar common toxicity criteria (CTC v3) system. A study comparing the RTOG/EORTC scoring to a validated patient-reported XQ in patients who had received IMRT for HN cancer found a modest agreement among the various observers in the RTOG/EORTC scores, low correlation with the salivary output, and an underestimation by the observers of the severity of xerostomia, compared with that reported by patients (Meirovitz et al. 2006). The lack of robust agreement and underestimation were possibly due to the inherent difficulties faced by observers assessing the severity of someone else's symptoms.

The likely explanation of the discrepancy between the preserved salivary output and patient-reported xerostomia is that the sparing of the parotid glands alone is not sufficient. This is related to the composition of the parotid saliva, which is devoid of mucins. Mucins serve as mucosal lubricants and as a selective permeability barrier of the mucosa. They bind water effectively and their presence on the mucous membrane surfaces helps maintain these tissues in hydrated state and contribute to patient's subjective sense of hydration (EISBRUCH et al. 2001a, b; TABAK 1995). Mucin-secreting glands such as the minor salivary glands, which are dispersed in the oral cavity, produce less than 10% of the total volume of the saliva but contribute the majority of the total mucins (MILNE and DAWES 1973). Another source of mucins is the submandibular glands. The importance of the mucin-producing glands in determining the severity of xerostomia was demonstrated in studies that correlated the RT doses to these glands, as well as their output, and patient-reported xerostomia (EISBRUCH et al. 1996; SCHILSTRA and MEERTENS 2001; CHAO et al. 2001a, b). It is likely that sparing the mucin-rich glands will further improve xersotomia compared with sparing the parotid glands alone. Sparing the minor salivary glands is achieved by reducing the doses to the noninvolved oral cavity (EISBRUCH et al. 2001a, b). Sparing of the submandibular glands by IMRT has recently been demonstrated (SAARILANTI et al. 2006; MURDOCH KINCH et al. 2008). MURDOCH-KINCH et al. (2008) have assessed prospectively dose–response relationships in the submandibular glands of close to 150 patients treated with IMRT for HN cancer, using selective measurements of the submandibular gland output. They found an exponential reduction of output as mean dose increased through mean dose 39 Gy, above which there was little output. The output increased during the 2 years after therapy if the mean dose was less than 39 Gy. IMRT replanning was performed in patients with HN cancer receiving bilateral neck RT and in whom contralateral level I was not a target. Reducing mean contralateral submandibular gland dose to less than 39 Gy was introduced to the cost function of the plan, and it achieved substantial reduction of gland doses without target underdosing. The conclusions of this study were that submandibular salivary flow rates depended on mean dose with recovery over time up to a threshold of 39 Gy. Substantial gland dose reduction to below this threshold and without target underdosing was feasible in some patients, at the expense of modestly higher doses to some other organs. The clinical benefits associated with these trade-offs need to be assessed. Other future efforts that require clinical assessment include improving even further salivary gland sparing by new technology such as intensity-modulated proton RT, and adding salivary protectants to salivary gland sparing.

12.6
Efforts to Reduce Dysphagia Related to Chemo-RT of Head and Neck Cancer

Intensification of the therapy for HN cancer, by altered fractionated RT or the addition of concurrent chemotherapy, has resulted in improved tumor control rates. The main late sequel following treatment intensification has been increasing rates and severity of long-term dysphagia. Evidence has recently emerged that aspiration pneumonia is associated with dysphagia after intensive chemo-RT, and that it constitutes an underreported sequel of therapy (EISBRUCH et al. 2002; NGUYEN et al. 2006). Improvements in target dose conformity may reduce the rate and severity of dysphagia following intensive therapy, if these improvements can sufficiently reduce the doses delivered to the anatomical structures whose malfunction after intensive chemo-RT causes dysphagia and aspiration. Identifying these structures is not trivial. Swallowing is a complex process that involves voluntary and involuntary stages which are coordinated through several cranial nerves and a multitude of muscles that control the function of the oral cavity, the pharynx, the larynx, hyoid bone, and esophagus. In recent years, studies assessing which are the relevant anatomical structures have been conducted, and dose–response relationships for these structures are emerging.

Laryngopharyngeal disorders resulting in late dysphagia and aspiration are not regimen-specific and are the result of edema and fibrosis (PAULOSKI et al. 1994; GOLDSMITH 2003; LOGEMANN 1998). To correlate the relationship of radiation-dose–volume–effect, it is critical to know the relative importance of the organs involved in swallowing physiology. (PAULOSKI et al. 1994; GOLDSMITH 2003; LOGEMANN 1998). evaluated the "organ at risk" in 170 patients. Laryngeal elevation, tongue-base retraction, and the cricopharyngeal opening consistently predicted patients' ability to swallow different food consistencies. EISBRUCH et al. (2004) reviewed the literature and identified the structures that, if damaged, could potentially cause abnormal swallowing physiology. From their study of 26 patients assessed with videofluoroscopy, direct endoscopy, and CT scans, they identified pharyngeal constrictors (PC) and glottic and supraglottic larynx (GSL) as dysphagia – and/or aspiration-related structures. In a prospective study, FENG et al. (2007) assessed dose–volume–effect relationship for the swallowing structures in 36 patients treated with chemotherapy concurrent with IMRT aiming to spare the swallowing structures. A strong correlation was observed between the mean doses to the swallowing structures and dysphagia end points. Aspiration was observed when the PC mean dose exceeded 60 Gy and the dose–volume threshold was V40 = 90%, V50 = 80%, V60 = 70%, and V65 > 50%. For aspiration to occur, the GSL dose–volume threshold was V50 > 50% (>50% of volume receiving 50 Gy). For stricture, a mean dose of ≥66 Gy and a dose–volume threshold of V50 = 85%, V60 = 70%, and V65 = 60% for PC was observed. The mean dose to the PC and esophagus was correlated with liquid swallowing, while only the mean dose to PC was correlated with solid swallowing on patient-reported and observer-rated swallowing scores.

In a retrospective study of 25 patients managed with radiation alone, JENSEN et al. (2007) studied the dose–volume–effect relationship using QOL questionnaires EORTC. In this study, radiation dose to base of tongue and PC did not correlate with swallowing endpoints. However, doses <60 Gy to the supraglottic area, larynx, and upper esophageal sphincter resulted in a low risk of aspiration.

DORNFELD et al. (2007) reported on 27 patients with HN cancer who were treated with IMRT radiation with chemotherapy and were free of disease for at least 1 year following treatment. Swallowing difficulties and the type of diet tolerated decreased progressively with radiation doses >50 Gy to the aryepiglottic folds, false vocal cords, and lateral pharyngeal walls near the false cord.

LEVENDAG et al. (2007) reported on 81 patients with oropharyngeal carcinoma treated with 3D CRT or IMRT with or without brachytherapy ± chemotherapy. A significant correlation was observed between the mean dose to the superior and middle pharyngeal constrictor muscles and patient complaints of severe dysphagia. A median dose of 50 Gy predicted a 20% probability of dysphagia. This probability increased significantly beyond a mean dose of 55 Gy, with an increase of 19% associated with each additional 10 Gy to superior and middle constrictors.

DOORNAERT et al. (2007) correlated the mean dose to the pharyngeal wall structures, including mucosa and pharyngeal constrictor muscles and swallowing outcome. They reported a steep dose–effect relationship beyond 45 Gy to pharyngeal wall structure and concluded that a mean dose of 45 Gy is the optimal threshold dose for predicting swallowing difficulties.

COGLAR et al. (2007) in a study of 96 patients with HN cancer treated using IMRT with or without chemotherapy observed no aspiration when the mean radiation dose to the larynx and inferior pharyngeal constrictor was ≤48 and ≤54 Gy, respectively. A dose–volume–effect was observed. At V50 = 21% for the larynx and V50 = 51% for the inferior constrictor, no aspiration or stricture were observed. No stricture was observed if the mean dose to the inferior constrictors was kept below 54 Gy.

O'MEARA et al. (2007) retrospectively reviewed the data of HN cancer patients treated with two-dimensional (2D) radiation with concurrent chemotherapy. They observed an association between the median dose to the inferior hypopharynx (pharyngoesophageal inlet) and severe late toxicity (grade ≥3 pharyngolaryngeal dysfunction). The incidence was 46%. The median dose to the inferior hypopharynx was 58 Gy among patients with severe late dysphagia, compared to 50 Gy in patients without severe dysphagia.

The differences between dose–volume–effect relationship and organs at risk between various studies could be due to lack of uniformity in dose reporting, differences in organ contouring, use of 2D vs. 3D data for treatment planning, dose optimization, and the endpoints used to measure swallowing dysfunctions.

12.7
Using IMRT to Reduce the Doses to the Swallowing Structures

Using current technologies, it is possible to reduce the radiation doses and the volume of critical structures involved in swallowing without compromising the target. EISBRUCH et al. (2004) identified the larynx and PC as playing an important role. By decreasing radiation to these structures using IMRT, they were able to reduce the incidence of aspiration and swallowing disorders (FENG et al. 2007, 2008). The main assumption enabling the sparing of the PCs was that only lateral, but not medial, retropharyngeal nodes are at risk, based on literature search (FENG et al. 2007). Thus far no out-of-target recurrences were observed in 107 patients with advanced oropharyngeal or nasopharyngeal cancer treated with chemo-IMRT sparing the swallowing structures and defining the retropharyngeal targets as the lateral nodes only (FENG et al. 2008). In a long-term follow-up of these patients it was noted that dysphagia improved continuously through 2-year follow-up and the rate of grade ≥ 2 dysphagia was rare (2/107). Notably, pharyngeal transit time has not been lengthened compared with pretherapy measurements in these patients, representing a potentially important improvement compared with previous data from patients treated with conventional RT.

12.8

Effects of Highly Conformal RT on Broad Aspects of QOL

Whether the reduction in xerostomia and potential reduction in dysphagia may have affected broader aspects of QOL has been examined in few studies.

LIN et al. (2003) assessed prospectively associations between xerostomia and QOL in patients receiving parotid-sparing RT at the University of Michigan. Patients were given a validated XQ, and a validated head-and-neck cancer-related QOL questionnaire consisting of four multi-item domains: Eating, Communication, Pain, and Emotion. The questionnaires and measurements of salivary output from the major glands were completed before RT started (pre-RT) and at 3, 6, and 12 months after RT. The XQ scores worsened significantly at 3 months compared with the pre-RT scores, but later they improved gradually through 12 months ($p = 0.003$), in parallel with an increase in the salivary output from the spared salivary glands. After 3 months, statistically significant improvement was noted in the summary QOL scores for all patients, through 12 months after RT ($p = 0.01$). The XQ and QOL summary scores did not correlate before RT but were significantly correlated at each post-RT point ($p < 0.01$). At these points, the XQ scores also correlated significantly with the scores of each of the individual QOL domains ($p \leq 0.01$), including the domains Pain and Emotion, which did not contain any xerostomia-related question. These results suggested that the efforts to improve xerostomia using IMRT may yield improvements in broad aspects of QOL.

In a subsequent study, a matched analysis of patients receiving IMRT or conventional RT was reported (JABBARI et al. 2005). During the initial months after therapy, the XQ and Head and Neck Quality of Life (HNQOL) summary scores worsened significantly in both groups compared with the pretherapy scores. Starting at 6 months, improvements of both XQ and HNQOL scores were found over time in the IMRT patients, compared with no trend of improvement in the standard RT patients. The trend of improvement over time in QOL in the IMRT patients was noted in most of the HNQOL domains (eating: $p = 0.07$, pain: $p = 0.05$, emotion: $p = 0.04$, and communication: $p = 0.13$), compared with no trend of improvement in most of the domains in the standard RT patients. As the scores of the IMRT (but not the standard RT) patients improved over time, the differences between the groups in the mean XQ and HNQOL summary scores widened. At 12 months, median XQ and HNQOL scores were lower (better) in the IMRT compared with the standard RT patients by 19 and 20 points, respectively, adjusted for the pretherapy values. It was concluded that after initial posttherapy declines in both groups, QOL improved over time after IMRT but not after standard RT, and that the potential benefits gained from IMRT in xerostomia or in QOL, compared with standard RT, are best reflected late (≥ 6 months) after therapy.

A study by YAO et al. (2007) from the University of Iowa confirmed these results. They compared retrospectively 26 patients with oropharyngeal cancer treated using IMRT and 27 similar patients treated using conventional RT. The IMRT group had higher mean Head and Neck Cancer Inventory scores (which represent better outcomes) for each of the four head-and-neck cancer-specific domains, including eating, speech, aesthetics, and social disruption, at 12 months after treatment. A significantly greater percentage of patients in the conventional RT group had restricted diets compared with those in the IMRT group.

A randomized study of IMRT vs. conventional RT for early nasopharyngeal cancer reported by Pow et al. (2006) included a QOL questionnaire delivered at baseline and periodically after therapy. Head-and-neck-specific QOL questionnaire (EORTC QLQ-HN35) revealed significantly better swallowing, speech, dry mouth, and sticky saliva, in the IMRT compared with the conventional RT group. Global health scores, assessed by the EORTC SF-36 questionnaire, improved over time in both groups; however, after 12 months, subscale scores for role-physical, bodily pain, and physical function, were significantly higher in the IMRT group, indicating a better condition, in parallel with improved patient-reported xerostomia.

In conclusion, the gains in xerostomia and dysphagia achieved by IMRT improve broad aspects of

QOL after therapy of HN cancer. Future improvements are likely to be achieved by reducing acute mucosal toxicity, and its consequential late morbidity, by selective radiosensitization and by better radioprotection of chemo-RT effects.

References

Brizel DM, Wasserman TH, Henke M et al. (2000) Phase III randomized trial of amifostine as a radioprotector in head and neck cancer. J Clin Oncol 18:339–3345

Butler EB, Teh BS, Grant WS et al. (1999) SMART (simultaneous modulated accelerated radiation therapy) boost: a new accelerated fractionation schedule for the treatment of head and neck cancer with intensity modulated radiotherapy. Int J Rad Onc Biol Phys 45:21–32

Chao KSC, Deasy JO, Markman J et al. (2001a) A prospective study of salivary function sparing in patients with head and neck cancers receiving intensity-modulated or three-dimensional radiation therapy: initial results. Int J Rad Onc Biol Phys 51:938–946

Chao KSC, Low D, Perez CA et al. (2000) Intensity-modulated radiation therapy in head and neck cancer: the Mallincrodt experience. Int J Cancer 90:92–103

Chao KSC, Majhail N, Huang CJ et al. (2001b) Intensity modulated radiation therapy reduces late salivary toxicity without compromising tumor control in patients with oropharyngeal carcinoma: a comparison with conventional techniques. Radiother Oncol 61:275–280

Coglar HB, Allen AM, Othus M et al. (2007) Dose to the larynx predicts for swallowing complications following IMRT and chemotherapy [Abstract #95]. Int J Radiat Oncol Bio Phys 69(suppl):53

De Neve W, De Gersem W, Derycke S (1999) Clinical delivery of IMRT for relapsed or second-primary head and neck cancer using a multileaf collimator with dynamic control. Radiother Oncol 50:301–314

Doornaert P, Slotman BJ, Rietveld DHF et al. (2007) The mean radiation dose in pharyngeal structures is a strong predictor of acute and persistent swallowing dysfunction and quality of life in head and neck radiotherapy [Abstract #97]. Int J Radiat Oncol Biol Phys 69(suppl):55

Dornfeld K, Simmons JR, Karnell L et al. (2007) Radiation doses to structures within and adjacent to the larynx are correlated with long-term diet– and speech–related quality of life. Int J Radiat Oncol Biol Phys 68:750–757

Eisbruch A, Kim HM, Ten Haken R et al. (1999) Dose, volume and function relationships in parotid glands following conformal and intensity modulated irradiation of head and neck cancer. Int J Radiat Oncol Biol Phys 45:577–587

Eisbruch A, Kim HM, Terrell JE et al. (2001a) Xerostomia and its predictors following parotid-sparing irradiation of head and neck cancer. Int J Radiat Oncol Biol Phys 50:695–704

Eisbruch A, Lyden T, Bradford CR et al. (2002) Objective assessment of swallowing dysfunction and aspiration after radiation concurrent with chemotherapy for head-and-neck cancer. Int J Radiat Oncol Biol Phys 53:23–28

Eisbruch A, Marsh LH, Martel MK et al. (1998) Comprehensive irradiation of head and neck cancer using conformal multisegmental fields: assessment of target coverage and noninvolved tissue sparing. Int J Rad Onc Biol Phys 41:559–568

Eisbruch A, Schwartz M, Rasch C et al. (2004) Dysphagia and aspiration after chemoradiotherapy for head and neck cancer: which anatomic structures are affected and can they be spared by IMRT? Int J Radiat Oncol Biol Phys 60:1425–1439

Eisbruch A, Ship JA, Kim HM et al. (2001b) Partial irradiation of the parotid gland. Semin Radiat Oncol 11:234–239

Eisbruch A, Ship JA, Martel MK et al. (1996) Parotid gland sparing in patients undergoing bilateral head and neck irradiation: techniques and early results. Int J Radiat Oncol Biol Phys 36:469–480

Feng FY, Kim H, Lyden T et al. (2008) Long-term results of IMRT of head and neck cancer aimed at sparing the swallowing structures. ASTRO Int J Rad Onc Biol Phys 2008;72 (Suppl. 1);71 (Abstr.)

Feng FY, Kim HM, Lyden TH et al. (2007) Intensity-modulated radiotherapy of head and neck cancer aiming to reduce dysphagia: early dose-effect relationships for the swallowing structures. Int J Radiat Onco Biol Phys 68:1289–1298

Franzen L, Funegard U, Ericson T et al. (1992) Parotid gland function during and following radiotherapy of malignancies in the head and neck. Eur J cancer 28:457–462

Goldsmith T (2003) Videofluroscopic evaluation of oropharyngeal swallowing. In: Som PM, Curtin HD (eds) Head and neck imaging, 4th edn. Mosby, St. Louis, pp 1727–1753

Hazuka MB, Martel MK, Marsh L et al. (1993) Preservation of parotid function after external beam irradiation in head and neck cancer patients: a feasibility study using 3-dimensional treatment planning. Int J Radiat Oncol Biol Phys 27:731–737

Hunt MA, Zelefsky MJ, Wolden S et al. (2001) Treatment planning and delivery of intensity-modulated radiation therapy for primary nasopharyngeal cancer. Int J Radiat Oncol Biol Phys 49:623–632

Jabbari S, Kim HM, Feng M et al. (2005) Quality of life and xerostomia following standard vs. intensity modulated irradiation: a matched case–control comparison. Int J Radiat Oncol Biol Phys 63:725–731

Jensen K, Lambertsen K, Grau C (2007) Late swallowing dysfunction and dysphagia after radiotherapy for pharynx cancer: frequency, intensity, and correlation with dose and volume parameters. Radiother Oncol 85:74–82

Kam MK, Leung SF, Zee B et al. (2007) Prospective randomized study of IMRT for nasopharyngeal cancer. J Clin Oncol 25:4873–4879

Lee N, Xia P, Quivey JM et al. (2002) Intensity modulated radiotherapy in the treatment of nasopharyngeal carcinoma: an update of the UCSF experience. Int J Radiat Oncol Biol Phys 53:12–22

Leslie MD, Dische S (1994) The early changes in salivary gland function during and after radiotherapy given for head and neck cancer. Radiother Oncol 30:26–32

Levandag PC, Teguh DN, Voet P et al. (2007) Dysphagia disorders in patients with cancer of the oropharynx are significantly affected by the radiation therapy dose to the superior and middle constrictor muscle: a dose–effect relationship. Radiother Oncol 85:64–73

Lin A, Kim HM, Terrell JE et al. (2003) Quality of life following parotid-sparing IMRT of head and neck cancer: a prospective longitudinal study. Int J Radiat Oncol Biol Phys 57:61–70

Logemann J (1998) Evaluation and treatment of swallowing disorders. PRO-ED, Austin, TX.

Maes A, Weltens C, Flamen P et al. (2002) Preservation of parotid function with uncomplicated conformal radiotherapy. Radiother Oncol 63:203–211

Malouf JG, Aragon C, Eisbruch A et al. (2003) Influence of parotid-sparing radiotherapy on xerostomia in head and neck cancer patients. Cancer Detect Prev 27:305–310

Marks JE, Davis CC, Gottsman VL et al. (1981) The effects of radiation on parotid salivary function. Int J Radiat Oncol Biol Phys 7:1013–1019

Meirovitz A, Murdoch-Kinch CA, Schipper M et al. (2006) Grading xerostomia by physicians or by patients after IMRT of head and neck cancer. Int J Radiat Oncol Biol Phys 66:445–453

Milne RW, Dawes C (1973) The relative contribution of different salivary glands to the blood group activity of whole saliva in humans. Vox Sang 25:298–307

Murdoch Kinch CA, Kim HM, Vineberg K et al. (2008) Dose–effect relationships for the submandibular glands and implications for their sparing by intensity modulated radiotherapy. Int J Radiat Oncol Biol Phys 72(2): 373–382

Nguyen NP, Frank C, Moltz CC et al. (2006) Aspiration rate following chemoradiation for head and neck cancer: an underreported occurrence. Radiother Oncol 80:302–306

O'Meara EA, Machtay M, Moughan J et al. (2007) Association between radiation doses to pharyngeal regions and severe late toxicity in head and neck cancer patients treated with concurrent chemoradiotherapy—An RTOG analysis [Abstract no. 96]. Int J Radiat Oncol Biology Phys 69(suppl):54

O'Sullivan B, Warde P, Grice B et al. (2001) The benefits and pitfalls of ipsilateral radiotherapy in carcinoma of the tonsillar region. Int J Radiat Oncol Biol Phys 51:332–343

Osoba D, Rodrigues G, Myles J et al. (1998) Interpretation of the significance of changes in health-related quality of life scores. J Clin Oncol 16:139–144

Pauloski BR, Logemann JA, Rademaker AW et al. (1994) Speech and swallowing function after oral and oropharyngeal resections: one-year follow-up. Head Neck 16:313–322

Pauloski BR, Rademaker AW, Logemann JA et al. (2006) Relationship between swallow motility disorders on videofluorography and oral intake in patients treated for head and neck cancer with radiotherapy with or without chemotherapy. Head Neck 28:1069–1076

Roesink JM, Moerland MA, Battersmann JJ et al. (2001) Quantitative dose–volume response analysis of changes in parotid gland function after radiotherapy in the head and neck region. Int J Radiat Oncol Biol Phys 51:938–946

Saarilanti K, Kouri M, Collan J et al. (2006) Sparing of the submandibular glands by intensity modulated radiotherapy in the treatment of head and neck cancer. Radiother Oncol 78:270–275

Schilstra C, Meertens H (2001) Calculation of the uncertainty in complication probability for various dose–response models, applied to the parotid gland. Int J Radiat Oncol Biol Phys 50:147–158.

Tabak LA (1995) In defense of the oral cavity: structure, biosynthesis, and function of salivary mucins. Annu Rev Physiol 57:547–564

Van Acker F, Flamen P, Lambin P et al. (2001) The utility of SPECT in determining the relationship between radiation dose and salivary gland dysfunction after radiotherapy. Nucl Med Commun 11:225–231

Vineberg KA, Eisbruch A, Coselmon MM et al. (2002) Is uniform target dose possible in IMRT plans in the head and neck? Int J Radiat Oncol Biol Phys 52:1159–1172

Withers HR, Taylor JMG, Maciejewski B (1988) Treatment volume and tissue tolerance. Int J Radiat Oncol Biol Phys 14:751–759

Wu Q, Manning M, Schmidt-Ullrich R et al. (2000) The potential for sparing of parotids and escalation of biologically equivalent dose with intensity modulated radiation treatments of head and neck cancers: a treatment design study. Int J Radiat Oncol Biol Phys 46:195–205

Yao M, Karnell LH, Funk GF et al. (2007) Health-related quality-of-life outcomes following IMRT versus conventional radiotherapy for oropharyngeal squamous cell carcinoma. Int J Radiat Oncol Biol Phys 69:1354–1360

Advantages of Proton Beam Therapy in Functional Preservation and Quality of Life in Head and Neck Radiotherapy

13

ANNIE W. CHAN, NORBERT J. LIEBSCH, and ALEXEI TROFIMOV

CONTENTS

13.1 History of Proton Beam Therapy *156*

13.2 Rationale of using Proton Beam Therapy for Head and Neck Cancers *156*

13.3 Intensity-Modulated Radiation Therapy vs. Intensity-Modulated Proton Therapy *156*

13.4 Proton Beam Therapy for Sinonasal Malignancies *157*

13.5 Proton Beam Therapy for Nasopharyngeal Carcinoma *158*

13.6 Proton Beam Therapy for Oropharyngeal Carcinoma *159*

13.7 Cost-Effectiveness of Proton Beam Therapy *160*

13.8 Future Directions *160*

References *160*

KEY POINTS

- Owing to the anatomical location of head and neck cancers, photon therapy can be associated with significant treatment-related toxicity such as xerostomia, swallowing dysfunction, hearing loss, or vision loss.
- The dose from a photon decreases exponentially with depth in the irradiated tissues. In contrast, proton beam has a finite range without an exit dose.
- With proton beam therapy, a smaller volume of normal tissues is irradiated than is feasible with any photon technique.
- Intensity-modulated proton therapy is a powerful delivery technique that results in improved dose distribution, compared to that with intensity-modulated radiation therapy.
- Initial clinical experience from single institutions with proton beam therapy in the treatment of head and neck cancers is very promising.
- Prospective clinical trials are underway to define the role of proton beam therapy in the treatment of head and neck cancers.

ANNIE W. CHAN, MD
NORBERT J. LIEBSCH, MD
ALEXEI TROFIMOV, MD
Department of Radiation Oncology, Massachusetts General Hospital, Francis H. Burr Proton Therapy Center, Harvard Medical School, 55 Fruit Street, Boston, MA, USA

13.1

History of Proton Beam Therapy

Proton beam therapy has been used to treat tumors for more than 50 years. The University of California at Berkeley began treating cancer patients in 1954, following the construction of the cyclotron at Lawrence Berkeley Laboratory. Massachusetts General Hospital (MGH)/Harvard Cyclotron Laboratory pioneered modern proton beam therapy, with more than 11,000 patients treated between 1961 and 2007. As of 2007, more than 65,000 patients have been treated with proton beam therapy worldwide (http://ptcog. web.psi.ch/ptcentres.html).

The use of proton beam therapy in the treatment of cancer will increase substantially in the near future. At present, there are 29 proton beam facilities in operation worldwide (http://ptcog.web.psi.ch/ptcentres. html). In the United States, there are currently five proton centers in operation, and at least another five are under development. Smaller and less costly models, which are currently under investigation, may further expand the clinical application of proton beam therapy. The role of proton beam therapy in the treatment of cancer will continue to be investigated through single- and multi-institutional trials.

13.2

Rationale of using Proton Beam Therapy for Head and Neck Cancers

The goal of modern radiation therapy is to treat the tumor with minimal dose to the surrounding normal tissues and thereby reducing toxicity and improving quality of life. Proton beam therapy, with its superior physical properties, provides an invaluable tool to achieve this goal. With proton beam therapy, a smaller volume of normal tissues is irradiated than is feasible with any photon technique. The dose from a photon decreases exponentially with depth in the irradiated tissues. In contrast, protons have a finite range. Protons deposit most of their radiation energy in what is known as the Bragg peak, which occurs at the point of maximum penetration of the protons in tissue. The exact depth to which protons penetrate, and at which the Bragg peak occurs, is dependent on the energy of the proton beam. This energy can be very precisely controlled to place the Bragg peak within a tumor that is targeted to receive the radiation dose. Because the

protons are absorbed at this point without an exit dose, normal tissues beyond the target receive very little or no radiation (Suit 2003; Suit et al. 2003).

Owing to the anatomical location of the head and neck and skull base tumors, two-dimensional or three-dimensional radiation therapy can be associated with significant treatment-related toxicity such as xerostomia, swallowing dysfunction, hearing loss, vision loss, and encephalopathy. When radiation is combined with concurrent chemotherapy, the acute and long-term side effects can be even more pronounced. Proton beam therapy with its superior dose distribution properties allows higher doses to be delivered to the tumor and lower doses to the surrounding normal structures. This potentially improves the tumor control probability and decreases acute and late toxicities.

13.3

Intensity-Modulated Radiation Therapy vs. Intensity-Modulated Proton Therapy

Intensity-modulated radiation therapy (IMRT) consists of radiation portals in which the intensity of photon (X-ray) radiation varies throughout the field. It has been increasingly applied in the treatment of head and neck tumors. To achieve dose conformality for tumor targets and avoid critical normal structures, dose to nontarget structures has to be increased. The "dose bath" received by the normal tissues could potentially result in unwanted acute and late side effects.

As protons are absorbed in the Bragg peak within the tumor, this "dose bath" phenomenon seen in IMRT does not occur with proton beam therapy (Lomax 2007). As the intensity of conventional photon radiation can be modulated to produce IMRT, the intensity of the proton radiation can also be modulated to produce intensity-modulated proton therapy (IMPT). This is achieved by a pencil beam scanning technique in which a small circular beam is scanned across the defined treatment field with the energy and intensity varying so that the dose in each voxel can be optimized. IMRT can only allow two-dimensional optimization, with modulation of the fluence occurring in the plane orthogonal to the beam direction. IMPT, in contrast, allows modulation of the fluence and the position of the Bragg peak. IMPT is therefore a three-dimensional optimization technique (Lomax 2007). In a dosimetric comparison study, IMPT has been shown to have a better ability to spare organs at risk than IMRT for the same

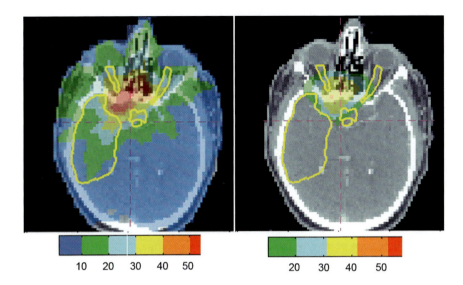

Fig. 13.1. Comparison of an intensity-modulated radiation therapy plan (IMRT, *left*) with an intensity modulated proton therapy plan (IMPT, *right*) in the treatment for a patient with T4 nasopharyngeal carcinoma. Note the unnecessary dose delivered to the brain and optic structures with the use of IMRT. The typical large dose bath of IMRT is not seen in IMPT

dose homogeneity. IMPT also significantly reduced the estimated risk of secondary cancer induction from radiation (STENEKER et al. 2006).

Figure 13.1 demonstrates the superiority of IMPT over IMRT in sparing critical and normal tissues of a patient with nasopharyngeal carcinoma. With IMRT, the nontarget structures such as the optic nerves, optic chiasm, orbits, and the brain received unnecessary low and moderate dose of radiation. The typical large dose bath of IMRT is not seen in IMPT. The long-term risk of neurocognitive dysfunction and radiation-induced brain tumor from this large radiation dose bath that is routinely seen with IMRT is not known.

13.4 Proton Beam Therapy for Sinonasal Malignancies

For most sinonasal malignancies, a combination of radical surgery and postoperative radiation constitutes standard treatment. Total maxillectomy is the most commonly performed surgical operation for maxillary sinus cancers. Transfacial medial maxillectomy or craniofacial resection is used when the disease involves the ethmoid sinuses. Despite such aggressive therapy, the outcome is poor, with fewer than half of the patients surviving at 5 years. In advanced tumors that involve the skull base, survival is further reduced. Treatment failure at the primary site is the main pattern of failure, ranging from 30 to 100% (KIM et al. 1999; LAVERTU et al. 1989; MENDENHALL et al. 2004; VIKRAM et al. 1984). Owing to the lack of any successful salvage treatment, patients eventually die from local tumor progression. Alternative treatment strategies are clearly needed for sinonasal malignancies with skull base involvement. Although it has been shown that higher radiation doses are associated with improved local control (GARDEN et al. 1995; VIKRAM et al. 1984), the surrounding critical normal tissues in the skull base preclude the delivery of adequate tumoricidal doses.

Owing to the proximity of the optic structures to the tumors in the paranasal sinuses and skull base, radiation-induced late ocular/visual toxicity such as retinopathy or optic neuropathy is very common. At the University of Florida, 27% of patients developed unilateral blindness secondary to radiation retinopathy or optic neuropathy, and 5% developed bilateral blindness because of optic neuropathy (KATZ et al. 2002). TAKEDA et al. (1999) also reported similar incidence of radiation retinopathy in their patients with malignancies of the nasal cavity and paranasal sinuses without tumor invasion of the eyes. WALDRON et al. (1998) reported the risk of unilateral or bilateral blindness in 41% and visual impairment in 24% of patients with ethmoid sinus cancer treated with conventional RT. Other radiation-induced ocular/visual toxicities such as neovascular glaucoma, cataract, and dry eye syndrome are also common after treatment with conventional radiation therapy for sinonasal malignancies (PARSONS et al. 1994; TAKEDA et al. 1999).

Newer radiation techniques that would allow decreased dose to the optic and ocular structures while at the same time delivering tumoricidal dose to the tumor target are extremely critical in minimizing these severe debilitating toxicities. Three-dimensional conformal radiation therapy or IMRT, though initially promising, has not been shown to improve the local control or survival for patients with sinonasal malignancies, although they have reduced toxicity (CHEN et al. 2007; DALY et al. 2007; HOPPE et al. 2007).

Between 1991 and 2002, 102 patients with advanced sinonasal cancers received proton radiation therapy at the MGH. There were 33 squamous cell carcinomas, 30 carcinomas with neuroendocrine differentiation, 20 adenoid cystic carcinomas, 13 soft tissue sarcomas, and 6 adenocarcinomas. The median dose was 71.6 Gy. Twenty percent of patients had undergone complete resection before proton radiation therapy. With a median follow-up of 6.6 years, the 5-year actuarial local control is 86% (CHAN et al. 2004; POMMIER et al. 2006). Distant metastasis was the predominant pattern of relapse for squamous cell, neuroendocrine, and adenoid cystic carcinomas. These results compare very favorably to those achieved by IMRT or three-dimensional conformal radiation therapy (CHEN et al. 2007; DALY et al. 2007; HOPPE et al. 2007).

The long-term ocular and visual toxicity in a group of patients treated with accelerated hyperfractionated proton radiation therapy at the MGH was reported (WEBER et al. 2006). The median dose to the gross tumor target was 70 Gy. Three percent of patients developed grade I retinal vasculopathy after treatment, with no associated visual loss. There was no vascular glaucoma, retinal detachment, or optic neuropathy. These data show that proton beam therapy allow the delivery of tumoricidal doses with minimal ocular/visual complications.

13.5
Proton Beam Therapy for Nasopharyngeal Carcinoma

Concurrent chemoradiation is the standard of care for patients with advanced nasopharyngeal carcinoma since the publication of the landmark Intergroup 0099 study (AL-SARRAF et al. 1998). The optimal radiation technique used alone or in combination with chemotherapy, however, still needs to be defined.

Recently, the outcome of a randomized study comparing two-dimensional radiation therapy and IMRT in patients with T1–2b N0–1 M0 nasopharyngeal carcinoma was reported (KAM et al. 2007). This randomized study showed that there was significantly less physician-rated severe xerostomia after

IMRT treatment compared with two-dimensional radiation therapy. This was observed at 1-year postradiation and paralleled by a significant difference in both the stimulated parotid flow rate and stimulated whole saliva flow rate between the two arms. There was, however, no significant difference in patient-reported xerostomia outcome between the two arms.

At the MGH, proton beam therapy has been used to treat very advanced NPC, particularly T4 (PATEL et al. 2007). Between 1990 and 2002, 17 patients with newly diagnosed T4 N0–3 tumors received combined conformal proton and photon radiation. Twelve patients (71%) had WHO type II or III histology. The median prescribed dose to the gross target volume was 73.6 Gy (range, 69.0–76.8 Gy). Eleven patients had accelerated hyperfractionated radiation therapy. Ten patients received chemotherapy (induction or concurrent). Only one patient failed to complete the planned concurrent chemotherapy and radiation course. With a median follow-up time of 43 months, only one patient developed local recurrence and two patients developed distant recurrence. No neck nodal recurrences were observed. The actuarial locoregional control and relapse-free survival rates at 3 years were 92 and 79%, respectively. The 3-year overall survival rate was 74%. This preliminary experience suggests that proton radiation therapy is effective in the treatment of T4 nasopharyngeal carcinoma. The promising result has led to a phase II study at MGH investigating the use of proton beam therapy for the treatment of nasopharyngeal carcinoma. In addition to locoregional and survival outcome as the primary end points of the trial, the other primary objective of the study is to assess health related quality-of-life outcomes after proton beam therapy using objective measurements and validated quality-of-life instruments.

To achieve tumor conformity and parotid sparing, IMRT always results in increased dose delivered to the oral cavity as compared to that of two-dimensional radiation therapy and proton beam therapy. Figure 13.2 compares the dose distribution between IMRT and IMPT in a patient with nasopharyngeal carcinoma. As noted, the dose bath in the oral cavity routinely seen in IMRT is not present in IMPT. IMPT allows sparing of the parotid glands as well as the sublingual glands and the minor salivary glands in the oral cavity. It would be important to determine whether the sparing of the oral cavity achieved by IMPT would result in improved physician-rated and patient-reported quality of life.

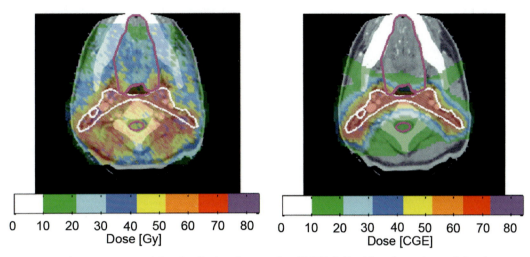

Fig. 13.2. Comparison of an intensity-modulated radiation therapy plan (IMRT, *left*) with an intensity modulated proton therapy plan (IMPT, *right*) in the treatment for nasopharyngeal carcinoma. Note the significant difference in dose delivered to the oral cavity between the two techniques

13.6
Proton Beam Therapy for Oropharyngeal Carcinoma

With the availability and widespread use of IMRT, oropharyngeal carcinoma is increasingly treated with IMRT. The results of IMRT from retrospective single institution studies are very promising (Chao et al. 2004; Garden et al. 2007; Lee et al. 2006) and have led to the investigation of the use of IMRT nationwide. The Radiation Therapy Oncology Group (RTOG) conducted a prospective single arm phase II multi-institutional trial investigating the use of IMRT alone for stage I–III oropharyngeal carcinoma. In the study, 69 patients were treated with IMRT to a total dose of 66 Gy in 2.2 Gy/fraction without chemotherapy. The primary end point was acute xerostomia grade 2 or higher. Acute xerostomia was grade 2 in 49% and grade 3 in 1.5%. Other major acute grade 2, 3, and 4 toxicities were mucositis – 30, 25, and 1.5%; and skin – 19, 10, and 0%, respectively. The worst late grade 2, 3, and 4 toxicities included skin – 11, 0, and 0%; mucous membranes – 15, 0, and 5%; and esophageal toxicity – 8, 3, and 0%, respectively. The worst late xerostomia scores were observed at median 5.7 months after radiation started: 63 and 5% grade 2 and 3, respectively. Xerostomia improved over time, and the xerostomia incidences were 20 and 1.5% for grade 2 and 3, respectively, at median 13.3 months after radiation started. At a median follow-up of 1.6 years, three patients had persistent or recurrent locoregional disease (Eisbruch et al. 2006).

The experience in the use of proton beam therapy for the treatment of oropharyngeal carcinoma is limited. Investigators at Loma Linda University Medical Center (LLUMC) conducted an accelerated hyperfractionation study for stage II–IV oropharyngeal carcinoma using a technique similar to the MD Anderson concomitant boost technique (Slater et al. 2005). The LLUMC trial differed from the concomitant boost trial in a number of factors, including a higher total dose of 75.9 Gy that was delivered in a shorter overall time of 28 treatment days. Only 25.5 Gy of the total dose was given with proton, with the rest delivered with the opposed lateral photon technique. None of the patients received concurrent chemotherapy. The intent of the study was not only to increase tumor control probability by increasing the total dose and decreasing the treatment time, but also to simultaneously decrease treatment-related morbidity by exploiting the dosimetric advantages of protons.

Over a period of more than 10 years, 29 patients were accrued to the study. All patients completed the prescribed dose without any interruption. With a median follow-up of 28 months, the 2-year locoregional control and disease-free survival rates were 93 and 81%, respectively. The 2-year actuarial incidence of late RTOG grade 3 toxicity was 16%. This small study was performed over a prolonged period of time without the use of chemotherapy and used proton radiation therapy for only 35% of the total dose. Further studies of proton beam therapy for oropharyngeal cancer are needed.

13.7
Cost-Effectiveness of Proton Beam Therapy

Estimation of the cost of proton vs. X-ray therapy must be based on comparable technology for the proton and the photon treatments. This would include patient evaluation, treatment planning, and delivery of planned dose, use of intensity modulation (IMRT and IMPT), quality assurance, and other factors. A valid cost analysis of proton or photon therapy should consider all of the relevant parameters and not only the cost of the technical aspects of treatment. That is, estimates of cost need to include those dealing with local regrowth and of treatment-related complication, acute and late. The predicted cost of these latter two factors needs to assess not only the direct medical costs but also the time, effort, cost of missed work, and the psychological impact of the regrowth or the developing complication. This depth of analysis of cost of management of cancer patients is not common, even though obviously important (SUIT et al. 2008).

13.8
Future Directions

Proton beam therapy, especially IMPT, results in significantly less dose delivered to the normal tissues in the treatment of head and neck cancers. It will be important to determine whether the decrease in normal tissue dose delivered by proton beam therapy will result in improved quality of life. For tumors such as sinonasal tumors with poor treatment outcome with conventional radiation, it will be important to determine whether increased dose can be delivered to the tumor, thereby increasing tumor control probability without increasing treatment toxicity.

References

Al-Sarraf M, LeBlanc M, Fu KK et al. (1998) Chemoradiotherapy versus radiotherapy in patients with advanced nasopharyngeal cancer: Phase III randomized Intergroup study 0099. J Clin Oncol 16:1310–1317

Chan AW, Pommier P, Deschler DG et al. (2004) Change in patterns of relapse after combined proton and photon irradiation for locally advanced paranasal sinus cancer. Int J Radiat Oncol Biol Phys 60:S320

Chao KS, Ozyigit G, Blanco AI et al. (2004) Intensity-modulated radiation therapy for oropharyngeal carcinoma: impact of tumor volume. Int J Radiat Oncol Biol Phys 59:43–50

Chen AM, Daly ME, Bucci MK et al. (2007) Carcinomas of the paranasal sinuses and nasal cavity treated with radiotherapy as a single institution over five decades: Are we making improvement? Int J Radiat Oncol Biol Phys 69:141–147

Daly ME, Chen AM, Bucci MK et al. (2007) Intensity-modulated radiation therapy for malignancies of the nasal cavity and paranasal sinuses. Int J Radiat Oncol Biol Phys 67:151–157

Eisbruch A, Harris J, Garden A et al. (2006) Phase II multi-institutional study of IMRT for oropharyngeal cancer (RTOG 00-22): early results. Int J Radiat Oncol Biol Phys 66:S46

Garden AS, Morrison WH, Wong PF et al. (2007) Disease-control rates following intensity-modulated radiation therapy for small primary oropharyngeal carcinoma. Int J Radiat Oncol Biol Phys 67:438–444

Garden AS, Weber RS, Morrison WH et al. (1995) The influence of positive margins and nerve invasion in adenoid cystic carcinoma of the head and neck treated with surgery and radiation. Int J Radiat Oncol Biol Phys 32:619–626

Hoppe BS, Stegman LD, Zelefsky MJ et al. (2007) Treatment of nasal cavity and paranasal sinus cancer with modern radiotherapy techniques in the postoperative setting – The MSKCC experience. Int J Radiat Oncol Biol Phys 67:691–702

Kam MK, Leung SF, Zee B et al. (2007) Prospective randomized study of intensity-modulated radiotherapy on salivary gland function in early-stage nasopharyngeal carcinoma patients. J Clin Oncol 25:4873–4879

Katz TS, Mendenhall WM, Morris CG et al. (2002) Malignant tumors of the nasal cavity and paranasal sinuses. Head Neck 24:821–829

Kim GE, Park HC, Keum KC et al. (1999) Adenoid cystic carcinoma of the maxillary antrum. Am J Otolaryngol 20:77–84

Lavertu P, Roberts JK, Kraus DH et al. (1989) Squamous cell carcinoma of the paranasal sinuses: the Cleveland clinic experience 1977–1986. Laryngoscope 99:1130–1136

Lee NY, de Arruda FF, Puri DR et al. (2006) A comparison of intensity-modulated radiation therapy and concomitant boost radiotherapy in the setting of concurrent chemotherapy for locally advanced oropharyngeal carcinoma. Int J Radiat Oncol Biol Phys 66:966–974

Lomax AJ (2007) Intensity-modulated proton therapy. In: Delaney T, Kooy H (eds) Proton and heavier charged particle radiotherapy. Lippincott Williams and Wilkins, Philadelphia, PA, pp 98–107

Mendenhall WM, Morris CG, Amdur RJ et al. (2004) Radiotherapy alone or combined with surgery for adenoid cystic carcinoma of the head and neck. Head Neck 26:154–162

Parsons JT, Bova FJ, Fitzgerald CR et al. (1994) Severe dry-eye syndrome following external beam irradiation. Int J Radiat Oncol Biol Phys 30:775–780

Particle therapy facilities in operation (inl. patient statistics) (2008). Particle Therapy Co-Operative Group. Retrieved 21 August 2008, from http://ptcog.web.psi.ch/ptcentres.html

Patel S, Adams JA, Busse PM et al. (2007) Nasopharynx. In: Delaney T, Kooy H (eds) Proton and heavier charged particle radiotherapy. Lippincott Williams and Wilkins,Philadelphia, PA, pp 98–107

Pommier P, Liebsch N, Deschler DG et al. (2006) Proton beam radiation therapy for skull base adenoid cystic carcinoma. Arch Otolaryngol Head Neck Surg 132:1242–1249

Slater JD, Yonemoto LT, Mantik DW et al. (2005) Proton radiation for treatment of cancer of the oropharynx: early experience at Loma Linda University Medical Center using a concomitant boost technique. Int J Radiat Oncol Biol Phys 62:494–500

Steneker M, Lomax A, Schneider U (2006) Intensity modulated photon and proton therapy for the treatment of head and neck tumors. Radiother Oncol 80:263–267

Suit HD (2003) Protons to replace photons in external beam radiation therapy? Clin Oncol (R Coll Radiol) 15:S29–S31

Suit HD, Goldberg S, Niemierko A et al. (2003) Proton beams to replace photon beams in radical dose treatments. Acta Oncol 42:800–808

Suit H, Kooy H, Trofimov A et al. (2008) Should positive phase III clinical trial data be required before proton beam therapy is more widely adopted? No Radiother Oncol 86:148–153

Takeda A, Shigematsu N, Suzuki S et al. (1999) Late retinal complications of radiation therapy for nasal and paranasal malignancies: relationship between irradiated-dose area and severity. Int J Radiat Oncol Biol Phys 44:599–605

Vikram B, Strong EW, Shah JP et al. (1984) Radiation therapy in adenoid cystic carcinoma. Int J Radiat Oncol Biol Phys 10:221–223

Waldron JN, O'Sullivan B, Warde P et al. (1998) Ethmoid sinus cancer: twenty-nine cases managed with primary radiation therapy. Int J Radiat Oncol Biol Phys 41:361–369

Weber DC, Chan AW, Lessell S et al. (2006) Visual outcome of accelerated fractionated radiation for advanced sinonasal malignancies employing photons/protons. Radiother Oncol 81:243–249

Target Definition and Delineation
CT/MRI/PET-Guided Targets

XAVIER GEETS and VINCENT GRÉGOIRE

CONTENTS

14.1 Introduction 164

14.2 Selection and Delineation of Nodal CTV 164
14.2.1 Evaluation of the Neck Node Status 164
14.2.2 Selection and Delineation of Nodal CTVs in the Node-Negative Neck 165
14.2.2.1 Guidelines for the Selection of the Target Volumes in the N0 Neck 165
14.2.2.2 Guidelines for the Delineation of the Target Volumes in the N0 Neck 166
14.2.3 Selection and Delineation of Nodal CTVs in the Node-Positive and Postoperative Neck 167

14.3 Delineation of Primary Tumor GTV with Multimodality Imaging 170

14.4 Selection and Delineation of the Primary Tumor CTV 172

14.5 Conclusion 172

References 173

XAVIER GEETS, MD, PhD
VINCENT GRÉGOIRE, MD, PhD, Hon FRCR
Radiation Oncology Department and Center for Molecular Imaging and Experimental Radiotherapy, Université Catholique de Louvain, St-Luc University Hospital, 10 Avenue Hippocrate, 1200 Brussels, Belgium

KEY POINTS:

- The implementation of IMRT for head and neck tumors requires proper selection of target volumes for the neck nodes and the primary tumors, and accurate 3D delineation of the selected volumes to avoid tumor geographic misses and/or overdosage of normal tissues.
- For CTV selection and delineation in the N0 neck, collaborative works led to the elaboration of consensus recommendations for the delineation of levels I to VI, which offer a unique set of unambiguous and easily identifiable boundaries on CT/MRI axial sections.
- Adjustments of these guidelines have been proposed for target volume delineation in positive and post-operative necks.
- FDG-PET outperforms anatomical imaging modalities (CT-MRI) for the delineation of the primary tumor GTV and leads to smaller and more accurate volumes in pharyngo-laryngeal SCC, but strict methodology and tools are required for PET images segmentation of the primary GTV.
- Refinements of GTV delineation brought by FDG-PET impact on the dose distribution with subsequent normal tissues sparing.
- The selection of the CTV for the primary tumors is a more complex task. The general principle is that the microscopic spread of tumor cells follows anatomical compartments bounded by anatomical barriers; this principle should govern the elaboration of recommendation for the selection of the primary CTV.
- The implementation of guidelines for the selection and 3D-delineation of target volumes on modern imaging modalities should contribute to reduce variations in GTV and CTV delineation for both the primary tumors and the neck nodes.

14.1

Introduction

Intensity-modulated radiation therapy (IMRT) has become more and more popular in head and neck radiotherapy. Its ability to generate complex-shaped and tight dose gradients between the targets and the surrounding organs at risk (OARs) brings an undeniable dosimetrical advantage over nonmodulated external-beam two-dimensional (2D) and three-dimensional (3D) radiation techniques. This makes IMRT especially suitable to confine the prescribed high doses to the target volumes (TVs), limiting thus the dose delivered to the OARs.

Maximizing the therapeutic index by such technique however requires optimal and precise selection and delineation of both TVs and OARs. Indeed, incomplete TVs coverage may lead to marginal tumor recurrence, thus possibly compromising patient's outcome. On the other hand, overestimation of the TVs would potentially lead to an overdosage of normal tissues with a possible increase in complication probability. In this regard, clinicians may have different opinion on how to balance the risk of potentially missing part of the TVs and the risk of excessive normal tissue irradiation. This may account for some of the differences among physicians on how conservatively they delineate targets. This issue partially explains the large interobserver variability in both selecting and outlying the targets, these interobserver differences in these tasks surpassing physical dose coverage deficiencies of the targets or dose uncertainties due to setup variations (Hong et al. 2004).

On the other hand, the identification and selection of the normal tissues, whose sparing may achieve significant gain in reducing the incidence and severity of both acute and late radiation-induced toxicities, is of prime importance in functional preservation strategies. Besides spinal cord, parotid gland, and mandible, the in-depth understanding of functional physiological processes suggests that potential gain would be expected from sparing other organs. For example, the patient-related xerostomia not only depends on the salivary flow, but also on the saliva quality influenced by the mucin-producing minor salivary and submandibular glands. This partially explains why parotid sparing alone is not enough to fully prevent xerostomia (Eisbruch 2007) and justifies the implementation of more specific sparing approaches. Similarly, some structures such as the pharyngeal constrictor muscle and the glottic/supraglottic larynx have been shown to be involved in the post chemo–radiation related dysphagia (Eisbruch et al. 2002a, b; Eisbruch 2004). As dose–volume–effect relationships for these structures exist (Feng et al. 2007), their partial sparing could potentially benefit patients (Eisbruch et al. 2004b, 2007).

Today, various imaging modalities are at the disposal of the radiation oncologist community to assist them in the diagnosis and the treatment planning tasks. Relying on different physical and biological principles, they present specific intrinsic characteristics that may significantly impact on the image interpretation and targets selection/delineation. Consequently, their uses in the treatment planning process should be carefully assessed and strict methodologies have to be defined, particularly for the primary tumor segmentation task. The purpose of the present chapter is to provide literature-based recommendations on the selection of the primary tumors and neck nodes gross target volume (GTV) and clinical target volume (CTV), and accurate multimodality-imaging-based 3D delineation of the selected volumes.

14.2

Selection and Delineation of Nodal CTV

14.2.1
Evaluation of the Neck Node Status

The clinical staging of the neck node relies on the available diagnostic information from the clinical examination of the neck and from the various imaging modalities, which depict more or less accurately the true tumor extent. The main difficulty with imaging modalities is that none of them has sensitivity or specificity of 100%, thus meaning that false-negative and false-positive results for depicting neoplastic node involvement occur. With anatomical imaging such as CT and MRI, a short-axis above 1 cm and/or central necrosis are typically used as criteria to define involved neck nodes; for CT, sensitivity and specificity ranging from 36 to 86% and 56 to 100%, respectively, have been reported (Laubenbacher et al. 1995; McGuirt et al. 1995; Benchaou et al. 1996; Stokkel et al. 2000; Stuckensen et al. 2000; Dammann et al. 2005). In these series, where the surgical lymph node specimen was used as the gold standard, CT and 18F-fluoro-deoxyglucose positron emission tomography (FDG-PET) performed with comparable diagnosis accuracy. More recent data showed that combining morphological and biological information from PET–CT improved accuracy for evaluating neck node in HNSCC, in comparison with FDG-PET or CT alone (Jeong et al. 2007). Another study has prospectively assessed the use of FDG-PET for the primary staging of 250 patients with HNSCC (not yet published). Although the accuracy of the neck staging was slightly improved over CT or MRI, the identification of unknown distant metastasis by the use of FDG-PET was the most important parameter influencing the management of these patients.

A potentially interesting use of FDG-PET is for staging patients with node-negative on anatomical imaging modalities, in which the issue could be to avoid unnecessary treatment of the neck if FDG-PET examination was negative. However, data clearly showed that in this specific situation, the sensitivity of FDG-PET only reached 70% (Stuckensen et al. 2000). These data are not surprising in light of the fact that in node-negative patients, microscopic infiltration can be observed in up to 30% of the cases after prophylactic neck node dissection. The limited spatial and contrast resolutions of PET indeed preclude the detection of microscopic disease.

In conclusion, FDG-PET has no, or only marginal, benefit in the evaluation of the neck node status in comparison with CT or MRI, and therefore FDG-PET is not likely to be superior for the selection of the neck nodes TVs.

14.2.2
Selection and Delineation of Nodal CTVs in the Node-Negative Neck

The selection of the volumes of tissues at risk of harboring subclinical disease that should be prophylactically irradiated (CTV) relies on the knowledge of the probability of microscopic invasion and the pattern of the lymphatic drainage for each tumor location and stage, since available imaging modalities fail to demonstrate potential microscopic disease. As the pattern of lymphatic drainage is predicable in previously untreated neck for oral cavity, larynx, and pharynx, several authors have advocated the concept of limited treatment, i.e., selective

neck dissection or irradiation. Indeed, data of pathological results and recurrence patterns accumulated over many years strongly suggest that more selective neck treatments might lead to substantial reduction in the dose inflicted on critical OARs, such as the parotid gland, without jeopardizing locoregional control (Eisbruch et al. 2004a; Dawson et al. 2000; Chao et al. 2003). The application of such selective treatments however requires standardization of the terminology and procedures.

14.2.2.1
Guidelines for the Selection of the Target Volumes in the N0 Neck

Large series on clinical and pathological neck node distributions and on neck recurrence after selective dissection procedures led to the elaboration of guidelines for the selection of the appropriate neck node levels to be treated. Although it is beyond the scope of this chapter to discuss these data at length, some general principles may be pointed up (Grégoire et al. 2000) for N0 patients, including (Table 14.1) the following:

- A selective treatment of the neck is appropriate for HNSCC of oral cavity, oropharynx, larynx, and hypopharynx.
- As a general rule, neck node levels I–III should be treated for oral cavity tumors, while levels II–IV have to be selected for oropharyngeal, hypopharyngeal, and laryngeal tumors.
- In addition to the levels I–III, level IV should be included in tumors from the mobile tongue due to the high incidence of skip metastases (Byers et al. 1997).
- No prophylactic nodal irradiation is needed for glottic T1 tumors since there is no lymphatic drainage originating from the true vocal cord.
- Elective treatment of level IIb could be omitted for N0 patients with a primary tumor in the oral cavity, larynx, or hypopharynx.
- For subglottic tumors, tumors with subglottic or transglottic extension, or hypopharyngeal tumors with esophageal extension, nodes in level VI (pretracheal, paratracheal, and recurrent nodes) should be included in the treated volume.
- For nasopharyngeal tumors, levels I–V and retropharyngeal nodes (RPNs) need to be treated, even in N0 patients.

Table 14.1. Guidelines for the selection of neck node levels to be treated for patients with head and neck squamous cell carcinomas

Location of primary tumor	Appropriate node levels to be treated	
	Stage N0–N1	Stage N2a–N2b
Oral cavity	I, II, and III (+IV for anterior tongue tumors)	I, II, III, IV, and V[a]
Oropharynx	II,[b] III, and IV (+RPNs for posterior pharyngeal wall tumors)	I, II, III, IV, V, and RPNs
Hypopharynx	II,[b] III, and IV (+VI for esophageal extension)	I, II, III, IV, V, and RPNs (+VI for esophageal extension)
Larynx[c]	II,[b] III, and IV (+VI for transglottic and subglottic tumors)	(I), II, III, IV, and V (+VI for transglottic and subglottic tumors)
Nasopharynx	II, III, IV, V, and RPNs	II, III, IV, V, and RPNs

[a]May be omitted if only levels I–III are involved
[b]Nodes in level IIb could be omitted for N0 patients
[c]T1 glottic cancer excluded

- In N0 patients with posterior pharyngeal wall tumor, RPNs should always be treated irrespective of the staging of the neck in the other levels.
- The treatment of the contralateral neck is more debated. As a rule, its inclusion within the TVs depends on the tumor location and extent. Typically, well-lateralized tumors (e.g., lateral border of the tongue, retromolar trigone) may be spared from contralateral neck treatment. To the contrary, midline tumors, tumors originating from or extending to a site that has bilateral lymphatic drainage (base of tongue, vallecula, posterior pharyngeal wall) are thought to benefit from a contralateral treatment.
- For contralateral neck irradiation, the selection of the node levels to be treated follows rules similar to those for the ipsilateral neck.
- Similar guidelines may be recommended for N1 patients without suspicion of extracapsular infiltration (Byers 1985).

The accurate selection of the targets to be irradiated is of prime importance, and the benefit of curing the patient has to be weighted against the possible overtreatment, with subsequent unnecessary radiation-related toxicities. It is widely accepted that a risk of subclinical invasion below 5–10% does not justify any prophylactic irradiation. If most of the situations are clear, some borderline cases exist. These include stage T2N0 glottic tumors, where the risk of neck lymph node metastases approaches 10%. The prophylactic nodal irradiation will lead to unnecessary additional toxicity in 90% of patients, while the

exclusion of such targets may result in potential treatment failure in about 10% of cases. Another gray zone refers to the contralateral neck irradiation in tonsillar or buccal SCC. In cases of N0 early primary cancers, the contralateral neck is often excluded from the areas to be irradiated (O'Sullivan et al. 2001). However, as the risk of contralateral node metastases increases with tumor extension into sites with bilateral lymphatic drainage (base of tongue, soft palate) or with advanced ipsilateral neck metastases, locally advanced stages certainly require bilateral neck irradiation (Lin et al. 2008a).

14.2.2.2
Guidelines for the Delineation of the Target Volumes in the N0 Neck

The first recommendations aiming at unifying neck node treatment came from the committee for Head and Neck Surgery and Oncology of the American Academy for Otolaryngology – Head and Neck Surgery. Popularized by Robbins, they were based on a systematic classification of the neck nodes into six levels (levels I–VI), bounded by identifiable anatomical structures such as blood vessels, nerves, muscles, bones, and cartilages (Robbins 1998, 1999). These recommendations have later been updated with refinements of some boundaries using radiological landmarks and further definition of sublevels (i.e., IIa–IIb, Va–Vb). Collaborative works between radiation oncologists, surgeons, and radiologists have led to the publication in 2004 of consensus recommendations for the delineation of levels I–VI on CT or MRI axial sections (GRÉGOIRE et al. 2003a, b). DAHANCA, EORTC, GORTEC, NCIC, and RTOG have endorsed these new recommendations that provide a unique set of unambiguous and identifiable boundaries. Regarding these consensus guidelines, the collaborative work translates as accurately as possible the surgical recommendations into radiological criteria on axial CT sections, and defined unambiguous boundaries to minimize differences among observers. A summary of these consensus guidelines is presented in Table 14.2. A typical CTV delineation of these levels is also illustrated in Fig. 14.1.

Again, an accurate choice and delineation of the boundaries of the various neck node levels and the exclusion of very-low-risk targets determine the ability to spare neighboring crucial tissues. As an example, the refinement in the definition of the cranial limit of the level II for node-negative patients, which moves from the jugular foramen at the base of skull (SOM et al. 1999) to the caudal edge of the lateral process of C1 in the recommendation from GREGOIRE et al. (2003). This has a significant benefit regarding the parotid gland sparing on that side of neck in N0 patients. The use of such boundary for the upper limit of level II has proved to be a safe procedure (EISBRUCH et al. 2004a).

14.2.3
Selection and Delineation of Nodal CTVs in the Node-Positive and Postoperative Neck

The recommendation guidelines provided by the above-mentioned consensus (GRÉGOIRE et al. 2003a, b) only concerned the node-negative neck, and some adjustments were required for positive and postoperative necks to take into account the specificities of these situations. Among these, the neoplastic invasion of node(s) may induce a retrograde lymph flow, thus carrying tumor cells in nodes not deemed to be typically invaded in the N0 neck, either higher up in the neck (i.e., more cranially than the lateral process of C1) or lower than the caudal limit of level IV or Vb. These hypotheses are supported by the data from EISBRUCH (2004a) that showed marginal recurrences in the node-positive neck near the base of skull above the upper limit of delineation for the N0 neck. Another important factor to consider in the node-positive neck is the risk of extracapsular extension, which is directly proportional to the size of the lymph

node and may be up to 95% in bulky lymph node more than 3 cm (CHAO et al. 2002). In case of extracapsular extension, tumor cells typically infiltrate in fatty space within 1 cm for small nodes (APISARNTHANARAX et al. 2006), but for bulky nodes or evidences of muscular infiltration on CT or MRI, additional adjacent structures may be at risk of tumoral infiltration, such as the sterno-cleido-mastoid and the paraspinal muscles. Based on the few data available, recommendations can be proposed for the selection and delineation of the nodal CTV in node-positive necks as follows:

- For patients with multiple unilateral nodes (N2b), the nodal targets should encompass levels I–V (Table 14.1). Level I could however be excluded for laryngeal tumors, and level V for oral cavity tumors with neck node involvement confined to levels I–III. The RPNs always needs to be included for oro- or hypopharyngeal tumors. The inclusion of the level VI in laryngeal or hypopharyngeal tumors follows the rules of N0 patients (Table 14.1).
- In case of involvement of upper level IIa or IIb with node(s), the retrostyloid space should be included up to the base of skull (Table 14.2, Fig. 14.2).
- In case of involvement of level IV or Vb with node, the lower border should be extended to include the supraclavicular fossa (Table 14.2, Fig. 14.2).
- In case of lymph node abutted to a muscle and/or radiological indication of muscular infiltration, it is recommended to include this muscle at least for the entire invaded level.
- When an involved node is located at the boundary with another level, it is recommended to extend the CTV to include this adjacent level, even if it was not intended to be part of CTV.
- For patients with bilateral neck nodes, one proposal is to consider each side of the neck separately, although there are no data available for this specific case.

In postoperative situation, there are even fewer data to build firm recommendations on the selection and delineation of neck targets, and these two steps should follow institutional guidelines to guarantee treatment consistency and avoid either over- or undertreatment. As a proposition, the entire surgical bed should be covered to take into account potential tumor cell spilling during the surgical procedure. Comparably to the node-positive neck, the nodal CTV should be extended to the retrostyloid space, supraclavicular fossa, adjacent muscle, or adjacent

Table 14.2. Consensus guidelines for the radiological boundaries of the neck node levels and spaces

Level/ space	Anatomical boundaries					
	Cranial	Caudal	Anterior	Posterior	Lateral	Medial
Ia	Geniohyoid m., plane tangent to basilar edge of mandible	Plane tangent to body of hyoid bone	Symphysis menti, platysma m.	Body of hyoid bone	Medial edge of anterior belly of digastric m.	NA[a]
Ib	Mylohyoid m., cranial edge of submandibular gland	Plane through central part of hyoid bone	Symphysis menti, platisma m.	Posterior edge of submandibular gland	Basilar edge/ innerside of mandible, platysma m., skin	Lateral edge of anterior belly of digastric m.
IIa	Caudal edge of lateral process of C1	Caudal edge of the body of hyoid bone	Posterior edge of submandibular gland; anterior edge of int. carotid: posterior edge of posterior belly of digastric m.	Posterior border of int. jugular vein	Medial edge of SCM	Medial edge of int. carotid, paraspinal m.
IIb	Caudal edge of lateral process of C1	Caudal edge of the body of hyoid bone	Posterior border of int. jugular vein	Posterior border of the SCM	Medial edge of the SCM	Medial edge of int. carotid paraspinal m.
III	Caudal edge of the body of hyoid bone	Caudal edge of cricoid cart	Postero-lateral edge of sternohyoid m., ant edge of SCM	Posterior edge of the SCM	Medial edge of the SCM	Int. edge of carotid, paraspinal m.
IV	Caudal edge of cricoid cartilage	2 cm cranial to sternoclavicular joint	Anteromedial edge of the SCM	Posterior edge of the SCM	Medial edge of the SCM	Medial edge of internal carotid, paraspinal m.
V	Cranial edge of body of hyoid bone	CT slice encompassing the transverse cervical vessels	Posterior edge of the CM	Anterolateral border of the trapezius m.	Platysma m., skin	Paraspinal m.
VI	Caudal edge of body of thyroid cartilage[b]	Sternal manubrium	Skin; platysma m.	Separation between trachea and esophagus[c]	Medial edges of thyroid gland, skin and antero-medial edge of the SCM	n.a.
RPNs	Base of skull	Cranial edge of the body of hyoid bone	Fascia under the pharyngeal mucosa	Prevertebral m.	Medial edge of the internal carotid	Midline
Retro-styloid	Base of skull (jugular foramen)	Upper limit of level II	Parapharyngeal space	Vertebral body/ base of skull	Parotid space	Lateral edge of RP nodes
Supraclavicular fossa	Lower border of level IV/Vb	Sterno-clavicular joint	SCM, skin, clavicle	Anterior edge of posterior scalene m.	Lateral edge of posterior scalenus m.	Thyroid gland/trachea

SCM sterno-cleido-mastoid muscle; *RPNs* retropharyngeal nodes
[a]Midline structure lying between the medial borders bellies of the digastric muscles
[b]For paratracheal and recurrent nodes, the cranial border is the caudal edge of the cricoid cartilage
[c]For pretracheal nodes, trachea, and anterior edge of cricoid cartilage

Target Definition and Delineation CT/MRI/PET-Guided Targets 169

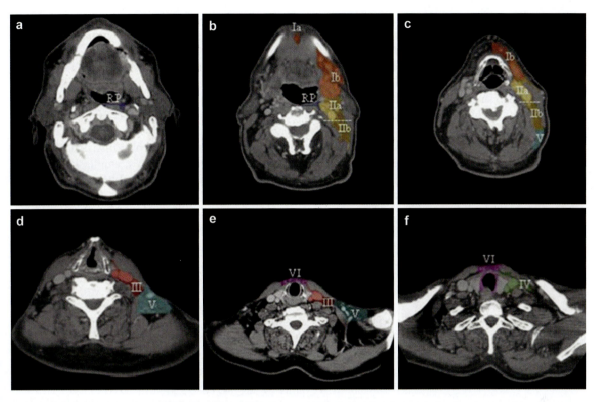

Fig. 14.1. Neck node levels I–VI delineated on axial CT slices using the radiological boundaries detailed in Table 14.2. The CT imaging comes from a patient with a T1N0M0 glottic SCC. The CT sections were selected at the level of the bottom edge of C1 (**a**), the upper edge of C3 (**b**), mid C4 (**c**), the bottom edge of C6 (**d**), the bottom edge of C7 (**e**), and mid D1 (**f**)

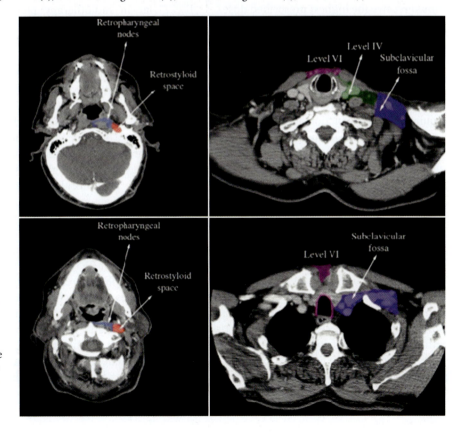

Fig. 14.2. Axial CT images from the same patient as in Fig. 14.1. The radiological boundaries defined on Table 14.2 were used for the delineation of the retrostyloid space (*left panels*) and the supraclavicular fossa (*right panels*)

node level in similar conditions. Lateral RPNs should also be included in the CTV in case of pharyngeal tumors with pathological node involvement.

The extension of nodal CTV into adjacent levels or structures needs to be weighed against an increased risk of treatment-induced morbidity. For example, the inclusion of level I de facto induces submandibular gland irradiation, with subsequent xerostomia. Similarly, the cranial extension of the level II to the retrostyloid space may be deleterious for parotid glands sparing. However, a generous selection and delineation of targets in clinically or pathologically involved necks is justified to avoid locoregional recurrences, at least until more data are available on the pattern of recurrence after selective neck treatment.

14.3
Delineation of Primary Tumor GTV with Multimodality Imaging

The accurate evaluation of the true primary tumor and its extensions still remains a challenging and difficult task for the radiation oncologist. However, this issue is crucial since the GTV represents the volume including the highest tumor cell density that should receive the highest prescribed dose.

The GTV delineation mainly relies on a precise physical examination and the use of optimal imaging modalities, but also requires sound clinical judgment and in-depth knowledge of the tumor spread pathways and the head and neck anatomy. Precise and reproducible GTV delineation from various imaging modalities requires accurate depiction of the tumor and its extension on a 3D basis. The imaging modalities currently available can offer anatomic (e.g., CT and MRI) or functional (e.g., PET) information, but they all present limitations in terms of spatial or contrast resolutions, and in terms of sensitivity and specificity. These limitations may significantly impact on the image interpretation and the subsequent tumor delineation.

In HNSCC, both TVs and OARs are typically delineated on planning CT. Although CT presents numerous advantages, including its availability, acceptable cost, high spatial resolution, and intrinsic information on the electronic density used for dose calculation, it lacks contrast resolution for soft tissues and tumor extent; it is sensitive to metallic artifacts from dental filling, which limits its performance in assessing oropharyngeal and oral cavity tumors. These limitations make the accurate distinction between the tumor and its environment problematic. This partially explains the large interobserver variability observed in many studies (BREEN et al. 2007; RIEGEL et al. 2006; HERMANS et al. 1997; COOPER et al. 2007; JEANNERET-SOZZI et al. 2006), which remains one of the major sources of inaccuracy in GTV delineation. The use of contrast-enhanced CT and basic delineation guidelines provided to the physicians have already been shown to improve consistency between observers (GEETS et al. 2005), emphasizing on the importance of image quality and guidelines for delineation criteria.

In comparison with CT, MRI offers better soft tissue contrast, which improves the delineation of GTV near the base of skull, such as in nasopharyngeal or paranasal sinus cancers (SOM 1997). However, in pharyngo-laryngeal tumors, several studies have failed to show any added value of MRI over CT on volumetric and reproducibility aspects, even when optimal MRI sequences with high spatial resolution were used (DAISNE et al. 2004; GEETS et al. 2005, 2006, 2007b). Consequently, we do not recommend the use of MRI in the routine treatment planning process of pharyngo-laryngeal SCC.

Besides these anatomical imaging modalities, the use of FDG-PET, which provides unique information on cellular functions, becomes more and more popular in radiotherapy planning. In a pioneer work, DAISNE et al. (2004) have demonstrated that the introduction of FDG-PET in the delineation procedure of pharyngo-laryngeal SCC led to significantly smaller GTVs compared with those delineated on CT or MRI. Of interest, a comparison with surgical laryngeal specimens showed that GTVs delineated from FDG-PET were the closest to the pathological GTV, while the use of CT or MRI led on average to an overestimation of the true tumor volume by 40 and 47%, respectively. This highlights that the lack of specificity of these anatomical imaging modalities may result in inadequate target definition with possible consequences on dose distribution. Although FDG-PET seems to be a good candidate in radiotherapy planning process, its optimal use is not a trivial task. The physics of PET, including the poor statistics and spatial resolution, results in high level of noise and blurred images that may severely affect the accurate determination of the volume and shape of the tumors.

Strict and validated methodologies are definitely required for the outlining of FDG-positive tissue. In this context, various methods have been proposed for patients with HNSCC. The visual interpretation of PET images and delineation of the tumor by an experienced physician is the easiest method (Ashamalla et al. 2007; Ciernik et al. 2003; Nishioka et al. 2002), but it is highly subjective and affected by the display windowing. This necessarily leads to unacceptable intra- and interobserver variations, precluding the use of such an approach. By contrast, threshold-based methods offer an objective and reproducible way for segmenting PET images (Black et al. 2004; Paulino et al. 2005). If the use of a fixed threshold, either relative or absolute, has been made popular by its simplicity, data from phantoms (Daisne et al. 2003) and patients (Gregoire et al. 2005) clearly demonstrated that the threshold to be applied to adequately fit the true volume largely varied from case to case. Reinforced by the absence of validation study, these data clearly illustrated that fixed threshold methods are not adequate for accurately segmenting HNSCC. More sophisticated methods include adaptive threshold-based approaches. Among these, segmentation techniques that account for the background activity in the threshold value to be applied have been shown to provide accurate delineation on phantom material (Daisne et al. 2003) and laryngeal tumors (Daisne et al. 2004). Although validated as objective and reliable, these methods require calibrations curves based on phantom acquisitions, which vary according to many parameters (e.g., the PET camera, reconstruction algorithms, filters), hindering thus the generalization of the method. In addition, threshold-based segmentation tools are not suitable for images with low signal-to-background ratios, as encountered in inflammatory situations or with images acquired during the course of radiotherapy. From a methodological point of view, the use of threshold-based methods was mainly motivated by the intrinsically low quality of PET images, i.e., the high level of noise and blurred images, that prevents the use of gradient-based methods. Such a method was however made possible by the implementation of specific image restoration tools, i.e., edge-preserving filters for denoising, and deconvolution algorithm for deblurring. This segmentation technique has been proved to be more accurate and reliable than threshold-based methods (Geets et al. 2007a), especially in segmenting images acquired during radiotherapy (Geets et al. 2007b).

With these adequate segmentation tools in hand, FDG-PET appears very promising since it provides smaller, more accurate and reproducible GTVs in comparison with CT or MRI (Daisne et al. 2004). More important, refining the GTV delineation by means of FDG-PET imaging ultimately led to more optimal dose distributions within PTVs and surrounding tissues (Geets et al. 2006, 2007b). Indeed, the reduction of the primary tumor TVs allowed by such an approach translated into significant decreases of the volumes receiving the highest dose using either 3D-confromal RT (Geets et al. 2006) or IMRT with helical tomotherapy (Geets et al. 2007b), as illustrated in Fig. 14.3. A prospective multicentric phase II study is currently being carried out to clinically validate this concept in HNSCC.

The impressive progresses performed in imaging, dose calculation, and delivery techniques have recently opened avenues for new treatment opportunities such

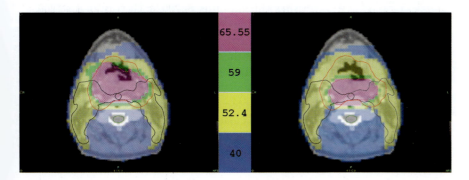

Fig. 14.3. Axial CT slices from a patient with a T4 N0 hypopharyngeal SCC treated with adaptive simultaneous integrated boost IMRT on a Tomotherapy® machine. Planning CT and FDG-PET were acquired before treatment. A prophylactic dose of 55.5 Gy (30 fractions of 1.85 Gy) was delivered on the nodal prophylactic PTV (*black line*) delineated on the planning CT. A therapeutic dose of 69 Gy (30 fractions of 2.3 Gy) was delivered on the PTV (*red line*) associated with the primary tumor CTV and GTV. The PTV was the CTV plus a 4-mm margin in every direction, except the skin direction. The CTV was the GTV plus a 5-mm margin in all directions. The primary tumor TVs were delineated based on contrast-enhanced CT (*left panel*) or FDG-PET (*right panel*) images. The comparison of the two plans shows a smaller volume of high dose in the FDG-PET-based plan compared with the CT-based plan

as adaptive radiation therapy and dose-painting approaches. Adaptive radiation therapy consists in reassessing the tumor volume after a given dose of radiation has been delivered and boosting the residual imaged tumor. Preliminary studies have already demonstrated the feasibility and usefulness of such approaches in pharyngo-laryngeal SCC, and showed significant tumor shrinkages using both anatomical and functional imaging (Geets et al. 2007b). Selection of small volumes for dose escalation strategies, even more when high dose by fraction is prescribed such as in simultaneous integrated boost IMRT, is mandatory to prevent unacceptable damages of critical structures embedded within the boost volumes. Another appealing approach is the integration of biological information from molecular imaging modalities with the purpose of targeting radiation-resistant regions inside the tumor, such as high clonogen density, proliferation, or hypoxia, hypothesizing that the regionally variable radiosensitivity may require heterogeneous dose distribution to achieve optimal tumor control. This approach, termed "dose painting" by Ling (Ling et al. 2000), has already been investigated in HNSCC with various tracers (Chao et al. 2001; Lin et al. 2008b; Grosu et al. 2007; Madani et al. 2007; Vanderstraeten et al. 2006). Although promising, these new treatment strategies are at their infancies and still need active research to solve important issues.

If imaging plays a growing role in the target definition in radiotherapy, one should keep in mind that the macroscopic modalities available will fail to depict subtle tumor extension, and in particular the mucosal extent of the disease. As shown by Daisne et al. (2004), if both CT/MRI and FDG-PET overestimated the GTV in most dimensions, all three imaging modalities failed in accurately assessing the mucosal invasion visualized on the macroscopic specimen. In this context, a careful physical examination, including endoscopy and palpation, still remains the best tool for the appreciation of the mucosal extent of HNSCC.

14.4
Selection and Delineation of the Primary Tumor CTV

The selection and delineation on a 3D basis of the primary tumor CTV is a complex issue, which remains mainly unresolved. A general principle that

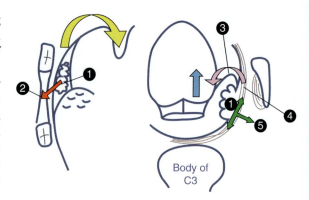

Fig. 14.4. Illustration of the microscopic oropharyngeal tumor spread pathways on a coronal view (*left panel*) and transverse slice through the body of C3 (*right panel*). Typical tumor spreads from tonsillar fossa (1) include the soft palate (*yellow arrow*), the glossotonsilar sulcus towards the retromolar trigone (2), the pharyngeal constrictor muscles (4), and when the pharyngobasilar raphe is transgressed, the parapharyngeal space (*green arrows*). Glossotonsillar sulcus (3) tumors extend to the base of tongue and to tonsillar fossa (*pink arrow*), while base of tongue tumor typically spreads into mobile tongue and floor of mouth muscles (*blue arrow*)

should govern the elaboration of recommendations is that the microscopic spread of SCC of the head and neck region follows anatomical compartments (e.g., paralaryngeal, parapharyngeal, and pre-epiglottic spaces) bounded by strong anatomical barriers (e.g., bone cortex, muscular facia, ligaments). Unless transgressed, such barriers would limit the local primary tumor spread and help at defining anatomical compartments for the primary tumor CTV. On the basis of those general principles, operational guidelines have been proposed for the major head and neck sites (Eisbruch et al. 2002a; Grégoire et al. 2003a). An example of local spread pathways is illustrated in Fig. 14.4 for the oropharynx. The main difficulty is related to those tumor locations where there is no barrier, such as in the tongue muscles or fatty spaces (i.e., parapharyngeal and submandibular spaces) that compose the head and neck region. On those structures, data are unfortunately lacking to determine whether a margin of 1, 1.5, 2 cm or more should be taken beyond the GTV.

14.5
Conclusion

The implementation of guidelines for the selection of the target volumes to be irradiated, as well as standardized rules for delineation of these volumes based on modern imaging modalities should contribute to reduce variations in GTV and CTV delineation for both primary tumors and neck nodes. This should contribute to increase homogeneity in treatment delivery on a patient and institution basis, and hence help to conduct multi-institutional clinical trials.

References

Apisarnthanarax S, Elliott DD, El-Naggar AK et al. (2006) Determining optimal clinical target volume margins in head-and-neck cancer based on microscopic extracapsular extension of metastatic neck nodes. Int J Radiat Oncol Biol Phys 64(3):678–683

Ashamalla H, Guirguis A, Bieniek E et al. (2007) The impact of positron emission tomography/computed tomography in edge delineation of gross tumor volume for head and neck cancers. Int J Radiat Oncol Biol Phy 68(2): 388–395

Benchaou M, Lehmann W, Slosman DO et al. (1996) The role of FDG-PET in the preoperative assessment of n-staging in head and neck cancer. Acta Otolaryngol 116(2):332–335

Black QC, Grills IS, Kestin LL et al. (2004) Defining a radiotherapy target with positron emission tomography. Int J Radiat Oncol Biol Phys 60(4):1272–1282

Breen SL, Publicover J, De Silva S et al. (2007) Intraobserver and interobserver variability in GTV delineation on FDG-PET-CT images of head and neck cancers. Int J Radiat Oncol Biol Phys 68(3):763–770

Byers RM (1985) Modified neck dissection. A study of 967 cases from 1970 to 1980. Am J Surg 150(4):414–421

Byers RM, Weber RS, Andrews T et al. (1997) Frequency and therapeutic implications of "skip metastases" in the neck from squamous carcinoma of the oral tongue. Head Neck 19(1):14–19

Chao KS, Bosch WR, Mutic S et al. (2001) A novel approach to overcome hypoxic tumor resistance: Cu-Atsm-guided intensity-modulated radiation therapy. Int J Radiat Oncol Biol Phys 49(4):1171–1182

Chao KS, Ozyigit G, Tran BN et al. (2003) Patterns of failure in patients receiving definitive and postoperative IMRT for head-and-neck cancer. Int J Radiat Oncol Biol Phys 55(2):312–321

Chao KS, Wippold FJ, Ozyigit G et al. (2002) Determination and delineation of nodal target volumes for head-and-neck cancer based on patterns of failure in patients receiving definitive and postoperative IMRT. Int J Radiat Oncol Biol Phys 53(5):1174–1184

Ciernik IF, Dizendorf E, Baumert BG et al. (2003) Radiation treatment planning with an integrated positron emission and computer tomography (PET/CT): a feasibility study. Int J Radiat Oncol Biol Phys 57(3):853–863

Cooper JS, Mukherji SK, Toledano AY et al. (2007) An evaluation of the variability of tumor-shape definition derived by experienced observers from CT images of supraglottic carcinomas (ACRIN protocol 6658). Int J Radiat Oncol Biol Phys 67(4):972–975

Daisne JF, Duprez T, Weynand B et al. (2004) Tumor volume in pharyngolaryngeal squamous cell carcinoma: comparison at CT, MR imaging, and FDG PET and validation with surgical specimen. Radiology 233(1):93–100

Daisne JF, Sibomana M, Bol A et al. (2003) Tri-dimensional automatic segmentation of PET volumes based on measured source-to-background ratios: influence of reconstruction algorithms. Radiother Oncol 69(3):247–250

Dammann F, Horger M, Mueller-Berg M et al. (2005) Rational diagnosis of squamous cell carcinoma of the head and neck region: comparative evaluation of CT, MRI, and 18FDG PET. AJR Am J Roentgenol 184(4):1326–1331

Dawson LA, Anzai Y, Marsh L et al. (2000) Patterns of local-regional recurrence following parotid-sparing conformal and segmental intensity-modulated radiotherapy for head and neck cancer. Int J Radiat Oncol Biol Phys 46(5): 1117–1126

Eisbruch A (2004) Dysphagia and aspiration following chemo-irradiation of head and neck cancer: major obstacles to intensification of therapy. Ann Oncol 15(3):363–364

Eisbruch A (2007) Reducing xerostomia by IMRT: what may, and may not, be achieved. J Clin Oncol 25(31):4863–4864

Eisbruch A, Foote RL, O'Sullivan B et al. (2002a) Intensity-modulated radiation therapy for head and neck cancer: emphasis on the selection and delineation of the targets. Semin Radiat Oncol 12(3):238–249

Eisbruch A, Levendag PC, Feng FY et al. (2007) Can IMRT or brachytherapy reduce dysphagia associated with chemo-radiotherapy of head and neck cancer? The Michigan and Rotterdam experiences. Int J Radiat Oncol Biol Phys 69(2 Suppl):S40–S42

Eisbruch A, Lyden T, Bradford CR et al. (2002b) Objective assessment of swallowing dysfunction and aspiration after radiation concurrent with chemotherapy for head-and-neck cancer. Int J Radiat Oncol Biol Phys 53(1):23–28

Eisbruch A, Marsh LH, Dawson LA et al. (2004a) Recurrences near base of skull after IMRT for head-and-neck cancer: implications for target delineation in high neck and for parotid gland sparing. Int J Radiat Oncol Biol Phys 59(1):28–42

Eisbruch A, Schwartz M, Rasch C et al. (2004b) Dysphagia and aspiration after chemoradiotherapy for head-and-neck cancer: which anatomic structures are affected and can they be spared by IMRT? Int J Radiat Oncol Biol Phys 60(5):1425–1439

Feng FY, Kim HM, Lyden TH et al. (2007) Intensity-modulated radiotherapy of head and neck cancer aiming to reduce dysphagia: early dose–effect relationships for the swallowing structures. Int J Radiat Oncol Biol Phys 68(5): 1289–1298

Geets X, Daisne JF, Arcangeli S et al. (2005) Inter-observer variability in the delineation of pharyngo-laryngeal tumor, parotid glands and cervical spinal cord: comparison between ct-scan and MRI. Radiother Oncol 77(1):25–31

Geets X, Daisne JF, Tomsej M et al. (2006) Impact of the type of imaging modality on target volumes delineation and dose distribution in pharyngo-laryngeal squamous cell carcinoma: comparison between pre- and per-treatment studies. Radiother Oncol 78(3):291–297

Geets X, Lee JA, Bol A et al. (2007a) A gradient-based method for segmenting FDG-PET images: methodology and validation. Eur J Nucl Med Mol Imaging 34(9):1427–1438

Geets X, Tomsej M, Lee JA et al. (2007b) Adaptive biological image-guided IMRT with anatomic and functional imaging in pharyngo-laryngeal tumors: IMPACT on target volume delineation and dose distribution using helical tomotherapy. Radiother Oncol 85(1):105–115

Grégoire V, Coche E, Cosnard G et al. (2000) Selection and delineation of lymph node target volumes in head and neck conformal radiotherapy. Proposal for standardizing terminology and procedure based on the surgical experience. Radiother Oncol 56(2):135–150

Gregoire V, Daisne JF, Geets X (2005) Comparison of CT- and FDG-PET-defined GT: in regard to paulino et al. (Int J Radiat Oncol Biol Phys 2005;61:1385–1392). Int J Radiat Oncol Biol Phys 63(1):308–309; author reply 309

Grégoire V, Daisne JF, Geets X et al. (2003a) Selection and delineation of target volumes in head and neck tumors: beyond ICRU definition. Rays 28(3):217–224

Grégoire V, Levendag P, Ang KK et al. (2003b) Ct-based delineation of lymph node levels and related CTVs in the node-negative neck: DAHANCA, EORTC, GORTEC, NCIC, RTOG consensus guidelines. Radiother Oncol 69(3):227–236

Grosu AL, Souvatzoglou M, Röper B et al. (2007) Hypoxia imaging with FAZA-PET and theoretical considerations with regard to dose painting for individualization of radiotherapy in patients with head and neck cancer. Int J Radiat Oncol Biol Phys 69(2):541–551

Hermans R, Van der Goten A, Baert AL (1997) Image interpretation in CT of laryngeal carcinoma: a study on intra- and interobserver reproducibility. Eur Radiol 7(7):1086–1090

Hong TS, Chappell RJ, Harari PM (2004) Variations in target delineation for head and neck IMRT: an international multi-institutional study. Int J Radiat Oncol Biol Phys 60:S157

Jeanneret-Sozzi W, Moeckli R, Valley JF et al. (2006) The reasons for discrepancies in target volume delineation: a SASRO study on head-and-neck and prostate cancers. Strahlenther Onkol 182(8):450–457

Jeong HS, Baek CH, Son YI et al. (2007) Use of integrated 18F-FDG PET/CT to improve the accuracy of initial cervical nodal evaluation in patients with head and neck squamous cell carcinoma. Head Neck 29(3):203–210

Laubenbacher C, Saumweber D, Wagner-Manslau C et al. (1995) Comparison of fluorine-18-fluorodeoxyglucose PET, MRI and endoscopy for staging head and neck squamous-cell carcinomas. J Nucl Med 36(10):1747–1757

Lin CY, Lee LY, Huang SF et al. (2008a) Treatment outcome of combined modalities for buccal cancers: unilateral or bilateral neck radiation? Int J Radiat Oncol Biol Phys 70(5):1373–1381

Lin Z, Mechalakos J, Nehmeh S et al. (2008b) The influence of changes in tumor hypoxia on dose-painting treatment plans based on 18F-FMISO positron emission tomography. Int J Radiat Oncol Biol Phys 70(4):1219–1228

Ling CC, Humm J, Larson S et al. (2000) Towards multidimensional radiotherapy (MD-CRT): biological imaging and biological conformality. Int J Radiat Oncol Biol Phys 47(3):551–560

Madani I, Duthoy W, Derie C et al. (2007) Positron emission tomography-guided, focal-dose escalation using intensity-modulated radiotherapy for head and neck cancer. Int J Radiat Oncol Biol Phys 68(1):126–135

McGuirt WF, Williams DW, Keyes JW et al. (1995) A comparative diagnostic study of head and neck nodal metastases using positron emission tomography. Laryngoscope 105 (4 Pt 1):373–375

Nishioka T, Shiga T, Shirato H et al. (2002) Image fusion between 18FDG-PET and MRI/CT for radiotherapy planning of oropharyngeal and nasopharyngeal carcinomas. Int J Radiat Oncol Biol Phys 53(4):1051–1057

O'Sullivan B, Warde P, Grice B et al. (2001) The benefits and pitfalls of ipsilateral radiotherapy in carcinoma of the tonsillar region. Int J Radiat Oncol Biol Phys 51(2):332–43 (erratum in Int J Radiat Oncol Biol Phys 2001;51(5):1465).

Paulino AC, Koshy M, Howell R et al. (2005) Comparison of CT- and FDG-PET-defined gross tumor volume in intensity-modulated radiotherapy for head-and-neck cancer. Int J Radiat Oncol Biol Phys 61(5):1385–1392

Riegel AC, Berson AM, Destian S et al. (2006) Variability of gross tumor volume delineation in head-and-neck cancer using CT and PET/CT fusion. Int J Radiat Oncol Biol Phys 65(3):726–732

Robbins KT (1998) Classification of neck dissection: current concepts and future considerations. Otolaryngol Clin North Am 31(4):639–655

Robbins KT (1999) Integrating radiological criteria into the classification of cervical lymph node disease. Arch Otolaryngol Head Neck Surg 125(4):385–387

Som PM (1997) The present controversy over the imaging method of choice for evaluating the soft tissues of the neck. AJNR Am J Neuroradiol 18(10):1869–1872

Som PM, Curtin HD, Mancuso AA (1999) An imaging-based classification for the cervical nodes designed as an adjunct to recent clinically based nodal classifications. Arch Otolaryngol Head Neck Surg 125(4):388–396

Stokkel MP, ten Broek FW, Hordijk GJ et al. (2000) Preoperative evaluation of patients with primary head and neck cancer using dual-head 18fluorodeoxyglucose positron emission tomography. Ann Surg 231(2):229–234

Stuckensen T, Kovács AF, Adams S et al. (2000) Staging of the neck in patients with oral cavity squamous cell carcinomas: a prospective comparison of PET, ultrasound, CT and MRI. J Craniomaxillofac Surg 28(6):319–324

Vanderstraeten B, Duthoy W, De Gersem W et al. (2006) [18F] fluoro-deoxy-glucose positron emission tomography ([18F] FDG-PET) voxel intensity-based intensity-modulated radiation therapy (IMRT) for head and neck cancer. Radiother Oncol 79(3):249–258

Advanced Techniques for Setup Precision and Tracking

Wolfgang A. Tomé

15

CONTENTS

15.1 Introduction *176*

15.2 Some Means to Control for Interfraction Patient Motion in Head and Neck IMRT *176*

15.3 Some Means to Control for Intrafraction Patient Motion in Head and Neck IMRT *176*

15.4 Possible Consequences of Not Controlling for Inter-and Intrafraction Patient Motion Using Tracking in Head and Neck IMRT *177*

15.5 Optical Tracking in Head and Neck IMRT *179*

15.6 Summary *181*

References *181*

KEY POINTS

- Owing to variations in daily patient setup and patient motion during treatment a distinction between "planned" and "delivered" IMRT plans must be made.
- Treatment-delivery-induced cold spots in target volumes can significantly decrease expected local tumor control because of inter- and intrafraction patient motion.

Wolfgang A. Tomé, PhD
Department of Human Oncology, University of Wisconsin School of Medicine and Public Health, CSC K4/314, 600 Highland Avenue, Madison, WI 53705, USA

- Treatment-delivery-induced hot spots in critical structures due to inter- and intrafraction patient motion can lead to normal tissue complications and hence contribute to decreased quality of life of head and neck cancer patients after intensity-modulated radiotherapy.
- Therefore, rigorous immobilization and daily patient setup verification using pretreatment volumetric image guidance, or optical tracking are necessary for the delivery of high-quality head and neck IMRT in order to obtain the intended local tumor control and to decrease normal tissue toxicity.
- Daily volumetric pretreatment image guidance using either MVCT or cone beam kV-CT allows one to correct for patient motion during the dynamic process of patient treatment.
- Subsequent patient motion cannot be corrected for using MVCT or cone beam kV-CT, since they are preformed on timescales that would make their use during treatment delivery unfeasible.
- Therefore, for intrafraction patient setup monitoring a different approach such as tracking the patient position in real time must be pursued.
- The ideal patient tracking system should be minimally invasive, have a high update frequency, have a high correlation to the object being tracked, and should give no additional ionizing radiation dose to the patient.
- For head and neck cancer patients optical tracking systems fulfill all the above requirements, and therefore represent an ideal patient tracking system for this patient population.

15.1

Introduction

The primary goals of radiation therapy are to deliver a tumorcidal dose, while avoiding severe normal tissue effects. Therefore, the planned dose distribution should be delivered as accurately as possible to maximize the expected local tumor control and the intended sparing of organs at risk. Two of the effects that impact on the accuracy with which a planned isodose distribution is delivered from treatment fraction to treatment fraction and during a treatment fraction are interfraction and intrafraction patient motion. Recently, several reports have been published that describe the possible dosimetric impact of interfraction and intrafraction patient and/or organ motion for a variety of anatomical sites (BORTFELD et al. 2002, 2004; COOLENS et al. 2006; EHLER et al. 2007; HONG et al. 2005; KIM et al. 2004; LITZENBERG et al. 2006; ORTON and TOME 2004; SCHALY et al. 2005; WU et al. 2006).

15.2

Some Means to Control for Interfraction Patient Motion in Head and Neck IMRT

Interfraction differences of patient setup position in head and neck IMRT can be handled using either pretreatment stereoscopic planar imaging or by using volumetric pretreatment imaging. When using stereoscopic imaging for interfraction patient setup correction one can only correct for the misalignment of boney anatomy. This technique of interfraction patient setup management may suffice when using conventional parallel opposed lateral head and neck treatment fields encompassing the entire anatomy in question. This treatment approach however is associated with significant normal tissue toxicity and a decreased quality of life for many head and neck cancer patients. Using more conformal treatment techniques, such as IMRT or helical tomotherapy, in which dose is tightly conformed to target volumes and normal critical structures are either avoided or treated to a dose that is below the tolerance dose for these structures, much of the toxicity of the conventional treatment regimen can be avoided. However, when using such a highly conformal treatment technique, the use of volumetric pretreatment imaging, or implanted electromagnetic

transponders when using an RF signal detection device is necessary to correct for any interfraction fraction motion (LITZENBERG et al. 2006; TOME et al. 2007; SHARPE et al. 2007; SHIRATO et al. 2007; WILLOUGHBY et al. 2006). It is important to note that volumetric pretreatment image guidance using either MVCT or cone beam kV-CT allows one to correct for patient motion at one point during the dynamic process of patient treatment. Any subsequent patient motion cannot be corrected using these methods of volumetric image guidance since they are preformed on timescales that would make their use during treatment delivery unfeasible. Furthermore, since it takes several minutes to acquire, process, and correlate a volumetric image data set to its corresponding baseline planning image data set to derive setup corrections when using in-room CT localization techniques such as CT on rails, kV or MV cone beam CT, or megavoltage helical CT, the setup position of the patient one is trying to correct may already have changed, and one therefore might be constantly forced to react to changes in patient position without being able to make a meaningful correction. Moreover, once interfraction patient motion has been corrected one has to wrestle with intrafraction patient motion. Several real time patient motion tracking methods are now in clinical use that allow one to monitor and correct for intrafraction patient motion.

15.3

Some Means to Control for Intrafraction Patient Motion in Head and Neck IMRT

As pointed out above, volumetric imaging techniques, except for magnetic resonance imaging and 3D-ultrasound, operate on time scales that prohibit their use for real time patient monitoring during treatment. To be able to monitor and to act on changes in patient position with minimal delay during head and neck IMRT treatment delivery, one needs a tracking system that has a high measurement update frequency. The ideal patient tracking system should be minimally invasive, have a high measurement update frequency, have a high correlation to the object being tracked, and should give no additional ionizing radiation dose to the patient. Several different tracking systems that approximate such an ideal patient tracking system using various technologies or combinations thereof, such as optical tracking, the tracking of electromagnetic transponders, and the X-ray tracking of implanted fiducials, have been clinically implemented for intrafraction patient tracking (BARONI et al. 2007; BOVA et al. 1997; LITZENBERG et al. 2007; MEEKS et al. 1998, 2005; TOME et al. 2000; WAGNER et al. 2007; WILLOUGHBY et al. 2006)

15.4
Possible Consequences of Not Controlling for Inter- and Intrafraction Patient Motion Using Tracking in Head and Neck IMRT

HONG et al. (2005) have studied the consequences of treatment-induced hot spots in organs at risk and treatment-induced cold spots in target volumes for head and neck IMRT dose distributions using actual patient setup histories obtained from ten patients treated with parallel opposed lateral fields. In their study they applied each of these ten patient setup histories on a fraction for fraction basis to head and neck IMRT treatment plans for various head and neck cancers. An example of the effects induced by inter- and intrafraction patient motion on the expected IMRT isodose distribution is shown in Fig. 15.1. The panel on the left shows the IMRT dose distribution that would be delivered if a patient's position is tracked in real time and if any offsets from the desired position will be corrected before and during treatment; on the other hand, the panel on the right shows the composite IMRT dose distribution the patient would have received if she would have been treated with the isocenter offset history shown.

To study the consequences of these offset histories on the realized EUD for hypothetical patients treated using any of these ten offset histories, the realized EUD was calculated for each of them. Figure 15.2 summarizes their findings in a graphical manner for a hypothetical patient having tonsil cancer, showing the resulting realized EUD values for the following

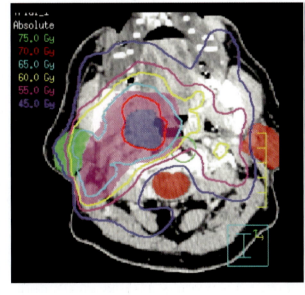
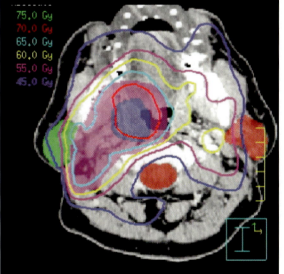
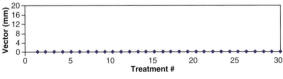
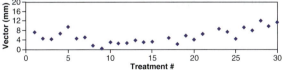

Fig. 15.1. Comparison of the composite dose distributions obtained for the case of optical tracking and standard patient localization using an aquaplast mask. The panel on the *left* shows the dose distribution that will be delivered when the patient's position is tracked in real time and any changes form the desired position are being corrected before and during treatment, while the panel on the *right* shows the composite dose distribution the patient would receive if she would have been treated with the isocenter offset history shown

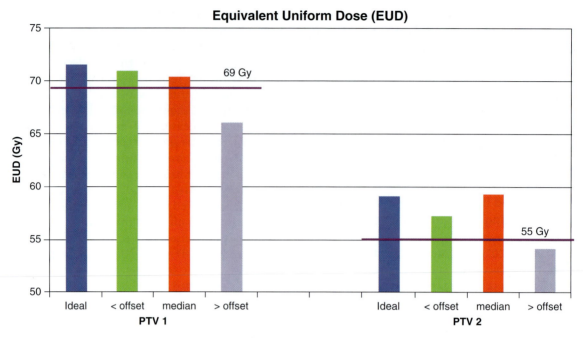

Fig. 15.2. The EUD values for four different setup histories are shown for the target structures PTV1 and PTV2. For each target structure the left most column corresponds to the setup history for no offsets from the indented treatment isocenter, followed by the one corresponding for the smallest offset, then for the median offset, and lastly the one corresponding to the largest offset from the indented treatment isocenter

four setup histories: Ideal (no offsets), the smallest offset, the median offset, and the largest offset from the intended treatment isocenter.

From Fig. 15.2 it can be seen that the treatment plans corresponding to the smallest and median offset yield EUD values that do not indicate a decrease in expected local tumor control since they are still larger than the intended prescription dose for both the PTV1 and PTV2, respectively (Tome and Fowler 2002). Only for the offset history corresponding to the largest offset do the resulting EUD values for the PTV1 and PTV2 fall below the prescription dose, and hence indicate that there is a treatment-induced loss in expected local tumor control if the patient would follow this treatment offset history when receiving head and neck IMRT.

Moreover, Hong et al. (2005) quantified the consequences of setup error on organs at risk. For the same patient, Fig. 15.3 depicts the impact that daily setup variations can have on the mean dose received by the to be spared parotid.

The results shown in Fig. 15.3 may at first appear counterintuitive since the setup histories with smallest and largest offsets are actually superior to the setup history corresponding to the ideal case of no offsets from the intended treatment isocenter. However, as indicated in Fig. 15.3 for these offset

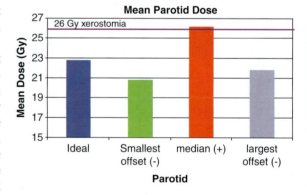

Fig. 15.3. The physical mean dose values for four different setup histories received by the spared parotid. The left most column corresponds to the ideal setup in which no offsets from the indented treatment isocenter are present, followed by the one corresponding to the smallest offset (−), then the one corresponding to the median offset (+), and finally the one corresponding to the largest offset (−) from the indented treatment isocenter. The plus sign (+) indicates that the direction of the overall offset was towards the spared parotid while the minus sign (−) indicates that the direction of the overall offset was away from the spared parotid

histories the overall resulting isocenter offset was away from the spared parotid and only for the isocenter offset history corresponding to the median offset the overall resulting offset was towards the spared parotid yielding a physical mean above 26 Gy as a result of the accumulated setup errors. This shows that if variation in patient setup is not controlled for on a daily basis using optical tracking or pretreatment volumetric image guidance one runs the risk of both losing expected local tumor control probability and inducing normal tissue complications one planned to avoid. Therefore, for the delivery of complex head and neck IMRT dose distributions that exhibit steep dose gradients daily patient setup verification using optical tracking or pretreatment volumetric image guidance is instrumental to achieve the desired outcome of local tumor control and the functional preservation of organs at risk.

15.5

Optical Tracking in Head and Neck IMRT

Optical tracking systems have been used in the treatment of intracranial lesions as well as head and neck cancer. These systems have been shown to allow submillimeter patient repositioning as well as the real time tracking of patients during treatment delivery (Bova et al. 1997; Meeks et al. 1998, 2000; Tome et al. 2000) In optically guided head and neck IMRT the stability of a patient's actual isocenter position is assured through tracking translations of and rotations around the patient's intended treatment isocenter. It is important to note, however, that optical tracking systems do not claim submillimeter treatment accuracy, but submillimeter patient repositioning accuracy from treatment fraction to treatment fraction as well as during treatment delivery. When used during radiation treatment for patient monitoring, these systems work very much like the gating systems used for motion management in radiotherapy, in the sense that the treatment beam is held off once the patient has moved out of a predetermined offset tolerance band (Bova et al. 1997; Meeks et al. 2000; Tome et al. 2000, 2001). Therefore, all errors that have been committed during the treatment preparation process are part of the ultimately achievable localization accuracy. These errors include but are not limited to patient motion during the acquisition of the treatment planning CT, target and normal structure delineation errors, uncertainties in image correlation when using a multimodality image-based target delineation process, and the finite voxel size of the underlying treatment planning CT. This last source of error can be minimized by choosing the smallest allowable field of view that contains the entire anatomy of interest, while the systematic error induced by patient motion during the acquisition treatment planning CT data set can be controlled for by encoding the passive optical markers attached to the fiducial bite block system into the treatment planning CT data set. This allows one to check for gross patient motion during the acquisition of the planning CT data set, if gross patient motion has occurred during the image acquisition process one will not be able to build a successful mathematical model of the fiducial array when selecting each of the passive optical markers to register the array in the control computer to enable one to optically track the patient for treatment setup and during treatment delivery. These sources of error put a lower bound on the patient localization accuracy that can ultimately be achieved with these systems. This lower bound has to be accounted for during treatment planning by adding an adequate PTV margin. Furthermore, optical tracking systems allow one in principle to reduce the random setup error to a minimum, namely into the submillimeter and subdegree range. Clearly being able to minimize the standard deviation for both the systematic and random setup error and being able to control residual patient motion during treatment in real time are clearly beneficial since they enter into the determination of the necessary treatment margin, and will therefore lead to a reduced treatment margin. The above discussion is of course applicable to other patient tracking systems as well (Van Herk 2004).

The first commercially available optical tracking system for radiation therapy was developed at the University of Florida (Bova et al. 1997; Meeks et al. 2000; Tome et al. 2000, 2001), which is commercially available under the trade name FreeTrack™ (Varian, Ashland, MA), and has been used for fractionated stereotactic radiotherapy, as well as intracranial and head and neck IMRT (Bova et al. 1997; Patel et al. 2002; Tome et al. 2000, 2001). Patient position tracking is accomplished using a hybrid Polaris position sensor unit (Northern Digital, Waterloo, Ontario), which consists of an array of two planar CCD cameras surrounded by a ring of infrared light emitting diodes, to optically track the position of either active or passive infrared markers arranged on a fiducial array that is attached to a bite block that links to a patient's upper dentition to form a fixed rigid body. For the Free Track system, the position sensor unit is permanently mounted to the ceiling of the treatment room at a distance of ~1.8 m from the isocenter of the treatment machine (cf. Fig. 15.4). The system is calibrated such that the optical tracking system has the isocenter of

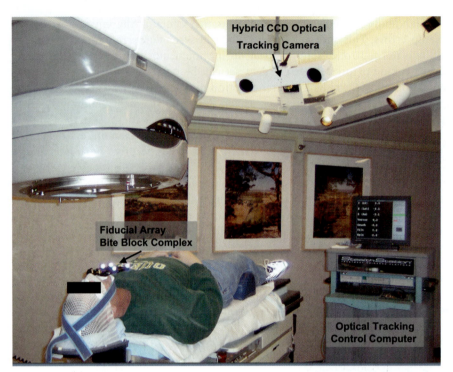

Fig. 15.4. Patient setup for head and neck IMRT using optical tracking. The difference between the actual patient position and the desired patient position is displayed on the screen of the optical tracking control computer

the treatment machine as its origin and uses the treatment machine coordinate system to determine the patient's position in the treatment room.

Patient localization is accomplished through detection of the optical fiducial array to which four passive markers are attached. This fiducial array as pointed out above is in turn attached to a custom bite plate that links to the upper dentition of the patient to form a rigid body. The patient position determined using optical guidance is then compared with the desired patient position (which has been decided on during treatment planning). During CT simulation, the biteplate-fiducial array is encoded into the treatment planning CT data set, and the image coordinates of the infrared light reflective markers are determined as part of the treatment planning process (cf. Fig. 15.5).

During treatment planning the desired isocenter coordinates are determined in CT space. As pointed out above, the spherical infrared light reflecting fiducial markers attached to the optical reference array are localized in the optical tracking control computer, thus determining their positions relative to the treatment isocenter, and hence defining a stereotactic coordinate system. After selecting the fiducials from the scan, the best fit between the image-defined coordinates of the fiducial array and the known geometry of the fiducial array are deter-

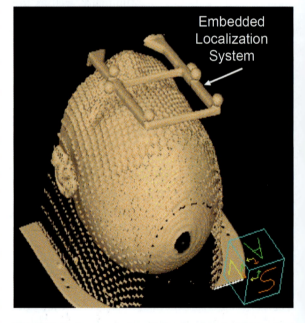

Fig. 15.5. Surface rendering of a head and neck IMRT patient showing the embedded fiducial array bite block complex

mined. The residual error between the image localization of the markers and the known geometry after the best fit is obtained is called the *mean registration error*, and is calculated for each patient. The mean registration error provides a quality assurance measure for optical tracking, since it ensures integrity of both the fiducial array and CT data set (MEEKS et al. 2000). Using optical tracking phantoms, it has consistently been shown that the mean registration error is ~0.3 mm, which is governed entirely by the finite size of the CT voxels. In head and neck IMRT the mean registration error can be maintained below 0.5 mm for patients who are not edentulous, while for edentulous patients it can be maintained below 0.7 mm. For a given CT data set, values larger than this are indicative of either patient motion during CT acquisition, spatial inaccuracies of the CT, or mechanical inaccuracy of the fiduicial array bite block complex.

For patient alignment, the FreeTrack™ system is used to determine the patient's position in real time and to report the displacement from the intended isocenter. As pointed out above, the optical tracking system reports translational misalignments from the isocenter as well as the rotational misalignment around the isocenter. In addition, the optical tracking system reports overall the *vector* error, which is the root mean square formed from the three translational misalignments, and hence, the magnitude of the displacement vector pointing from the treatment machine isocenter to the intended treatment isocenter. Patients are repositioned such that their desired isocenter position is within 0.3 mm vector misalignment and 0.3° of rotational misalignment about each axis from the treatment machine isocenter. During treatment delivery, patients are monitored in real time, in case that a patient moves out of the 0.5 mm vector offset tolerance sphere around the desired patient isocenter position, the treatment is interrupted and the patient is realigned. This process continues until all treatment fields are delivered.

15.6

Summary

Clearly, a distinction between "planned" and "delivered" IMRT plans must be made, since treatment-delivery-induced cold spots in target volumes can decrease the expected local tumor control because of possible inter- and intrafraction patient motion. Moreover, for complex head and neck IMRT dose distributions treatment-delivery-induced hot spots in critical structures due to possible inter- and intrafraction patient motion can lead to normal tissue complications one meant to avoid. Therefore,

rigorous immobilization and patient setup verification using daily pretreatment volumetric image guidance, or optical tracking is necessary for the delivery of high-quality head and neck IMRT in order to obtain the intended local tumor control and decrease in normal tissue toxicity. However, daily volumetric pretreatment image guidance using either MVCT or cone beam kV-CT allows one to correct for patient motion at one point during the dynamic process of patient treatment. Any subsequent patient motion cannot be corrected for using MVCT or cone beam kV-CT, since they are preformed on timescales that would make their use during treatment delivery unfeasible. Therefore, for intrafraction patient motion monitoring a different approach such as tracking a patient's position in real time using an optical tracking system needs to be pursued.

References

Baroni G, Riboldi M, Spadea MF et al. (2007) Integration of enhanced optical tracking techniques and imaging in IGRT. J Radiat Res (Tokyo) 48(Suppl A):A61–A74

Bortfeld T, Jiang SB, Rietzel E (2004) Effects of motion on the total dose distribution. Semin Radiat Oncol 14:41–51

Bortfeld T, Jokivarsi K, Goitein M et al. (2002) Effects of intrafraction motion on IMRT dose delivery: statistical analysis and simulation. Phys Med Biol 47:2203–2220

Bova FJ, Buatti JM, Friedman WA et al. (1997) The Univeristy of Florida frameless high-precision stereotactic radiotherapy system. Int J Radiat Oncol Biol Phys 38:875–882

Coolens C, Evans PM, Seco J et al. (2006) The susceptibility of IMRT dose distributions to intrafraction organ motion: an investigation into smoothing filters derived from four dimensional computed tomography data. Med Phys 33:2809–2818

Ehler ED, Nelms BE, Tome WA. (2007) On the dose to a moving target while employing different IMRT delivery mechanisms. Radiother Oncol 83:49–56

Hong TS, Tome WA, Chappell RJ et al. (2005) The impact of daily setup variations on head-and-neck intensity-modulated radiation therapy. Int J Radiat Oncol Biol Phys 61:779–788

Kim S, Akpati HC, Kielbasa JE et al. (2004) Evaluation of intrafraction patient movement for CNS and head & neck IMRT. Med Phys 31:500–506

Litzenberg DW, Balter JM, Hadley SW et al. (2006) Influence of intrafraction motion on margins for prostate radiotherapy. Int J Radiat Oncol Biol Phys 65:548–553

Litzenberg DW, Willoughby TR, Balter JM et al. (2007) Positional stability of electromagnetic transponders used for prostate localization and continuous, real-time tracking. Int J Radiat Oncol Biol Phys 68:1199–1206

Meeks SL, Bova FJ, Friedman WA et al. (1998) IRLED-based patient localization for linac radiosurgery. Int J Radiat Oncol Biol Phys 41:433–439

Meeks SL, Bova FJ, Wagner TH et al. (2000) Image localization for frameless stereotactic radiotherapy. Int J Radiat Oncol Biol Phys 46:1291–1299

Meeks SL, Tome WA, Willoughby TR et al. (2005) Optically guided patient positioning techniques. Semin Radiat Oncol 15:192–201

Orton, NP, Tome, WA (2004) The impact of daily shifts on prostate IMRT dose distributions. Med Phys 31:2845–2848

Patel RR, Tomé WA, Tannehill SP et al. (2002) Optically guided intensity modulated radiotherapy for the head and neck. Radiother Oncol 64:S248

Schaly B, Bauman GS, Song W et al. (2005) Dosimetric impact of image-guided 3D conformal radiation therapy of prostate cancer. Phys Med Biol 50:3083–3101

Sharpe MB, Craig T, Moseley DJ (2007) Image guidance: treatment target localization systems. Front Radiat Ther Oncol 40:72–93

Shirato H, Shimizu S, Kitamura K et al. (2007) Organ motion in image-guided radiotherapy: lessons from real-time tumor-tracking radiotherapy. Int J Clin Oncol 12:8–16

Tome WA, Fowler JF (2002) On cold spots in tumor subvolumes. Med Phys 29:1590–1598

Tome WA, Jaradat HA, Nelson IA et al. (2007) Helical tomotherapy: image guidance and adaptive dose guidance. Front Radiat Ther Oncol 40:162–178

Tome WA, Meeks SL, Buatti JM et al. (2000) A high-precision system for conformal intracranial radiotherapy. Int J Radiat Oncol Biol Phys 47:1137–1143

Tome WA, Meeks SL, McNutt TR et al. (2001) Optically guided intensity modulated radiotherapy. Radiother Oncol 61:33–44

Wagner TH, Meeks SL, Bova FJ et al. (2007) Optical tracking technology in stereotactic radiation therapy. Med Dosim 32:111–120

Willoughby TR, Kupelian PA, Pouliot J et al. (2006) Target localization and real-time tracking using the Calypso 4D localization system in patients with localized prostate cancer. Int J Radiat Oncol Biol Phys 65:528–534

Wu Q, Ivaldi G, Liang J et al. (2006) Geometric and dosimetric evaluations of an online image-guidance strategy for 3D-CRT of prostate cancer. Int J Radiat Oncol Biol Phys 64:1596–1609

Van Herk M (2004) Errors and Margins in radiotherapy. Semin Radiat Oncol 24:52–64

Adaptive Image-Guided Radiotherapy for Head and Neck Cancer

16

ULRIK VINDELEV ELSTROEM and CAI GRAU

CONTENTS

16.1 Introduction *183*

16.2 In-Room Image-Guidance Technologies for ART *184*

16.3 Impact of Anatomical Changes During Treatment *185*

16.4 Adaptation Strategies *187*

References *189*

KEY POINTS

- Anatomic changes during radiotherapy, due to tumor and tissue shrinkage and patient weight loss, occur frequently and may have dosimetric consequences.
- Adaptation to anatomical changes may improve target coverage and/or normal tissue sparing.
- In-room volumetric imaging has improved our ability to adapt radiation treatment to the changes in anatomy.
- A complete adaptive image-guided radiotherapy strategy involves daily imaging on the treatment couch, segmentation of structures, re-optimization, and treatment evaluation.
- It is still unknown whether it is safe (in terms of local-regional control) to decrease the size of the GTV during the course of fractionated RT.
- Clinical studies are needed to elucidate the benefit of various adaptation strategies.

16.1
Introduction

The natural goal for improvements in radiotherapy is to enhance locoregional control and reduce side effects. In recent years the technical developments in methods for tumor delineation and treatment delivery have improved both tumor coverage and healthy tissue sparing. Especially high precision conformal radiotherapy techniques such as intensity-modulated radiotherapy (IMRT) and stereotactic radiotherapy have enabled dose escalation to the target with decreased volume of healthy tissue irradiated to a high dose level. However, the consequence of the increasingly conformal dose distributions is enhanced sensitivity to changes in the patient from planning to

ULRIK VINDELEV ELSTROEM, MSc
CAI GRAU, MD, DMSc
Department of Oncology, Aarhus University Hospital, 44 Noerrebrogade, 8000 Aarhus C, Denmark

treatment and during the course of fractionated radiotherapy. Setup errors and anatomical changes may cause deviations between planned and delivered dose distribution, which can lead to underdosage of tumor volume and/or overdosage of normal tissue if not properly corrected for. Most setup errors can be avoided by conventional measures such as rigid patient immobilization, and MV port film, while the internal soft tissue deformations occurring because of weight loss, tissue shrinkage, breathing motion, or deformation of tumor/normal tissues require more sophisticated imaging and adaptive strategies. This may involve developing a new treatment plan on the basis of the new anatomic information. To this end, adaptive image-guided radiotherapy (IGRT) offers a possible solution and safety-net. The recent advances in treatment-room image-guidance technologies (as reviewed by DAWSON and JAFFRAY (2007)) have facilitated convenient and frequent imaging of the patient anatomy throughout the treatment course, and thus form a basis for treatment plan adjustments to shape and position of target and organs at risk on a regular basis. The adaptive radiotherapy (ART) process in which the subsequent delivery can be modified using a systematic feedback of the geometric and dosimetric information from previous fractions is still in an investigational phase of development for many tumor sites, including the head and neck region.

The present chapter will discuss the various technical aspects and challenges of adaptive IGRT of head and neck cancer. The first section will focus on image-guidance technologies, especially systems used in the treatment room. The second part will examine the anatomical changes observed during the fractionated treatment course and the dosimetric consequences for the outcome. Finally, replanning and adaptation strategies to maintain pretreatment objectives are addressed.

16.2

In-Room Image-Guidance Technologies for ART

Geometric uncertainties in target and sparing tissue volumes are influenced by errors in target delineation and localization, interfraction patient setup errors and organ motion, and intrafraction motion (e.g., patient movement and respiratory motion). All contributing factors have to be considered to determine the appropriate treatment margins (VAN HERK 2004; YAN et al. 2005). However, in the present context,

it is the interfraction errors that are of main interest, since the intrafractional movements in the head and neck region are neglectable for most cases, and accuracy in target definition is the subject of Chap. 14.

Patient/organ geometric variation in head and neck treatment has been traditionally quantified using rigid body displacement of bony anatomy using radiographs from the planning CT or a simulation as reference. Imaging utilizing the MV treatment X-ray beam itself was one of the first methods of visualizing internal anatomy at the time of treatment using film or flat-panel detectors. With electronic portal imaging devices (EPID) integrated in the standard linear accelerator it has become feasible to apply off-line correction strategies aiming at reducing systematic setup errors and margins in dose escalation protocols (DE BOER et al. 2001). The inherent better contrast in kV imaging compared with MV has facilitated developments in accelerator- or room-mounted kV X-ray systems to improve imaging at the time of treatment delivery. In-room kV imaging thus provides improved patient positioning for less radiation exposure (PASANI et al. 2000), and systems with automated couch adjustment enable efficient work flow of value for daily online correction. However, as treatment progresses many head and neck cancer patients undergo anatomic changes in response to the treatment, e.g., due to tumor shrinkage and weight loss. Clearly, planar imaging based on bony contrast is insufficient for monitoring these effects, and volumetric imaging providing soft-tissue visualization of target and critical structures is needed.

Complete 3D volumetric information on soft tissue can be obtained in the treatment room using ultrasound, CT, or MRI. For dose-plan verification and replanning, CT has been most widely used and different solutions will be presented. A CT scan of diagnostic quality of the patient in the treatment position can be obtained in conjunction with daily treatment by installing the imaging device in the treatment room, and using a turntable or similar translation technique. Using a CT-on-rails system, significant changes have been reported for head and neck cancer patients (BARKER et al. 2004), as discussed in the next section.

A novel and versatile CT technique is kV cone-beam CT (CBCT). CBCT integrates the kV tube and flat panel detector on the gantry of the linear accelerator, so the same axis of rotation is shared between kV imaging and MV treatment beams (JAFFRAY et al. 2002). In a single rotation around the patient, 2D projections are recorded and immediately reconstructed to 3D-volumetric images similar to conventional CT, thus providing both setup and anatomic information of the patient on the couch prior to treatment. As mentioned by XING et al. (2007), the linear-accelerator-based CBCT has made ART practicality feasible. However, some pending problems are still to be solved to improve the application in ART of head and neck cancer. The limited gantry speed results in a relatively long acquisition time (~1 min), which makes the images prone to patient motion artifacts due to, e.g., coughing or swallowing. The influence of scatter radiation is more severe in CBCT than in conventional fan-beam CT because of the X-ray beam geometry which leads to increased image noise and reduced image contrast (SIEWERDSEN and JAFFRAY 2001). The various artifacts degrade image quality and introduce errors in the Hounsfield unit values of the 3D reconstruction, thereby distorting the dose-computational performance (YANG et al. 2007). Finally, limited scan range in the superior–inferior direction will for many clinical cases prevent imaging of the complete treatment volume.

Megavoltage cone-beam CT (MVCBCT) can be constructed from projections of the radiation beam detected by the electronic portal imaging device during the gantry rotation (POULIOT et al. 2005). MVCBCT has inherently somewhat poorer soft tissue contrast than does kV CBCT, but has been shown to be feasible to estimate the dosimetric impact on changing anatomy in the head and neck region (MORIN et al. 2007). A helical megavoltage CT (MVCT) is an integrated imaging part of the tomotherapy delivery system (MACKIE 2006). In spite of the poorer low-contrast resolution, the MVCT images provide sufficient contrast to follow anatomic changes in soft-tissue organs during RT (HAN et al. 2008). For dose computations, the negligible contribution of photoelectric effect to the attenuation of radiation at megavoltage energies makes the CT number to electron density calibration simpler than for kV images (LANGEN et al. 2005).

16.3

Impact of Anatomical Changes During Treatment

Even though daily adjustment of the patient position at treatment to reduce systematic and random setup errors has become more and more routine clinical practice, such procedures may be inadequate to prevent geometrical errors in the delivery if the anatomy changes as treatment progresses. Especially with crit-

ical normal tissues such as spinal cord, optic nerves, and salivary glands in close proximity to high-dose tumor volume, significant anatomic changes will acquire adaptive planning to fulfill the desired treatment goal. Dose–volume constraints and penalty weights are used to optimize dose plans, e.g., maximum spinal cord dose of 45 Gy to reduce the risk of radiation injury (MARUCCI et al. 2004), mean parotid dose below 26 Gy to reduce risk of xerostomia (EISBRUCH et al. 1999), mean dose below 60 Gy to the supraglottic region, the larynx, and upper esophageal sphincter to reduce risk of aspiration (JENSEN et al. 2007). Following the developments in volumetric imaging, the consequences of anatomic variation has become the subject of a number of investigations.

BARKER et al. (2004) used an integrated CT-linear accelerator system to examine changes in target and normal tissue during the treatment course in 14 head and neck cancer patients. CT images were acquired three times a week and contours were manually delineated. Shrinkage of the primary gross tumor volume was observed with a median volume reduction of 70% at the last treatment fraction (range, 10–92%). The rate of volume loss correlated highly with initial tumor size, indicating that this might be a predictive parameter in an adaptive treatment strategy. Besides shrinkage, the tumor positions changed over time by 3 mm (median value, range 0–17 mm). The volumes of the parotid glands showed a median loss of 28% at the end of treatment and the center of mass positions shifted medially by 3 mm (median, range 0–10 mm). The latter observation was highly correlated with weight loss during the RT course. Figure 16.1 illustrates the geometrical changes of the parotid glands and the dosimetric consequence near the end of treatment of a patient with cancer in the oral cavity imaged using kV CBCT.

A few studies have examined the dosimetric impact of anatomic changes during IMRT of head and neck cancer and the effect of replanning. In a retrospective study by HANSEN et al. (2006) 13 patients underwent a second CT scan followed by replanning during the IMRT course (19 fractions delivered on average), the indication being weight loss and/or tumor shrinkage. Between the two CT scans, the mean volume of parotid glands decreased by 16% (right) and 22% (left), whereas a minor difference between the PTVs was observed. Replanning using the second CT scan showed a significant reduction in dose to normal tissue and an increase in target volume dose compared with recalculation of the original plan on

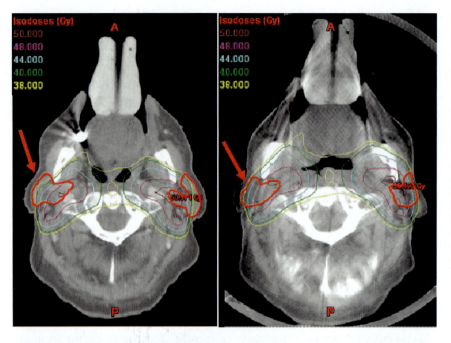

Fig. 16.1. The dosimetric consequence of changes in anatomy for the case of the parotid glands. From the planning CT (*left*) to a CBCT (*right*) recorded in week 6 (50 days elapsed, fraction 30) the right parotid (indicated by *red arrow*) was reduced 45% in volume and the center-of-mass moved 3 mm medially with reference to the vertebra (C2), resulting in an increase in mean dose from 19.5 to 28.9 Gy. The same but less pronounced effect was observed for the left parotid gland (ELSTROEM et al. 2007)

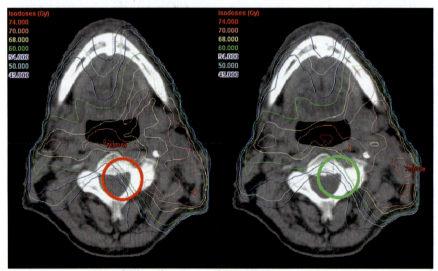

Fig. 16.2. Example of IMRT replanning during treatment of a hypopharyngeal cancer patient. CT in week 5 of treatment with recalculation of the original treatment plan shows potential over-dosage of 55 Gy to the spinal cord (*left, red circle*). Replanning re-established a maximum dose below 50 Gy (*right, green circle*) (ELSTROEM et al. 2006)

the new anatomy. Figure 16.2 shows a clinical case of a hypopharyngeal cancer patient who underwent replanning during treatment. In a prospective study enrolling ten nasopharyngeal cancer patients treated with IMRT, Kuo et al. (2006) reported the effect of regression of enlarged lymph nodes on parotid dose. As treatment progressed, the nodal regression caused a shift of the parotid glands into the high-dose region. A second CT and replanning after 45 Gy of delivery led to a reduction of more than 3 Gy in the mean dose to parotid glands, compared with original plan. As pointed out by the authors, recontouring of large lymph nodes that regress during therapy results in a risk of underdosing microscopic disease. This issue constitutes one of the future challenges in ART of head and neck cancer, and should be carefully studied in prospective clinical trials.

The actual dose delivered to target and critical structures during radiotherapy play a central role in the evaluation of the importance of changes in the patient. Conducting two weekly CT scans with an in-room CT scanner over the IMRT treatment course of 11 head and neck cancer patients, O'DANIEL et al. (2007) investigated the difference between planned and delivered dose. The clinical IMRT plans were recalculated on the multiple CT image sets after alignment with either external markers or bony anatomy. Deformable registration was finally applied to map the consecutive recalculated dose distributions to the original treatment plan to facilitate a calculation of the cumulative delivered dose. It was observed that in 45% of the patients, setup using external markers led to increases in the parotid gland mean dose above the planned dose by 5–7 Gy (median, 3 and 1 Gy ipsilateral and contralateral, respectively). If bone alignment was used instead (e.g., as with application of daily setup correction), reductions relative to the above in 91% of patients were reported (median, 2 Gy; range, 0.3–8.3 Gy); however, the parotid dose was still 1.0 Gy (median) greater than planned. No significant change in dose to spinal cord and target volumes was found with either approach.

Clearly, the significant discrepancy between planned and delivered parotid mean dose reported by O'DANIEL et al. (2007) can have consequences for the design and interpretation of parotid sparing IMRT protocols. The deformable dose-mapping technique applied in the study to accumulate dose from multiple volumetric images enabled an examination of the dosimetric effect of both setup uncertainty and anatomical changes (e.g., weight loss, parotid shrinkage and medial motion, as discussed earlier). Another approach was reported by HAN et al. (2008) in a retrospective study including five nasopharyngeal cancer patients treated with helical tomotherapy. The patients were imaged daily using MVCT with subsequent registration to the planning CT for setup error correction. Contours of the spinal cord and parotid glands were manually drawn on the volumetric image sets at regular intervals, facilitating a calculation of the delivered dose at the respective treatment fractions. The results showed a significant decrease in the average parotid gland volume over the treatment course from 20.5 to 13.2 cm³, which led to a significant increase in average median parotid dose from 83 to 142.6 cGy/treatment fraction. To evaluate the significance of daily setup corrections on the spinal cord dose, the dose distributions with and without random setup errors were simulated (i.e., the latter case only including systematic errors). Without daily setup correction, the total D_{max} increased 7.6% on average (range, 3.3–15.5%) compared with daily adjustment using MVCT image registration. The latter approach also gave rise to much smaller variation in D_{max} for the spinal cord.

As seen from the reported studies, anatomic changes can lead to significant deviations between planned and delivered dose to target and normal organs. However, it is also clear from the published data that there exists a large heterogeneity among patients with respect to the size and consequences of the changes observed in these relative small cohorts.

Besides changes in anatomy, the contributions from setup uncertainties to geometrical variation in RT of head and neck cancer have been a subject of numerous studies (the subject of Chap. 15). The gain in accuracy of delivery by daily image-guidance was mentioned by O'DANIEL et al. (2007) and HAN et al. (2008). In a retrospective study of 24 head and neck patients, ZEIDAN et al. (2007) have assessed the dependence of the residual setup error on the frequency of pretreatment IG using MVCT. Reducing image-guidance from daily to every second day resulted in 11% of all treatments to be subject to a misalignment error of at least 5 mm. A similar result was observed for approximately one-third of the treatments if a weekly image-guidance protocol was used. Another source of residual setup errors is the variation in the head inclination. Owing to head rotations and/or nonrigid movement between rigid structures, ZHANG et al. (2006) have reported differences in the range of 2–6 mm between multiple regions of interest depending on image registration site. The size and consequence of patient setup error and deformation depend to a high degree on setup procedures and type of immobilization used at each institution and should be reflected in the treatment margins applied.

16.4
Adaptation Strategies

The concept of ART was introduced by YAN et al. (1997, 2005) in the treatment of prostate cancer. The process consisted of acquisition of multiple daily CT image sets to estimate the patient-specific geometric variations and subsequently determine a PTV to account for these, with modification of the treatment plan accordingly. This is an example of an offline adaptive strategy in which the processing of the image feedback and treatment adaptation are conducted at a later stage in the treatment course. Opposed to this, an online adaptive approach applies the basic functions of imaging, planning, and treatment at each fraction. There is a huge difference in timescale between the two schemes going from days to minutes with increased complexity due to the repeated execution of the workflow. However, the basic processes involved are the same, and it requires the combination of many steps, such as recontouring, re-optimization, plan evaluation, dose reconstruction, and dose accumulation. The usability of ART depends in several ways on the quality of the volumetric imaging behind it. As mentioned previously, the recent advances in treatment-room volumetric imaging systems have brought ART forward.

A clinical realization of ART requires a robust inverse planning strategy to be feasible. Recently, DE LA ZERDA et al. (2007) have categorized the basic strategies for adaptation into two separate classes. In the first class are those adapting to changing geometry which takes organ deformations into account just before treatment. An example has been reported by MOHAN et al. (2005) describing a method that uses deformation of the intensity distributions of each beam in the original IMRT plan based on the deformation in anatomy relative to the planning CT, thereby avoiding time consuming full-fledged replanning. The second class includes those adapting to geometry and delivered dose; i.e., the dose distribution is optimized by adapting to both anatomic changes and the dose-delivery history. DE LA ZERDA et al. (2007) further divided these into immediately correcting and prudent correcting strategies. Very briefly, the former aims at compensating dosimetric discrepancies in each voxel between planned and previously delivered dose online at the current fraction. In the latter, on the other hand, the dose compensation is accomplished by spreading the previous dosimetric errors over a number of subsequent fractions. Although preferable, this offline scheme is not dependant on daily volumetric imaging prior to treatment and would be applicable for many head and neck cases in which the variation of the anatomy may not be notable from day to day but over a larger time span. Tumor shrinkage and weight loss are initiated by the treatment itself, and for many patients a plan modification will probably not be required before one or more weeks into the fractionated treatment course.

The ability to accumulate delivered dose to specific volumes over multiple 3D image sets plays an important role in any dose-based adaptation strategy. Image-registration algorithms aim at determining the transformation that performs a voxel to voxel mapping between two image data sets, e.g., from time-of-treatment images to planning CT. This enables an identification of structures and a monitoring of their changes in shape and position. Furthermore, if the daily delivered dose is recalculated on the treatment CT, it can be mapped back to the planning CT to compute the cumulative dose distribution as the treatment course progresses. Comparing this with the planned distribution form the basis for evaluation of treatment performance and decision-making of whether to adjust the treatment plan as discussed previously. However, as seen in Sect. 16.3, the significant anatomical changes in head and neck cancer patients require nonrigid or deformable registration in which the transformation between image sets contains voxel-dependant distortion. Figure 16.3 shows an example of rigid vs. deformable registration between planning CT and a CBCT conducted close to end of treatment. Deformable registration algorithms are still in an early stage of development and various models have been proposed but none of them are reliable enough for routine clinical application yet (see XING et al. (2007) for summary of deformable registration approaches). Not only dose accumulation will emerge from this active area of research, and YANG et al. (2007) have reported the use of deformable registration to map electron density information from the initial planning CT to CBCT images acquired prior to treatment. In this way the dose calculation is performed on a deformed planning CT (i.e., anatomy from CBCT) which circumvents the inherent problems with image artifacts in CBCT as mentioned in Sect. 16.2. A final application of deformable registration important for the clinical feasibility of adaptive IGRT is in the development of image segmentation. The increasing amount of volumetric images for replanning in ART requires delineation of target and normal structures. Since the temporal anatomical changes in the head and neck region evolve smoothly these cases might be well suited for creating computational algorithms for automatic segmentation, based on the original organ contouring.

The clinical benefits of adaptive IGRT in the head and neck region are potentially huge, since it may at the same time secure optimal target coverage, allow dose-painting of resistant subvolumes, and enable even better normal tissue sparing than IMRT. However, the clinical evidence to support its usefulness is still to be seen. It will take large clinical series to show the benefit. Whether bullet-proof phase III evidence will ever be produced is questionable, since the widespread introduction of IMRT has shown that it is difficult to motivate clinicians and patients to test new technology in randomized trials.

Despite the technical achievements, there are still a number of open questions, which need to be addressed.

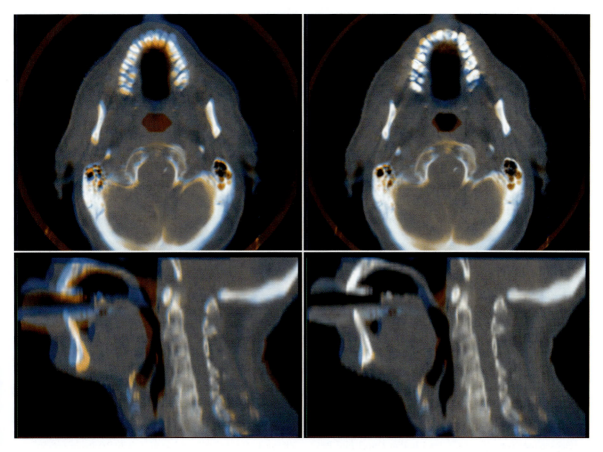

Fig. 16.3. *Red/blue* visualization of the difference between the rigid registration (*left*) and the deformable registration (*right*) of a CBCT image set from week 6 of treatment to the planning CT. A saggital slice and an axial slice are shown for each registration. Improved alignment around the oral cavity is obtained by deformable registration as depicted to the right (NOE et al. 2008)

First of all, it should be remembered that our current dose–volume constraints basically stem from the pre-IMRT era. So collection and correlation of clinical data to dosimetric information will continue to be an important scientific issue. Secondly, it must be documented that adapting the treatment fields is safe in terms of local-regional control, since such a strategy may result in missing microscopic disease. Finally, logistics for segmentation, re-optimization, and decision-making should be elaborated in order to make dynamic adaptive image-guided feasible on a routine basis.

References

Barker JL, Garden AS, Ang KK et al. (2004) Quantification of volumetric and geometric changes occurring during fractionated radiotherapy for head-and-neck cancer using an integrated CT/linear accelerator system. Int J Radiat Oncol Biol Phys 59:960–970

Dawson L, Jaffray DA (2007) Advances in image-guided radiation therapy. J Clin Oncol 25:938–946

de Boer HCJ, van Sornsen de Koste JR, Creutzberg CL et al. (2001) Electronic portal image assisted reduction of systematic set-up errors in head and neck irradiation. Radiother Oncol 61:299–308

de la Zerda A, Armbruster B, Xing L (2007) Formulating adaptive radiation therapy planning into closed-loop control framework. Phys Med Biol 52:4137–4153

Eisbruch A, Ten Haken RK, Kim HM et al. (1999) Dose, volume, and function relationships in parotid salivary glands following conformal and intensity-modulated irradiation of head and neck cancer. Int J Radiat Oncol Biol Phys 45:577–587

Elstroem UV, Buus S, Muren LP et al. (2007) Cone-beam CT assessed changes in volume and dose parameters for salivary glands during parotid sparing IMRT for head and neck cancer. Radiother Oncol 84(Suppl 1):S165–S166 (abstract 368)

Elstroem UV, Petersen JB, Poulsen PR et al. (2006) Feasibility of adaptive image-guided IMRT for head and neck cancer using cone-beam CT obtained at the treatment couch. Radiother Oncol 81(Suppl 1):S219 (abstract 528)

Han C, Chen YJ, Liu A et al. (2008) Actual dose variation of parotid gland and spinal cord for nasopharyngeal cancer patients during radiotherapy. Int J Radiat Oncol Biol Phys 70:1256–1262

Hansen EK, Bucci MK, Quivey JM et al. (2006) Repeat CT imaging and replanning during the course of IMRT for head-and-neck cancer. Int J Radiat Oncol Biol Phys 64:355–362

Jaffray DA, Siewerdsen JH, Wong JW et al. (2002) Flat-panel cone-beam computed tomography for image-guided radiation therapy. Int J Radiat Oncol Biol Phys 53:1337–1349

Jensen K, Lambertsen K, Grau C (2007) Late swallowing dysfunction and dysphagia after radiotherapy for pharynx cancer: frequency, intensity and correlation with dose and volume parameters. Radiother Oncol 85:74–82

Kuo YC, Wu TH, Chung TS et al. (2006) Effect of regression of enlarged neck lymph nodes on radiation doses received by parotid glands during intensity-modulated radiotherapy for head and neck cancer. Am J Clin Oncol 29:600–605

Langen KM, Meeks SL, Poole DO et al. (2005) The use of megavoltage CT (MVCT) images for dose recomputations. Phys Med Biol 50:4259–4276

Mackie TR (2006) History of tomotherapy. Phys Med Biol 51:R427–R453

Marucci L, Niemierko A, Leibsch NJ et al. (2004) Spinal cord tolerance to high-dose fractionated 3D conformal proton-photon irradiation as evaluated by equivalent uniform dose and dose volume histogram analysis. Int J Radiat Oncol Biol Phys 59:551–555

Mohan R, Zhang X, Wang H et al. (2005) Use of deformed intensity distributions for on-line modification of image-guided IMRT to account for interfractional anatomic changes. Int J Radiat Oncol Biol Phys 61:1258–1266

Morin O, Chen J, Aubin M et al. (2007) Dose calculation using megavoltage cone-beam CT. Int J Radiat Oncol Biol Phys 67:1201–1210

Noe KØ, De Senneville BD, Elstroem UV et al. (2008) Acceleration and validation of optical flow based deformable registration for image-guided radiotherapy. Acta Oncol 47(7):1286–1293

O'Daniel JC, Garden AS, Schwartz DL et al. (2007) Parotid gland dose in intensity-modulated radiotherapy for head and neck cancer: is what you plan what you get? Int J Radiat Oncol Biol Phys 69:1290–1296

Pasani L, Lockman D, Jaffray DA et al. (2000) Setup error in radiotherapy: on-line correction using electronic kilovoltage and megavoltage radiographs. Int J Radiat Oncol Biol Phys 47:825–839

Pouliot J, Bani-Hashemi A, Chen J et al. (2005) Low-dose megavoltage cone-beam CT for radiation therapy. Int J Radiat Oncol Biol Phys 61:552–560

Siewerdsen J, Jaffray DA (2001) Cone-beam computed tomography with a flat-panel imager: magnitude and effects of X-ray scatter. Med Phys 28:220–231

van Herk M (2004) Errors and margins in radiotherapy. Semin Radiat Oncol 14:52–64

Xing L, Siebers J, Keall P (2007) Computational challenges for image-guided radiation therapy: framework and current research. Semin Radiat Oncol 17:245–257

Yan D, Lockman D, Martinez A et al. (2005) Computed tomography guided management of interfractional patient variation. Semin Radiat Oncol 15:168–179

Yan D, Vicini F, Wong J et al. (1997) Adaptation radiation therapy. Phys Med Biol 42:123–132

Yang Y, Schreibmann E, Li T et al. (2007) Evaluation of onboard kV cone beam CT (CBCT)-based dose calculation. Phys Med Biol 52:685–706

Zeidan OA, Langen KM, Meeks SL et al. (2007) Evaluation of image-guidance protocols in the treatment of head and neck cancer. Int J Radiat Oncol Biol Phys 67:670–677

Zhang L, Garden AS, Lo J et al. (2006) Multiple regions-of-interest analysis of setup uncertainties for head-and-neck cancer radiotherapy. Int J Radiat Oncol Biol Phys 64:1559–1569

Improving Form and Function

Through Surgical Care in Head and Neck Squamous Cell Carcinoma

GREG HARTIG and SCOTT CHAIET

CONTENTS

17.1 Introduction *191*

17.2 Oral Cavity *192*
17.2.1 Guiding Principles *192*
17.2.2 Free Tissue Transfer *192*
17.2.3 Oral Tongue *192*
17.2.4 Anterior and Lateral
Mandible Defects *193*
17.2.5 Implants and Prosthetics *194*

17.3 Oropharynx *194*
17.3.1 Guiding Principles *194*
17.3.2 Transoral Microscopic Laser Techniques *195*
17.3.3 Open Approaches *195*

17.4 Larynx and Hypopharynx *196*
17.4.1 Trends *196*
17.4.2 Open Partial Methods/Supracricoid
Laryngectomy *196*
17.4.3 Transoral Laser
Endoscopic Techniques *196*

**17.5 Paranasal Sinuses
and Skull Base** *197*
17.5.1 Guiding Principles *197*
17.5.2 Multidisciplinary
Resection/Reconstruction *197*
17.5.3 Endoscopic and Image Guidance
Technology *198*
17.5.4 Robotic Technology *198*

17.6 Neck *198*
17.6.1 Guiding Principles *198*
17.6.2 History and Trends *198*
17.6.3 Sentinel Node Techniques and Imaging *199*

17.7 Conclusions *199*

References *199*

GREG HARTIG, MD, FACS
Department of Surgery, H4/750 CSC, University of Wisconsin School of Medicine, 600 Highland Avenue, Madison WI 53792, USA
SCOTT CHAIET, MD
Otolaryngology-Head and Neck Surgery UW Health, 600 Highland Avenue, Madison WI 53792, USA

> **KEY POINTS**
>
> - Increased use of free tissue transfer has greatly improved aesthetic and functional results for persons undergoing resection of oral cavity carcinomas.
> - Recent advancements in laser technology and improvements in the operating microscope have allowed more accurate transoral surgical management of select oropharyngeal carcinomas with less morbidity and more rapid recoveries.
> - Using both open and newer endoscopic partial laryngectomy techniques, many patients have the option of laryngeal preservation through surgical as well as nonsurgical treatment options.
> - With an interdisciplinary surgical team, including otolaryngologists, neurosurgeons, ophthalmologists, and reconstructive surgeons, malignancies of the paranasal sinuses, orbit, anterior, and middle cranial fossa skull base are now amenable to safe oncologic resection.
> - Through careful assessment of nodal metastasis patterns and appropriate utilization of postoperative radiotherapy, most neck dissection procedures can be accomplished with sparing of spinal accessory nerve function. Improved imaging and use of sentinel node biopsy techniques will allow more selective use of lymphadenectomy in the future.

17.1

Introduction

Mucosal squamous cell carcinoma of the head and neck is a heterogeneous disease best managed through the efforts and talents of a multidisciplinary team, including radiation oncology, medical oncology, head and neck surgical oncology, neuroradiology, pathology, dentistry, and speech-language pathology. The successes of primary radiotherapy and chemoradiotherapy have raised the bar with regard to the oncologic, functional, and aesthetic results expected when primary surgery is used. In this chapter, we provide a summary of the most important surgical advances in recent past with an emphasis on those efforts that improve the functional and aesthetic outcomes of our patients geared toward preservation of quality of life.

17.2
Oral Cavity

17.2.1
Guiding Principles

In contrast to many other head and neck sites, oral cavity carcinomas are almost uniformly managed surgically. Effective surgical extirpation of oral cavity carcinomas begins with an accurate assessment of tumor extent and expected defect size when the tumor is resected with a 10–15 mm oncologic margin. Appreciation of the anticipated defect helps guide the process of considering reconstructive options. Goals in reconstruction are to optimize appearance and function. Functional considerations include speech, mastication, bolus manipulation, and swallowing. For every patient, it is important to systematically review all reconstructive options from simple to complex, including the following: healing by secondary intent, primary closure, skin grafting, local and regional tissue transfer, and free tissue transfer.

Significant advancements in major oral cavity reconstruction have been made in the past 30 years. In 1979, Ariyan described the pectoralis major flap for head and neck reconstruction (Ariyan 1979). Over the next 10–15 years, the pectoralis major myocutaneous (PMC) transfer became the most commonly used solution for major oral cavity reconstruction. The PMC transfer offered an easy harvest of large volumes of well-vascularized soft tissue. This allowed reconstruction of almost any oral cavity soft tissue defect. However, the bulk of the PMC flap often limited functional and aesthetic results. For example, the remaining tongue would often be tethered downward by the PMC flap preventing optimal speech and swallowing function. Also, these regional tissue transfers could not

adequately address the problem of boney reconstruction that is so often encountered in major oral cavity resection with mandibular or maxillary involvement.

17.2.2
Free Tissue Transfer

The use of microvascular free tissue transfer, or free flaps, for head and neck reconstruction was first performed by Daniel and Taylor (1973). Initially, popularity was limited by concern over the risks of the operation and the specialized training and instrumentation required to perform these complex procedures. In the past 20 years, the pendulum has shifted dramatically toward increased use of free flaps and away from the remaining techniques. Although free tissue transfer remains challenging, the substantial improvements in aesthetic and functional results achieved have driven utilization. Overall, the availability of surgeons trained and experienced to perform these procedures has increased, thereby decreasing complication rates and further improving functional and aesthetic results. Concerns over increased costs of free flaps stemming from longer operative procedures are offset by shorter hospital stays and decreased rehabilitation efforts.

The following examples of oral tongue reconstruction and mandibular reconstruction illustrate these concepts.

17.2.3
Oral Tongue

The first goal in reconstructing the oral tongue is to create a safe, healthy barrier between the contaminated oral cavity and the neck below. This requires a body of soft tissue that will remain healthy within the oral cavity to separate these two sites. Schusterman et al. (1991) found a 14% incidence of at least partial flap necrosis with pectoralis flaps used in oral cavity reconstruction. In contrast, free tissue transfer has overall success rates of more than 95% in most series (Spiegel et al. 2007).

Assuming we can create a safe wound at low risk of complications such as breakdown or fistula formation, our second goal is to optimize function. This is accomplished through avoidance of tethering, weighting down, or distorting shape of the nonresected tongue. The radial forearm free flap (RFFF) has become the most popular option for reconstructing moderately large defects of the oral tongue. First described for oral cavity reconstruction in the early 1980s by Soutar, this fasciocutaneous flap has become widely used throughout the head and neck because of its many favorable characteristics – easily harvested, large quantity of healthy thin tissue, and a consistent large caliber vascular supply for microvascular anastamoses (SOUTAR et al. 1983). For reconstruction, the RFFF can be shaped and folded to reconstitute the original shape of the tongue. For example, a bilobed shape allows the restoration of tongue bulk and coverage of adjacent floor of mouth and gingival defect (URKEN and BILLER 1994).

Recently, SU et al. (2003) examined speech and swallowing function in persons reconstructed with the radial forearm flap as compared with the pectoralis major flap for oral tongue and tongue base defects. Persons with radial forearm flap reconstruction had better intelligibility scores, presumably because of greater tongue mobility. See Fig. 17.1 for an example of a radial forearm flap used for a hemiglossectomy defect.

Advancements in chemoradiation have reduced the need for total glossectomy, especially for lesions at the base of tongue. However, certain advanced, nonsquamous, and recurrent cancers will require near total glossectomy, for which free tissue transfer can again dramatically improve functional results (DE BREE et al. 2008). The primary goal of these reconstructions is to build a large convex oral mound that approximates the size and shape of the native tongue. The myocutaneous rectus abdominus, as well as lattissimus dorsi transfer, provides thick subcutaneous tissue, low donor site morbidity, and well-vascularized skin for reconstruction of total glossectomy defects. In a majority of cases, persons resume an oral diet and achieve intelligible speech (LYOS et al. 1999).

17.2.4
Anterior and Lateral Mandible Defects

Resection of the anterior mandible without reconstruction results in loss of lower third facial support with consequent oral incompetence, severe impairment in speech and swallowing, sleep apnea, and a much distorted appearance. Historically, this was one of the most disabling deformities sustained by head and neck cancer patients.

In contrast, resection of the lateral mandible is much less deforming and debilitating. Removing the lateral mandible results in unbalanced forces in the muscles of mastication. The more powerful pterygoid muscles pull the remaining mandible to the side of the resection with resultant crossbite malocclusion. Similarly, any remnant of the upper mandible on the side of the resection will be pulled inward and superiorly. Even so, the functional and cosmetic consequences of lateral mandibular loss are much less severe than anterior loss. In fact, free flap reconstruction of the lateral mandible was controversial as little as a decade ago. Primary closure or skin graft reconstruction was the preferred option at the University of Pittsburgh into the mid-1990s (ALVI and MYERS 1996). It is now generally agreed that reconstruction with vascularized bone offers the best result in most patients. See Fig. 17.2 for an example of lateral mandibular defect reconstructed with fibular free flap.

With free tissue transfer using osteocutaneous flaps, a number of vascularized bone grafts are now available from donor sites such as fibula, scapula, iliac crest, rib, and radius. Fibular free flap reconstruction is generally the most popular given the

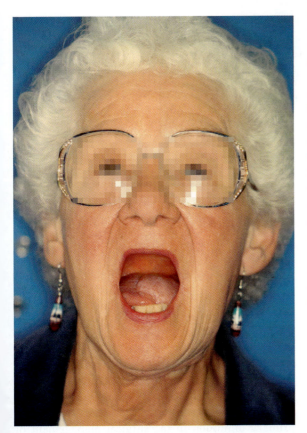

Fig. 17.1. Patient with hemiglossectomy reconstruction

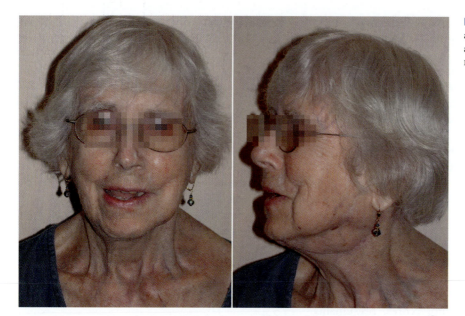

Fig. 17.2. Anterior (*left*) and lateral (*right*) views of a patient with lateral reconstruction

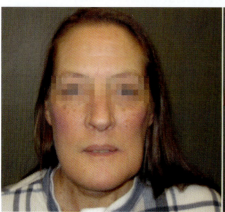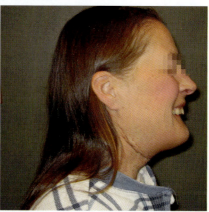

Fig. 17.3. Anterior (*left*) and lateral (*right*) views of a patient with anterior reconstruction

long healthy bone stock available, the ease of two team surgery, and the very limited donor site morbidity resulting from loss of the bone (CORDEIRO et al. 1999). In cases where lower extremity vascular supply is poor or aberrant, a scapular or iliac crest flap is used. See Fig. 17.3 for an example of anterior mandibular reconstruction with fibular free flap.

17.2.5
Implants and Prosthetics

Implants and prostheses are an important adjunct to surgical reconstruction of the oral cavity. Reconstruction of hard or soft palatal defects have traditionally employed the use of an obturator, or prosthetic. Use of dental implants can greatly improve the appearance and masticator ability of those undergoing mandibular reconstruction. Ideally these implants can even be placed at the time of the primary reconstruction.

17.3
Oropharynx

17.3.1
Guiding Principles

Given the highly effective nature of primary radiotherapy and concurrent chemo-radiation therapy for the management of oropharyngeal lesions, the use of primary surgery has decreased. Traditionally, the primary limitation in the surgical management of oropharyngeal carcinomas related to the trade-off between tumor visualization and the morbidity associated with the approach. The surgeon can achieve excellent visualization with the lip split and paramedian mandibular split but creates a significant aesthetic issue of scarring through the midline of the lip. Using the lingual release or the lateral pharyngotomy approaches, this lip scar can be avoided, representing a significant advancement. However, these options necessitated disruption of motor and sensory function in nonresected pharyngeal tissues, adding physiological dysfunction apart from the tumor resection. As a result, speech and, in particular, swallowing rehabilitation can be quite delayed. Hospitalization is also prolonged since free tissue transfers are typically required for closure, and a longer period of time must be allowed for its healing before swallowing rehabilitation can begin, given the risks of fistula formation if an oral diet is initiated too early.

17.3.2
Transoral Microscopic Laser Techniques

In contrast to the surgical morbidity of the open approach for oropharyngeal tumors, a transoral approach to the oropharynx avoids many of these problems. Traditionally, these transoral approaches were limited by poor visualization at the most inferior and posterior aspect of the resection. This in turn limited oncologic confidence. However, improvements in operating microscopes, advances in surgical laser technology, and increases in surgical experience gained through laryngeal endoscopic resections have created new interest in transoral microscopic laser resection of oropharyngeal carcinomas.

Well-defined lesions of the tongue base and palatine tonsil can be transorally resected with less morbidity and with more rapid recovery, compared with traditional open approaches. Oncologic and functional results compare favorably with nonsurgical strategies. In a recent case series analysis by GRANT et al. (2006), 59 persons with squamous cell carcinoma of the tongue base with stages 1 through 4 were treated with primary transoral CO_2 laser resection. Approximately one half received adjuvant radiotherapy based on nodal status, presence or absence of extra-capsular extension, T stage, and margin status. A 5-year local control rate of 90% compared well with nonoperative series; duration of recovery and functional results were much improved over those seen with open approaches.

However, as with free tissue transfer expertise in its early years, the availability of surgeons experienced in these transoral microscopic laser excisions is limited. For this reason, at present, primary radiotherapy and chemo-radiotherapy remain the dominant strategies for oropharyngeal carcinomas. Surgery is reserved for scenarios of persistent and recurrent disease.

Novel minimally invasive techniques will continue to grow from successes of transoral microscopic laser excisions. The University of Pennsylvania group is currently applying robotic technology, well established in other surgical specialties, to the oropharynx. Initial published results from a prospective trial on three tongue base cancer excisions show benefits over open approaches and possibly even over transoral microscopic laser excisions (O'MALLEY and WEINSTEIN 2007).

17.3.3
Open Approaches

Surgical salvage for failed nonoperative therapy is in general more challenging than primary surgery for oropharyngeal carcinomas. Confirmation of disease is the first challenge. In the patient with no visible evidence of disease, but development of recurrent symptoms and declining performance status, the use of FDG-PET imaging has become very helpful in providing prognostic information (ENOMOTO et al. 2008). Secondly, these salvage resections typically require the broad exposure of an open approach and generous resections to encompass the original nontreated tumor volume to provide the best assurance that the disease has been cleared.

In situations where the patient still has adequate vasculature for microvascular anastomosis, the broad spectrum of options provided with free tissue transfer have been invaluable. Using the RFFF reconstruction, excellent speech and swallow outcomes have been shown after resection of the tongue base (RIEGER et al. 2007) and in resections of up to one half of the soft palate (SEIKALY et al. 2003). Please see Fig. 17.4 of hemipalatal reconstruction with radial forearm flap. When prior surgery and radiotherpay have failed, the PMC flap again becomes useful in reconstructing large salvage surgical defects (ZOU et al. 2007). Clearly, these procedures involve a trade-off of quality of life for the opportunity for cure. Many but not all patients will remain at least partially gastrostomy-tube-dependent. However, most are even decannulated and will achieve good quality speech and aesthetics.

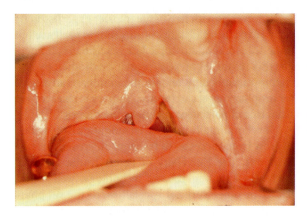

Fig. 17.4. Hemipalatal reconstruction

17.4
Larynx and Hypopharynx

17.4.1
Trends

Since the first good description of the total laryngectomy procedure by Billroth in 1873, the surgical management of laryngeal squamous cell carcinoma has focused on preserving laryngeal function without sacrificing disease control. Historically, surgery took the form of an array of open conservation procedures that were advanced in the 1950s through the 1970s. Many of these open techniques, especially in the management of supraglottic cancers, were limited by the need for good patient performance status and strong pulmonary reserve. Although these techniques still have a role in preserving laryngeal function, they are less frequently used because of the increased use of both nonsurgical strategies and transoral surgical techniques, both of which are applicable to patients with more compromised health and performance status.

17.4.2
Open Partial Methods/Supracricoid Laryngectomy

In 1913 Wilfred Trotter described an open lateral pharyngotomy approach to access smaller carcinomas of the supraglottic larynx and pharynx. Through the 1920s and 1930s, he popularized this technique and showed that much of the laryngeal framework could be removed with preservation of function. This experience laid the ground work for the concept of conservation surgery of the laryngopharynx. In 1946, Justo M. Alonso described the original horizontal supraglottic laryngectomy and his early experience with it (Rubin and Silver 1992). This procedure, which classically involves removal of the epiglottis, pre-epiglottic space, and false vocal folds and is used in the management of T1–T3 carcinomas of the supraglottic larynx, gained popularity in the United States and internationally in the decades that followed.

The primary limitation of the supraglottic laryngectomy was related to the need for reasonable pulmonary reserve and the more prolonged rehabilitation of swallowing function. However, it remains a useful and effective option for select patients with supraglottic carcinomas. It allows for avoidance of a tracheostomy and preservation of speech and swallowing.

The supracricoid partial laryngectomy procedure, an extension of the supraglottic partial laryngectomy procedure, consists of removing the supraglottic larynx and also the vocal folds and paraglottic space of the larynx, preserving the cricoid ring and one or both arytenoids. Initially described in 1959 by Austrian surgeons Majer and Rieder (Barretto 1975), it became defined and refined by Henri and Ollivier Laccourreye, who then with the help of Greg Weinstein presented their techniques and results in the English literature in 1990 (Holsinger et al. 2005; Laccourreye et al. 1990a). Similar to the supraglottic laryngectomy, this procedure has both high local control rates and a more prolonged recovery interval. Particularly when performed in conjunction with the cricohyoidoepiglottopexy reconstruction, this technique provides excellent speech and swallowing function (Laccourreye et al. 1990b).

17.4.3
Transoral Laser Endoscopic Techniques

Transoral laser microsurgical removal of laryngeal squamous cell carcinoma was first described for glottic carcinomas by Strong and Jako in 1972 (Strong and Jako 1972) and for supraglottic carcinomas by Vaughan in 1978 (Vaughan 1978). The popularity of transoral resection of both glottic and supraglottic carcinomas has grown in recent years. Its utilization has been augmented by better instrumentation such as more accurate microspot CO_2 lasers, fiber delivery lasers such as the thulium laser, improved operating microscopes, and better laryngoscopes allowing broader visualization and working areas for the procedure. Surgeons such as Wolfgang Steiner have done much in the last two decades to expand the indications for transoral laser resection of laryngeal and pharyngeal carcinomas. The concept of sectional removal of these lesions with microscopic margin control has been a key difference in the resection of larger lesions that were previously felt to be poorly suited for an endoscopic approach. The advantages of this transoral approach as opposed to an open conservation approach lay in the more rapid recovery of speech and swallowing function and the ability to safely perform these procedures on individuals with poorer pulmonary reserve. In addition, tracheotomy is often avoided.

Most believe that open conservation procedures such as the supraglottic and supracricoid operations are preferred for some T3 and select T4 lesions, whereas transoral procedures have been shown to compare favorably to open conservation procedures for T1–T2 glottic and supraglottic carcinomas. For those lesions amenable to either open or endoscopic approaches, T1–T2N0, the larger literature review published by the American Cancer Society shows results for both approaches that compare favorably with primary radiation therapy (MENDENHALL et al. 2004).

The primary limitation in the increased utilization of successful transoral laser resection techniques lies in the difficulty individual surgeons have in gathering the experience necessary to obtain the better results reported in the literature. The newly available use of flexible fiberoptic (thulium laser) or flexible mirror (CO_2) delivery of the laser energy simplifies endoscopic removal by allowing the surgeon to more easily and broadly vary the angle of cutting with the laser. As this technology becomes widely available, the advancement should result in greater ease and more favorable results for those with more modest experience.

17.5
Paranasal Sinuses and Skull Base

17.5.1
Guiding Principles

Malignancies of the skull base and paranasal sinuses are rare and histologically a more heterogeneous group than malignancies of other mucosal head and neck sites. Although dominated by squamous cell carcinoma, other epithelial malignancies within the nose and paranasal sinuses include adenoid cystic carcinomas, adenocarcinomas, and more rarely esthesioneuroblastomas, sinonasal undifferentiated carcinomas, melanoma, and others. Nonepithelial malignancies, primarily sarcomas such as osteogenic, rhabdomyosarcomas, and chondrosarcomas occur at a higher proportion in the nose and paranasal sinuses than for other sites in the head and neck. Prognosis for this group of malignancies is poor with frequent local failure. However, newer technologies and operative strategies have allowed for more successful resections with less morbidity while maintaining low complication rates.

17.5.2
Multidisciplinary Resection/Reconstruction

Traditional open surgical approaches include variations of ethmoidectomy, maxillectomy, and more recently the craniofacial resection for tumors of the anterior skull base. The interdisciplinary surgical team of a neurosurgeon and otolaryngologist, as well as ophthalmologists and reconstructive surgeons, now allows for resections of advanced lesions with intracranial involvement of the skull base, once deemed unresectable. CUMMINGS (2005) stated that "[T]he boundary between resectability and unresectability for advanced skull base malignancy is ill defined." Even with more aggressive surgical management, collaborative data published in 2005 on large craniofacial resections across 17 institutions show low mortality (4.7%) and complication rates (36.3%) (GANLY et al. 2005).

Reconstruction again commonly uses microvascular free tissue transfer in place of pedicled flaps historically used to provide volume to maintain the shape of the overlying face, provide support for the brain and orbit, and separate the CNS from the aerodigestive track (PUSIC et al. 2007).

Recent advances in the area of open surgical resection of paranasal sinus malignancy have focused on decreasing the use of large facial incisions in the approach for these tumors. The evolution to the subcranial approach to the skull base allows a more complete visualization of the paranasal sinuses from the traditional frontal craniotomy approach. This in turn has allowed the avoidance of facial incisions such as the lateral rhinotomy incision and Weber Fergusson incision that had been in common usage for decades. One key difference in philosophy allowing resection through limited incisions has been the move away from attempts at en bloc resection and towards greater use of a stepwise or piecemeal approach to resection. Removal of one part of the tumor then allowed improved visualization and removal of the next part, etc. This evolution fit well with endoscopic tools concurrently developed for paranasal sinus surgery for inflammatory disease.

In reality, en-bloc resection of paranasal sinus malignancies was always harder to achieve in practice than it was for other head and neck sites. Comparisons of these sectional approach procedures compared with a traditional en-bloc procedure show no significant difference in local control (WELLMAN et al. 1999). Multiple authors have also reported large series comparing endoscopic resections with open techniques, and again, results are similar (BUCHMANN et al. 2006; NICOLAI et al. 2008).

17.5.3
Endoscopic and Image Guidance Technology

For lesions that do not invade the dura or brain parenchyma, endoscopic techniques have become increasingly utilized in an effort to minimize operative morbidity and risk. Initially developed in the early 1990s, these endoscopic techniques were utilized for benign neoplastic diseases such as inverting papilloma. More recently, strict endoscopic or combination of endoscopic and open techniques for cases with dural or parenchymal involvement has been utilized for malignancies. The development of image guidance technologies, widely utilized in neurosurgery and otolaryngology, also improve accuracy and safety for these procedures.

17.5.4
Robotic Technology

Minimally invasive endoscopic image-guided surgery of the paranasal sinuses and skull base avoids large incisions and preserves bone. However, a major disadvantage is the inability to provide a watertight dural closure during reconstruction. This limitation may be addressed through development of robotic technology for skull base resections (HANNA et al. 2007). A number of skull base centers are now experimenting with the use of robotic techniques in managing lesions via the sphenoid sinus (BUMM et al. 2005), parapharyngeal space, and infratemporal fossa (O'MALLEY and WEINSTEIN 2007), furthering the safety of these minimally invasive resections.

17.6
Neck

17.6.1
Guiding Principles

In the absence of distant disease, the presence of cervical nodal metastasis is the single most important prognostic factor for survival in mucosal squamous cell carcinoma of the head and neck. The presence of lymph node metastasis decreases the probability of survival by ~50% (SHAH 1996). The adequate management of overt and occult nodal disease has been an area of interest and debate among clinicians for decades.

17.6.2
History and Trends

For nearly 100 years, the radical neck dissection procedure was considered the procedure of choice for known nodal disease. From the 1960s forward, the trend has been to evaluate the efficacy of less aggressive procedures, most often ones that spare the posterior triangle (level 5) lymph nodes. This group of lymph nodes is much less commonly involved in head and neck squamous cell carcinoma with the exception of nasopharyngeal carcinoma. In preserving level 5, loss of the spinal accessory nerve and consequent trapezius weakness, the most significant morbidity of the radical neck dissection procedure, is significantly diminished.

Similarly, the use of neck dissections sparing the submandibular and submental triangles (level 1) is typical when managing carcinomas of the pharynx and larynx. Avoidance of this level 1 dissection spares salivary function through preservation of the submandibular gland and avoids the aesthetic risk of marginal mandibular nerve injury with consequent loss of lower lip depressor function. These neck dissections preserving low risk neck levels are referred to as selective neck dissections (SND). The equivalent therapeutic value of SND has been clearly established for elective neck dissections with regional recurrence rates of around 5% (BYERS 1985; BYERS et al. 1988; CLAYMAN and FRANK 1998; SPIRO et al. 1996). When pathology shows positive nodal disease, a combination of SND with postoperative radiotherapy is recommended (BYERS et al. 1999).

Also, an increasing body of evidence suggests that these less aggressive SND procedures are safe even for those who have overt nodal disease undergoing primary surgical therapy. One of the larger series by Ambrosch et al. in 2001 reported on subjects who were clinically N0 and N1 undergoing elective and therapeutic SND, respectively. Among 254 pathologically N+ dissections, there was a 5 and 12% regional recurrence rate for pN1 and pN2 disease respectively, similar to control, achievable with the modified radical neck dissection (AMBROSCH et al. 2001). In these individuals, the use of SND must be considered carefully. The use of the more aggressive modified radical or radical neck dissection procedures are generally reserved for those situations where patients have gross extracapsular nodal disease invading surrounding structures such as the sternocliedomastoid or internal jugular vein.

The safe utilization of SND techniques for many with lesser volume N1–N2b disease is dependent on the efficacy of postoperative radiotherapy. In most series, regional recurrences are most commonly located within the field of the SND, not in the levels that were left behind by performing less than a comprehensive dissection (LOHUIS et al. 2004; ANDERSEN et al. 2002; CHEPEHA et al. 2002).

17.6.3
Sentinel Node Techniques and Imaging

In malignant melanoma, it is common to use sentinel node biopsy techniques to select those individuals who would benefit from more comprehensive lymphadenectomy. The use of sentinel node techniques for mucosal squamous cell carcinoma is being investigated. Although sentinel node techniques have not been consistently feasible for floor of mouth cancers given the proximity of the primary site injection with the at-risk nodal basin, this technique has shown value for other oral cavity, oropharyngeal, and even laryngeal sites. A multi-institutional trial completed in 2008 examining pathological results of sentinel node biopsy with subsequent elective neck dissection for selected squamous cell carcinoma of the oral cavity provided a negative predictive value of 96% (CIVANTOS et al. 2008). Whether or not these patients with negative sentinel node biopsies will have equivalent regional control rates to those who are N0 after SND remains to be seen.

Advancements in imaging have made it possible to avoid lymphadenectomy in many patients with N2 disease being treated with primary chemoradiation therapy. In the past, these individuals would have typically undergone postchemoradiotherapy neck dissection. The use of CT/FDG-PET fusion imaging for this group has proven to be an accurate way of selecting those who would benefit by neck dissection. In a study by YAO et al. (2007), the negative predictive value of a negative CT/FDG-PET fusion study was 100%. Future studies that support this finding will give surgeons confidence to defer unneeded surgical management.

17.7
Conclusions

Modern surgical management of head and neck squamous cell carcinoma has focused on optimizing functional and aesthetic results through reducing the morbidity of resection with endoscopic, microscopic, and transoral resection techniques, and through improving reconstruction results with greater and more refined use of free tissue transfer. Improvements in assessing disease status and staging through better imaging and less invasive methods of operative staging such as sentinel node biopsy will also result in overall improvements in form and function for our patients.

References

Alvi A, Myers EN (1996) Skin graft reconstruction of the composite resection defect. Head Neck 18:538–543

Ambrosch P, Kron M, Pradier O et al. (2001) Efficacy of selective neck dissection: a review of 503 cases of elective and therapeutic treatment of the neck in squamous cell carcinoma of the upper aerodigestive tract. Otolaryngol Head Neck Surg 124:180–187

Andersen PE, Warren F, Spiro J et al. (2002) Results of selective neck dissection in management of the node-positive neck. Arch Otolaryngol Head Neck Surg 128:1180–1184

Ariyan S (1979) The pectoralis major myocutaneous flap. A versatile flap for reconstruction in the head and neck. Plast Reconstr Surg 63:73–81

Barretto PM (1975) Panel discussion: the historical development of laryngectomy. IV. The South American contribution to the surgery of laryngeal cancer. Laryngoscope 85: 299–321

Buchmann L, Larsen C, Pollack A et al. (2006) Endoscopic techniques in resection of anterior skull base/paranasal sinus malignancies. Laryngoscope 116:1749–1754

Bumm K, Wurm J, Rachinger J et al. (2005) An automated robotic approach with redundant navigation for minimal invasive extended transsphenoidal skull base surgery. Minim Invasive Neurosurg 48:159–164

Byers RM (1985) Modified neck dissection. A study of 967 cases from 1970 to 1980. Am J Surg 150:414–421

Byers RM, Wolf PF, Ballantyne AJ (1988) Rationale for elective modified neck dissection. Head Neck Surg 10:160–167

Byers RM, Clayman GL, McGill D et al. (1999) Selective neck dissections for squamous carcinoma of the upper aerodigestive tract: patterns of regional failure. Head Neck 21:499–505

Chepeha DB, Hoff PT, Taylor RJ et al. (2002) Selective neck dissection for the treatment of neck metastasis from squamous cell carcinoma of the head and neck. Laryngoscope 112:434–438

Civantos F, Jr, Zitsch R, Bared A et al. (2008) Sentinel node biopsy for squamous cell carcinoma of the head and neck. J Surg Oncol 97:683–690

Clayman GL, Frank DK (1998) Selective neck dissection of anatomically appropriate levels is as efficacious as modified radical neck dissection for elective treatment of the clinically negative neck in patients with squamous cell carcinoma of the upper respiratory and digestive tracts. Arch Otolaryngol Head Neck Surg 124:348–352

Cordeiro PG, Disa JJ, Hidalgo DA et al. (1999) Reconstruction of the mandible with osseous free flaps: a 10-year experience with 150 consecutive patients. Plast Reconstr Surg 104:1314–1320

Cummings CW (2005) Cummings otolaryngology head & neck surgery, 4th edn. Elsevier Mosby, Philadelphia, PA

Daniel RK, Taylor GI (1973) Distant transfer of an island flap by microvascular anastomoses. A clinical technique. Plast Reconstr Surg 52:111–117

de Bree R, Rinaldo A, Genden EM et al. (2008) Modern reconstruction techniques for oral and pharyngeal defects after tumor resection. Eur Arch Otorhinolaryngol 265:1–9

Enomoto K, Inohara H, Higuchi I et al. (2008) Prognostic value of FDG-PET in patients with oropharyngeal carcinoma treated with concurrent chemoradiotherapy. Mol Imaging Biol 10:224–229

Ganly I, Patel SG, Singh B et al. (2005) Complications of craniofacial resection for malignant tumors of the skull base: report of an International Collaborative Study. Head Neck 27:445–451

Grant DG, Salassa JR, Hinni ML et al. (2006) Carcinoma of the tongue base treated by transoral laser microsurgery, part one: untreated tumors, a prospective analysis of oncologic and functional outcomes. Laryngoscope 116:2150–2155

Hanna EY, Holsinger C, DeMonte F et al. (2007) Robotic endoscopic surgery of the skull base: a novel surgical approach. Arch Otolaryngol Head Neck Surg 133:1209–1214

Holsinger FC, Laccourreye O, Weinstein GS et al. (2005) Technical refinements in the supracricoid partial laryngectomy to optimize functional outcomes. J Am Coll Surg 201:809–820

Laccourreye H, Laccourreye O, Weinstein G et al. (1990a) Supracricoid laryngectomy with cricohyoidoepiglottopexy: a partial laryngeal procedure for glottic carcinoma. Ann Otol Rhinol Laryngol 99:421–426

Laccourreye H, Laccourreye O, Weinstein G et al. (1990b) Supracricoid laryngectomy with cricohyoidopexy: a partial laryngeal procedure for selected supraglottic and transglottic carcinomas. Laryngoscope 100:735–741

Lohuis PJ, Klop WM, Tan IB et al. (2004) Effectiveness of therapeutic (N1, N2) selective neck dissection (levels II to V) in patients with laryngeal and hypopharyngeal squamous cell carcinoma. Am J Surg 187:295–299

Lyos AT, Evans GR, Perez D et al. (1999) Tongue reconstruction: outcomes with the rectus abdominis flap. Plast Reconstr Surg 103:442–447; discussion 448–449

Mendenhall WM, Werning JW, Hinerman RW et al. (2004) Management of T1–T2 glottic carcinomas. Cancer 100:1786–1792

Nicolai P, Battaglia P, Bignami M et al. (2008) Endoscopic surgery for malignant tumors of the sinonasal tract and adjacent skull base: a 10-year experience. Am J Rhinol 22:308–316

O'Malley BW, Jr, Weinstein GS (2007) Robotic skull base surgery: preclinical investigations to human clinical application. Arch Otolaryngol Head Neck Surg 133:1215–1219

Pusic AL, Chen CM, Patel S et al. (2007) Microvascular reconstruction of the skull base: a clinical approach to surgical defect classification and flap selection. Skull Base 17:5–15

Rieger JM, Zalmanowitz JG, Li SY et al. (2007) Functional outcomes after surgical reconstruction of the base of tongue using the radial forearm free flap in patients with oropharyngeal carcinoma. Head Neck 29:1024–1032

Rubin JS, Silver CE (1992) Surgical approach to submucosal lesions of the supraglottic larynx: the supero-lateral thyrotomy. J Laryngol Otol 106:416–419

Schusterman MA, Kroll SS, Weber RS et al. (1991) Intraoral soft tissue reconstruction after cancer ablation: a comparison of the pectoralis major flap and the free radial forearm flap. Am J Surg 162:397–399

Seikaly H, Rieger J, Wolfaardt J et al. (2003) Functional outcomes after primary oropharyngeal cancer resection and reconstruction with the radial forearm free flap. Laryngoscope 113:897–904

Shah JP (1996) Head and neck surgery, 2nd edn. Mosby-Wolfe, New York

Soutar DS, Scheker LR, Tanner NS et al. (1983) The radial forearm flap: a versatile method for intra-oral reconstruction. Br J Plast Surg 36:1–8

Spiegel JH, Polat JK (2007) Microvascular flap reconstruction by otolaryngologists: prevalence, postoperative care, and monitoring techniques. Laryngoscope. 117(3):485–490.

Spiro RH, Morgan GJ, Strong EW et al. (1996) Supraomohyoid neck dissection. Am J Surg 172:650–653

Strong MS, Jako GJ (1972) Laser surgery in the larynx. Early clinical experience with continuous CO2 laser. Ann Otol Rhinol Laryngol 81:791–798

Su WF, Hsia YJ, Chang YC et al. (2003) Functional comparison after reconstruction with a radial forearm free flap or a pectoralis major flap for cancer of the tongue. Otolaryngol Head Neck Surg 128:412–418

Urken ML, Biller HF (1994) A new bilobed design for the sensate radial forearm flap to preserve tongue mobility following significant glossectomy. Arch Otolaryngol Head Neck Surg 120:26–31

Vaughan CW (1978) Transoral laryngeal surgery using the CO2 laser: laboratory experiments and clinical experience. Laryngoscope 88:1399–1420

Wellman BJ, Traynelis VC, McCulloch TM et al. (1999) Midline anterior craniofacial approach for malignancy: results of en bloc versus piecemeal resections. Skull Base Surg 9:41–46

Yao M, Luo P, Hoffman HT et al. (2007) Pathology and FDG PET correlation of residual lymph nodes in head and neck cancer after radiation treatment. Am J Clin Oncol 30:264–270

Zou H, Zhang WF, Han QB et al. (2007) Salvage reconstruction of extensive recurrent oral cancer defects with the pectoralis major myocutaneous flap. J Oral Maxillofac Surg 65:1935–1939

The Contribution of Chemotherapy

18

Michalis V. Karamouzis, Michael K. Gibson, and Athanassios Argiris

CONTENTS

18.1   Introduction   *203*

18.2   Chemotherapy in Multimodality
       Treatment   *204*

18.3   Organ Preservation Considerations   *204*

18.4   The Emerging Role of Cetuximab   *206*

18.5   Treatment-Related Toxicities   *207*
18.5.1   Acute Toxicities   *207*
18.5.2   Late and Chronic Toxicities   *210*

18.6   Conclusions   *211*

References   *212*

- As treatment has been intensified, it becomes increasingly important to measure and address the impact of treatment-related toxicities on quality of life parameters.
- The incorporation of targeted systemic agents, such as the epidermal growth factor receptor inhibitors, and of radioprotectants into combined modality treatments offers the potential for improving the risk to benefit ratio.
- Future clinical research should focus on how to ameliorate acute and late treatment-related toxicities and improve quality of life while maintaining therapeutic efficacy.

KEY POINTS

- Concomitant chemoradiotherapy has been shown to improve locoregional control, organ preservation, and/or survival over radiotherapy alone and has emerged as a standard treatment for patients with locally advanced squamous cell carcinoma of the head and neck.
- The addition of chemotherapy to radiotherapy can worsen acute radiation-induced toxicities, including mucositis and dermatitis, and result in chemotherapy predominantly-related toxicities, such as myelosuppression, neuropathy, nausea and vomiting.

Michalis V. Karamouzis, MD
Michael K. Gibson, MD
Athanassios Argiris, MD
Division of Hematology-Oncology, University of Pittsburgh School of Medicine, UPMC Cancer Pavilion, 5th Floor, 5150 Centre Avenue, Pittsburgh, PA 15232, USA

18.1
Introduction

Squamous cell carcinomas of the head and neck (SCCHN) are a heterogeneous group of malignancies that originate in the epithelium of the nasal cavity, sinuses, pharynx, oral cavity, and larynx. They are frequently diagnosed at advanced stages with extension of the primary tumor to adjacent structures and/or regional spread to neck lymph nodes. Since SCCHN and its treatment can affect organs and systems critical for important functions, such as speaking, breathing, and swallowing, patients with SCCHN may develop a variety of symptoms and impairments, including mouth or neck pain, difficulties in chewing and swallowing resulting in malnutrition and aspiration, hoarseness or loss of natural voice, problems in breathing, head and neck deformities, and others. Given the risk for potential functional deficits from potentially curative treatment, not only cure but organ preservation, functional outcomes, and quality of life (QOL) are of foremost importance in the management of patients with SCCHN.

Therapeutic options for the treatment of locally advanced SCCHN have evolved over the past two decades as a result of developments in the area of combined modality strategies. Historically, standard therapy for locally advanced SCCHN involved surgical resection with or without postoperative radiotherapy for resectable disease or radiation therapy alone for unresectable tumors. In an effort to increase the probability of organ preservation and survival, chemotherapy was evaluated as a component of combined modality approaches. The contribution of induction, concomitant, and/or adjuvant chemotherapy was studied in a large number of phase III randomized clinical trials. On the basis of this cumulative experience, concomitant chemoradiotherapy (CRT) emerged as a standard treatment for improving survival and/or achieving organ preservation in locally advanced SCCHN. However, with treatment intensification, mostly related to the addition of chemotherapy to radiotherapy in a concurrent fashion, complications of treatment are seen in increased frequency. This chapter aims to concisely review the efficacy and toxicity of current combined modality approaches with a focus on functional outcomes and the potential impact on QOL.

18.2
Chemotherapy in Multimodality Treatment

Patients with locally advanced SCCHN (i.e., AJCC stages III/IVA–B) have a potentially curable disease that requires multidisciplinary evaluation and management. A major step forward in the treatment of locally advanced SCCHN was the introduction of the concurrent administration of chemotherapy and radiotherapy. Numerous randomized clinical trials demonstrated that concomitant CRT yields improved locoregional control and/or survival than either radiotherapy alone or the sequential administration of chemotherapy and radiotherapy (Table 18.1). A meta-analysis of individual patient data from nearly 11,000 participants in 63 trials conducted between 1965 and 1993 (Meta-analysis of Chemotherapy in Head and Neck Cancer [MACH-NC]) demonstrated that the addition of chemotherapy to locoregional treatment, as induction, concomitant, or adjuvant

treatment, confers an absolute survival benefit of 4% at 5 years (Pignon et al. 2000). Most of the benefit was seen with concomitant CRT; however, there was a relatively large heterogeneity in this subgroup of trials. An updated analysis that included 24 additional studies and a total of 9,615 patients treated with concomitant CRT confirmed that it produces an absolute survival improvement of 8% at 5 years (Bourhis et al. 2004). The survival advantage with concomitant CRT over radiotherapy alone was predominantly a result of improved locoregional control, whereas only a minor impact on distant recurrence was evident. The survival benefit documented in multiple randomized clinical trials and meta-analyses supported the use of concomitant CRT as a standard-of-care treatment of stage III/IV SCCHN (Argiris et al. 2008).

Although many regimens of CRT have been used, platinum-based concomitant CRT is widely accepted as standard. High-dose cisplatin ($100\,mg\,m^{-2}$ every 3 weeks for three cycles) is the regimen that has been studied the most and has yielded positive results in multiple cooperative group phase III trials in locally advanced SCCHN (Adelstein et al. 2003; Al-Sarraf et al. 1998; Bernier et al. 2004; Cooper et al. 2004; Forastiere et al. 2003). Cisplatin or carboplatin plus 5-fluorouracil (5-FU) has also been extensively utilized (Calais et al. 1999; Wendt et al. 1998).

Induction chemotherapy with the addition of taxanes (docetaxel or paclitaxel) to cisplatin and 5-FU was shown to improve survival (Hitt et al. 2005; Vermorken et al. 2007; Posner et al. 2007) or organ preservation outcomes (Calais et al. 2006) over cisplatin and 5-FU alone in phase III randomized clinical trials. This led to a renewed interest in the role of induction chemotherapy in locally advanced SCCHN. A number of ongoing randomized trials are evaluating the potential survival advantage when cisplatin, docetaxel, and 5-FU are added to concomitant CRT. As regimens that incorporate induction are increasingly utilized, the potential of cumulative or repeated toxicities over a prolonged treatment period should be taken into consideration (Trotti et al. 2007).

18.3
Organ Preservation Considerations

Major factors affecting the choice of primary treatment modality include tumor resectability and the desire for organ preservation as well as the ability of

The Contribution of Chemotherapy 205

Table 18.1. Selected phase III trials of primary concomitant CRT vs. RT alone in locally advanced SCCHN

References	Number of patients analyzed	Primary sites and resectability	Radiotherapy regimen (Gy)	Chemotherapy regimen	Overall survival (%)
JEREMIC et al. (2000)	130	Nasopharynx, oral cavity, oropharynx, larynx, hypopharynx; unresectable	Std fxn 70	Cisplatin 6 mg m^{-2} day^{-1} Carboplatin 25 mg m^{-2} day^{-1}	32[*] 28[*] RT alone: 15 (5-year)
AL-SARRAF et al. (1998)	147	Nasopharynx	Std fxn 70	Cisplatin 100 mg m^{-2} days 1, 22, 43	CRT: 78[*] RT alone: 47 (3-year)
ADELSTEIN et al. (2003)	271	Oral cavity, oropharynx, larynx, hypopharynx; unresectable	Std fxn 70 Split course to 70	Cisplatin 100 mg m^{-2} days 1, 22, 43 Cisplatin 75 mg m^{-2} days 1, 29, 57 + 5-FU 1,000 mg m^{-2} day^{-1} CI for 96 h	37[*] 27 (NS) RT alone: 23 (3-year)
DENIS et al. (2004)	222	Oropharynx; resectability not specified	Std fxn 70	Carboplatin 70 mg m^{-2} day^{-1} days 1–4, 22–26, 43–47 5-FU 600 mg m^{-2}/CI day^{-1} days 1–4, 22–26, 43–47	CRT: 22[*] RT alone: 16 (5-year)
WENDT et al. (1998)	270	Oral cavity, oropharynx, larynx, hypopharynx; unresectable	Three courses, 13 fxns each, 1.8 b.i.d., total dose 70.2	Cisplatin 60 mg m^{-2} day 1 and 5-FU 350 mg m^{-2} bolus day 2 + LV 50 mg m^{-2} i.v. bolus day 2 and 5-FU 350 mg m^{-2} days 2–5 + LV 100 mg m^{-2} day^{-1} CI days 2–5 Repeat days 22 and 44	CRT: 48[*] RT alone: 24 (3-year)
FORASTIERE et al. (2003)	518	Larynx; resectable	Std fxn 70	RT alone Induction CT (cisplatin 100 mg m^{-2} + 5-FU 1,000 mg m^{-2} day^{-1} CI for 120 h; Q21 days) × 2–3 cycles then RT/surgery Cisplatin 100 mg m^{-2} days 1, 22, 43 concurrent with RT	No differences in overall survival Laryngeal preservation rate was superior in Arm C

[*]Statistically significant difference in survival
CRT chemoradiotherapy; *RT* radiotherapy; *Std fxn* standard fractionation; *CI* continuous infusion

the patient to comply with and tolerate treatment. Although an important treatment goal is organ preservation, physicians recognize that such attempts might leave an anatomically intact but dysfunctional organ. No conclusive data exist regarding QOL in surgical vs. nonsurgical approaches. In general, oral cavity primaries are usually treated with surgery, followed by postoperative concomitant CRT on the basis of high-risk pathological features, since the cosmetic and functional results are regarded as satisfactory.

However, locally advanced oropharyngeal primaries are usually treated with CRT with good efficacy and functional results. Patients with locally advanced hypopharyngeal and laryngeal primaries should be considered for organ preserving treatment (ARGIRIS et al. 2008).

Preservation of natural voice by retaining an intact larynx is the best example of an organ preservation goal. It has been suggested that long-term QOL in patients undergoing CRT is better than in those who underwent total laryngectomy (Boscolo-Rizzo et al. 2008). Total laryngectomy is widely recognized as one of the surgical procedures most feared by SCCHN patients. Social isolation, job loss, and depression are common consequences. The development of active chemotherapy regimens has prompted an era of intensive clinical research. Induction chemotherapy followed by radiotherapy in a subset of patients with responsive tumors has been shown to allow laryngeal preservation in about two thirds of patients with locally advanced laryngeal or hypopharyngeal primaries, without compromising survival. The landmark Department of Veterans Affairs Laryngeal Cancer Study first established a role for induction chemotherapy followed by radiotherapy for organ preservation in advanced laryngeal cancer (The Department of Veterans Affairs Laryngeal Cancer Study Group 1991). This approach was also confirmed in the setting of hypopharyngeal cancer in a phase III randomized study conducted by the European Organization for Research and Treatment of Cancer (EORTC) (Lefebvre et al. 1996). Following the VA larynx study, the US Intergroup carried out a phase III randomized trial (RTOG 91-11) to determine the best nonsurgical treatment for achieving laryngeal preservation in patients with resectable laryngeal SCCHN (Forastiere et al. 2003) (Table 18.1). A total of 547 patients were randomized to one of three treatment groups: induction chemotherapy with cisplatin and 5-FU followed by radiotherapy, concomitant CRT with cisplatin, or radiotherapy alone. The majority of patients had T3N0–1 disease representing an intermediate stage patient population. Although overall survival was almost identical between the three arms, the laryngeal preservation rate at 5 years was highest with concomitant CRT (84%) vs. 70% with induction ($p = 0.0029$) and 66% with radiotherapy alone ($p = 0.00017$) (Forastiere et al. 2006). Laryngectomy-free survival was better in the chemotherapy arms (47% with concomitant CRT and 45% with induction followed by radiotherapy) vs. radiotherapy alone. There was a trend for reduced rate of distant metastases in the two chemotherapy treatment groups (14 and 13%) compared with radiotherapy alone (22%). It should be noted that toxicity was substantially increased in both chemotherapy-treated groups, compared with those randomized to radiotherapy alone (Forastiere et al. 2003).

The implementation of laryngeal-preserving treatment requires evaluation and decision-making by a specialized multidisciplinary team (Pfister et al. 2006). Functional outcomes in terms of speech quality appear to be good after nonsurgical management. Speech does not appear to be affected to the same degree as swallowing in patients who have undergone organ preservation techniques (Lefebvre 2006). Intelligibility of speech is reported to be primarily unaffected by organ preservation techniques. However, subtle chronic voice changes may be evident after organ-sparing CRT (Rieger et al. 2006).

18.4
The Emerging Role of Cetuximab

A more recent addition to the armamentarium against SCCHN is the epidermal growth factor receptor (EGFR) inhibitors, a class of novel agents that are potent radiosensitizers. The EGFR is a type I tyrosine kinase membrane receptor that regulates key cellular functions and is overexpressed in SCCHN. Various methods are clinically available for the inhibition of EGFR and its downstream signaling pathways (Karamouzis et al. 2007). Cetuximab, a chimeric IgG1 monoclonal antibody against the extracellular ligand-binding domain of EGFR, is the prototype anti-EGFR agent and the first molecularly targeted agent to obtain regulatory approval for the treatment of patients with locally advanced SCCHN. In a pivotal phase III trial conducted by Bonner et al., the combination of radiation and cetuximab was compared with radiation alone in a total of 424 patients with locally advanced SCCHN. Significant improvements in locoregional control (47 vs. 34% at 3 years, $p < 0.01$), progression-free survival (42 vs. 31% at 3 years, $p = 0.04$), and overall survival (55 vs. 45% at 3 years, $p = 0.03$) were identified (Bonner et al. 2006). Perhaps more notably, survival gain did not occur at the cost of increased in-field side effects. In particular, common radiation-related effects such as mucositis and dermatitis were not worse in the experimental arm. Furthermore, cetuximab is not associated with common cisplatin-related toxicities that include myelosuppression, nephrotoxicity, and neuropathy. However, cetuximab-specific toxicities, such as acneiform rash and infusion reactions, were observed in the cetuximab arm. In the context of this phase III randomized trial, QOL was assessed using the EORTC Quality of Life Questionnaire C30 (EORTC QLQ-C30) and EORTC QLQ Head-and-Neck-Cancer-Specific Module. It was demonstrated that QOL worsened during treatment and improved after cessation of treatment, reaching baseline levels at 12 months, but there were no significant differences in QOL scores between the two treatment arms (CURRAN et al. 2007).

The efficacy results with cetuximab are comparable to those achieved with platinum-based regimens; however, no randomized trial has yet compared cetuximab with cisplatin each given concurrently with radiation. A main focus of ongoing research is the incorporation of cetuximab in platinum-based CRT. An ongoing phase III trial sponsored by the Radiation Therapy Oncology Group (RTOG 0122) is comparing concurrent radiotherapy and cisplatin with or without cetuximab.

18.5
Treatment-Related Toxicities

18.5.1
Acute Toxicities

Combined modality therapy of SCCHN is usually associated with multiple acute complications. Frequently seen acute side effects include mucositis, dysphagia, aspiration, hoarseness, and dermatitis (TROTTI et al. 2003; GARCIA-PERIS et al. 2007; ROSENTHAL et al. 2006). Xerostomia and taste impairment may occur early during the course of radiotherapy but can be chronic (RUO REDDA and ALLIS 2006). In general, the acute toxicities of radiotherapy are exacerbated during concomitant CRT because of the radiosensitizing properties of chemotherapy. The rate of severe mucositis is approximately doubled with the addition of chemotherapy to radiotherapy, whereas the duration of mucositis and other acute toxicities is also longer in patients receiving CRT (BRIZEL et al. 1998). Patients receiving CRT experience more weight loss and more frequently require a feeding tube during therapy. Hospitalizations are also increased, and chemotherapy dose reductions are commonly needed. In addition to the in-field locoregional effects of radiotherapy, chemotherapy-specific, nonhematologic toxicities, such as nausea, vomiting, neuropathy, nephropathy, and ototoxicity may occur. Acute nonhematologic toxicity rates were consistently higher in the CRT arms in randomized clinical trials that compared concomitant CRT to radiotherapy alone despite interobserver variability and disparate reporting of rates of nonhematologic

acute toxicities across studies (BENTZEN and TROTTI 2007) (Table 18.2). Although hematologic toxicities are seldom observed with radiotherapy alone, the addition of chemotherapy often causes significant myelosuppression (Table 18.2). Toxicities of concomitant CRT with high-dose cisplatin given every 3 weeks for three cycles, a standard CRT regimen, are shown in Table 18.3. Treatment-related toxicities may result in treatment delays and dose reductions, compromising treatment delivery. At least one third of patients do not receive the third cycle of cisplatin with this regimen (ADELSTEIN et al. 2003; AL-SARRAF et al. 1998; BERNIER et al. 2004; COOPER et al. 2004; FORASTIERE et al. 2003).

Swallowing dysfunction is a major cause of morbidity in SCCHN patients undergoing multimodality treatment (FROWEN and PERRY 2006). Swallowing function usually deteriorates during treatment, and the effect of CRT may be more pronounced than that of radiotherapy alone (BLEIER et al. 2007; EISBRUCH et al. 2002; LOGEMANN et al. 2008). Silent aspiration and aspiration pneumonia are frequent (EISBRUCH et al. 2002). Poor oral intake due to loss of taste and appetite, mucositis, and dysphagia leads to malnutrition and may compromize treatment efficacy and diminish QOL. Feeding tubes are often used to compensate for reduced oral intake. Percutaneous endoscopic gastrostomy tubes are generally preferred over nasogastric tubes (CADY 2007). Although prophylactic placement of feeding tubes is supported by many, it is possible that swallowing function is better preserved when patients continue to swallow during treatment (ROSENTHAL et al. 2006).

Many agents, including granulocyte-macrophage-colony stimulating factor or granulocyte-colony stimulating factor, have been tested for their effect on reducing the severity of radiation-induced mucositis without conclusive results (STAAR et al. 2001; RYU et al. 2007). Keratinocyte growth factor is a fibroblast growth factor that stimulates many cellular events, among them detoxification of reactive oxygen. Recombinant human keratinocyte growth factor (palifermin) is approved for use in patients with hematologic malignancies receiving myelotoxic therapy requiring hematopoietic stem cell support. The use of palifermin in patients with SCCHN undergoing concurrent CRT is being tested in terms of ameliorating acute mucositis, although the most efficacious dosing schedule has not yet been identified (BRIZEL et al. 2008).

Although multimodality treatment is generally associated with increased acute toxicity, the addition

Table 18.2. Acute toxicities in phase III randomized trials of concomitant CRT in SCCHN

Primary tumor site	CRT regimen	Non-hematologic toxicity grade 3–4	Hematologic toxicity grade 3–4	References
Postoperative CRT vs. RT				
OC, OP, HP, L	RT (66 Gy) + cisplatin (100 mg m^{-2}) days 1, 22, 43	Mucositis: 41 vs. 21% Dysphagia: 10 vs. 12% Skin toxicity: 1 vs. 2% Nausea/vomiting: 11 vs. 0%	Neutropenia: 13 vs. 0%	BERNIER et al. (2004)
OC, OP, HP, L	RT (60–66 Gy) + cisplatin (100 mg m^{-2}) days 1,22,43	Mucositis: 30 vs. 18% Dysphagia: 24.5 vs. 15% Skin toxicity: 7 vs. 10% Nausea/vomiting: 20 vs. 0% Infection: 6 vs. 1% Neurologic: 5 vs. 0% Renal: 2.5 vs. 0% Others: 16 vs. 2%	Hematologic: 38 vs. 0% Anemia: 3 vs. 0%	COOPER et al. (2004)
OC, OP, HP, L	RT (50–64 Gy) + cisplatin (20 mg m^{-2})/5-FU (600 mg m^{-2}) days 1–5, 29–33	Mucositis: 21 vs. 13% Skin toxicity: 13 vs. 9% Renal: 6.5 vs. 1% Infection: 9 vs. 7%	Leukopenia: 4.5 vs. 0% Thrombopenia: 2 vs. 0%	FIETKAU et al. (2006)
Primary CRT vs. standard RT				
NP	RT (70 Gy) + cisplatin (100 mg m^{-2}) days 1, 22, 43	Mucositis: 37 vs. 28% Vomiting: 14 vs. 3% Skin toxicity: 2.5 vs. 4.5% Infection: 2.5 vs. 1.5%	Neutropenia: 6 vs. 0%	AL-SARRAF et al. (1998)
OP	RT (70 Gy) + Cb (70 mg m^{-2} days 1–4)/5-FU (600 mg m^{-2} days 1–4) for three cycles	Mucositis: 71 vs. 39% Skin toxicity: 40 vs. 42% Weight loss: 13 vs. 5% Feeding tube: 33 vs. 13% Toxic death: 1 vs. 0%	Neutropenia: 4 vs. 0% Thrombopenia: 5.5 vs. 1% Anemia: 3 vs. 0%	CALAIS et al. (1999)
OC, OP, HP, L	RT (66–72 Gy) + cisplatin (20 mg m^{-2} days 1–4)/5-FU (1,000 mg m^{-2} days 1–4) for two cycles	Mucositis: 84 vs. 26% Skin toxicity: 44 vs. 10% Weight loss: 70 vs. 28% Feeding tube: 58 vs. 32% Nausea/vomiting: 6 vs. 0%	Neutropenia: 38 vs. 0% Neutropenic fever needing hospitalization: 36 vs. 0% Thrombopenia: 16 vs. 0%	ADELSTEIN et al. (2000)
L	RT (70 Gy) + cisplatin (100 mg m^{-2}) days 1, 22, 43	Mucositis: 43 vs. 24% Dysphagia: 35 vs. 19% Skin toxicity: 7 vs. 9% Nausea/vomiting: 20 vs. 0%	Hematologic: 47 vs. 3%	FORASTIERE et al. (2003)

(Continued)

Table 18.2. (Continued)

Primary tumor site	CRT regimen	Non-hematologic toxicity grade 3–4	Hematologic toxicity grade 3–4	References
		Renal: 4 vs. 0%		
		Neurologic: 5 vs. 0%		
		Infection: 4 vs. 1%		
Primary CRT vs. altered fractionation RT				
OC, OP, HP, L	RT 3 courses, 13 fxns each, 1.8 Gy b.i.d., total dose 70.2 Gy Cisplatin 60 mg m^{-2}, and 5-FU 350 mg m^{-2} i.v. bolus day 2 and LV 50 mg m^{-2} bolus D2; 5-FU 350 mg m^{-2} day^{-1} CI days 2–5 + LV 100 mg m^{-2} day^{-1} CI days 2–5. Repeat days 22 and 44	Mucositis: 38 vs. 17% Skin toxicity: 17 vs. 7%	Leukopenia: 15 vs. 0% Thrombopenia: 1.5 vs. 0% Anemia: 1.5 vs. 0%	WENDT et al. (1998)
OC, OP, HP, L	RT (1.25 cGy b.i.d. to 70 Gy) + cisplatin (12 mg m^{-2}d^{-1} days 1–5) + 5-FU (600 mg m^{-2} day^{-1} days 1–5) weeks 1 and 6. RT dose 75 Gy in control arm.	Mucositis: 77 vs. 75% Feeding tube: 44 vs. 29% Sepsis: 14 vs. 4% Toxic death: 2 vs. 0%	NR	BRIZEL et al. (1998)
OC, OP, HP, L	Hfx RT (77 Gy) + cisplatin (6 mg m^{-2}) daily	Mucositis: 49 vs. 42% Dysphagia: 25 vs. 18% Nausea/vomiting: 6 vs. 0% Renal: 5 vs. 0%	Leukopenia: 12 vs. 0% Thrombopenia: 8 vs. 0%	JEREMIC et al. (2000)
OP	RT (66–70 Gy) + Cb (75 mg m^{-2} day^{-1} days 1–4) + 5-FU (1,000 mg m^{-2} day^{-1} CI for 96 h) every 28 days for 3 cycles	Mucositis: 48 vs. 15% Dysphagia: 24 vs. 11% Skin toxicity: 16 vs. 4% Renal: 1 vs. 0%	Leukopenia: 23 vs. 0% Thrombopenia: 4.5 vs. 0% Anemia: 2 vs. 0%	OLMI et al. (2003)
OC, OP, HP, L	Hfx RT (1.2 Gy b.i.d. to 74.4 Gy) + cisplatin (20 mg m^{-2} day^{-1} days 1–5) on weeks 1 and 5	Mucositis: 60 vs. 62% Dysphagia: 55 vs. 46% Nausea/vomiting: 7.5 vs. 0% Renal: 2 vs. 0% Ototoxicity: 2 vs. 0% Infection: 8.5%	Hematologic: 3 vs. 0%	HUGUENIN et al. (2004)
OC, OP, HP	Hfx Acc RT (70.6 Gy) + 5-FU (600 mg m^{-2} day^{-1} for 120 hrs) + MMC (10 mg m^{-2} bolus) days 5 and 36. RT dose 77.6 Gy in control arm	Mucositis: 66 vs. 76% Dysphagia: 72 vs. 72% Dysgeusia: 10 vs. 14% Skin toxicity: 32 vs. 46%	Leukopenia: 8.5 vs. 0% Thrombopenia: 2 vs. 0% Anemia: 3 vs. 0%	BUDACH et al. (2005)
OP, HP	RT (80.4 Gy – 1.2 Gy twice daily – OP and 75.6 Gy – 1.2 Gy twice daily – HP) + cisplatin (100 mg m^{-2} days 1, 22, 43) + 5-FU (750 mg m^{-2} day^{-1} days 1–5 cycle 1; 430 mg m^{-2} day^{-1} cycles 2 and 3)	Mucositis: 83 vs. 70% Skin toxicity: 38 vs. 27% Nausea/vomiting: 6 vs. 0%	Neutropenia: 33 vs. 2%	BENSADOUN et al. (2006)

OC oral cavity; *OP* oropharynx; *HP* hypopharynx; *L* larynx; *NP* nasopharynx; *CDDP* cisplatin; *Cb* carboplatin; *5-FU* fluorouracil; *LV* leucovorin; *MMC* mitomycin-C; *RT* radiation; *Hfx* hyperfractionated; *Acc* accelerated; *fxn* fraction; *NR* not reported

Table 18.3. Grade 3–5 toxicities with radiation plus high-dose cisplatin (combined data from 5 randomized trials (ADELSTEIN et al. 2003; AL-SARRAF et al. 1998; BERNIER et al. 2004; COOPER et al. 2004; FORASTIERE et al. 2003))

Toxicity	Radiotherapy + Cisplatin 100 mg m^{-2} every 3 weeks × 3 (%)	Radiotherapy alone (%)
Leukopenia	16–42	1
Nausea/vomiting	12–20	0–7%
Renal	2–8	0–1
Infection	1–6	0–3
Dermatitis/skin	3–7	4–10
Stomatitis/mucositis	37–45	21–32
Death	0–5	0–3

of novel, molecularly targeted agents, such as cetuximab, to radiotherapy has the potential to enhance efficacy without increasing in-field toxicities or worsen QOL parameters (BONNER et al. 2006; CURRAN et al. 2007). Although the future role of cetuximab has not been fully explored and may involve its addition to platinum-based chemotherapy, radiotherapy and cetuximab represents a viable alternative for patients who cannot receive or tolerate concomitant CRT.

Appropriate patient selection for CRT and aggressive supportive care during treatment is critical. Comorbidities play an important role in the choice of the therapeutic regimen. The outcome of elderly patients with head and neck cancer is particularly affected by comorbidities (SANABRIA et al. 2007). Furthermore, the benefit of concomitant CRT has been found to decrease with increasing age (BOURHIS et al. 2006). The increasing risk of death with increasing age may result from a combination of death from therapy-related complications and intercurrent illnesses.

18.5.2
Late and Chronic Toxicities

In addition to causing acute toxicities, multimodality treatment can be potentially associated with nonresolving, chronic toxicities or late occurring side effects with an onset of several months after completion of radiation. Late toxicities are predominantly attributed to the effect of radiation, and include osteoradionecrosis (ZBAREN et al. 2006), dental caries (KIELBASSA et al. 2006), subcutaneous fibrosis, trismus (LOUISE KENT et al. 2008), thyroid dysfunction (JERECZEK-FOSSA et al. 2004), pharyngeal or esophageal stenosis (LEE et al. 2006), myelitis, and sensorineural hearing loss (JERECZEK-FOSSA et al. 2003). Up to 100% of patients may develop at least one late toxicity of any grade, as shown in a study of 44 five-year survivors (DENIS et al. 2003).

A few randomized clinical trials that compared CRT with radiotherapy alone have provided reports of late toxicities with sufficient detail. There are certainly many challenges in collecting data years after treatment completion and completeness of reporting as well as grading definitions are variable. From the available data, it is uncertain whether the addition of chemotherapy increases the frequency of late toxicities (DENIS et al. 2004; JEREMIC et al. 2000; BUDACH et al. 2005) (Table 18.4). An exception is that sensorineural hearing loss is more frequent in patients with nasopharyngeal cancer treated with radiotherapy plus cisplatin than with radiotherapy alone (LOW et al. 2006). Other chemotherapy-related toxicities, such as neuropathy and renal failure, may also be chronic.

Xerostomia is the most frequent late toxicity in patients who undergo radiation or CRT, as it is observed in almost all long-term survivors (DENIS et al. 2003; NORDGREN et al. 2008). Several strategies are used or are under evaluation for preventing treatment-related xerostomia, among them surgical salivary gland transfer (JHA et al. 2003), concomitant cytoprotectants (e.g., amifostine) (JELLEMA et al. 2006), and salivary-gland-sparing novel radiation techniques, such as intensity-modulated radiation therapy (PACHOLKE et al. 2005). Oral care includes good oral hygiene with fluoride agents and antimicrobials to prevent dental caries and oral infections (e.g., chlorexidine, hexitidine), saliva substitutes to relieve symptoms, and sialogenic agents to stimulate saliva production from remaining intact gland tissue (e.g., pilocarpine) (GRAFF et al. 2007). However, it should be noted that all of these preventive and treatment options are ineffective in the vast majority of patients.

As one examines QOL aspects, it is important to correlate QOL and clinical outcomes in order to provide meaningful data to clinicians (MURPHY et al. 2007). Baseline QOL has been shown to be an independent prognostic factor of treatment efficacy in patients

Table 18.4. Severe (grade 3–4) late toxicities reported in selected phase III randomized studies with concomitant CRT in SCCHN

References	No. of patients	Follow-up	Xerostomia (%)		Bone/ osteoradion-ecrosis (%)		Skin fibrosis (%)		Subcutane-ous fibrosis (%)		Mucosa (%)		Taste alteration (%)	
			CRT	RT	CRT	RT	CRT	RT	CRT	RT	CRT	RT	CRT	RT
DENIS et al. (2004)*	44	All 5-year survivors	15	18	6	0	7	6	NR	NR	15	18	19	6
JEREMIC et al. (2000)	130	Median 6.6 years	22	15	6	5	11	8	12	6	NR	NR	NR	NR
BUDACH et al. (2005)	373	Results at 5 years	28.5	26	6	5	18	14	NR	NR	6	8	42	4

The study by BUDACH et al. used hyperfractionated accelerated radiotherapy in both arms. *CRT* chemoradiotherapy; *RT* radio-therapy; *NR* not reported
*$p > 0.05$ for all comparisons

with locally advanced SCCHN (SIDDIQUI et al. 2008). Moreover, the severity of comorbidities in patients with SCCHN predicts survival (PICCIRILLO et al. 2002). Many patients with locally advanced SCCHN may not be good candidates for potentially curative concomitant CRT because of older age, multiple comorbidities, and/or compromised performance status. However, in appropriately selected patients, an aggressive treatment approach is usually justifiable. Patients rank cure as the most important treatment objective that overshadows the priority of potential toxicities (LIST et al. 2000). Nevertheless, it is possible that when cure is achieved QOL assumes a greater importance. In general, QOL declines during treatment but returns toward baseline in ~1 year after completion of treatment (MURPHY et al. 2007; LIST et al. 1999).

Most swallowing disorders after organ preservation treatment are associated with movement impairment of the structures related to swallowing, such as decreased movement of the base of tongue, pharyngeal dysmotility, and reduced laryngeal elevation, which may result in episodes of aspiration (RIEGER et al. 2006). Several studies have reported that swallowing dysfunction improves gradually in the first year postteatment (LAZARUS et al. 2007), and despite the majority of patients requiring enteral feeding tube support during treatment, about 80–90% of patients may become tube-free at the end of the first year (RIEGER et al. 2006; AKST et al. 2004). However, recovery may never be complete. Swallowing difficulties that are first noted as acute complications during treatment may become chronic and irreversible. Approximately 8–18% of long-term survivors are

enteral feeding tube dependent (RIEGER et al. 2006; AGARWALA et al. 2007). Higher doses of radiation therapy have been associated with higher rates of long-term enteral feeding (RIEGER et al. 2006; CHOONG and VOKES 2008). Moreover, the onset of late toxicities, such as osteoradionecrosis, myelitis, pharyngeal or esophageal stenosis, soft tissue fibrosis, and others, can affect QOL permanently.

Permanent defects in functions, such as speech, chewing, swallowing, and appearance deformities may lead to unanticipated social and psychological problems that impact QOL (MURPHY et al. 2007). As a further indicator of the deep impact of the chronic losses, SCCHN patients have higher suicide rate compared with the general population and the overall population of cancer patients (ZELLER 2006; KENDAL 2007). As such, SCCHN patients should be cautiously monitored and should be encouraged to participate in long-term supportive care programs while providers should continue to search for ways to reduce long-term impairments.

18.6
Conclusions

Current multimodality treatment approaches, and predominantly the use of concomitant CRT, have led to improved organ preservation rates and survival but at the same time have increased the frequency of acute treatment-related complications. After years of stagnation, the field of SCCHN therapeutics is being enriched with the addition of new molecularly targeted agents that can be incorporated into multimodality treatment strategies. However, advances in therapeutics and treatment intensification should be balanced against functional consequences and acute and late toxicities that affect QOL. Assessment of QOL parameters should be an essential component of prospective clinical trials in SCCHN. Moreover, future investigations need to explore novel ways to ameliorate treatment-induced toxicity. Additionally, the understanding of the molecular changes governing SCCHN development may allow for the identification of valid biomarkers that will guide for the individualization of treatment approaches in patients with SCCHN.

References

Adelstein DJ, Lavertu P, Saxton JP et al. (2000) Mature results of a phase III randomized trial comparing concurrent chemoradiotherapy with radiation therapy alone in patients with stage III and IV squamous cell carcinoma of the head and neck. Cancer 88:876–883

Adelstein DJ, Li Y, Adams GL et al. (2003) An intergroup phase III comparison of standard radiation therapy and two schedules of concurrent chemoradiotherapy in patients with unresectable squamous cell head and neck cancer. J Clin Oncol 21:92–98

Agarwala SS, Cano E, Heron DE et al. (2007) Long-term outcomes with concurrent carboplatin, paclitaxel and radiation therapy for locally advanced, inoperable head and neck cancer. Ann Oncol 18:1224–1229

Akst LM, Chan J, Elson P et al. (2004) Functional outcomes following chemoradiotherapy for head and neck cancer. Otolaryngol Head Neck Surg 131:950–957

Al-Sarraf M, LeBlanc M, Giri PG et al. (1998) Chemoradiotherapy versus radiotherapy in patients with advanced nasopharyngeal cancer: phase III randomized intergroup study 0099. J Clin Oncol 16:1310–1317

Argiris A, Karamouzis MV, Raben D et al. (2008) Head and neck cancer. Lancet 371:1695–1709

Bensadoun RJ, Benezery K, Dassonville O et al. (2006) French multicenter phase III randomized study testing concurrent twice-a-day radiotherapy and cisplatin/5-fluorouracil chemotherapy (BiRCF) in unresectable pharyngeal carcinoma: results at 2 years (FNCLCC-GORTEC). Int J Radiat Oncol Biol Phys 64:983–994

Bentzen SM, Trotti A (2007) Evaluation of early and late toxicities in chemoradiation trials. J Clin Oncol 25:4096–4103

Bernier J, Domenge C, Ozsahin M et al. (2004) Postoperative irradiation with or without concomitant chemotherapy for locally advanced head and neck cancer. N Engl J Med 350:1945–1952

Bleier BS, Levine MS, Mick R et al. (2007) Dysphagia after chemoradiation: analysis by modified barium swallow. Ann Otol Rhinol Laryngol 116:837–841

Bonner JA, Harari PM, Giralt J et al. (2006) Radiotherapy plus cetuximab for squamous-cell carcinoma of the head and neck. N Engl J Med 354:567–578

Boscolo-Rizzo P, Maronato F, Marchiori C et al. (2008) Long-term quality of life after total laryngectomy and postoperative radiotherapy versus concurrent chemoradiotherapy for laryngeal preservation. Laryngoscope 118:300–306

Bourhis J, Amand C, Pignon JP (2004) Update of MACH-NC (meta-analysis of chemotherapy in head & neck cancer) database focused on concomitant chemoradiotherapy. J Clin Oncol 22(14S):5505

Bourhis J, Le Maitre A, Pignon J (2006) Impact of age on treatment efficacy in locally advanced head and neck cancer (HNC): two individual patient data meta-analyses. J Clin Oncol 24:5501

Brizel DM, Albers ME, Fisher SR et al. (1998) Hyperfractionated irradiation with or without concurrent chemotherapy for locally advanced head and neck cancer. N Engl J Med 338:1798–1804

Brizel DM, Murphy BA, Rosenthal DI et al. (2008) Phase II study of palifermin and concurrent chemoradiation in head and neck squamous cell carcinoma. J Clin Oncol 26:2489–2496

Budach V, Stuschke M, Budach W et al. (2005) Hyperfractionated accelerated chemoradiation with concurrent fluorouracil-mitomycin is more effective than dose-escalated hyperfractionated accelerated radiation therapy alone in locally advanced head and neck cancer: final results of the radiotherapy cooperative clinical trials group of the German Cancer Society 95–06 Prospective Randomized Trial. J Clin Oncol 23:1125–1135

Cady J (2007) Nutritional support during radiotherapy for head and neck cancer: the role of prophylactic feeding tube placement. Clin J Oncol Nurs 11:875–880

Calais G, Alfonsi M, Bardet E et al. (1999) Randomized trial of radiation therapy versus concomitant chemotherapy and radiation therapy for advanced-stage oropharynx carcinoma. J Natl Cancer Inst 91:2081–2086

Calais G, Pointreau Y, Alfonsi M et al. (2006) Randomized phase III trial comparing induction chemotherapy using cisplatin (P) fluorouracil (F) with or without docetaxel (T) for organ preservation in hypopharynx and larynx cancer. Preliminary results of GORTEC 2000–01. J Clin Oncol 24(18S):5506

Choong N, Vokes E (2008) Expanding role of the medical oncologist in the management of head and neck cancer. CA Cancer J Clin 58:32–53

Cooper JS, Pajak TF, Forastiere AA et al. (2004) Postoperative concurrent radiotherapy and chemotherapy for high-risk squamous-cell carcinoma of the head and neck. N Engl J Med 350:1937–1944

Curran D, Giralt J, Harari PM et al. (2007) Quality of life in head and neck cancer patients after treatment with high-dose radiotherapy alone or in combination with cetuximab. J Clin Oncol 25:2191–2197

Denis F, Garaud P, Bardet E et al. (2003) Late toxicity results of the GORTEC 94-01 randomized trial comparing radiotherapy with concomitant radiochemotherapy for advanced-stage oropharynx carcinoma: comparison of LENT/SOMA, RTOG/EORTC, and NCI-CTC scoring systems. Int J Radiat Oncol Biol Phys 55:93–98

Denis F, Garaud P, Bardet E et al. (2004) Final results of the 94–01 French Head and Neck Oncology and Radiotherapy

Group randomized trial comparing radiotherapy alone with concomitant radiochemotherapy in advanced-stage oropharynx carcinoma. J Clin Oncol 22:69–76

Eisbruch A, Lyden T, Bradford CR et al. (2002) Objective assessment of swallowing dysfunction and aspiration after radiation concurrent with chemotherapy for head-and-neck cancer. Int J Radiat Oncol Biol Phys 53:23–28

Fietkau R, Lautenschläger C, Sauer R et al. (2006) Postoperative concurrent radiochemotherapy versus radiotherapy in high-risk SCCA of the head and neck: results of the German phase III trial ARO 96–3. J Clin Oncol 24(Suppl 18):5507

Forastiere AA, Goepfert H, Maor M et al. (2003) Concurrent chemotherapy and radiotherapy for organ preservation in advanced laryngeal cancer. N Engl J Med 349:2091–2098

Forastiere AA, Maor M, Weber RS et al. (2006) Long-term results of Intergroup RTOG 91-11: a phase III trial to preserve the larynx – induction cisplatin/5-FU and radiation therapy versus concurrent cisplatin and radiation therapy versus radiation therapy. ASCO Annual Meeting Proceedings Part I, Jun 20 Suppl, Abstract no. 5517 [J Clin Oncol 24(18S)]

Frowen JJ, Perry AR (2006) Swallowing outcomes after radiotherapy for head and neck cancer: a systematic review. Head Neck 28:932–944

Garcia-Peris P, Paron L, Velasco C et al. (2007) Long-term prevalence of oropharyngeal dysphagia in head and neck cancer patients: impact on quality of life. Clin Nutr 26:710–717

Graff P, Lapeyre M, Desandes E et al. (2007) Impact of intensity-modulated radiotherapy on health-related quality of life for head and neck cancer patients: matched-pair comparison with conventional radiotherapy. Int J Radiat Oncol Biol Phys 67:1309–1317

Hitt R, Lopez-Pousa A, Martinez-Trufero J et al. (2005) Phase III study comparing cisplatin plus fluorouracil to paclitaxel, cisplatin, and fluorouracil induction chemotherapy followed by chemoradiotherapy in locally advanced head and neck cancer. J Clin Oncol 23:8636–8645

Huguenin P, Beer KT, Allal A et al. (2004) Concomitant cisplatin significantly improves locoregional control in advanced head and neck cancers treated with hyperfractionated radiotherapy. J Clin Oncol 22:4665–4673

Jellema AP, Slotman BJ, Muller MJ et al. (2006) Radiotherapy alone, versus radiotherapy with amifostine 3 times weekly, versus radiotherapy with amifostine 5 times weekly: a prospective randomized study in squamous cell head and neck cancer. Cancer 107:544–553

Jereczek-Fossa BA, Alterio D, Jassem J et al. (2004) Radiotherapy-induced thyroid disorders. Cancer Treat Rev 30:369–384

Jereczek-Fossa BA, Zarowski A, Milani F et al. (2003) Radiotherapy-induced ear toxicity. Cancer Treat Rev 29:417–430

Jeremic B, Shibamoto Y, Milicic B et al. (2000) Hyperfractionated radiation therapy with or without concurrent low-dose daily cisplatin in locally advanced squamous cell carcinoma of the head and neck: a prospective randomized trial. J Clin Oncol 18:1458–1464

Jha N, Seikaly H, Harris J et al. (2003) Prevention of radiation induced xerostomia by surgical transfer of submandibular salivary gland into the submental space. Radiother Oncol 66:283–289

Karamouzis MV, Grandis JR, Argiris A (2007) Therapies directed against epidermal growth factor receptor in aerodigestive carcinomas. JAMA 298:70–82

Kendal W (2007) Suicide and cancer: a gender-comparative study. Ann Oncol 18:381–387

Kielbassa AM, Hinkelbein W, Hellwig E et al. (2006) Radiation-related damage to dentition. Lancet Oncol 7:326–335

Lazarus C, Logemann JA, Pauloski BR et al. (2007) Effects of radiotherapy with or without chemotherapy on tongue strength and swallowing in patients with oral cancer. Head Neck 29:632–637

Lee WT, Akst LM, Adelstein DJ et al. (2006) Risk factors for hypopharyngeal/upper esophageal stricture formation after concurrent chemoradiation. Head Neck 28:808–812

Lefebvre JL (2006) Laryngeal preservation in head and neck cancer: multidisciplinary approach. Lancet Oncol 7:747–755

Lefebvre JL, Chevalier D, Luboinski B et al.; for EORTC Head and Neck Cancer Cooperative Group (1996) Larynx preservation in pyriform sinus cancer: preliminary results of a European Organization for Research and Treatment of Cancer phase III trial. J Natl Cancer Inst 88:890–899

List MA, Siston A, Haraf D et al. (1999) Quality of life and performance in advanced head and neck cancer patients on concomitant chemoradiotherapy: a prospective examination. J Clin Oncol 17:1020–1028

List MA, Stracks J, Colangelo L et al. (2000) How do head and neck cancer patients prioritize treatment outcomes before initiating treatment? J Clin Oncol 18:877–884

Logemann JA, Pauloski BR, Rademaker AW et al. (2008) Swallowing disorders in the first year after radiation and chemoradiation. Head Neck 30:148–158

Louise Kent M, Brennan MT, Noll JL et al. (2008) Radiation-induced trismus in head and neck cancer patients. Support Care Cancer 16:305–309

Low WK, Toh ST, Wee J et al. (2006) Sensorineural hearing loss after radiotherapy and chemoradiotherapy: a single, blinded, randomized study. J Clin Oncol 24:1904–1909

Murphy BA, Ridner S, Wells N et al. (2007) Quality of life research in head and neck cancer: a review of the current state of the science. Crit Rev Oncol Hematol 62:251–267

Nordgren M, Hammerlid E, Bjordal K et al. (2008) Quality of life in oral carcinoma: a 5-year prospective study. Head Neck 30:461–470

Olmi P, Crispino S, Fallai C et al. (2003) Locoregionally advanced carcinoma of the oropharynx: conventional radiotherapy vs. accelerated hyperfractionated radiotherapy vs. concomitant radiotherapy and chemotherapy – a multicenter randomized trial. Int J Radiat Oncol Biol Phys 55:78–92

Pacholke HD, Amdur RJ, Morris CG et al. (2005) Late xerostomia after intensity-modulated radiation therapy versus conventional radiotherapy. Am J Clin Oncol 28:351–358

Pfister DG, Laurie SA, Weinstein GS et al. (2006) American Society of Clinical Oncology clinical practice guideline for the use of larynx-preservation strategies in the treatment of laryngeal cancer. J Clin Oncol 24:3693–3704

Piccirillo JF, Lacy PD, Basu A et al. (2002) Development of a new head and neck cancer-specific comorbidity index. Arch Otolaryngol Head Neck Surg 128:1172–1179

Pignon JP, Bourhis J, Domenge C et al.; for MACH-NC Collaborative Group (2000) Chemotherapy added to locoregional treatment for head and neck squamous-cell carcinoma: three meta-analyses of updated individual data. Lancet 355:949–955

Posner MR, Hershock DM, Blajman CR et al. (2007) Cisplatin and fluorouracil alone or with docetaxel in head and neck cancer. N Engl J Med 357:1705–1715

Rieger JM, Zalmanowitz JG, Wolfaardt JF (2006) Functional outcomes after organ preservation treatment in head and neck cancer: a critical review of the literature. Int J Oral Maxillofac Surg 35:581–587

Rosenthal DI, Lewin JS, Eisbruch A (2006) Prevention and treatment of dysphagia and aspiration after chemoradiation for head and neck cancer. J Clin Oncol 24:2636–2643

Ruo Redda MG, Allis S (2006) Radiotherapy-induced taste impairment. Cancer Treat Rev 32:541–547

Ryu JK, Swann S, Leveque F et al. (2007) The impact of concurrent granulocyte macrophage-colony stimulating factor on radiation-induced mucositis in head and neck cancer patients: a double-blind placebo-controlled prospective phase III study by Radiation Therapy Oncology Group 9901. Int J Radiat Oncol Biol Phys 67:643–650

Sanabria A, Carvalho AL, Vartanian JG et al. (2007) Comorbidity is a prognostic factor in elderly patients with head and neck cancer. Ann Surg Oncol 14:1449–1457

Siddiqui F, Pajak TF, Watkins-Bruner D et al. (2008) Pretreatment quality of life predicts for locoregional control in head and neck cancer patients: a radiation therapy oncology group analysis. Int J Radiat Oncol Biol Phys 70:353–360

Staar S, Rudat V, Stuetzer H et al. (2001) Intensified hyperfractionated accelerated radiotherapy limits the additional benefit of simultaneous chemotherapy – results of a multicentric randomized German trial in advanced head-and-neck cancer. Int J Radiat Oncol Biol Phys 50:1161–1171

The Department of Veterans Affairs Laryngeal Cancer Study Group. (1991) Induction chemotherapy plus radiation compared with surgery plus radiation in patients with advanced laryngeal cancer. N Engl J Med 324:1685–1690

Trotti A, Bellm LA, Epstein JB et al. (2003) Mucositis incidence, severity and associated outcomes in patients with head and neck cancer receiving radiotherapy with or without chemotherapy: a systematic literature review. Radiother Oncol 66:253–262

Trotti A, Pajak TF, Gwede CK et al. (2007) TAME: development of a new method for summarising adverse events of cancer treatment by the Radiation Therapy Oncology Group. Lancet Oncol 8:613–624

Vermorken JB, Remenar E, van Herpen C et al. (2007) Cisplatin, fluorouracil, and docetaxel in unresectable head and neck cancer. N Engl J Med 357:1695–1704

Wendt TG, Grabenbauer GG, Rodel CM et al. (1998) Simultaneous radiochemotherapy versus radiotherapy alone in advanced head and neck cancer: a randomized multicenter study. J Clin Oncol 16:1318–1324

Zbaren P, Caversaccio M, Thoeny HC et al. (2006) Radionecrosis or tumor recurrence after radiation of laryngeal and hypopharyngeal carcinomas. Otolaryngol Head Neck Surg 135:838–843

Zeller JL (2006) High suicide risk found for patients with head and neck cancer. JAMA 296:1716–1717

Contributions of Targeted Agents

19

DERIC L. WHEELER, TIEN HOANG, and PAUL M. HARARI

CONTENTS

19.1 Introduction *215*

19.2 **Molecular Targeting Agents in HNSCC** *216*
19.2.1 Epidermal Growth Factor Receptor–EGFR Biology *216*
19.2.2 EGFR Blockade *216*
19.2.3 Vascular Endothelial Growth Factor–VEGF/VEGFR Biology *218*
19.2.4 Bevacizumab *218*

19.3 **Promising Molecular Targets** *218*
19.3.1 HER Family Members *218*
19.3.2 Src Family Kinases *219*
19.3.3 Insulin-Like Growth Factor-I Receptor *219*
19.3.4 Aurora Kinase *219*
19.3.5 Mammalian Target of Rapamycin *219*

19.4 **Toxicity, Morbidity, and Quality of Life with Molecular Targeting Agents** *219*
19.4.1 Hypersensitivity Reactions *220*
19.4.2 Skin Toxicities *220*
19.4.3 Gastrointestinal Toxicities *220*
19.4.4 Hemorrhagic Toxicities *221*
19.4.5 Other Toxicities *221*

References *222*

DERIC L. WHEELER, PhD, ASSISTANT PROFESSOR
PAUL M. HARARI, MD, Jack Fowler Professor and Chairman
Department of Human Oncology, University of Wisconsin School of Medicine and Public Health, 600 Highland Ave, K4/336 CSC, Madison, WI 53792
TIEN HOANG, MD, Assistant Professor
Department of Medicine, University of Wisconsin School of Medicine and Public Health, 600 Highland Ave, K6/566 CSC, Madison, WI 53792, USA

KEY POINTS

- The cellular growth receptors epidermal growth factor receptor (EGFR) and vascular endothelial growth factor receptor (VEGFR) play a strong role in the biology of head and neck squamous cell carcinoma (HNSCC).
- A series of promising molecularly targeting agents that impact EGFR and VEGFR signaling are under active preclinical and clinical investigation in HNSCC.
- Toxicity profiles are generally less with molecular targeting agents than with conventional cytotoxic chemotherapy.
- It may prove possible to substitute selected molecular inhibitors for cytotoxic agents, thereby lessening toxicity and enhancing quality of life.
- Personalized cancer treatment strategies that derive from molecular biology and genetics of individual tumors are within our future reach.

19.1
Introduction

The dominant pattern of spread and recurrence for head and neck squamous cell carcinoma (HNSCC) is locoregional; therefore, surgery and radiation have historically played the central role in curative treatment. More recently, a beneficial role for cytotoxic chemotherapy in both the curative and palliative setting for patients with HNSCC has become better defined. However, even with this aggressive multidisciplinary approach, the overall survival rate for advanced HNSCC has only begun to show modest improvement. In addition, modern treatment regimens used for HNSCC are quite toxic, and often result in compromised functional status and impaired quality of life (QOL). Therefore, the development of novel therapeutic alternatives to standard therapy is highly desired. Recent advances in targeted molecular therapy have identified the epidermal growth factor receptor (EGFR) and the vascular endothelial growth factor (VEGF) and its receptor (VEGFR) as highly promising therapeutic targets. This chapter focuses on current molecular targeting agents used in HNSCC, promising molecular targets in HNSCC and the impact molecular targeting agents may have on patient QOL.

19.2
Molecular Targeting Agents in HNSCC

19.2.1
Epidermal Growth Factor Receptor – EGFR Biology

The EGFR is a member of the HER (human epidermal growth factor receptor) family of receptor tyrosine kinases and consists of four members: EGFR (ErbB1/HER1), HER2/neu (ErbB2), HER3 (ErbB3), and HER4 (ErbB4). Stimulation of the receptor through ligand binding leads to receptor oligomerization at the plasma membrane. This activates the receptor tyrosine kinase and thereby causes autophosphorylation of tyrosine residues in the cytoplasmic tail. These phosphorylated tyrosines serve as docking sites for various proteins that contain Src homology domains and phosphotyrosine binding domains. These events lead to the activation of several signaling cascades most notably the Ras/RAF/MEK/ERK, phosphotidylinositol-3-kinase (PI3K)-Akt, Stat, and phospholipase C gamma pathways (Fig. 19.1). The activation of these pathways ultimately promotes tumor cell proliferation, survival, invasion, and angiogenesis. Aberrant expression or activity of the EGFR is identified as a central regulator of proliferation and progression in many human cancers, including HNSCC, non-small cell lung cancer (NSCLC), metastatic colorectal cancer (mCRC), and brain cancer. Therefore, the EGFR is considered a promising molecular target for therapeutic modulation in oncology.

19.2.2
EGFR Blockade

Targeting the EGFR with molecular inhibitors has been intensely pursued in the last decade as a cancer treatment strategy. Two primary strategies have been developed to target the EGFR, including anti-EGFR monoclonal antibodies (mAbs) and small molecule tyrosine kinase inhibitors (TKI) (Table 19.1). Dating back to the early 1980s, Mendelsohn and colleagues purified a series of mAbs to the EGFR to test these agents as inhibitors of tumor growth. Born out of these efforts, cetuximab (IMC-C225, Erbitux) was developed to target the extracellular ligand binding domain of the EGFR and thereby block natural ligand binding. Cetuximab prevents receptor activation and dimerization and ultimately induces receptor internalization and downregulation. Cetuximab exhibits promising antitumor activity as monotherapy or in combination with chemotherapy and/or radiation.

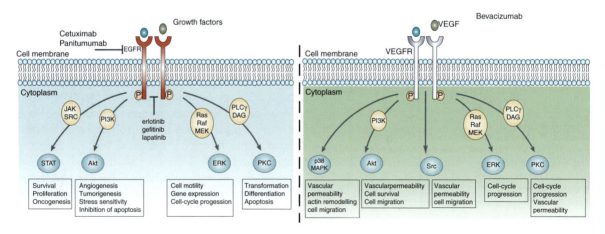

Fig. 19.1. EGFR and VEGFR signaling pathways

Table 19.1. EGFR targeting agents studied in HNSCC

Agent	Type	Phase of development in HNSCC
Cetuximab	Chimeric antibody	III
Erlotinib	TKI	III
Gefitinib	TKI	III
panitumumab	Humanized antibody	II
Lapatinib	EGFR, HER2TKI	I/II
h-R3/nimot uzumab	Humanized antibody	I/II
EKB-569	EGFR TKI	I

In a phase III clinical trial using cetuximab in locally advanced HNSCC, Bonner et al. (2006) compared the efficacy of radiotherapy alone to radiotherapy plus cetuximab. The results of this trial showed an improvement in overall survival and progression-free survival by 20 and 5 months, respectively, with the addition of cetuximab. Locoregional control was also improved by a median of 9.5 months with the addi-

tion of cetuximab to radiotherapy. The results of this phase III trial demonstrating significant improvement in locoregional control, overall survival, and progression-free survival by the addition of cetuximab to radiotherapy led to the Food and Drug Administration (FDA) approval of cetuximab for use in HNSCC in combination with radiation in 2006. Several other trials, at various phases, further investigating the role of cetuximab have also been reported (Table 19.2).

A second approach of EGFR inhibition involves the use of TKIs, which bind to the ATP-binding site in the tyrosine kinase domain of the EGFR. These agents inhibit EGFR autophosphorylation and ultimately lead to blockade of downstream signaling and cellular proliferation. Three anti-EGFR TKIs, erlotinib (OSI-774, Tarceva), gefitinib (ZD1839, Iressa), and Lapatinib (GW572016, Tykerb) are now approved by the FDA for use in oncology, with erlotinib and gefitinib being the most studied to date in HNSCC. These agents have been studied in phase I and II clinical trials in both the recurrent and metastatic HNSCC setting. Trials investigating gefitinib in this setting have shown an overall survival of 6–8 months, with response rates ranging from 3 to 10% (Cohen et al. 2003, 2005; Wheeler et al. 2005). Studies using erlotinib in a phase I/II trial with recurrent or metastatic

Table 19.2. EGFR monoclonal antibody clinical trials in HNSCC

Study/phase	Regimen	No. of patients	Outcome
Stage III/IV recurrent metastatic HNSCC (Trigo et al. 2004)	Cetuximab	103	PFS = 2.3 months, OS = 5.9 months
III locally advanced HNSCC (Bonner et al. 2006)	Cetuximab + RT	211	PFS = 17.1 months, OS = 49 months
	RT	213	PFS = 12.4 months, OS = 29.3 months
II cisplatin refractory HNSCC (Baselga et al. 2005)	Cetuximab	96	PFS = 2.2 months, OS = 5.2 months
II cisplatin refractory HNSCC (Herbst et al. 2005)	Cetuximab	76	RR = 10%, PFS = 2.8 months, OS = 6.1 months
III Metastatic/recurrent HNSCC (Burtness et al. 2005)	Cetuximab + chemo	57	PFS = 4.2 months, OS = 9.2 months
	Placebo + chemo	60	PFS = 2.7 months, OS = 8 months
II metastatic/recurrent HNSCC) (Vermorken et al. 2007)	Cetuximab	60	CP + PR + SD = 46%, TTP = 70 day
	Cetuximab + chemo	53	CR + PR + SD = 26%, TTP = 50 day

PFS progression-free survival; *OS* overall survival; *RR* overall response rate; *RT* radiotherapy; *Chemo* chemotherapy; *CR* complete response; *PR* partial response; *SD* stable disease; *TTP* time to progression

HNSCC showed overall survival of 6 months and a response rate of 4% (Soulieres et al. 2004). There are no published results of phase III studies to date with EGFR TKIs in HNSCC.

19.2.3
Vascular Endothelial Growth Factor – VEGF/VEGFR Biology

The VEGF comprises a family (VEGF-A, VEGF-B, VEGF-C, VEGF-D and the virally encoded VEGF-E) of endothelial specific mitogens, which regulate angiogenesis during nonpathological and pathological processes. These effects are mediated through a family of VEGF tyrosine kinase receptors, namely, VEGFR-1, VEGFR-2, and VEGFR-3. Activation of these receptors results in the activation of several downstream signaling cascades, including Src, phospholipase C gamma, p38 MAPK, PI3K/Akt, and Ras/RAF/MEK/ERK pathways (Fig. 19.1) (Olsson et al. 2006). The activation of these signaling pathways leads to multiple proangiogenic activities, including endothelial cell proliferation, expression of proteases, microvasculature leakage, and increased hexose transport believed to be necessary for higher energy demands. Altered expression of VEGF has been observed in multiple human diseases, including diabetic retinopathy, rheumatoid arthritis, psoriasis, and tumor angiogenesis. HNSCC tumors commonly overexpress VEGF, and angiogenesis has been shown to be critical for the development and growth of these tumors. VEGF overexpression also correlates with poor prognosis in HNSCC, and therefore targeted therapies against the VEGF signaling pathway have drawn interest.

19.2.4
Bevacizumab

Bevacizumab (Avastin™) is a humanized monoclonal antibody directed against VEGF. Bevacizumab has undergone investigation in many solid tumor types, including lung, gastrointestinal, ovarian, and breast and has gained FDA approval in mCRC, NSCLC, and breast cancer. Overexpression of VEGF has been tightly linked to patients with HNSCC (Lothaire et al. 2006), and strong efforts are being made to test the efficacy of bevacizumab as a clinical strategy in HNSCC. It has recently been established that tumors that are dependent on the EGFR have upregulated VEGF and this has been strongly correlated with resistance to EGFR targeting agents in HNSCC (Charoenrat et al. 2000). This finding led to a phase I/II study combining bevacizumab with the anti-EGFR TKI erlotinib in patients with recurrent metastatic HNSCC (Vokes et al. 2005). This study found that at the recommended dose of $15\,mg\,kg^{-1}$ of bevacizumab every 3 weeks and 150 mg of erlotinib daily 2 patients (4%) out of 48 had complete response and 5 (10%) had partial response. Median progression-free survival and overall survival were 4 and 7 months, respectively. Bevacizumab is currently being studied in a phase II trial in combination with cetuximab in recurrent/metastatic HNSCC. Other studies in the HNSCC setting using bevacizumab include (1) a phase II trial using pemetrexed and bevacizumab without platinum compounds in the recurrent metastatic setting (Karamouzis et al. 2007), (2) a phase II trial in stage IV locally advanced HNSCC combining radiation in combination with weekly concurrent docetaxel, along with biweekly bevacizumab (Savvides et al. 2007), and (3) a randomized phase II trial of concomitant chemoradiation with 5-fluorouracil and hydroxyurea with or without bevacizumab in intermediate stage HNSCC (Choong et al. 2007).

19.3
Promising Molecular Targets

19.3.1
HER Family Members

Looking beyond EGFR and VEGF, several other promising molecular targets are emerging for HNSCC. One of these targets, HER2, is a receptor tyrosine kinase (RTK) related to the EGFR. Inhibition of HER2 using lapatinib, a dual EGFR and HER-2 receptor TKI, demonstrated promising preclinical activity in HNSCC models (Rusnak et al. 2001). These findings led to a phase II trial with 42 patients with recurrent/metastatic HNSCC. This trial was broken into two arms, 27 without prior exposure to an EGFR inhibitor and 15 with prior exposure (Abidoye et al. 2006). Stable disease was seen in 37% of individuals without prior exposure and in 20% with prior exposure to EGFR inhibitors. The conclusions from this trial suggested that lapatinib as a sole agent has no significant antitumor activity on tumors that have or have not been previously treated with EGFR inhibitors.

Despite the lack of single agent activity in recurrent/metastatic HNSCC, lapatinib was further explored in combination with radiotherapy. Bourhis and colleagues performed a phase I trial of lapatinib in combination with standard fractionation radiation therapy and full dose concurrent cisplatin in 19 patients with locally advanced HNSCC (HARRINGTON et al. 2006). The authors reported that 14 patients (74%) achieved complete responses and 5 (26%) achieved partial responses.

One highly promising molecule that resides within the HER family is HER3. Themes have emerged in the last 2 years that escape from therapies targeting the EGFR involves equilibrium shifts in HER family signaling via HER3 (ENGELMAN et al. 2007; SERGINA et al. 2007; WHEELER et al. 2008). Several laboratories are designing antibodies that will block HER3 hetero-dimerization with EGFR or HER2 to prevent signals transduced to the PI(3)K/ Akt survival pathway.

19.3.2
Src Family Kinases

Src family kinases (SFKs) are nonreceptor cytoplasmic tyrosine kinases that play critical roles in regulating cellular invasion, adhesion, motility, migration, proliferation, and survival. SFKs regulate signals from cell surface molecules, including growth factor receptors (EGFR, PDGFR, FGFR) and G-protein-coupled receptors. Preclinical analysis demonstrated a strong rationale for targeting SFKs in HNSCC. SFK inhibition using dasatinib (BMS-354825) in HNSCC cell lines led to cell cycle arrest and apoptosis (JOHNSON et al. 2005). Inhibitors of SFKs such as dasatinib, AZD0530, and bosutinib (SKI-606) are currently undergoing phase I/II evaluations in advanced solid tumors, including HNSCC (TABERNERO et al. 2007).

19.3.3
Insulin-Like Growth Factor-I Receptor

Signaling through the insulin-like growth factor-I receptor (IGF-IR) leads to cellular proliferation, apoptosis, metastasis, and resistance to cytotoxic cancer therapies. Recent work combining the fully humanized anti-IGF-IR monoclonal antibody A12 (ImClone Systems, New York, NY) with radiation resulted in pronounced antitumor growth compared with either agent alone (ALLEN et al. 2007). In addition, TKIs directed against the IGF-IR are now in phase I trials. These results suggest IGF-IR signal

transduction blockade as a promising strategy to improve radiation therapy efficacy in human tumors, forming a basis for future clinical trials in HNSCC.

19.3.4
Aurora Kinase

Aurora kinases are serine/threonine kinases that are essential for cell proliferation by controlling spindle formation during mitosis. Studies investigating the relationship between aurora kinases and HNSCC found a strong correlation between the upregulation of aurora kinase A mRNA and distant metastases, poor disease-free and overall survival (REITER et al. 2006). Several aurora kinase A inhibitors (MP529, MLN8054) and aurora kinase B inhibitors (AZD1152) are under clinical development.

19.3.5
Mammalian Target of Rapamycin

The mammalian target of rapamycin (mTOR) is a serine/threonine protein kinase that regulates cell growth, cell proliferation, cell motility, cell survival, protein synthesis, and transcription. Further, it has recently been implicated in the pathogenesis of HNSCC and therefore serves as a promising molecular target (HAY and SONENBERG 2004). mTOR is activated by Akt and ultimately blocks apoptosis and increases proliferative potential of cancer cells. Several mTOR inhibitors are being investigated (Rapamycin, CI-779, RAD001 and AP23753).

19.4
Toxicity, Morbidity, and Quality of Life with Molecular Targeting Agents

Cytotoxic chemotherapy has become an integral modality in the treatment of HNSCC. In patients with locally advanced, unresectable disease, concurrent chemoradiation is considered the standard of care, albeit at the expense of increased toxicity. In an effort to improve local and distant tumor control further, investigators have advocated for even more agressive chemotherapy regimens as well as intensified, altered radiation schedules, which can result in more serious morbidities that may compromise patient QOL. Therefore, the development of the molecular targeting agents has created a new hope. By targeting specific molecules or biologic processes critical for the development and survival of HNSCC tumors, these molecular drugs are anticipated to improve the therapeutic window by maximizing the antitumor activity with diminished toxicities in normal tissues. As a proof of this concept, the pivotal trial of radiation in combination with or without cetuximab in HNSCC shows a clear survival advantage without an increase in the overall toxicity profile associated with radiation (BONNER et al. 2006).

However, despite the generally more tolerable toxicity profile in comparison to cytotoxic chemotherapy drugs, molecular-targeted agents can cause undesired, and sometimes fatal, adverse events. Those toxicities generally derive from effects of the drug on their molecular target in normal tissue compartments, such as cutaneous events associated with anti-EGFR agents, or vascular events related to anti-angiogenic drugs. There are also events related to the molecular structure of the compounds rather than to their specific biologic targets, such as hypersensitive reactions seen in patients treated with antibody drugs such as cetuximab.

19.4.1
Hypersensitivity Reactions

Cetuximab currently is the only targeted drug approved for use in HNSCC, either with radiation for locoregionally advanced disease or as monotherapy for recurrent or metastatic disease after platinum-based therapy failure. According to cetuximab prescribing information, serious grade 3 or 4 hypersensitivity reactions to this antibody, which could present as acute airway obstruction with bronchospasm and stridor, hypotension, and anaphylaxis, were observed in 2–5% of 1,373 patients, with fatal outcome in one patient. However, reports on the incidence from different geographic regions in the USA appear to vary significantly, with lower rates (<1%) seen in the Northeast, while higher rates were reported in North Carolina, Arkansas, Missouri, Virginia, and Tennessee (CHUNG et al. 2008; O'NEIL et al. 2007). In fact, serious cetuximab-related infusion reactions were reported as high as 22% in 88 patients treated in trials at two academic institutions in North Carolina and Tennessee (O'NEIL et al. 2007). Recently, a research group has identified the mechanism of hypersensitivity reaction to cetuximab as due to the presence of preexisting IgE antibodies against galactose-α-1,3-galactose, an oligosaccharide present on the Fab portion of the recombinant antibody molecule (CHUNG et al. 2008). In clinical practice, it is recommended to premedicate patients with an H1 antagonist such as diphenhydramine (50 mg, i.v.) 30–60 min before cetuximab infusion. In addition, patients need to be monitored for at least 1 h after infusion. Nevertheless, most of the severe reactions still manifest with the first treatment despite premedication.

19.4.2
Skin Toxicities

Cutaneous toxicites such as papulopustular rash, dry skin, fissuring, hair and nail alterations, and periungual inflammation are among the most common side effects seen with mAbs and TKIs targeting EGFR pathway, affecting 45–100% of patients (LACOUTURE 2006). The drugs are thought to block the EGFR signaling in keratinocytes in the basal layer of the epidermis and outer layers of the hair follicle, leading to apoptosis of the keratinocytes, inflammatory reactions, and pathological skin manifestations. Rash usually develops within the first 2 weeks of therapy, primarily in the face, neck, and upper body, which could be a concern in patients undergoing radiation for their head and neck cancer. Fortunately, cetuximab-related skin toxicities are not severe in majority of the patients, and it appears that cetuximab does not increase the incidence and severity of radiation-induced reactions (BONNER et al. 2006). Nevertheless, these adverse events could lead to sequelae such as discomfort, pain, infection, and psychosocial effects. Therefore, patient counseling on avoidance of direct sun exposure and wearing sunscreen, as well as early management with topical corticosteroids or antibiotic application, even oral antibiotics are recommended.

19.4.3
Gastrointestinal Toxicities

Diarrhea is another common side effect seen with anti-EGFR therapy, in particular EGFR-TKIs. The underlying mechanism of diarrhea is unclear. In large phase III clinical studies with gefitinib or erlotinib, diarrhea was reported in 27–55% of the patients, although only 3–6% experienced severe, grade ≥ 3 symptoms (SHEPHERD et al. 2005; THATCHER et al.

2005). The diarrhea incidence appears much lower in patients treated with the anti-EGFR monoclonal antibody cetuximab (19%) (Bonner et al. 2006). In addition, this adverse event was also observed quite commonly with small molecule TKIs such as lapatinib (EGFR/ErbB2 inhibitor), CI-1033 (pan-ErbB inhibitor), and vandetanib (VEGFR/EGFR inhibitor) (Burris et al. 2005; Janne et al. 2007; Miller et al. 2005), as well as in other multitarget TKIs with or without antiangiogenic activity such as sorafenib, sunitinib, and imatinib (Demetri et al. 2002; Escudier et al. 2007; Motzer et al. 2007). That suggests a complex mechanism underlying diarrhea associated with TKIs. If left untreated, this adverse event greatly affects patient QOL and can result in dehydration. Fortunately, it is easily managed with best supportive measures in majority of patients, although dose reduction is needed in some cases.

19.4.4
Hemorrhagic Toxicities

A major concern with anti-angiogenic/vascular targeting therapy is the potential risk of bleeding. Experimental data of antiangiogenic agents in HNSCC are still limited. However, extensive experience in other diseases has demonstrated that hemorrhage, an uncommon event, can occur and can be fatal. In the randomized phase II trial of bevacizumab in combination with chemotherapy in untreated NSCLC patients, which demonstrated the promising therapeutic value of bevacizumab, life-threatening bleeding described as hemoptysis and hematemesis were observed in 6 of 67 patients, resulting in four deaths (Johnson et al. 2004). These major bleeding events were associated with squamous cell histology, tumor necrosis and cavitation, and tumor location close to major blood vessels. A milder and more common hemorrhagic event was grade 1/2 epistaxis, which was seen in up to 44% of patients. In the subsequent large phase III NSCLC study which excluded patients with squamous cell subtype and significant hemoptysis history, grade ≥ 3 bleeding events overall occurred more often in the bevacizumab-containing arm compared with the control arm (4.4 vs. 0.7%, $p < 0.001$) (Sandler et al. 2006). In this selected patient population, fatal hemoptysis was reduced to 1.2% in patients receiving bevacizumab. Beside hemoptysis, other hemorrhagic events (grade 3 or higher) such as brain hemorrhage, hematemesis, and melena were uncommon (<1% for each event). On the basis of this study, the approved indication for the use of bevacizumab in NSCLC is to include only patients with nonsquamous NSCLC. Of note, in the randomized phase III studies leading to the approval of bevacizumab in colon cancer and breast cancer, the incidence of severe bleeding was not higher with the treatment of this monoclonal antibody, and no fatal bleeding was reported (Hurwitz et al. 2004; Miller et al. 2007). The bleeding risk has also been observed closely in clinical trials involving small molecule TKIs with anti-VEGFR activity. Indeed, fatal pulmonary hemorrhage was reported in patients with squamous cell lung carcinoma in two separate phase II studies using single agent sunitinib and sorafenib (Gatzemeier et al. 2006; Socinski et al. 2006). Result from large phase III studies involving antiangiogenic TKIs are awaited.

19.4.5
Other Toxicities

Several other uncommon, but detrimental adverse events related to molecularly targeted agents have been reported. Those toxicities seem to be associated with certain groups of drugs. In trials with bevacizumab, gastrointestinal perforation and fistula, and intra-abdominal abscess occurred in 2.4% of colon cancer patients. Risk of nongastrointestinal fistula (tracheoesophageal, biliary, vagina, and bladder) in <0.3% is also included in the bevacizumab label warnings. In addition, cardiovascular events such as hypertension, myocardial ischemia, and arrhythmias were also observed in studies involving antiangiogenic or vascular targeting drugs.

In summary, molecularly targeted agents are generally well tolerated in comparison with cytotoxic chemotherapy. Common side effects associated with molecular agents are usually manageable with available supportive treatment. However, clinicians and patients should be aware of certain toxicities, which, albeit uncommon, can influence morbidity, quality of life and mortality. A desired goal with targeted therapies is to select those patients most likely to respond favorably to the drug and least likely to experience toxicities from treatment. This personalized cancer treatment approach is within our future reach, but will require expert systematic preclinical and clinical investigations and the development of an increasing array of highly selective molecular targeting agents.

References

Abidoye OO, Cohen EE, Wong SJ et al. (2006) A phase II study of lapatinib (GW572016) in recurrent/metastatic (R/M) squamous cell carcinoma of the head and neck (SCCHN). ASCO Meeting Proceedings, Jun 20, Abstract no. 5568

Allen GW, Saba C, Armstrong EA et al. (2007) Insulin-like growth factor-I receptor signaling blockade combined with radiation. Cancer Res 67:1155–1162

Baselga J, Trigo JM, Bourhis J et al. (2005) Phase II multicenter study of the antiepidermal growth factor receptor monoclonal antibody cetuximab in combination with platinum-based chemotherapy in patients with platinum-refractory metastatic and/or recurrent squamous cell carcinoma of the head and neck. J Clin Oncol 23:5568–5577

Bonner JA, Harari PM, Giralt J et al. (2006) Radiotherapy plus cetuximab for squamous-cell carcinoma of the head and neck. N Engl J Med 354:567–578

Burris HA, 3rd, Hurwitz HI, Dees EC et al. (2005) Phase I safety, pharmacokinetics, and clinical activity study of lapatinib (GW572016), a reversible dual inhibitor of epidermal growth factor receptor tyrosine kinases, in heavily pretreated patients with metastatic carcinomas. J Clin Oncol 23:5305–5313

Burtness B, Goldwasser MA, Flood W et al. (2005) Phase III randomized trial of cisplatin plus placebo compared with cisplatin plus cetuximab in metastatic/recurrent head and neck cancer: an Eastern Cooperative Oncology Group study. J Clin Oncol 23:8646–8654

Charoenrat PO, Rhys-Evans P, Modjtahedi H et al. (2000) Vascular endothelial growth factor family members are differentially regulated by c-erbB signaling in head and neck squamous carcinoma cells. Clin Exp Metastasis 18:155–161

Choong NW, Haraf DJ, Cohen EE et al. (2007) Randomized phase II study of concomitant chemoradiotherapy with 5-fluorouracil-hydroxyurea (FHX) compared to FHX and bevacizumab (BFHX) in intermediate stage head and neck cancer (HNC). ASCO Meeting Proceedings, Jun 20, Abstract no. 6034

Chung CH, Mirakhur B, Chan E et al. (2008) Cetuximab-induced anaphylaxis and IgE specific for galactose-alpha-1,3-galactose. N Engl J Med 358:1109–1117

Cohen EE, Kane MA, List MA et al. (2005) Phase II trial of gefitinib 250 mg daily in patients with recurrent and/or metastatic squamous cell carcinoma of the head and neck. Clin Cancer Res 11:8418–8424

Cohen EE, Rosen F, Stadler WM et al. (2003) Phase II trial of ZD1839 in recurrent or metastatic squamous cell carcinoma of the head and neck. J Clin Oncol 21:1980–1987

Demetri GD, von Mehren M, Blanke CD et al. (2002) Efficacy and safety of imatinib mesylate in advanced gastrointestinal stromal tumors. N Engl J Med 347:472–480

Engelman JA, Zejnullahu K, Mitsudomi T et al. (2007) MET amplification leads to gefitinib resistance in lung cancer by activating ERBB3 signaling. Science 316:1039–1043

Escudier B, Eisen T, Stadler WM et al. (2007) Sorafenib in advanced clear-cell renal-cell carcinoma. N Engl J Med 356:125–134

Gatzemeier U, Blumenschein G, Fosella F et al. (2006) Phase II trial of single-agent sorafenib in patients with advanced non-small cell lung carcinoma. ASCO Meeting Proceedings, Jun 20, Abstract no. 7002

Harrington KJ, Bourhis J, Nutting CM et al. (2006) A phase I, open-label study of lapatinib plus chemoradiation in patients with locally advanced squamous cell carcinoma of the head and neck (SCCHN). ASCO Meeting Proceedings, Jun 20, Abstract no. 5553

Hay N, Sonenberg N (2004) Upstream and downstream of mTOR. Genes Dev 18:1926–1945

Herbst RS, Arquette M, Shin DM et al. (2005) Phase II multicenter study of the epidermal growth factor receptor antibody cetuximab and cisplatin for recurrent and refractory squamous cell carcinoma of the head and neck. J Clin Oncol 23:5578–5587

Hurwitz H, Fehrenbacher L, Novotny W et al. (2004) Bevacizumab plus irinotecan, fluorouracil, and leucovorin for metastatic colorectal cancer. N Engl J Med 350:2335–2342

Janne PA, von Pawel J, Cohen RB et al. (2007) Multicenter, randomized, phase II trial of CI-1033, an irreversible pan-ERBB inhibitor, for previously treated advanced non small-cell lung cancer. J Clin Oncol 25:3936–3944

Johnson DH, Fehrenbacher L, Novotny WF et al. (2004) Randomized phase II trial comparing bevacizumab plus carboplatin and paclitaxel with carboplatin and paclitaxel alone in previously untreated locally advanced or metastatic non-small-cell lung cancer. J Clin Oncol 22:2184–2191

Johnson FM, Saigal B, Talpaz M et al. (2005) Dasatinib (BMS-354825) tyrosine kinase inhibitor suppresses invasion and induces cell cycle arrest and apoptosis of head and neck squamous cell carcinoma and non-small cell lung cancer cells. Clin Cancer Res 11:6924–6932

Karamouzis MV, Friedland D, Johnson R et al. (2007) Phase II trial of pemetrexed (P) and bevacizumab (B) in patients (pts) with recurrent or metastatic head and neck squamous cell carcinoma (HNSCC): an interim analysis. ASCO Meeting Proceedings, Jun 20, Abstract no. 6049

Lacouture ME (2006) Mechanisms of cutaneous toxicities to EGFR inhibitors. Nat Rev Cancer 6:803–812

Lothaire P, de Azambuja E, Dequanter D et al. (2006) Molecular markers of head and neck squamous cell carcinoma: promising signs in need of prospective evaluation. Head Neck 28:256–269

Miller K, Wang M, Gralow J et al. (2007) Paclitaxel plus bevacizumab versus paclitaxel alone for metastatic breast cancer. N Engl J Med 357:2666–2676

Miller KD, Trigo JM, Wheeler C et al. (2005) A multicenter phase II trial of ZD6474, a vascular endothelial growth factor receptor-2 and epidermal growth factor receptor tyrosine kinase inhibitor, in patients with previously treated metastatic breast cancer. Clin Cancer Res 11: 3369–3376

Motzer RJ, Hutson TE, Tomczak P et al. (2007) Sunitinib versus interferon alfa in metastatic renal-cell carcinoma. N Engl J Med 356:115–124

O'Neil BH, Allen R, Spigel DR et al. (2007) High incidence of cetuximab-related infusion reactions in Tennessee and North Carolina and the association with atopic history. J Clin Oncol 25:3644–3648

Olsson AK, Dimberg A, Kreuger J et al. (2006) VEGF receptor signalling – in control of vascular function. Nat Rev Mol Cell Biol 7:359–371

Reiter R, Gais P, Jutting U et al. (2006) Aurora kinase A messenger RNA overexpression is correlated with tumor progression and shortened survival in head and neck squamous cell carcinoma. Clin Cancer Res 12:5136–5141

Rusnak DW, Lackey K, Affleck K et al. (2001) The effects of the novel, reversible epidermal growth factor receptor/ErbB-2 tyrosine kinase inhibitor, GW2016, on the growth of human normal and tumor-derived cell lines in vitro and in vivo. Mol Cancer Therap 1:85–94

Sandler A, Gray R, Perry MC et al. (2006) Paclitaxel–carboplatin alone or with bevacizumab for non-small-cell lung cancer. N Engl J Med 355:2542–2550

Savvides P, Greskovich J, Bokar J et al. (2007) Phase II study of bevacizumab in combination with docetaxel and radiation in locally advanced squamous cell cancer of the head and neck (SCCHN). ASCO Meeting Proceedings, Jun 20, Abstract no. 6068

Sergina NV, Rausch M, Wang D et al. (2007) Escape from HER-family tyrosine kinase inhibitor therapy by the kinase-inactive HER3. Nature 445:437–441

Shepherd FA, Rodrigues Pereira J, Ciuleanu T et al. (2005) Erlotinib in previously treated non-small-cell lung cancer. N Engl J Med 353:123–132

Socinski MA, Novello S, Sanchez JM et al. (2006) Efficacy and safety of sunitinib in previously treated, advanced non-small cell lung cancer (NSCLC): preliminary results of a multicenter phase II trial. ASCO Meeting Proceedings, Jun 20, Abstract no. 7001

Soulieres D, Senzer NN, Vokes EE et al. (2004) Multicenter phase II study of erlotinib, an oral epidermal growth factor receptor tyrosine kinase inhibitor, in patients with recurrent or metastatic squamous cell cancer of the head and neck. J Clin Oncol 22:77–85

Tabernero J, Cervantes A, Hoekman K et al. (2007) Phase I study of AZD0530, an oral potent inhibitor of Src kinase: first demonstration of inhibition of Src activity in human cancers. ASCO Meeting Proceedings, Jun 20, Abstract no. 3520

Thatcher N, Chang A, Parikh P et al. (2005) Gefitinib plus best supportive care in previously treated patients with refractory advanced non-small-cell lung cancer: results from a randomised, placebo-controlled, multicentre study (Iressa survival evaluation in lung cancer). Lancet 366:1527–1537

Trigo J, Hitt R, Koralewski P et al. (2004) Cetuximab monotherapy is active in patients (pts) with platinum-refractory recurrent/metastatic squamous cell carcinoma of the head and neck (SCCHN): results of a phase II study. ASCO Meeting Proceedings, Jun 20, Abstract no. 5502

Vermorken JB, Trigo J, Hitt R et al. (2007) Open-label, uncontrolled, multicenter phase II study to evaluate the efficacy and toxicity of cetuximab as a single agent in patients with recurrent and/or metastatic squamous cell carcinoma of the head and neck who failed to respond to platinum-based therapy. J Clin Oncol 25:2171–2177

Vokes EE, Cohen W, Mauer AM et al. (2005) A phase I study of erlotinib and bevacizumab for recurrent or metastatic squamous cell carcinoma of the head and neck (HNC). ASCO Meeting Proceedings, Jun 20, Abstract no. 5504

Wheeler DL, Huang S, Kruser TJ et al. (2008) Mechanisms of acquired resistance to cetuximab: role of HER (ErbB) family members. Oncogene 27:3944–3956

Wheeler RH, Jones D, Sharma P et al. (2005) Clinical and molecular phase II study of gefitinib in patients (pts) with recurrent squamous cell cancer of the head and neck (H&N Ca). ASCO Meeting Proceedings, Jun 20, Abstract no. 5531

Toxicity, Quality of Life, Prevention, Rehabilitation, Supportive Care

Late Radiation-Induced Side Effects

20

Johannes A. Langendijk and Hendricus P. Bijl

C O N T E N T S

20.1 **Introduction** *227*

20.2 **Assessment of Radiation-Induced Side Effects** *228*

20.3 **The Impact of Radiation-Induced Toxicity on Quality of Life** *229*

20.4 **Xerostomia** *230*
20.4.1 Mechanisms of Radiation Damage to the Salivary Glands *230*
20.4.2 Prediction of Radiation-Induced Xerostomia *232*
20.4.3 Prevention of Xerostomia by Radio-Protective Agents *233*
20.4.3.1 Amifostine *233*
20.4.3.2 Pilocarpine *233*

20.5 **Swallowing Dysfunction** *234*
20.5.1 Evaluation of Swallowing Dysfunction *234*
20.5.2 Mechanisms of Swallowing Dysfunction After (Chemo)Radiation *234*
20.5.3 Prediction of Swallowing Dysfunction *236*
20.5.4 Prevention of Swallowing Dysfunction *237*
20.5.4.1 Radiation Delivery Techniques *237*
20.5.4.2 Preventive Swallowing Exercises *237*

20.6 **Summary and Conclusion** *237*

References *237*

KEY POINTS

- Xerostomia is the most frequently reported grade 2 or higher radiation-induced side effect.
- Swallowing dysfunction is the most frequently reported grade 3 or higher radiation-induced side effect after curative (chemo) radiation.
- In particular swallowing dysfunction and xerostomia have a negative impact on health-related quality of life.
- The probability of patient-rated xerostomia depends on the dose distribution in different salivary glands
- Amifostine reduces the probability on radiation-induced xerostomia, but the added value when combined with intensity-modulated radiotherapy remains to be determined.
- Pilocarpine is a cheap and safe drug with the potential of preventing xerostomia in well selected subset of patients.
- The probability of swallowing dysfunction depends on the dose distribution in a number of anatomical structures that are involved in swallowing, such as the pharyngeal constrictor muscles, the supraglottic and glottic larynx and the upper esophageal sphincter.

Johannes A. Langendijk, MD
Department of Radiation Oncology, University Medical Centre Groningen/University of Groningen, Groningen, The Netherlands
Hendricus P. Bijl, MD
Department of Radiation Oncology, University Medical Centre Groningen/University of Groningen, Groningen, The Netherlands

20.1

Introduction

In the last decade, there has been a growing interest in the evaluation of treatment-related side effects and health-related quality of life (HRQOL) of patients suffering from head and neck cancer (HNC). Traditionally, the primary goal of treatment in HNC patients is to achieve long-term locoregional tumor control and prolonged survival. New treatment strategies, either the delivery of radiotherapy (RT) with concomitant chemotherapy (CHRT) or altered fractionation schedules, have shown to improve tumor control and overall survival of HNC patients (Bourhis et al. 2006; Baujat et al. 2006; Langendijk et al. 2004). Despite these improvements in treatment outcome, clinicians as well as patients are increasingly concerned about the impact of standard and novel treatment approaches not only on the traditional endpoints, but also on treatment-related side effects and the impact that these side effects may have on HRQOL. There are a number of reasons for this increasing interest in side effects related to radiation treatment. First, most of these novel treatment approaches are associated with increased morbidity that are often persistent or even progressive in severity and may affect the long-term HRQOL of a cancer survivor or compromise the survival benefit from therapy. Second, there has been a clear shift from primary surgery to organ-preservation strategies in HNC. However, preservation of organ anatomy does not necessarily translate into preservation of organ function and many patients treated with organ-preservation protocols are dealing with devastating side effects such as severe swallowing dysfunction, aspiration and/ or problems with speech (Forastiere et al. 2003; Staar et al. 2001). Conversely, advances in RT such as intensity-modulated radiotherapy (IMRT), and the availability of more adequate staging techniques (e.g., PET) enable radiation oncologists to administer a high dose to the tumor and to other high-risk areas, while reducing the radiation dose significantly to the surrounding organs-at-risk (OARs). This results in a lower probability of early and late radiation-induced side effects. The result is that, for many patients, long-term irreversible side effects and the subsequent effects on HRQOL are an important consideration when selecting among the available treatment options.

In this chapter, we will extensively discuss those side effects that have the most impact on HRQL and are therefore most relevant from the patient's perspective. Finally, we will briefly overview the possibilities to prevent these most devastating radiation-induced side effects in HNC.

20.2
Assessment of Radiation-Induced Side Effects

The head and neck region contains a wide variety of anatomical structures with an even larger number of functions that may be affected when a curative dose of radiation either or not combined with systemic agents will be administered. Acute side effects generally occur during or within a few weeks after completion of RT, particularly in highly proliferative normal tissues, such as the mucosa and the skin. Typical late side effects become manifest after a certain latent period ranging from months to years and may include radiation-induced salivary dysfunction, soft tissue and muscular fibrosis, mucosal atrophy, vascular damage, neural damage, ulceration and (osteo)necrosis and endocrine effects. There are data emerging for a number of tissues that late side effects may be causally related to acute side effects, in particular in those organ systems in which a barrier against mechanical and/or chemical stress is established by the acutely responding component, e.g., confluent oral mucositis may result in chronic, nonhealing ulcers and necrosis. This phenomenon has been referred to as *consequential late effects* (Slonina et al. 2001; Peters et al. 1988; Dorr and Hendry 2001).

A number of toxicity grading systems have been developed for classifying late radiation-induced toxicity in which grading is ranked according to the severity of a given side effect. These classification systems include the Subjective, Objective, Management, Analytic/Late Effects Normal Tissue system (SOMA-LENT)(Anon 1995a, b), the Radiation Oncology Group/ European Organisation for Research and Treatment of Cancer system (RTOG/EORTC) (Cox et al. 1995), and more recently, the Common Terminology for Adverse Events version 3.0 (CTCAE v3.0). The CTCAE v3.0 grading system includes the definitions of a large set toxicity items and does not only take into account toxicity induced by RT but also side effects induced by other treatment modalities such as surgery and chemotherapy. Furthermore, assessments of both acute and late side effects are merged into one grading system.

Although the CTCAE v3.0 is currently the most frequently used grading system for treatment-related side effects in clinical trials, reports on late radiation-induced side effects have been and are still subject to a wide variability with regard to the frequency and severity of late side effects. Moreover, it has been generally recognized that in the majority of clinical studies, side effects are presumably underreported.

Besides the use of multiple grading systems, there are a number of other reasons that account for the variability in toxicity reporting. First, the grading of many items is defined in such a way, that reliable scoring requires investigations that are not carried out on a routine basis (e.g., grading of the item xerostomia requires both subjective and objective (salivary flow) assessment parameters, while in most institutions, salivary flow measurements are not performed on a routine basis). Second, reliable assessment of side effects sometimes requires special attention and additional questioning by health-care providers. This is nicely illustrated by an example in one of our own patients, who was asked whether he had any problems with swallowing. Although, he initially denied having any problems with swallowing (grade 0), it eventually turned out that he was not able to swallow anything and to be completely dependent on percutaneous endoscopic gastrostomy (grade 4), which he himself, however, did not experience as a problem. Third, irrespective of the grading system used, reliable assessment of side effects requires adequate follow up evaluations at regular intervals. In addition, as recently pointed out by BENTZEN and TROTTI (2007), there is still limited guidance or standards for safety data reporting, resulting in a wide variety in the way results with respect to late side effects are analyzed, reported, and presented in literature. Therefore, a reliable estimation of the incidence of late radiation-induced side effects in HNC remains difficult or even impossible.

To overcome part of these problems, the department of Radiation Oncology of the VU University Medical Center developed a Standard Follow up Program (SFP) which was clinically introduced in 1997 for all patients with HNC treated with primary and/or postoperative (chemo)radiation. To enhance the reliability of reporting, the radiation oncologists involved were trained to assess side effects using standardized checklists. At the same time points, HRQOL was evaluated, using the EORTC QLQ-C30 (version 3.0) (AARONSON et al. 1993) together with the HNC-specific module, the EORTC QLQ-H&N35 (BJORDAL and KAASA 1992).

The results regarding the prevalence of radiation-induced side effects up to 24 months after completion of RT among the first 500 patients included in this SFP are depicted in Fig. 20.1. Noteworthy is that the compliance to the SFP was >90% at all time points for all patients eligible. As expected, the prevalence for grade 2 or higher morbidity was highest for xerostomia. The prevalence of the other grade 2 or more toxicity varied between 11% for laryngeal reactions (at 24 months) and 44% for subcutaneous fibrosis (at 24 months). For late pharyngeal reactions (swallowing dysfunction), there was a trend towards improvement at longer intervals, while for subcutaneous fibrosis, an opposite trend was observed. Pharyngeal side effects were the most frequently reported grade 3 or higher side effects, which however improved from 21% at 6 months to 13% at 6 months.

20.3
The Impact of Radiation-Induced Toxicity on Quality of Life

We performed a prospective observational study to determine the impact of radiation-induced side effects on the general dimensions of HRQOL (LANGENDIJK et al. 2008). The study sample was composed of 458 disease-free patients included in the SFP. Of all the toxicity scales investigated, only two significantly affected self-reported HRQOL: xerostomia and swallowing dysfunction. Although xerostomia was reported most frequently, HRQOL was most affected by swallowing dysfunction (Table 20.1). Only little or moderate effects for grade 2 or higher xerostomia were found on most but not all HRQOL scales, while swallowing dysfunction affected all HRQOL scales significantly and moreover, these effects were classified as moderate to very much for grade 2 or more. The results indicated that swallowing dysfunction after curative (CH)RT had more effect on the more general dimensions of HRQOL than similar grades of xerostomia, in particular in the first 12 months after completion of treatment. Similar results were found by others (LIST et al. 1997, 1999; JENSEN et al. 2006; DIRIX et al. 2008; BRAAM et al. 2006). As the incidence of radiation-induced salivary dysfunction and xerostomia can be reduced by the use of new radiation techniques, such as IMRT (BRAAM et al. 2006; EISBRUCH et al. 1999, 2003; JABBARI et al. 2005; FANG et al. 2007; KAM et al. 2003, 2007; Pow et al. 2006; McMILLAN et al. 2006; WU et al. 2000), it is very likely that the problem

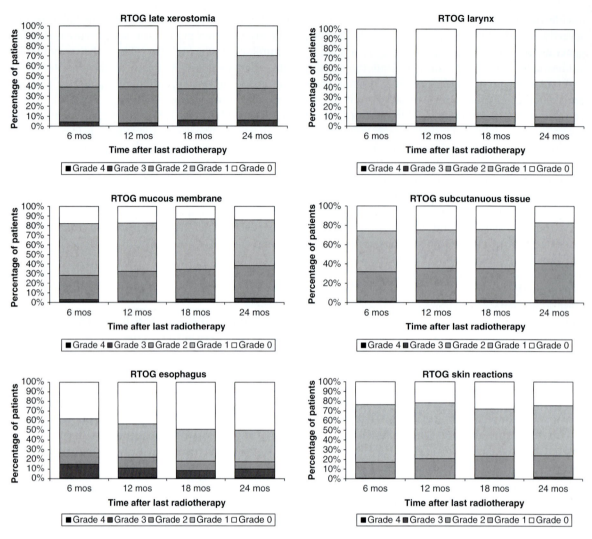

Fig. 20.1. Prevalence of late radiation-induced morbidity according to RTOG late radiation morbidity scoring system in 500 patients treated with bilateral 3D-conformal (chemo)-radiation treated at the VU University Medical Center, Amsterdam, The Netherlands

of swallowing dysfunction is becoming one of the most important side effects after curative (CH)RT.

20.4
Xerostomia

20.4.1
Mechanisms of Radiation Damage to the Salivary Glands

In a rat model, a four-phase pattern both in the submandibular and the parotid gland of the rat could be distinguished (ZEILSTRA et al. 2000; COPPES et al. 2001).

The first phase (0–10 days) is characterized by a rapid decline in flow rate without changes in amylase secretion or acinar cell number. The second phase (10–60 days) consists of a decrease in amylase secretion and is paralleled by acinar cell loss. Flow rate, amylase secretion and acinar cell numbers do not change in the third phase (60–120 days). The fourth phase (120–240 days) is characterized by a further deterioration of gland function but an increase in acinar cell number, albeit with poor tissue morphology. Comparable changes have been observed in rat submandibular tissue (ZEILSTRA et al. 2000; COPPES et al. 2002).

Within 3 days after irradiation with a single dose of 15 Gy, salivary flow reduces to near 50% from baseline (VISSINK et al. 1990; PETER et al. 1995; COPPES

Table 20.1. The impact of xerostomia and swallowing dysfunction according to the late RTOG toxicity scoring system at 6 months after (chem)radiation

	Xerostomia				
	Grade 0	Grade 1	Grade 2	Grade 3–4	*p*-value
Toxicity scale and QOL scales					
Physical functioning	81	82	75	71	<0.001
Role functioning	74	74	67	67	0.044
Emotional functioning	84	80	74	69	0. 001
Social functioning	88	85	79	64	<0.001
Global quality of life	73	75	65	55	<0.001
Fatigue	25	28	36	42	<0.001
Swallowing dysfunction					
Physical functioning	84	82	72	68	<0.001
Role functioning	77	76	62	55	0.044
Emotional functioning	84	80	70	69	0.001
Social functioning	91	83	73	68	<0.001
Global quality of life	78	72	63	56	<0.001
Fatigue	23	29	41	43	<0.001

The values indicate the mean values for the different HRQOL scales. Higher scores represent better functioning. The effects of swallowing dysfunction on the general dimensions of HRQOL were more pronounced compared with those of xerostomia. At 12 months, the impact of swallowing on HRQOL further increased bit gradually decreased at 18 and 24 months (data not shown)

et al. 1997, 1997, 2001; ZEILSTRA et al. 2000). This early effect is most probably due to the presence of non-removed dysfunctional cells at the level of membranes (PRATT and SODICOFF 1972; EL-MOFTY and KAHN 1981; VISSINK et al. 1992) and/or a disturbed intracellular signaling (FRANZEN et al. 1991; COPPES et al. 1997, 2000; VISSINK et al. 1991; HENRIKSSON et al. 1994; PAARDEKOOPER et al. 1998; ZEILSTRA et al. 2000). The late effects of radiation on the parotid and submandibular glands have been studied less extensively, and have been reported as a dose-dependent further decline in function (COPPES et al. 2001; NAGLER et al. 1993) and loss of acinar cells (HENRIKSSON et al. 1994; O'CONNELL et al. 1999). Unfortunately, in these studies the whole or half of the glands were irradiated. Therefore, indirect effects due to damage to other organs confound the interpretation with regards to salivary gland function (NAGLER 2001; KONINGS et al. 2001).

Also in human, a rapid decrease of the salivary flow rate has been observed during the first week of RT, after which there is a gradual decrease to less than 10% of the initial flow rate depending on the localization of the radiation portals (DREIZEN et al. 1976; SHANNON et al. 1978; LIU et al. 1990; FRANZEN et al. 1991; JONES et al. 1996; BURLAGE et al. 2001). Although in the older literature the submandibular gland was thought to be less radiosensitive than the parotid gland, both glands have been shown to be as sensitive to RT, at least with respect to their function (LIU et al. 1990; BURLAGE et al. 2001). In rats, it has been shown that the submandibular gland may be even more sensitive for the late effects of radiation because of the inability to restore the damage (COPPES et al. 2002).

The early (BURLAGE et al. 2001) and late (LIU et al. 1990) human data on the radiation-induced severe drop in flow rate of both the parotid and submandibular gland are somewhat in contradiction to the functional data derived from scintigraphic studies (VALDES OLMOS et al. 1994; LIEM et al. 1996). Some authors showed a failure of the major salivary glands to excrete saliva early postirradiation, and a decreased uptake of 99mTc-pertechnetate together with a loss of secretory function in the postirradiation stage. This effect was stronger in parotid than in submandibular glands, although the incidence of xerostomia did not correlate with the effects observed in the scintigraphic studies (LIEM et al. 1996), pointing to the obvious discrepancy between the actual salivary flow and the scintigraphic (LIEM et al. 1996) and morphological changes (VISSINK et al. 1991) induced by irradiation. Therefore, the combination of objective (measurement of salivary flow rate) and subjective (questionnaires) parameters still provides the best assessment with regard to the pattern of patients' complaints and the effects of various therapies on these complaints.

20.4.2
Prediction of Radiation-Induced Xerostomia

In order to optimize radiation treatment, it is of great importance to know which dose–volume histogram (DVH) parameters are most predictive for the development of radiation-induced xerostomia. In most studies, unstimulated or stimulated parotid flow has been used as the primary endpoint in relation to DVH parameters. The results of these studies point out that that the reduction of salivary flow (after stimulation) is best predicted by the mean parotid dose (EISBRUCH et al. 1999; CHAO et al. 2001; ROESINK et al. 2001, 2005). Recently, Semenenko and Li reported on the results of a systematic review, using a series of published clinical datasets regarding dose–response relationships for xerostomia. The primary endpoint was defined as a reduction of stimulated salivary flow below 25% from baseline within 6 months after RT. For this endpoint, a TD50 of 31.4 Gy was found (SEMENENKO and LI 2008).

Ship et al. observed the important role of the submandibular glands in the production of saliva in the nonstimulated state (SHIP et al. 1991). MURDOCH-KINCH et al. (2008) investigated the dose–response relationships for submandibular glands based on selective measurements of their output and their 3D dose distributions (MURDOCH-KINCH et al. 2008). They demonstrated an exponential reduction in salivary output as the mean dose increased beyond the threshold of 39 Gy. The salivary output gradually improved over the 2-year observation period when the mean dose did not exceed the threshold dose. This threshold dose of 39 Gy appears to be higher than the threshold for the stimulated parotid gland (26 Gy) as observed by EISBRUCH et al. (1999). Another recent study from Saarilahti et al. showed

the importance of sparing the submandibular gland (SAARILAHTI et al. 2006).

From a clinical point of view, patient-rated xerostomia may be more relevant than salivary flow. However, the results of a number of studies indicate that the prediction of patient-rated xerostomia is much more complex and does not only depend on the dose to the parotid glands but also to the dose to other major and minor salivary glands. This is supported by the findings of two prospective studies in which patients with nasopharyngeal carcinoma were randomly assigned to receive conventional RT vs. IMRT. In these two studies, salivary flow was significantly better among patients treated with IMRT, which however did not translate into a significant improvement of patient-rated xerostomia (POW et al. 2006; KAM et al. 2007).

JELLEMA et al. (2005) found that both the mean parotid and submandibular gland dose were significantly associated with patient-rated xerostomia. Moreover, the probability of developing moderate or severe xerostomia as a function of the mean parotid dose significantly increased with a higher mean dose in the submandibular glands. This was illustrated by the increasing steepness of the probability curves with increasing doses in the submandibular glands (Fig. 20.2).

The threshold dose for patient-rated xerostomia may also differ between unilaterally and bilaterally irradiated patients (JELLEMA et al. 2007). Patient-rated xerostomia is more pronounced among patients treated with bilateral irradiation than among those treated with unilateral irradiation and the mean dose to the contralateral parotid gland appears to be the most important prognostic factor for patient-rated xerostomia. The TD50 for moderate or severe patient-rated xerostomia increased from 23 Gy for bilaterally treated patients to 45 Gy for unilaterally treated patients (JELLEMA et al. 2007). The authors suggested that the spared salivary gland compensated for the loss of function of the irradiated parotid gland. The results regarding the importance of the oral cavity dose regarding patient-rated xerostomia are conflicting (JELLEMA et al. 2005; EISBRUCH et al. 2001).

All these findings clearly illustrate the complexity of predicting patient-rated xerostomia and also point out that the clinical introduction of IMRT only focusing on reducing the mean parotid dose is probably not sufficient to reduce the subjective findings of xerostomia in all cases.

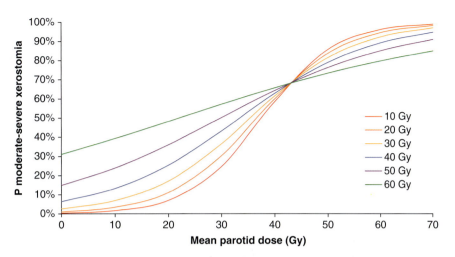

Fig. 20.2. The probability (p) on moderate to severe patient-rated xerostomia (EORTC QLQ-N&N35) as a function of the mean parotid dose. The different coloured curves indicate this relationship for the different mean doses administered to the submandibular glands. The results clearly show that the steepness of the curve in case of a low dose to the submandibular glands is higher compared to the curves with higher mean doses to the submandibular glands

20.4.3
Prevention of Xerostomia by Radio-Protective Agents

20.4.3.1
Amifostine

Amifostine is a thio-organic compound that was originally developed as a protector against radiation-induced toxicity in the event of nuclear war. Amifostine and its active metabolite, WR-1065, accumulate in many epithelial tissues with the highest concentrations found in the salivary glands, spleen, and kidneys (Tanaka et al. 1983). There are a number of normal tissues, which have been reported to be protected, particularly the salivary glands. In tumor bearing animals there was a selective cytoprotection of normal tissues from the irradiation without protection of the tumor (Phillips et al. 1973; Washburn et al. 1976; Yuhas et al. 1980). Brizel et al. conducted a large, prospective randomized multicenter trial for patients treated with RT for HNC (Brizel et al. 2000). Patients were randomized to receive RT alone vs. amifostine prior to RT. The incidence of grade ≥2 acute xerostomia significantly decreased from 78% without amifostine to 51% with amifostine, while the median dose at onset of xerostomia increased significantly from 42 Gy without amifostine to 60 Gy with amifostine. Similar results were found by other investigators (Jellema et al. 2006). Despite these positive results, amifostine has never been used on a large scale basis for a number of reasons, which include high costs, induction of side effects directly related to amifostine administration itself, the increasing use of competitive radiation techniques such as IMRT and the controversies with respect to the selectivity to the normal tissues of amifostine and the subsequent presumed protective effect on the tumor (Lindegaard and Grau 2000). Although amifostine certainly has a protective effect on salivary function, its value in combination with currently available advanced radiation techniques, such as IMRT, has never been confirmed in controlled studies.

20.4.3.2
Pilocarpine

Pilocarpine is well known for its largely parasympathetic stimulation which induces salivary secretion. The side effects are considered mild when used in low dosages of 2.5–5 mg up to four administrations a day. Histological studies on rat salivary glands have shown that prophylactic treatment with sialogogues (like pilocarpine) has some radio-protective potential (Norberg and Lundquist 1989; Kim et al. 1991). Coppes et al. (1997) showed that pretreatment with pilocarpine resulted in sparing of radiation-induced changes in rat salivary gland function (Coppes et al. 1997). Roesink et al. (1999) provided direct evidence that the effect of pilocarpine was not restricted to the irradiated gland but it also enhanced the flow rate in the contralateral, nonirradiated gland after single doses of 10–30 Gy (Roesink et al. 1999). Recently, Burlage et al. reported on a prospective, double blinded, placebo-controlled randomized trial, that investigated the protective effect of concomitant pilocarpine administration on parotid gland dysfunction, which was the first study on this subject with well-documented data on DVHs of irradiated parotid glands (Burlage et al. 2008). Overall, no significant differences were noted between placebo and pilocarpine regarding the parotid flow rate. However, in the subset of patients with a mean parotid dose >40 Gy, pilocarpine administration resulted in higher flow rates at 12 months after RT. In all other randomized clinical studies that investigated the value of pilocarpine to reduce xerostomia, information about the dose to the parotid glands and the volume irradiated was very limited or absent. Lajtman et al. (2000) only observed a positive effect of pilocarpine in the subset of patients treated with partial irradiation of the parotid glands. In the other positive study (Haddad and Karimi 2002), both parotid glands, including their upper part, were included within the irradiation fields with a minimum doses of 40 Gy. In the six "negative" studies, the volume of the irradiated parotid glands appeared to be higher than in the positive trials (Warde et al. 2002). These findings suggest that a certain level of damage has to be present before a beneficial effect of pilocarpine can be expected, which is in agreement with the results obtained from animal studies (Coppes et al. 1997, 2000; Roesink et al. 1999). On the other hand, if the damage exceeds beyond a certain level, no effect can be expected from concomitant pilocarpine administration, because of the lack of cells able to proliferate and restore radiation damage. Based on these results and given its low toxicity profile, concomitant pilocarpine administration can be considered whenever the mean dose to the parotid glands goes beyond a certain dose (e.g., 40 Gy).

20.5

Swallowing Dysfunction

20.5.1
Evaluation of Swallowing Dysfunction

Various methods are used to evaluate swallowing function including clinical evaluation (oral sensomotoric assessment and observing symptomatic aspiration), questionnaires on swallowing problems and objective assessment methods. For the objective assessment of swallowing function, there are two main instrumental studies, including videofluoroscopic evaluation (VF) and fiberoptic endoscopic evaluation of swallowing (FEES). VF is recognized as the gold-standard evaluation because it shows the entire oropharyngeal swallow which can be quantified. Information is provided regarding all events, allowing for the diagnosis of specific swallowing disorders and causes of aspiration (Dodds et al. 1990; Logemann 1993). Interventions appropriate to the disorder to allow safe oral alimentation can be used, and their immediate effectiveness can be verified (Logemann et al. 1998). FEES is a video-endoscopic tool (Aviv et al. 2000) sensitive to detect residuals, laryngeal penetration, and aspiration, and avoids radiation exposure (Hiss and Postma 2003). It does not show the oral phase, pharyngeal stripping, transit through the UES, or the extent of aspiration (Aviv et al. 2000). VF is currently the preferred objective assessment method in most institutions (McConnel and O'Connor 1994; Pauloski et al. 1994).

Besides objective methods to assess swallowing dysfunction, a number of instruments have been developed to assess patient-rated swallowing dysfunction. There are three commonly used and validated questionnaires specifically designed for subjective swallowing assessment, including the performance status scale for head and neck cancer patients (PSS-H&N) and the M.D. Anderson Dysphagia Inventory (MDADI). The PSS-H&N is a rapid, clinician-rated instrument consisting of three subscales: normalcy of diet, public eating, and understandability of speech (List et al. 1996). The MDADI is a more detailed patient-completed measure of function and HRQOL (Chen et al. 2001). In addition to these specific questionnaires, many investigators have been using the more general HNQOL questionnaires with or without their head and neck specific modules, containing a limited number of questions regarding swallowing function (e.g., the EORTC QLQ-H&N35) (Levendag et al. 2007).

20.5.2
Mechanisms of Swallowing Dysfunction After (Chemo)Radiation

Studies on swallowing using VF after (CH)RT for HNC revealed a large variety of motility disorders (Table 20.2) (Carrara-de et al. 2003; Hughes et al. 2000; Ku et al. 2007; Lazarus et al. 1996, 2000;

Table 20.2. Motility disorders assessed by videofluoroscopy after curative (chemo)radiation

Motility disorders	References
Increased bolus preparation	LEVENDAG et al. (2007)
Prolonged oral transit time	CARRARA-DE et al. (2003); HUGHES et al. (2000); KU et al. (2007)
Decreased tongue strength/control	LAZARUS et al. (1996, 2000)
Reduced tongue-based contact to the pharyngeal wall	NEWMAN et al. (2002); EISBRUCH et al. (2002); GOGUEN et al. (2006); GRANER et al. (2003); KOTZ et al. (2004); LAZARUS (1993)
Pharyngeal constrictor dysmotility	CARRARA-DE et al. (2003); HUGHES et al. (2000); GRANER et al. (2003); KOTZ et al. (2004); KU et al. (2007)
Changes in bolus prepulsion	LEVENDAG et al. (2007)
Velopharyngeal incompetence	CARRARA-DE et al. (2003); KU et al. (2007)
Decreased Laryngeal elevation	LEVENDAG et al. (2007); CARRARA-DE et al. (2003); EISBRUCH et al. (2002); GOGUEN et al. (2006); GRANER et al. (2003); KOTZ et al. (2004)
Decreased laryngeal vestibular closure	GRANER et al. (2003)
Laryngeal penetration	GOGUEN et al. (2006); GRANER et al. (2003); KOTZ et al. (2004); NEWMAN et al. (2002); KU et al. (2007)
Reduced hyoid movement	EISBRUCH et al. (2002)
Epiglottic dysmotility	NEWMAN et al. (2002); KOTZ et al. (2004)
Increased pharyngeal residue	LEVENDAG et al. (2007); NEWMAN et al. (2002); KOTZ et al. (2004)
Abnormal function upper esophageal sphincter	NEWMAN et al. (2002); EISBRUCH et al. (2002)

NEWMAN et al. 2002; EISBRUCH et al. 2002; GOGUEN et al. 2006; GRANER et al. 2003; KOTZ et al. 2004; LAZARUS 1993; SMITH et al. 2000; WU et al. 2000; YU et al. 2003). Furthermore, these swallowing disorders can lead to clinically apparent as well as silent aspiration or continued alternate feeding such as placement of gastrostomy tube (PEG) (CARRARA-DE et al. 2003; GOGUEN et al. 2006; GRANER et al. 2003; HUGHES et al. 2000; NGUYEN et al. 2004, 2006; SMITH et al. 2000; WU et al. 2000). The type of swallowing disorders observed after RT are largely similar as observed after CHRT.

Many of these VF-abnormalities may be the result of fibrosis of the pharyngeal musculature after (CH) RT. Radiation causes fibrosis of the soft tissues which impairs laryngeal elevation (EISELE et al. 1991). Other investigators found a tendency for laryngeal elevation to worsen over time (SMITH et al. 2000) or an increasing impact over time of reduced cricopharyngeal opening on oral intake (PAULOSKI et al. 2006). Because cricopharyngeal opening is dependent on hyolaryngeal elevation and anterior movement to pull open the relaxed sphincter, the appearance of reduced cricopharyngeal opening in conjunction with reduced laryngeal elevation at the later time

points suggests the progression of fibrosis of the pharyngeal muscles to be the basis of swallowing problems after (CH)RT. Recently, EISBRUCH et al. (2004) suggested that the pharyngeal constrictors and laryngeal adductors, which lie close to the submucosa, are primarily affected by the inflammatory processes in the mucosa and submucosa. These processes include the accumulation of macrophages and increased local levels of proinflammatory cytokines (HANDSCHEL et al. 2001; SONIS et al. 2000), producing edema and fibrosis that may, in addition, affect the underlying muscles.

The results of studies on the correlation between patient-rated dysphagia and objective assessments of dysphagia yielded conflicting results (HORNER and MASSEY 1988; LITVAN et al. 1997; NEWTON et al. 1994; PAULOSKI et al. 2002; WITTERICK et al. 1995). In HNC, it was found that patients expressing subjective swallowing complaints demonstrated significantly worse objective swallowing functions and aspiration (PAULOSKI et al. 2002). In another study, objective swallowing disorders were found in patients with and without swallowing complaints (KENDALL et al. 1998). These results emphasize the importance of assessing both objective swallowing function and subjective swallowing complaints among patients with and without these complaints in order to get more understanding of the nature of the anatomical and pathophysiological changes after (CH)RT that actually result into clinically relevant swallowing dysfunction.

20.5.3
Prediction of Swallowing Dysfunction

To improve radiation delivery techniques, in particular to prevent swallowing dysfunction, it is essential to determine the relationships between the radiation dose distribution in anatomical structures that are involved in swallowing and the probability on swallowing dysfunction. A number of authors tried to identify these so-called swallowing organs at risk (Table 20.3) (DORNFELD et al. 2007; FENG et al. 2007; LEVENDAG et al. 2007; JENSEN et al. 2007; POULSEN et al. 2008; CAGLAR et al. 2008). The results of these studies suggest that dose distributions in a number of anatomical structures, such as the pharyngeal constrictor muscles, the supraglottic and glottic larynx as well as the upper esophageal sphincter can be considered as OAR. However, all these studies can be criticized for a number of reasons, such as the small size, the use of different kind of endpoints, lack of baseline evaluations and lack of longitudinal assessments.

Table 20.3. Overview of studies aiming at identifying organs at risk for swallowing dysfunction after curative (chemo) radiation

References	Number of patients	Study design	Treatment	Assessments	Findings regarding dose effect relationships
DORNFELD et al. (2007)	27	Prospective cohort study	IMRT	HNCI	Dose to the supraglottic region (aryepiglottic folds, false vocal cords) and lateral pharyngeal walls associated with restrictive diet and weight loss
FENG et al. (2007)	36	Prospective cohort study	IMRT	HNQOL + UWQOL + VF	Dose to the pharyngeal constrictors (in particular the superior) and supraglottic region associated with VF aspiration Mean dose to pharyngeal constrictors and esophagus associated with patient-rated liquid swallowing
LEVENDAG et al. (2007)	81	Cross-sectional study	EBRT ± CHT or brachytherapy	PSS + MDADI + EORTC H&N35	Mean dose in middle and superior constrictor muscles associated with severe patient-rated dysphagia (univariate analysis)
JENSEN et al. (2007)	35	Cross-sectional study	EBRT	EORTC H&N35 + FEES	Doses<60 Gy to the supraglottic region, larynx, and UES associated with aspiration index.
POULSEN et al. (2008)	345	Prospective cohort study	EBRT	Dische swallowing toxicity score	Craniocaudal length of the treatment field associated with grade 4 toxicity
CAGLAR et al. (2008)	96	Posttreatment swallowing evaluation	EBRT ± CHT	SPS and addi-tional VF when SPS-score >1	Volume of larynx and volume of inferior constrictor muscles receiving ≥50 Gy associated with strictures and aspiration

EBRT external beam radiotherapy; *CHT* chemotherapy; *SPS* swallowing performance scale; *PSS* performance status scale; *MDADI* M.D. Anderson dysphagia inventory; *VF* videofluoroscopy; *FEES* functional endoscopic evaluation of swallowing; *UES* upper esophageal sphincter; *HNCI* head and neck cancer inventory; *HNQOL* head and neck quality of life questionnaire; *UWQOL* University of Washington head and neck-related quality of life

Therefore, the exact DVH-parameters and subsequent threshold values for these parameters remain to be determined.

20.5.4
Prevention of Swallowing Dysfunction

20.5.4.1
Radiation Delivery Techniques

The existence of relationships between the dose distributions in certain anatomical structures and swallowing dysfunction suggest that advanced radiation techniques such as IMRT, will result in better outcome with regard to swallowing function. However, clinical data confirming this assumption remain very scarce. Some authors (EISBRUCH et al. 2004, 2007) demonstrated that swallowing structure sparing IMRT is feasible, but the value of this technique with respect to the reduction of swallowing dysfunction after definitive (CH)RT remains to be determined. Others suggested that reducing the dose in these structures by brachytherapy, might result in a significant and clinically relevant reduction of swallowing dysfunction (EISBRUCH et al. 2007; LEVENDAG et al. 2007).

20.5.4.2
Preventive Swallowing Exercises

Swallowing rehabilitation can help to reduce swallowing problems (MITTAL et al. 2003). Rehabilitation consists of promotor exercises (to increase the strength and mobility of the lips, tongue, and mandible), swallow manoeuvres (to facilitate swallowing function and to prevent aspiration), and compensation techniques (adjusting posture, adjusting food consistency). Despite the overwhelming amount of evidence of swallowing problems after treatment for oral or oropharyngeal cancer, no controlled studies on efficacy of swallowing rehabilitation are documented.

Recently, Carroll et al. reported on the results of a retrospective case control study. In this study, nine patients received pretreatment swallowing exercises prior to CHRT, and nine patients received swallowing exercises during routine posttreatment management (CARROLL et al. 2008). Swallowing function was objectively evaluated using VF approximately 3 months after completion of treatment. The patients who received pretreatment swallowing exercises showed significantly better swallowing function, including better epiglottis inversion and better tongue-based contact to the pharyngeal wall than patient that were subjected to the routine posttreatment management. However, there were no significant differences regarding PEG tube removal between the two groups.

20.6
Summary and Conclusion

Definitive (CH)RT in HNC may result in a wide variety of toxicities of which xerostomia and swallowing dysfunction are the most frequently reported. In addition, these two side effects have the most impact on HRQOL. New radiation delivery techniques such as IMRT are able to spare most important OARs from these side effects. However, for some endpoints, in particular regarding swallowing dysfunction and patient-rated xerostomia, the exact DVH-constraints for the different OAR's remain to be determined.

References

Aaronson NK, Ahmedzai S, Bergman B et al. (1993) The European Organization for Research and Treatment of Cancer QLQ-C30: a quality-of-life instrument for use in international clinical trials in oncology. J Natl Cancer Inst 85(5):365–376

Anon (1995a) LENT SOMA scales for all anatomic sites. Int J Radiat Oncol Biol Phys 31(5):1049–1091

Anon (1995b) LENT SOMA tables. Radiother Oncol 35(1):17–60

Aviv JE, Parides M, Fellowes J et al. (2000) Endoscopic evaluation of swallowing as an alternative to 24-hour pH monitoring for diagnosis of extraesophageal reflux. Ann Otol Rhinol Laryngol Suppl 184:25–27

Baujat B, Audry H, Bourhis J et al. (2006) Chemotherapy in locally advanced nasopharyngeal carcinoma: an individual patient data meta-analysis of eight randomized trials and 1753 patients. Int J Radiat Oncol Biol Phys 64(1):47–56

Bentzen SM (2007) Trotti A. Evaluation of early and late toxicities in chemoradiation trials. J Clin Oncol 25(26):4096–4103

Bjordal K, Kaasa S (1992) Psychometric validation of the EORTC Core Quality of Life Questionnaire, 30-item version and a diagnosis-specific module for head and neck cancer patients. Acta Oncol 31(3):311–321

Bourhis J, Overgaard J, Audry H et al. (2006) Hyperfractionated or accelerated radiotherapy in head and neck cancer: a meta-analysis. Lancet 368(9538):843–854

Braam PM, Terhaard CH, Roesink JM et al. (2006) Intensity-modulated radiotherapy significantly reduces xerostomia compared with conventional radiotherapy. Int J Radiat Oncol Biol Phys 66(4):975–980

Brizel DM, Wasserman TH, Henke M et al. (2000) Phase III randomized trial of amifostine as a radioprotector in head and neck cancer. J Clin Oncol 18(19):3339–3345

Burlage FR, Coppes RP, Meertens H et al. (2001) Parotid and submandibular/sublingual salivary flow during high dose radiotherapy. Radiother Oncol 61(3):271–274

Burlage FR, Roesink JM, Kampinga HH et al. (2008) Protection of salivary function by concomitant pilocarpine during radiotherapy: a double-blind, randomized, placebo-controlled study. Int J Radiat Oncol Biol Phys 70(1):14–22

Caglar HB, Tishler RB, Othus M et al. (2008) Dose to larynx predicts for swallowing complications after intensity-modulated radiotherapy. Int J Radiat Oncol Biol Phys 72(4):1110–1118

Carrara-de AE, Feher O, Barros AP et al. (2003) Voice and swallowing in patients enrolled in a larynx preservation trial. Arch Otolaryngol Head Neck Surg 129(7):733–738

Carroll WR, Locher JL, Canon CL et al. (2008) Pretreatment swallowing exercises improve swallow function after chemoradiation. Laryngoscope 118(1):39–43

Chao KS, Deasy JO, Markman J et al. (2001) A prospective study of salivary function sparing in patients with head-and-neck cancers receiving intensity-modulated or three-dimensional radiation therapy: initial results. Int J Radiat Oncol Biol Phys 49(4):907–916

Chen AY, Frankowski R, Bishop-Leone J et al (2001) The development and validation of a dysphagia-specific quality-of-life questionnaire for patients with head and neck cancer: the M. D. Anderson dysphagia inventory. Arch Otolaryngol Head Neck Surg 127(7):870–876

Coppes RP, Roffel AF, Zeilstra LJ et al. (2000) Early radiation effects on muscarinic receptor-induced secretory responsiveness of the parotid gland in the freely moving rat. Radiat Res 153(3):339–346

Coppes RP, Vissink A, Konings AW (2002) Comparison of radiosensitivity of rat parotid and submandibular glands after different radiation schedules. Radiother Oncol 63(3):321–328

Coppes RP, Vissink A, Zeilstra LJ et al. (1997) Muscarinic receptor stimulation increases tolerance of rat salivary gland function to radiation damage. Int J Radiat Biol 72(5):615–625

Coppes RP, Zeilstra LJ, Kampinga HH et al. (2001) Early to late sparing of radiation damage to the parotid gland by adrenergic and muscarinic receptor agonists. Br J Cancer 85(7):1055–1063

Coppes RP, Zeilstra LJ, Vissink A et al. (1997) Sialogogue-related radioprotection of salivary gland function: the degranulation concept revisited. Radiat Res 148(3):240–247

Cox JD, Stetz J, Pajak TF (1995) Toxicity criteria of the Radiation Therapy Oncology Group (RTOG) and the European Organization for Research and Treatment of Cancer (EORTC). Int J Radiat Oncol Biol Phys 31(5):1341–1346

Dirix P, Nuyts S, Vander PV et al. (2008) The influence of xerostomia after radiotherapy on quality of life: results of a questionnaire in head and neck cancer. Support Care Cancer 16(2):171–179

Dodds WJ, Logemann JA, Stewart ET (1990) Radiologic assessment of abnormal oral and pharyngeal phases of swallowing. AJR Am J Roentgenol 154(5):965–974

Dornfeld K, Simmons JR, Karnell L et al. (2007) Radiation doses to structures within and adjacent to the larynx are correlated with long-term diet- and speech-related quality of life. Int J Radiat Oncol Biol Phys 68(3):750–757

Dorr W, Hendry JH (2001) Consequential late effects in normal tissues. Radiother Oncol 61(3):223–231

Dreizen S, Brown LR, Handler S et al. (1976) Radiation-induced xerostomia in cancer patients. Effect on salivary and serum electrolytes. Cancer 38(1):273–278

Eisbruch A, Dawson LA, Kim HM et al (1999) Conformal and intensity modulated irradiation of head and neck cancer: the potential for improved target irradiation, salivary gland function, and quality of life. Acta Otorhinolaryngol Belg 53(3):271–275

Eisbruch A, Kim HM, Terrell JE et al. (2001) Xerostomia and its predictors following parotid-sparing irradiation of head-and-neck cancer. Int J Radiat Oncol Biol Phys 50(3):695–704

Eisbruch A, Levendag PC, Feng FY et al (2007) Can IMRT or brachytherapy reduce dysphagia associated with chemoradiotherapy of head and neck cancer? The Michigan and Rotterdam experiences. Int J Radiat Oncol Biol Phys 69 (2 Suppl):S40–S42

Eisbruch A, Lyden T, Bradford CR et al. (2002) Objective assessment of swallowing dysfunction and aspiration after radiation concurrent with chemotherapy for head-and-neck cancer. Int J Radiat Oncol Biol Phys 53(1):23–28

Eisbruch A, Schwartz M, Rasch C et al. (2004) Dysphagia and aspiration after chemoradiotherapy for head-and-neck cancer: which anatomic structures are affected and can they be spared by IMRT? Int J Radiat Oncol Biol Phys 60(5):1425–1439

Eisbruch A, Ship JA, Dawson LA et al (2003) Salivary gland sparing and improved target irradiation by conformal and intensity modulated irradiation of head and neck cancer. World J Surg 27(7):832–837

Eisbruch A, Ten Haken RK, Kim HM et al. (1999) Dose, volume, and function relationships in parotid salivary glands following conformal and intensity-modulated irradiation of head and neck cancer. Int J Radiat Oncol Biol Phys 45(3):577–587

Eisele DW, Koch DG, Tarazi AE et al. (1991) Case report: aspiration from delayed radiation fibrosis of the neck. Dysphagia 6(2):120–122

El-Mofty SK, Kahn AJ (1981) Early membrane injury in lethally irradiated salivary gland cells. Int J Radiat Biol Relat Stud Phys Chem Med 39(1):55–62

Fang FM, Tsai WL, Chen HC et al. (2007) Intensity-modulated or conformal radiotherapy improves the quality of life of patients with nasopharyngeal carcinoma: comparisons of four radiotherapy techniques. Cancer 109(2):313–321

Feng FY, Kim HM, Lyden TH et al. (2007) Intensity-modulated radiotherapy of head and neck cancer aiming to reduce dysphagia: early dose-effect relationships for the swallowing structures. Int J Radiat Oncol Biol Phys 68(5):1289–1298

Forastiere AA, Goepfert H, Maor M et al. (2003) Concurrent chemotherapy and radiotherapy for organ preservation in advanced laryngeal cancer. N Engl J Med 349(22):2091–2098

Franzen L, Funegard U, Sundstrom S et al. (1991) Fractionated irradiation and early changes in salivary glands. Different effects on potassium efflux, exocytotic amylase release and gland morphology. Lab Invest 64(2):279–283

Goguen LA, Posner MR, Norris CM et al (2006) Dysphagia after sequential chemoradiation therapy for advanced head and neck cancer. Otolaryngol Head Neck Surg 134(6):916–922

Graner DE, Foote RL, Kasperbauer JL et al (2003) Swallow function in patients before and after intra-arterial chemoradiation. Laryngoscope 113(3):573–579

Haddad P, Karimi M (2002) A randomized, double-blind, placebo-controlled trial of concomitant pilocarpine with head and neck irradiation for prevention of radiation-induced xerostomia. Radiother Oncol 64(1):29–32

Handschel J, Sunderkotter C, Prott FJ et al. (2001) Increase of RM3/1-positive macrophages in radiation-induced oral mucositis. J Pathol 193(2):242–247

Henriksson R, Frojd O, Gustafsson H et al (1994) Increase in mast cells and hyaluronic acid correlates to radiation-induced damage and loss of serous acinar cells in salivary glands: the parotid and submandibular glands differ in radiation sensitivity. Br J Cancer 69(2):320–326

Hiss SG, Postma GN (2003) Fiberoptic endoscopic evaluation of swallowing. Laryngoscope 113(8):1386–1393

Horner J, Massey EW (1988) Silent aspiration following stroke. Neurology 38(2):317–319

Hughes PJ, Scott PM, Kew J et al (2000) Dysphagia in treated nasopharyngeal cancer. Head Neck 22(4):393–397

Jabbari S, Kim HM, Feng M et al. (2005) Matched case-control study of quality of life and xerostomia after intensity-modulated radiotherapy or standard radiotherapy for head-and-neck cancer: initial report. Int J Radiat Oncol Biol Phys 63(3):725–731

Jellema AP, Doornaert P, Slotman BJ et al. (2005) Does radiation dose to the salivary glands and oral cavity predict patient-rated xerostomia and sticky saliva in head and neck cancer patients treated with curative radiotherapy? Radiother Oncol 77(2):164–171

Jellema AP, Slotman BJ, Doornaert P et al. (2007) Unilateral versus bilateral irradiation in squamous cell head and neck cancer in relation to patient-rated xerostomia and sticky saliva. Radiother Oncol 85(1):83–89

Jellema AP, Slotman BJ, Muller MJ et al. (2006) Radiotherapy alone, versus radiotherapy with amifostine 3 times weekly, versus radiotherapy with amifostine 5 times weekly: a prospective randomized study in squamous cell head and neck cancer. Cancer 107(3):544–553

Jensen K, Bonde JA, Grau C (2006) The relationship between observer-based toxicity scoring and patient assessed symptom severity after treatment for head and neck cancer. A correlative cross sectional study of the DAHANCA toxicity scoring system and the EORTC quality of life questionnaires. Radiother Oncol 78(3):298–305

Jensen K, Lambertsen K, Grau C (2007) Late swallowing dysfunction and dysphagia after radiotherapy for pharynx cancer: frequency, intensity and correlation with dose and volume parameters. Radiother Oncol 85(1):74–82

Jones RE, Takeuchi T, Eisbruch A et al. (1996) Ipsilateral parotid sparing study in head and neck cancer patients who receive radiation therapy: results after 1 year. Oral Surg Oral Med Oral Pathol Oral Radiol Endod 81(6):642–648

Kam MK, Chau RM, Suen J et al. (2003) Intensity-modulated radiotherapy in nasopharyngeal carcinoma: dosimetric advantage over conventional plans and feasibility of dose escalation. Int J Radiat Oncol Biol Phys 56(1):145–157

Kam MK, Leung SF, Zee B et al. (2007) Prospective randomized study of intensity-modulated radiotherapy on salivary gland function in early-stage nasopharyngeal carcinoma patients. J Clin Oncol 25(31):4873–4879

Kendall KA, McKenzie SW, Leonard RJ et al. (1998) Structural mobility in deglutition after single modality treatment of head and neck carcinomas with radiotherapy. Head Neck 20(8):720–725

Kim KH, Kim JY, Sung MW et al. (1991) The effect of pilocarpine and atropine administration on radiation-induced injury of rat submandibular glands. Acta Otolaryngol 111(5):967–973

Konings AW, Vissink A, Coppes RP (2001) Comments on: extended-term effects of head and neck irradiation in a rodent. Eur J Cancer 37:1938–1945; Eur J Cancer 2002; 38(6):851–852

Kotz T, Costello R, Li Y et al. (2004) Swallowing dysfunction after chemoradiation for advanced squamous cell carcinoma of the head and neck. Head Neck 26(4):365–372

Ku PK, Yuen EH, Cheung DM et al (2007) Early swallowing problems in a cohort of patients with nasopharyngeal carcinoma: symptomatology and videofluoroscopic findings. Laryngoscope 117(1):142–146

Lajtman Z, Krajina Z, Krpan D et al. (2000) Pilocarpine in the prevention of postirradiation xerostomia. Acta Med Croatica 54(2):65–67

Langendijk JA, Doornaert PAH, Verdonck-de Leeuw IM et al. (2008) The impact of late treatment-related toxicity on quality of life (EORTC QLQ-C30) among patients with head and neck cancer treated with radiotherapy. J Clin Oncol 26(22):3770–3776

Langendijk JA, Leemans CR, Buter J et al. (2004) The additional value of chemotherapy to radiotherapy in locally advanced nasopharyngeal carcinoma: a meta-analysis of the published literature. J Clin Oncol 22(22):4604–4612

Lazarus CL (1993) Effects of radiation therapy and voluntary maneuvers on swallow functioning in head and neck cancer patients. Clin Commun Disord 3(4):11–20

Lazarus CL, Logemann JA, Pauloski BR et al (1996) Swallowing disorders in head and neck cancer patients treated with radiotherapy and adjuvant chemotherapy. Laryngoscope 106(9 Pt 1):1157–1166

Lazarus CL, Logemann JA, Pauloski BR et al (2000) Swallowing and tongue function following treatment for oral and oropharyngeal cancer. J Speech Lang Hear Res 43(4): 1011–1023

Levendag PC, Teguh DN, Voet P et al (2007) Dysphagia disorders in patients with cancer of the oropharynx are significantly affected by the radiation therapy dose to the superior and middle constrictor muscle: a dose-effect relationship. Radiother Oncol 85(1):64–73

Liem IH, Olmos RA, Balm AJ et al (1996) Evidence for early and persistent impairment of salivary gland excretion after irradiation of head and neck tumours. Eur J Nucl Med 23(11):1485–1490

Lindegaard JC, Grau C (2000) Has the outlook improved for amifostine as a clinical radioprotector? Radiother Oncol 57(2):113–118

List MA, D'Antonio LL, Cella DF et al. (1996) The Performance Status Scale for Head and Neck Cancer Patients and the Functional Assessment of Cancer Therapy-Head and Neck Scale. A study of utility and validity. Cancer 77(11): 2294–2301

List MA, Mumby P, Haraf D et al (1997) Performance and quality of life outcome in patients completing concomitant chemoradiotherapy protocols for head and neck cancer. Qual Life Res 6(3):274–284

List MA, Siston A, Haraf D et al (1999) Quality of life and performance in advanced head and neck cancer patients on concomitant chemoradiotherapy: a prospective examination. J Clin Oncol 17(3):1020–1028

Litvan I, Sastry N, Sonies BC (1997) Characterizing swallowing abnormalities in progressive supranuclear palsy. Neurology 48(6):1654–1662

Liu RP, Fleming TJ, Toth BB et al. (1990) Salivary flow rates in patients with head and neck cancer 0.5 to 25 years after radiotherapy. Oral Surg Oral Med Oral Pathol 70(6):724–729

Logemann JA (1993) The dysphagia diagnostic procedure as a treatment efficacy trial. Clin Commun Disord 3(4):1–10

Logemann JA, Rademaker AW, Pauloski BR et al. (1998) Normal swallowing physiology as viewed by videofluoroscopy and videoendoscopy. Folia Phoniatr Logop 50(6):311–319

McConnel FM, O'Connor A (1994) Dysphagia secondary to head and neck cancer surgery. Acta Otorhinolaryngol Belg 48(2):165–170

McMillan AS, Pow EH, Kwong DL et al (2006) Preservation of quality of life after intensity-modulated radiotherapy for early-stage nasopharyngeal carcinoma: results of a prospective longitudinal study. Head Neck 28(8):712–722

Mittal BB, Pauloski BR, Haraf DJ et al. (2003) Swallowing dysfunction–preventative and rehabilitation strategies in patients with head-and-neck cancers treated with surgery, radiotherapy, and chemotherapy: a critical review. Int J Radiat Oncol Biol Phys 57(5):1219–1230

Murdoch-Kinch CA, Kim HM, Vineberg KA et al. (2008) Dose-effect relationships for the submandibular salivary glands and implications for their sparing by intensity modulated radiotherapy. Int J Radiat Oncol Biol Phys 72(2):373–382

Nagler RM (2001) Extended-term effects of head and neck irradiation in a rodent. Eur J Cancer 37(15):1938–1945

Nagler RM, Baum BJ, Fox PC (1993) Acute effects of X irradiation on the function of rat salivary glands. Radiat Res 136(1):42–47

Newman LA, Robbins KT, Logemann JA et al (2002) Swallowing and speech ability after treatment for head and neck cancer with targeted intraarterial versus intravenous chemoradiation. Head Neck 24(1):68–77

Newton HB, Newton C, Pearl D et al. (1994) Swallowing assessment in primary brain tumor patients with dysphagia. Neurology 44(10):1927–1932

Nguyen NP, Frank C, Moltz CC et al (2006) Aspiration rate following chemoradiation for head and neck cancer: an underreported occurrence. Radiother Oncol 80(3):302–306

Nguyen NP, Moltz CC, Frank C et al (2006) Dysphagia severity following chemoradiation and postoperative radiation for head and neck cancer. Eur J Radiol 59(3):453–459

Nguyen NP, Moltz CC, Frank C et al (2004) Dysphagia following chemoradiation for locally advanced head and neck cancer. Ann Oncol 15(3):383–388

Norberg LE, Lundquist PG (1989) Aspects of salivary gland radiosensitivity: effects of sialagogues and irradiation. Arch Otorhinolaryngol 246(4):200–204

O'Connell AC, Redman RS, Evans RL et al. (1999) Radiation-induced progressive decrease in fluid secretion in rat submandibular glands is related to decreased acinar volume and not impaired calcium signaling. Radiat Res 151(2):150–158

Paardekooper GM, Cammelli S, Zeilstra LJ et al. (1998) Radiation-induced apoptosis in relation to acute impairment of rat salivary gland function. Int J Radiat Biol 73(6):641–648

Pauloski BR, Logemann JA, Rademaker AW et al (1994) Speech and swallowing function after oral and oropharyngeal resections: one-year follow-up. Head Neck 16(4):313–322

Pauloski BR, Rademaker AW, Logemann JA et al (2002) Swallow function and perception of dysphagia in patients with head and neck cancer. Head Neck 24(6):555–565

Pauloski BR, Rademaker AW, Logemann JA et al (2006) Relationship between swallow motility disorders on videofluorography and oral intake in patients treated for head and neck cancer with radiotherapy with or without chemotherapy. Head Neck 28(12):1069–1076

Peter B, Van Waarde MA, Vissink A et al. (1995) The role of secretory granules in radiation-induced dysfunction of rat salivary glands. Radiat Res 141(2):176–182

Peters LJ, Ang KK, Thames HD Jr. (1988) Accelerated fractionation in the radiation treatment of head and neck cancer. A critical comparison of different strategies. Acta Oncol 27(2):185–194

Phillips TL, Kane L, Utley JF (1973) Radioprotection of tumor and normal tissues by thiophosphate compounds. Cancer 32(3):528–535

Poulsen MG, Riddle B, Keller J et al. (2008) Predictors of acute grade 4 swallowing toxicity in patients with stages III and IV squamous carcinoma of the head and neck treated with radiotherapy alone. Radiother Oncol 87(2):253–259

Pow EH, Kwong DL, McMillan AS et al. (2006) Xerostomia and quality of life after intensity-modulated radiotherapy vs. conventional radiotherapy for early-stage nasopharyngeal carcinoma: initial report on a randomized controlled clinical trial. Int J Radiat Oncol Biol Phys 66(4):981–991

Pratt NE, Sodicoff M (1972) Ultrastructural injury following x-irradiation of rat parotid gland acinar cells. Arch Oral Biol 17(8):1177–1186

Roesink JM, Konings AW, Terhaard CH et al. (1999) Preservation of the rat parotid gland function after radiation by prophylactic pilocarpine treatment: radiation dose dependency and compensatory mechanisms. Int J Radiat Oncol Biol Phys 45(2):483–489

Roesink JM, Moerland MA, Battermann JJ et al. (2001) Quantitative dose-volume response analysis of changes in parotid gland function after radiotherapy in the head-and-neck region. Int J Radiat Oncol Biol Phys 51(4):938–946

Roesink JM, Schipper M, Busschers W et al. (2005) A comparison of mean parotid gland dose with measures of parotid gland function after radiotherapy for head-and-neck cancer: implications for future trials. Int J Radiat Oncol Biol Phys 63(4):1006–1009

Saarilahti K, Kouri M, Collan J et al (2006) Sparing of the submandibular glands by intensity modulated radiotherapy in the treatment of head and neck cancer. Radiother Oncol 78(3):270–275

Semenenko VA, Li XA (2008) Lyman-Kutcher-Burman NTCP model parameters for radiation pneumonitis and xerostomia based on combined analysis of published clinical data. Phys Med Biol 53(3):737–755

Shannon IL, Trodahl JN, Starcke EN (1978) Radiosensitivity of the human parotid gland. Proc Soc Exp Biol Med 157(1):50–53

Ship JA, Fox PC, Baum BJ (1991) How much saliva is enough? "Normal" function defined. J Am Dent Assoc 122(3):63–69

Slonina D, Hoinkis C, Dorr W (2001) Effect of keratinocyte growth factor on radiation survival and colony size of human epidermal keratinocytes in vitro. Radiat Res 156 (6):761–766

Smith RV, Kotz T, Beitler JJ et al. (2000) Long-term swallowing problems after organ preservation therapy with concomitant radiation therapy and intravenous hydroxyurea: initial results. Arch Otolaryngol Head Neck Surg 126(3):384–389

Sonis ST, Peterson RL, Edwards LJ et al (2000) Defining mechanisms of action of interleukin-11 on the progression of radiation-induced oral mucositis in hamsters. Oral Oncol 36(4):373–381

Staar S, Rudat V, Stuetzer H et al. (2001) Intensified hyperfractionated accelerated radiotherapy limits the additional benefit of simultaneous chemotherapy–results of a multicentric randomized German trial in advanced head-and-neck cancer. Int J Radiat Oncol Biol Phys 50(5):1161–1171

Tanaka Y, Akagi K, Hasegawa T et al. (1983) [Studies on the radioprotective effects of YM-08310 (=WR-2721) Part 1: Radioprotective effects of YM-08310 on normal and malignant tissues in mice]. Nippon Igaku Hoshasen Gakkai Zasshi 43(5):700–709

Valdes Olmos RA, Keus RB, Takes RP et al. (1994) Scintigraphic assessment of salivary function and excretion response in radiation-induced injury of the major salivary glands. Cancer 73(12):2886–2893

Vissink A, 's-Gravenmade EJ, Ligeon EE et al. (1990) A functional and chemical study of radiation effects on rat parotid and submandibular/sublingual glands. Radiat Res 124(3):259–265

Vissink A, Down JD, Konings AW (1992) Contrasting dose-rate effects of gamma-irradiation on rat salivary gland function. Int J Radiat Biol 61(2):275–282

Vissink A, Kalicharan D, Gravenmade EJ et al (1991) Acute irradiation effects on morphology and function of rat submandibular glands. J Oral Pathol Med 20(9):449–456

Warde P, O'Sullivan B, Aslanidis J et al. (2002) A Phase III placebo-controlled trial of oral pilocarpine in patients undergoing radiotherapy for head-and-neck cancer. Int J Radiat Oncol Biol Phys 54(1):9–13

Washburn LC, Rafter JJ, Hayes RL (1976) Prediction of the effective radioprotective dose of WR-2721 in humans through an interspecies tissue distribution study. Radiat Res 66(1):100–105

Witterick IJ, Gullane PJ, Yeung E (1995) Outcome analysis of Zenker's diverticulectomy and cricopharyngeal myotomy. Head Neck 17(5):382–388

Wu CH, Hsiao TY, Ko JY et al. (2000) Dysphagia after radiotherapy: endoscopic examination of swallowing in patients with nasopharyngeal carcinoma. Ann Otol Rhinol Laryngol 109(3):320–325

Wu Q, Manning M, Schmidt-Ullrich R et al. (2000) The potential for sparing of parotids and escalation of biologically effective dose with intensity-modulated radiation treatments of head and neck cancers: a treatment design study. Int J Radiat Oncol Biol Phys 46(1):195–205

Yu CL, Fielding R, Chan CL (2003) The mediating role of optimism on post-radiation quality of life in nasopharyngeal carcinoma. Qual Life Res 12(1):41–51

Yuhas JM, Spellman JM, Culo F (1980) The role of WR-2721 in radiotherapy and/or chemotherapy. Cancer Clin Trials 3(3):211–216

Zeilstra LJ, Vissink A, Konings AW et al. (2000) Radiation induced cell loss in rat submandibular gland and its relation to gland function. Int J Radiat Biol 76(3):419–429

Head and Neck Cancer Quality of Life Instruments

21

MARCY A. LIST

CONTENTS

21.1   Introduction   *243*

21.2   Definition of QOL   *244*

21.3   Available Tools for Measurement of QOL   *244*
21.3.1   Generic Measures   *244*
21.3.2   Cancer-Specific Measures   *245*
21.3.3   HNC-Specific Measures   *245*

21.4   Challenges in HNC QOL Assessment and Interpretation   *246*

21.5   Choosing Measures and Assessment Schedules   *247*
21.5.1   Schedule of Assessments   *247*

21.6   Summary   *248*

References   *248*

KEY POINTS

- Quality of life (QOL) may be defined as the patient's perception of the impact of illness and/or treatment across multiple dimensions.
- There are currently a wide range of QOL instruments available to researchers and clinicians and the measure selected for use in a given study should be based on the purpose of the assessment.
- Available QOL tools for head and neck cancer (HNC) range from general to cancer-specific to those designed to specifically measure the effects of HNC and its treatment.

MARCY A. LIST, PhD
University of Chicago, Cancer Research Center, 5841 S Maryland, MC 1140, Chicago, IL 60637, USA

- QOL assessment is labor-intensive and requires careful attention to, and analysis of, missing data.
- Recent QOL research has suggested guidelines for interpretation of QOL differences in terms of clinical relevance.
- Future research is needed to explore how QOL might be useful clinically for an individual patient as well as to calculate instrument-specific standardized scores that would in turn provide for easier comparison across measures and studies.

21.1

Introduction

Treatment end points for patients with malignant disease have historically been reflected by objective tumor response, overall survival, and/or disease-free survival. However, over the past three decades, with the introduction of multimodality treatments and the increasing number of cancer survivors, has come the growing awareness and concern for the psychosocial needs of patients with cancer. The loss of health and/or the consequences of treatment can result in physical or functional impairment, disruption of social and family interactions, and psychological distress, all of which affect quality of life (QOL). As a result, health-care interventions must be judged not only by their impact on survival, but also on QOL. Extending survival does not always correlate with improvements in QOL, and conversely, specific treatments may not necessarily prolong life but may enhance its quality. Understanding the patient's perception of his/her disease, and its treatment and symptoms, is critical to comprehensive cancer care, patient education, and the informed evaluation of therapeutic options.

For patients with head and neck cancer (HNC) in particular, appreciation of the full impact of the disease and its treatment is critical. Because the majority of patients with HNC are diagnosed with advanced stage disease, treatment tends to be aggressive with significant acute and long-term effects. Both the disease and the consequences of therapy interfere with basic human functions, including eating, speaking, and breathing. Such impairment has a marked influence on day-to-day activities and QOL.

21.2
Definition of QOL

Quality of life (QOL) may be defined as the *patient's perception* of the impact of illness and/or treatment. Note that, while we will refer to QOL throughout the chapter, the focus is on health-related QOL, not other aspects of the individual's circumstances. There are two fundamental premises of QOL:

- Multidimensionality, the concept that QOL encompasses a broad range of domains
- Subjectivity, the notion that two people may have substantially different reactions to a similar disability

These two elements distinguish QOL assessment from standard toxicity ratings or global functional ratings (e.g., the Karnofsky scale of performance status). Both standard toxicity ratings and global functional ratings are assessed by the health-care provider rather than by the patient, and only one area of functioning is described (e.g., somatic symptoms or performance). QOL differs from other traditional treatment end points such as response rate or survival in that it changes over time because of a variety of conditions and events. As a result, the general strategy of QOL evaluation is to examine these changes over the course of the disease and its treatment.

While specific definitions vary, QOL is generally considered to include at least three, and often four, domains (Cella 1997, 1998; Schipper and Levitt 1985; Schipper et al. 1996):

- Physical/somatic (e.g., pain, nausea, and fatigue)
- Functional (e.g., energy level, and activities of daily living)
- Social (e.g., maintenance of relationships with family and friends)
- Psychological/emotional (e.g., mood, anxiety, and depression)

As discussed in the next section with respect to measures, one must also distinguish between symptoms and symptom measures, and true QOL measures. The former, while reflecting the patient's experience, are limited to perceptions of specific physical sensations in contrast to QOL measures, which seek to obtain a comprehensive, multidimensional representation of the patient's overall perceived state. While the relationship between symptoms, function, and QOL is not always direct, symptoms may affect QOL and QOL measures often incorporate questions about symptoms.

21.3
Available Tools for Measurement of QOL

There are currently a wide range of QOL instruments available to researchers and clinicians, and the measure selected for use in a given study should be based on the purpose of the assessment. In general, QOL measures can be categorized as generic measures (i.e., applicable across diseases), or specific measures, which are disease-, site-, and treatment-modality-specific. The sections below briefly describe a number of the more frequently used measures in HNC evaluation. A recent review by Tschiesner et al. (2008) presents a content comparison of QOL measures based on the international classification of functioning, disability, and health. This analysis presents differences among measures and thus might assist with questionnaire interpretation or selection. Illustrative recent reviews of patient-reported outcome measures in HNC include a paper by Pusic et al. (2007), which focuses on surgery, and a broad review of QOL research in HNC by Murphy et al. (2006).

21.3.1
Generic Measures

Generic measures are useful if one is interested in comparing a cohort of HNC patients to groups of other, noncancer patients. Frequently used instruments include the medical outcomes study 36-item short form (MOS SF-36) (Ware and Sherbourne 1992) and the psychosocial adjustment to illness scale-self report (PAIS-SR) (Derogatis 1986) which evaluates a patient's overall adjustment to their illness. With questions such as "has your overall health significantly increased or decreased over the past month?" and "can you walk up a flight of stairs?" the use of a general health measure can capture the patient's opinion of whether the disease has substantially affected their overall physical and emotional health.

21.3.2
Cancer-Specific Measures

A second level of information can be obtained using measures that are specific to cancer, with the two most frequently used tools being the functional assessment of cancer therapy (FACT-G) (CELLA 1997; CELLA et al. 1993) and the European Organization for Research and Treatment of Cancer Quality of Life Questionnaire Core 30 Items (EORTC QLQ-30) (AARONSON et al. 1993; BJORDAL et al. 1994). These instruments address global QOL as well as the multitude of ways in which cancer and cancer treatments can affect patients. For example, they include items related to symptoms such as nausea and vomiting, fatigue, relationships with family and friends, and the ability to work and do normal activities. In general, individual items are collapsed and summarized as domain scores, including but not limited to physical, emotional, functional, and social well-being or function. These cancer-specific instruments allow for comparison among patients with different types of cancers.

FACT-G, now in version 4, is a 27-item compilation of questions divided into four primary domains: physical well-being, social/family well-being, emotional well-being, and functional well-being. It takes about 5 minutes to complete and has been well validated (CELLA et al. 1993). Using global rating of change scale as an anchor, CELLA et al. (2002b) have proposed that a clinically meaningful change corresponds to a total FACT-G raw score in the range of 5–7 points.

EORTC-QLQ-C30 (most current is version 3.0) is a 30-item questionnaire grouped into five functional subscales (role, physical, cognitive, emotional, and social functioning). In addition, there are three multi-item symptom scales (fatigue, pain, and nausea and vomiting), individual questions concerning common symptoms in cancer patients, and two questions assessing overall QOL (AARONSON et al. 1993). It takes about 10–15 min to complete. WYRWICH et al. (2005) suggest that for the total QOL and other QOL domains the difference between pretreatment and follow-up scores can be categorized into clinically significant improvement (positive difference > standard error of measurement), clinically significant

deterioration (negative difference < the standard error of measurement), and no change (difference fails to meet either criteria).

As noted by PUSIC et al. (2007), it is important to recognize that these various instruments are not interchangeable; although they all measure some aspect of QOL, they provide different information. As an example, one study administered both the QLQ-C30 and the FACT-G to 244 patients with breast cancer or Hodgkin lymphoma (KEMMLER et al. 1999). The two questionnaires covered markedly different aspects of QOL, and the overlap was not substantial enough to permit a direct comparison between the two instruments.

21.3.3
HNC-Specific Measures

Most cancers and cancer treatments have side effects, symptoms, and/or residual effects that are disease (e.g., swallowing related to HNC or lymphadema related to breast cancer) and/or modality (e.g., radiation-related side effects) specific. This section lists and describes a number of the most frequently used HNC-specific measures, whose reliability and validity have been well documented. The reader is referred to the reviews cited above for additional instruments.

FACT – Head and Neck (FACT-H&N) consists of the FACT-G, to which an 11-item site-specific, HNC subscale is added. The HN subscale evaluates the unique concerns of patients with HNC (e.g., swallowing, chewing) (LIST et al. 1996a, D'ANTONIO et al. 1996).

EORTC QLQ H&N35. A head and neck cancer module (H&N35) was designed to be used in conjunction with the QLQ-C30 (BJORDAL et al. 1994). This scale includes items assessing symptoms and side effects relevant to patients with HNC, and appears to be sensitive to temporal changes before, during, and after treatment with surgery, radiation therapy (RT), and chemotherapy (BJORDAL et al. 1999).

University of Washington. The University of Washington QOL (UW-QOL) questionnaire is a self-administered scale consisting of 15 questions assessing nine domains including pain, physical appearance, activity, recreation, employment, chewing, swallowing, speech, shoulder function, and overall QOL (HASSAN and WEYMULLER 1993). One study of 29 patients undergoing resection of oral cancer compared the EORTC QLQ H&N35 with the UW-QOL (ROGERS et al. 1998). The two scales were found to be complementary rather than duplicative. The authors concluded that although the UW-QOL provided less specific information compared with the EORTC QLQ H&N35, it was shorter and easier to use.

University of Michigan Head and Neck Quality-of-Life-Questionnaire (HNQOLQ). The HNQOLQ is a 20-item 5-point Likert questionnaire that was designed specifically to address problems incurred by patients with HNC. Items are summarized to generate four QOL domains: pain, communication, eating, and emotional well-being (TERRELL et al. 1997, 1998). Global symptoms, disability attributable to HNC and response to treatment are also assessed.

As previously discussed, in addition to the above measures which have a reasonably broad global QOL focus, there are a number of more targeted modality- (e.g., radiation) and/or symptom-specific measures (e.g., xerostomia, dysphagia). The following list illustrates some of these instruments.

FACT Head and Neck Symptom Index (FHNSI). The FHNSI is a recently developed ten-item more targeted symptom-focused approach to patient assessment. It was specifically designed to overcome some of the perceived barriers (resources, difficulties in interpretation described below) to incorporating longer multidimensional QOL measures in clinical practice. The FHNSI is composed of items extracted from the FACT H&N (CELLA et al. 2003). Comparison with full administration of the FACT H&N documented that the FHNSI is a reliable and valid symptom index, which can be administered alone or scored using items embedded within the FACT H&N (YOUNT et al. 2007).

QOL-RT instrument. A head and neck module has been developed for the QOL-RT instrument to more specifically address issues related to RT in patients with HNC (TROTTI et al. 1998). This instrument evaluates the impact of treatment on mucus production, saliva, taste, cough, and local pain.

The Head and Neck Radiotherapy Questionnaire. This is a patient-rated tool that was designed to measure early treatment-related effects in patients undergoing RT for HNC (BROWMAN et al. 1993). It consists of 22 questions that cover symptoms related to six domains: oral cavity, throat, skin, digestive function, energy, and psychosocial function.

Dysphagia-specific QOL instrument. The MD Anderson dysphagia inventory (MDADI) is a validated, self-administered questionnaire designed specifically to evaluate the impact of treatment-related dysphagia on QOL (CHEN et al. 2001). This instrument includes global, emotional, functional, and physical subscales.

Voice-related QOL measure. The voice-related QOL measure (V-RQOL) is a ten-item, self-administered validated voice outcome measure (HOGIKYAN and SETHURAMAN 1999). Scores are reported in two domains: social-emotional and physical-functioning, and a total score, all ranging from 1 to 100. A higher score indicates better voice-related QOL.

The University of Michigan Xerostomia-Related QOL Scale. This scale, which consists of 15 items, was developed to assess the impact of salivary gland dysfunction and xerostomia on four major domains of oral health-related QOL – physical functioning, personal/psychological functioning, social functioning, and pain/discomfort issues (HENSEN et al. 2001).

While it is presented here as a frequently used measure, it is important to note that the Performance Status Scale is not technically a QOL instrument. It was developed as a functional measure, similar to the Karnofsy and is rated by the interviewer.

Performance Status Scale. The Performance Status Scale for Head and Neck Cancer (PSS-HN) consists of three subscales: normalcy of diet, understandability of speech, and eating in public (LIST et al. 1990, 1996a, b). The interviewer rates the patient on each scale based on his or her response to targeted questions. Scores on each subscale range from 0 to 100, with higher scores indicating better performance. The PSS-HN has demonstrated good interrater reliability, sensitivity to changes over time (e.g., before, during, and posttreatment), and differences related to broad functional categories (LIST et al. 1996a).

21.4

Challenges in HNC QOL Assessment and Interpretation

QOL of life assessment and interpretation present many challenges to both clinicians and researchers. Practical barriers include time and resource constraints. Collection of patient-reported outcomes is extremely labor-intensive and, in contrast to traditional outcomes such as survival and/or disease-free survival, missing data (e.g., a missed assessment) cannot be retrieved. Assessing patterns, and controlling for missing data in analytic methods is critical. Interpreting QOL data in both the aggregate (e.g., group means and comparisons) as well as with respect to an individual patient is not always straightforward or obvious. The clinical meaningfulness of specific scores and differences, and the translation of

QOL data into treatment decisions (GILL and FEINSTEIN 1994; TAYLOR et al. 1996; MORRIS et al. 1998; BROWMAN 1999) are areas of current research. Differences in design across studies, in terms of measures used and time points assessed, make cross study comparisons difficult. HNC is a heterogeneous disease for which historically there has been considerable variability in approach to treatment both across and within modalities as well as fewer randomized trials. Recent years have seen a shift towards more conservative surgeries, more targeted RT techniques, and new chemoradiation therapy combinations including biologics. Thus, current outcomes may not be reflected in existing data.

In an effort to assist in the interpretation of QOL scores, a number of guidelines have been proposed (CELLA et al. 2002a). Investigators have begun to examine commonly used measurement tools to define changes in scores that are clinically significant or meaningful, that is, differences in scores that patients perceive as different and/or that are associated with differences on other parameters.

21.5
Choosing Measures and Assessment Schedules

Choice of measure will depend on the question being asked (e.g., comparing the specific effects of different radiation treatment regimens, a comprehensive assessment of the broad range of potential symptoms and side effects of a new treatment) and available resources. For instance, investigators at the University of Chicago have focused clinically on the refinement of chemoradiotherapy regimens for locoregionally advanced HNC patients. The purpose of the accompanying QOL research has been to examine both the acute and long-term effects of each of these regimens, for patient education as well as to inform the next iteration of trials (LIST et al. 1996b, 1999). This goal has necessitated a rather comprehensive assessment with longitudinal follow-up. Patients enrolled on specific protocols are assessed pretreatment, on-treatment, and at several time points posttreatment. Assessment includes overall QOL (FACT-G), HNC-specific functional status (PSS-HN eating, speaking, and socializing), HNC-specific symptoms (FACT H&N subscale), overall performance status (Karnofsky performance status scale), the specific effects of radiation therapy (RTQ), and a depression screen (CES-D). The entire assessment takes 10–20 min/assessment point.

21.5.1
Schedule of Assessments

The schedule of assessments is also dependent on the research question of interest. Because HNC patients may present with comorbidities related to alcohol abuse and because studies have shown that pretreatment QOL is the best predictor of posttreatment QOL (LIST et al. 1999; HAMMERLID and TAFT 2001; DE GRAEFF et al. 2000), the collection of baseline data is imperative. Posttreatment, the question of how often to assess patients requires striking a balance between the desire to closely track changes in patients' QOL over time and the financial, personnel, and analytic burdens of assessing patients too frequently. Studies often assess patients at baseline and the end of treatment, and then 1, 6, 12, and 24 months following treatment. Figure 21.1 below presents a schematic example of how the longitudinal collection of QOL data can be vital to truly differentiating the effect of two different types of treatments.

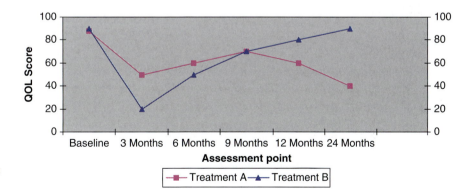

Fig. 21.1. QOL assessment schedule

In this illustration, the different lines represent different treatment arms. The QOL scores are shown on the *Y*-axis while the time since treatment is shown on the *X*-axis. At baseline groups have similar QOL scores; during treatment patients receiving treatment B show a more profound decline in QOL and by 6 months both groups have returned to about 50% of pretreatment levels. If one had stopped following patients at 3 months, however, one might have concluded that treatment B had more residual toxicity. If stopped at 6 months, treatments would have been considered equivalent. At 12 months it is beginning to appear that treatment B patients are doing better and at 24 months, treatment B patients have returned to their pretreatment levels while those receiving treatment A are declining.

21.6
Summary

While the past 5 years have shown many advances in the field of HNC QOL research, there are still a number of continued challenges that command attention. Mean QOL scores, that is, group averages, are adequate and sufficient for between-treatment comparisons. The extent to which, and how, the same data might be useful clinically for an individual patient, for example, to assist in decision-making is a relatively uncharted area of investigation. From a methodologic perspective, efforts are underway to calculate instrument-specific standardized scores that would in turn provide for easier comparison across measures and studies. Continued and expanded application of QOL data to the design of psychosocial or other interventions is now necessary and warranted.

References

Aaronson NK, Ahmedzai S, Bergman B et al. (1993) The European Organization for Research and Treatment of Cancer QLQ-C30: a quality-of-life instrument for use in international clinical trials in oncology. J Natl Cancer Inst 85:365–376
Bjordal K, Ahlner-Elmqvist M, Tollesson E et al. (1994) Development of a European Organization for Research and Treatment of Cancer (EORTC) questionnaire module to be used in quality of life assessments in head and neck cancer patients. EORTC Quality of Life Study Group. Acta Oncol 33:879–885

Bjordal K, Hammerlid E, Ahlner-Elmqvist M et al. (1999) Quality of life in head and neck cancer patients: validation of the European Organization for Research and Treatment of Cancer quality of life questionnaire-H&N35. J Clin Oncol 17:1008–1019
Browman GP (1999) Science, language, intuition, and the many meanings of quality of life. J Clin Oncol 17:1651–1653
Browman GP, Levine MN, Hodson DI et al. (1993) The head and neck radiotherapy questionnaire: a morbidity/quality-of-life instrument for clinical trials of radiation therapy in locally advanced head and neck cancer. J Clin Oncol 11:863–872
Cella D (1997, November) F.A.C.I.T. manual: manual of the functional assessment of chronic illness therapy (FACIT) scales – version 4. Center on Outcomes, Research and Education, Evanston Northwestern Hospital Health Care and Northwestern University, Evanston, IL
Cella D (1998) Quality of life. In: Holland J (ed) Psychooncology. Oxford University Press, New York, pp 1135–1146
Cella D, Bullinger M, Scott C et al. (2002a) Group vs individual approaches to understanding the clinical significance of differences or changes in quality of life. Mayo Clin Proc 77:384–392
Cella D, Hahn EA, Dineen K (2002b) Meaningful change in cancer-specific quality of life scores: differences between improvement and worsening. Qual Life Res 11:207–221
Cella D, Paul D, Yount S et al. (2003) What are the most important symptom targets when treating advanced cancer? A survey of providers in the National Comprehensive Cancer Network (NCCN). Cancer Invest 4:526–535
Cella DF, Tulsky DS, Gray G et al. (1993) The functional assessment of cancer therapy (FACT) scale: development and validation of the general measure. J Clin Oncol 11:570–579
Chen AY, Frankowski R, Bishop-Leone J et al. (2001) The development and validation of a dysphagia-specific quality-of-life questionnaire for patients with head and neck cancer: the M. D. Anderson dysphagia inventory. Arch Otolaryngol Head Neck Surg 127:870–876
D'Antonio LL, Zimmerman GJ, Cella DF, et al. (1996) Quality of life and functional status measures in patients with head and neck cancer. Arch Otolaryngol Head Neck Surg 122:482–487
de Graeff A, de Leeuw JR, Ros WJ et al. (2000) Long-term quality of life of patients with head and neck cancer. Laryngoscope 110:98–106
Derogatis LR (1986) The psychosocial adjustment to illness scale (PAIS). J Psychosom Res 30:77–91
Gill TM, Feinstein AR (1994) A critical appraisal of the quality of quality-of-life measurements. JAMA 272:619–626
Hammerlid E, Taft C (2001) Health-related quality of life in long-term head and neck cancer survivors: a comparison with general population norms. Br J Cancer 84:149–156
Hassan SJ, Weymuller EA, Jr (1993) Assessment of quality of life in head and neck cancer patients. Head Neck 15:485–496
Hensen BS, Inglehart MR, Eisbruch A et al. (2001). Preserved salivary output and xerostomia-related quality of life in head and neck cancer patients receiving parotid-sparing radiotherapy. Oral Oncol 37:84–93
Hogikyan ND, Sethuraman G (1999) Validation of an instrument to measure voice-related quality of life (V-RQOL). J Voice 13:557–569

Kemmler G, Holzner B, Kopp M et al. (1999) Comparison of two quality-of-life instruments for cancer patients: the functional assessment of cancer therapy-general and the European Organization for Research and Treatment of Cancer quality of life questionnaire-C30. J Clin Oncol 17:2932–2940

List MA, D'Antonio LL, Cella DF et al. (1996a) The performance status scale for head and neck cancer patients and the functional assessment of cancer therapy-head and neck scale. A study of utility and validity. Cancer 77:2294–2301

List MA, Ritter-Sterr C, Lansky SB (1990) A performance status scale for head and neck cancer patients. Cancer 66:564–569

List MA, Ritter-Sterr CA, Baker TM et al. (1996b) Longitudinal assessment of quality of life in laryngeal cancer patients. Head Neck 18:1–10

List MA, Siston A, Haraf D et al. (1999) Quality of life and performance in advanced head and neck cancer patients on concomitant chemoradiotherapy: a prospective examination. J Clin Oncol 17:1020–1028

Morris J, Perez D, McNoe B (1998) The use of quality of life data in clinical practice. Qual Life Res 7:85–91

Murphy BA, Ridner S, Wells N et al. (2006) Quality of life in head and neck cancer: a review of the current state of the science. Crit Rev Oncol Hematol 62:251–267

Pusic A, Liu JC, Chen CM et al. (2007) A systematic review of patient-reported outcome measures in head and neck cancer surgery. Otolaryngol Head Neck Surg 136:525–535

Rogers SN, Lowe D, Brown JS et al. (1998) A comparison between the University of Washington head and neck disease-specific measure and the medical short form 36, EORTC QOQ-C33 and EORTC head and neck 35. Oral Oncol 34:361–372

Schipper H, Levitt M (1985) Measuring quality of life: risks and benefits. Cancer Treat Rep 69:1115–1125

Schipper H, Clinch JJ, Olweny CLM (1996) Quality of life studies: definitions and conceptual issues. In: Spilker B (ed) Quality of life and pharmacoeconomics in clinical trials, 2nd edn. Lippincott-Raven, Philadelphia, pp 11–23

Taylor KM, Macdonald KG, Bezak A et al. (1996) Physicians' perspective on quality of life: an exploratory study of oncologists. Qual Life Res 5:5–14

Terrell JE, Fisher SG, Wolf GT (1998) Long-term quality of life after treatment of laryngeal cancer. Arch Otolaryngol Head Neck Surg 124:964–971

Terrell JE, Nanavati KA, Esclamado RM et al. (1997) Head and neck cancer-specific quality of life. Arch Otolaryngol Head Neck Surg 123:1125–1132

Trotti A, Johnson DJ, Gwede C et al. (1998) Development of a head and neck companion module for the quality of life-radiation therapy instrument (QOL-RTI). Int J Radiat Oncol Biol Phys 42:257–261

Tschiesner U, Rogers SN, Harréus U et al. (2008) Content comparison of quality of life questionnaires used in head and neck cancer based on the international classification of functioning, disability and health: a systematic review. Eur Arch Otorhinolaryngol 265:627–637

Ware JE, Jr, Sherbourne CD (1992) The MOS 36-item short-form health survey (SF-36). I. Conceptual framework and item selection. Med Care 30:473–483

Wyrwich KW, Bullinger M, Aaronson N et al. (2005) Estimating clinically significant differences in quality of life outcomes. Qual Life Res 14:285–295

Yount S, List M, Du H et al. (2007) A randomized validation study comparing embedded versus extracted FACT head and neck symptom index scores. Qual Life Res 16:1615–1626

Measuring and Reporting Toxicity

22

KENNETH JENSEN and CAI GRAU

CONTENTS

22.1   Introduction   251
22.1.1 Cause–Effect Chain   252

22.2   Methods for Measurement
        of Side Effects   252
22.2.1 Analytical End Points   253
22.2.2 Objective Signs   253
22.2.3 Observer-Scored Subjective
        Symptoms   253
22.2.4 Patient-Assessed Symptoms and
        Quality of Life   254

22.3   Comparison of Morbidity Measures   254

22.4   Reporting Toxicity   255

22.5   Conclusion   256

References   256

KEY POINTS

- Morbidity is as important as tumor effect when reporting and evaluating treatment result.
- Physical measures of local toxicity will often be the most specific measure of the effect of radiotherapy.
- Use accepted scoring systems.
- Use patient-based reporting of subjective end points.
- Observe for side effects sufficiently long to establish peak intensity, duration, recovery, or progression.

KENNETH JENSEN, MD, PhD
Department of Oncology, Aarhus University Hospital, Noerrebrogade 44, 8000 Aarhus C, Denmark
CAI GRAU, MD, DMSc, Professor
Department of Oncology, Aarhus University Hospital, Noerrebrogade 44, 8000 Aarhus C, Denmark

- Analyze and report using methods that take into account patients at risk and follow-up time.
- Report measures of cumulated toxicity.

22.1
Introduction

Advancements in radiotherapy come from improvements in the therapeutic ratio – the relationship between tumor effect and morbidity. Survival and local control are well defined and consensus exists on the proper analysis and reporting. On the other hand, side effects are often difficult to quantify and no consensus exists on analysis or reporting. Toxicity of multimodality treatment is increasingly complex to register, analyze, and report because the number of potential side effects is virtual infinite.

Physical measures of morbidity are seldom used and frequently are not very relevant to the patient. Semiquantitative measures are frequently used in the form of toxicity scoring systems. These systems are not validated and are often scored by an observer other than the patient, in spite of data that show observer-based scoring to be inferior to patient-based ratings of subjective symptoms (see below). Patient-based questionnaires exist that can be used to quantify subjective side effects. These instruments are often well validated and also provide measures of the overall consequences of disease and treatment. Nevertheless, data from patient-based questionnaires are often difficult to interpret and the correlation with clinically observable or measurable changes is not straightforward.

Data on morbidity are needed to compare different treatment strategies. Furthermore, the demand for morbidity data are increasing as quantitative data on radiosensitivity and volume dependency are exploited for the purposes of improving patient care with treatments that promise to increase normal tissue sparing and provide more treatment options.

Strategies for measurement and reporting of specific toxicities will not be provided in this chapter, but a general discussion and some examples illustrating the challenges and possibilities will be given.

22.1.1
Cause–Effect Chain

The molecular changes induced by radiotherapy may induce changes in organ function that are measurable and quantifiable. The cause–effect relationship is presented in Fig. 22.1, which also illustrates the patient-relevance and specificity of the different measures of a side effect. Examples are mentioned in Table 22.1. Few side effects are physically measurable, and the physical measures that do exist are often of limited relevance to the patient. In most studies only one or few side effects can be selected for this kind of investigation because of resources. Changes in organ function may produce a physiologic sensation interpreted by the patient in a patient-specific context and subsequently reported by the patient as a symptom and this may lead to patient-specific influence on overall measures of health and well-being. The overall effects on the life of the patient is the most relevant measure of toxicity but at the same time dependent on many factors such as biological and psychological "reserve-capacity" and adaptation, and

Table 22.1. Examples of the end points of Fig. 22.1

End point	Example
Physical changes	Residues in the pyriform sinus
Symptoms	The swallowing scale of EORTC QLQ-H&N35
Observer-scored subjective symptoms	Dysphagia scale of CTCAE 3.0
Overall function	Social eating scale of EORTC QLQ-H&N35
Quality of life	Quality of life scale of EORTC QLQ-C30

is therefore not very specific to the radiation-induced damage of organs. This trade-off between patient-relevance and specificity has been described by BENTZEN et al. (2003). An example is radiotherapy-induced damage of the salivary glands leading to measurable decrease in salivary flow. The degree to which this is registered as dry mouth depends on prior salivary flow, dental status, and mucosal damage. A dry mouth can seriously impair a patient's ability to eat and speak and may have consequential effects for the patient's employment, financial possibilities, social life, and overall quality of life. Sometimes radiation induces damage to major salivary glands without giving rise to any clinically significant effects either because the submucous glands of the oral cavity have been preserved, leading to sufficient lubrication of the mucous membranes between meals, or because the patient has adapted and drinks plenty of water with his meals. In these cases, relatively few subjective symptoms and a limited impact on overall quality of life will be registered.

22.2
Methods for Measurement of Side Effects

Radiotherapy can affect organ function in ways that are physically measurable, e.g., changes of organ size, flow, and biomechanical properties, potentially leading to overall changes in function and overall well-being. The methods for measuring side effects must cover this range of consequences in order to give a comprehensive insight into the side effects of radiotherapy.

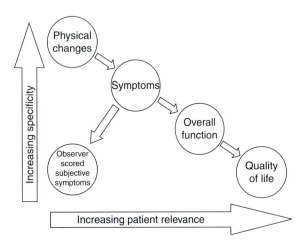

Fig. 22.1. Illustration of the cause–effect chain and the trade-off between relevance and specificity of different measures of side effects. Adapted from JENSEN (2007)

22.2.1
Analytical End Points

Generally, physical measurement using analytical end points should be carried out if a certain physiological effect or protection is aimed for, as it will establish the proof of principle with the greatest specificity and sensitivity. In the following, examples will be given on specific analytical end points. More unspecific end points measuring the overall strain from radiodiotherapy, such as body weight or albumin concentration in the blood, may also be highly relevant analytical end points.

Xerostomia is a clinically important end point and the parotid gland is a good example of a well-defined structure (the gland) with a well defined end point (saliva production), making it an ideal test case for volume sparing. Several relevant end points of salivary gland functions exist: whole mouth flow (NAVAZESH and CHRISTENSEN 1982) and gland-specific flow (JONES et al. 1996; TYLENDA et al. 1988). Gland-specific flow measurements are essential for establishing dose–volume–effect relationships, as other measures will depend on several variables. Irrespective of measurement methods, the inter- and intrasubject variations are high, especially for unstimulated flow (BURLAGE et al. 2005; NAVAZESH and CHRISTENSEN 1982). Comparing different methods of stimulation, ERICSON (1969) found only a moderate correlation. Regional assessment of salivary gland function using SPECT or PET and its correlation with radiation dose is an interesting research topic (BUUS et al. 2006; VAN ACKER et al. 2001). Since both subvolume and overall organ function can be measured directly, the dose–volume–effect relationship can theoretically be described without making any model assumptions.

Dysphagia is another clinically important end point. It is not reported as frequently as xerostomia, but might be of greater importance for health and quality of life (JENSEN et al. 2007b): Swallowing is a carefully orchestrated process depending on connective tissue, muscles, as well as motor- and sensory nerves. Changes in all involved structures and all processes have been described (HUGHES et al. 2000; LAZARUS 1993; PARISE et al. 2004; SHAKER et al. 2002; WU et al. 2000). The organ at risk for the development of dysphagia is a matter of debate (FENG et al. 2007; JENSEN et al. 2007a; LEVENDAG et al. 2007). No single organ or specific dysfunction has been shown to determine the overall swallowing process and the ability for protection of airways.

Swallowing is traditionally assessed using modified barium swallows (video-fluoroscopy (VF)). This method provides the observer with several quantitative measurements of speed and range of motion of the structures involved in the swallowing process as well as a quantitative estimate of residuals, penetration, and aspiration (LANGMORE 2003). Even though only semiquantitative measures are produced, functional endoscopic evaluation of swallowing (FEES) without or with sensory testing (FEESST) can also be used to assess swallowing objectively (AVIV 2000; AVIV et al. 2000; WU et al. 1997). It does not produce direct information on the oropharyngeal phase of swallowing but this type of information can be assessed indirectly. Furthermore, the method gives information on the sensitivity of the throat and aspiration of saliva. It is less costly to perform than VF and does not expose the patient to ionizing radiation (LANGMORE 2003; WU et al. 1997).

Thus, measuring specific organ functions is a difficult but important research area in that it allows us to gain knowledge on the etiology of side effects and relationship with radiotherapy.

22.2.2
Objective Signs

Semiquantitative, more or less arbitrary objective assessment scales, such as those assessing change from absent to severe, are available for a variety of end points. Several classical radiobiological end points belong to this category: fibrosis, atrophy, and mucositis. These signs are often scored using large manuals published by corporative groups (see below). Interpretation of auditory-evoked potentials (GRAU et al. 1992), speech (PAULOSKI et al. 1998), and cognitive changes (CHEUNG et al. 2000) are other examples of semi-quantitative objective end points relevant for research in side effects after radiotherapy.

22.2.3
Observer-Scored Subjective Symptoms

Systems for quantitatively scoring subjective and objective morbidity have been developed and are continuously evolving: Dische (DISCHE et al. 1989), WHO (MILLER et al. 1981), NCIC-CTG, EORTC/RTOG SOMA-LENT (COX et al. 1995; PAVY et al. 1995; RUBIN et al. 1995), DAHANCA (OVERGAARD et al. 2003), and CTCAE (TROTTI et al. 2003) are examples of authors or organizations that have included subjective symptoms in their scoring systems. These manuals contain an abundance of graded end points. They are constructed by consensus and rarely validated against other end points. Most scales have an observer-based scoring of symptom intensity or treatment of a given side effect. Most of our available knowledge of subjective side effects after radiotherapy is based on such systems, as they are relatively simple, fast, and inexpensive to use. The scoring systems have repeatedly been shown to be sensitive enough to detect differences in toxicity dependent on factors such as volume (JENSEN et al. 2007c), acceleration (SKLADOWSKI et al. 2006), fractionation (DISCHE et al. 1997), and concomitant chemotherapy (DENIS et al. 2003). Although grade III–IV morbidity seems to be the standard unit for reporting morbidity, irrespective of end point and scoring systems, the different scoring systems have only limited correlation with each other and cannot be used interchangeably (DENIS et al. 2003). Furthermore, many studies are underpowered to detect clinically relevant differences in occurrence of the relatively rare grade III and IV end points and other measures of cumulated toxicity should be therefore be applied (see below) (BENTZEN and TROTTI 2007). This is especially the case if treatment arms in a randomized study have qualitatively different important side effects.

Despite their weaknesses, toxicity should be scored according to generally accepted scoring systems because uniformity in the reporting of side effects strongly increases the value of data.

22.2.4
Patient-Assessed Symptoms and Quality of Life

Patient-assessed symptoms and quality of life are generally assessed by questionnaires. Several patient-administered, well-validated questionnaires exist. Cancer (AARONSON et al. 1993; BJORDAL et al. 1999; CELLA et al. 1993), head and neck (BJORDAL et al. 1999; D'ANTONIO et al. 1996; HASSAN and WEYMULLER 1993) as well as symptom-specific questionnaires (CHEN et al. 2001; HENSON et al. 2001) are available. The questionnaires provide information on overall measures of well-being and function, as well as very specific symptoms. As for observer-assessed morbidity, the key issue is to pick a well-validated measurement tool, well known to the scientific community. Two methods for measurement should not be expected

to produce comparable scores just because the name of their scales might be identical (ALLENBY et al. 2002; VELIKOVA et al. 2004).

22.3
Comparison of Morbidity Measures

Comparison of different end points can best be done if a gold standard exists. The gold standard for subjective end points is patient-assessed side effect. Observers other than the patient tend to underestimate both the frequency and degree of subjective side effects compared with patients themselves (Fig. 22.2).

Underestimation is probably not only a question of experience or training but an inherent problem. STEPHENS et al. (1997) compared physician ratings with patient-assessed symptoms using the Rotterdam Symptom Checklist in two randomized controlled trials. Physicians generally underestimated symptoms, but the degree of underestimation varied greatly between symptoms and between studies (treatment modality), but did not vary with the number of patients seen per center, indicating that training was not the reason for underestimation. An interesting finding was that concordance decreased as patient-reported symptom intensity increased. Quality of life data have impact on the interpretation of trial results. Data can be retrieved without insurmountable problems using methods such as a touch screens in the patient waiting areas. Therefore, physician-based scoring of subjective symptoms can mainly be justified by arguments of resources since it has inferior specificity and sensitivity.

Different methods for measuring toxicity do not always correlate and one measure can not be substituted with another: In CTCAE "objective" xerostomia is measured with whole mouth unstimulated flow as unstimulated flow (lubrication of the oral cavity between meals) is thought to be the best predictor of xerostomia. Nevertheless, the available data only partly support this simplistic correlation between salivary gland function and xerostomia (AMOSSON et al. 2003; EISBRUCH et al. 2001; JELLEMA et al. 2005; PARLIAMENT et al. 2004; ROESINK et al. 2005). When comparing other objective and subjective symptoms similar problems are observed: Objective assessment of cognitive function and sedation, using Mini Mental State Examination and

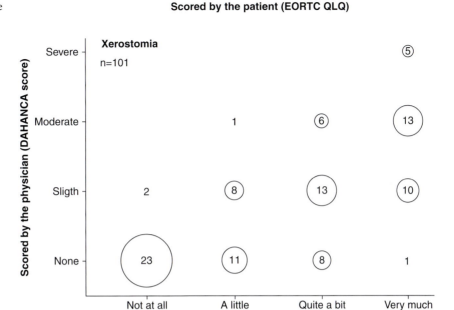

Fig. 22.2. The concordance between observer and patient-assessed xerostomia in head and neck cancer patients. The size of the circles represents the number of patients. From JENSEN et al. (2006)

Alertness/Sedation scale, were not correlated with self-reported cognitive function of the EORTC questionnaire in 29 palliative patients. Patient-reported swallowing problems have been compared with the findings of FEES, dental problems with a dental examination, and xerostomia with saliva flow in 35 pharynx cancer survivors (JENSEN et al. 2007b). A significant correlation for all end points was found, but patient-reported toxicity predicted observable morbidity with variable sensitivity and specificity. The correlation between physiological changes, symptoms, and a detrimental effect on quality of life is substantiated by the literature for many end points, but one measurement of a term of the cause–effect chain cannot be replaced by another. Correlation is not equality.

22.4
Reporting Toxicity

Local control and survival as well as side effects must be quantified in clinical studies to provide the scientific community with a relevant impression of clinical benefit. Not only must the relevant end points of morbidity be quantified and registered, but the data must also be analyzed and presented in a relevant manner. Side effects after radiotherapy often develop years after the end of therapy and measures of toxicity must therefore take both time and patients at risk into account in that patients often continue to be at risk of late toxicities (JUNG et al. 2001). Actuarial analysis has been suggested to be the method of choice for analyzing and reporting late effects because incidence measures underestimate the true risk of toxicity (DENIS et al. 2003, 2004). It is definitely the recommended method for irreversible end points such as telangiectasia and intestinal stenosis (BENTZEN et al. 1995). Nevertheless, some acute and late toxicities, such as xerostomia and perhaps skin fibrosis, are at least partially reversible, and therefore are not suited for actuarial analysis. In such situations, prevalence measures are the preferred end point (Fig. 22.3, data from JENSEN et al. (2007c)).

To compare treatments with different toxicity profiles, some measure of the overall strain on the patient is needed: Weight loss, number of patients finishing at planned time of finishing all treatment cycles, quality of life, and number of grade 3 and 4 events at any given time are previously used relevant measures. Adding the number of high-grade events has been further developed into the TAME concept (TROTTI et al. 2007). This system is potentially useful but has some unsolved problems with differences in interpretability depending on outcome and the quality of follow-up (GRAU et al. 2007).

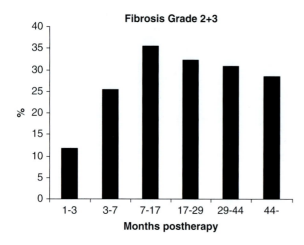

Fig. 22.3. Fibrosis in 139 patients with pharynx cancer

22.5
Conclusion

To gain the full benefit of the possibilities of more conformal radiotherapy, more specific morbidity data must be collected with the best available methods to gain information on dose and volume dependency. At the same time, radiotherapy is more often combined with other treatments. Each modality has its unique morbidity profile and new side effects will arise as a consequence of the combination of modalities. This poses new demands for methods that assess the overall strain on the patient and at the same time is adaptable and sensitive enough to allow registration of unexpected specific toxicities. All information must be collected prospectively and interpreted in the light of duration, progression, or reversibility. These challenges raise a number of important scientific and logistical questions that await an answer.

References

Aaronson NK, Ahmedzai S, Bergman B et al. (1993) The European Organization for Research and Treatment of Cancer QLQ-C30: a quality-of-life instrument for use in international clinical trials in oncology. J Natl Cancer Inst 85(5):365–376

Allenby A, Matthews J, Beresford J et al. (2002) The application of computer touch-screen technology in screening for psychosocial distress in an ambulatory oncology setting. Eur J Cancer Care (Engl) 11(4):245–253

Amosson CM, Teh BS, Van TJ et al. (2003) Dosimetric predictors of xerostomia for head-and-neck cancer patients treated with the smart (simultaneous modulated accelerated radiation therapy) boost technique. Int J Radiat Oncol Biol Phys 56(1):136–144

Aviv JE (2000) Prospective, randomized outcome study of endoscopy versus modified barium swallow in patients with dysphagia. Laryngoscope 110(4):563–574

Aviv JE, Kaplan ST, Thomson JE et al. (2000) The safety of flexible endoscopic evaluation of swallowing with sensory testing (FEESST): an analysis of 500 consecutive evaluations. Dysphagia 15(1):39–44

Bentzen SM, Dorr W, Anscher MS et al. (2003) Normal tissue effects: reporting and analysis. Semin Radiat Oncol 13(3):189–202

Bentzen SM, Trotti A (2007) Evaluation of early and late toxicities in chemoradiation trials. J Clin Oncol 25(26):4096–4103

Bentzen SM, Vaeth M, Pedersen DE et al. (1995) Why actuarial estimates should be used in reporting late normal-tissue effects of cancer treatment... now! Int J Radiat Oncol Biol Phys 32(5):1531–1534

Bjordal K, Hammerlid E, Ahlner-Elmqvist M et al. (1999) Quality of life in head and neck cancer patients: validation of the European Organization for Research and Treatment of Cancer Quality of Life Questionnaire-H&N35. J Clin Oncol 17(3):1008–1019

Burlage FR, Pijpe J, Coppes RP et al. (2005) Variability of flow rate when collecting stimulated human parotid saliva. Eur J Oral Sci 113(5):386–390

Buus S, Grau C, Munk OL et al. (2006) Individual radiation response of parotid glands investigated by dynamic 11C-methionine PET. Radiother Oncol 78(3):262–269

Cella DF, Tulsky DS, Gray G et al. (1993) The functional assessment of cancer therapy scale: development and validation of the general measure. J Clin Oncol 11(3):570–579

Chen AY, Frankowski R, Bishop-Leone J et al. (2001) The development and validation of a dysphagia-specific quality-of-life questionnaire for patients with head and neck cancer: the M. D. Anderson dysphagia inventory. Arch Otolaryngol Head Neck Surg 127(7):870–876

Cheung M, Chan AS, Law SC et al. (2000) Cognitive function of patients with nasopharyngeal carcinoma with and without temporal lobe radionecrosis. Arch Neurol 57(9):1347–1352

Cox JD, Stetz J, Pajak TF (1995) Toxicity criteria of the Radiation Therapy Oncology Group (RTOG) and the European Organization for Research and Treatment of Cancer (EORTC). Int J Radiat Oncol Biol Phys 31(5):1341–1346

D'Antonio LL, Zimmerman GJ, Cella DF et al. (1996) Quality of life and functional status measures in patients with head and neck cancer. Arch Otolaryngol Head Neck Surg 122(5):482–487

Denis F, Garaud P, Bardet E et al. (2003) Late toxicity results of the GORTEC 94-01 randomized trial comparing radiotherapy with concomitant radiochemotherapy for advanced-stage oropharynx carcinoma: comparison of LENT/SOMA, RTOG/EORTC, and NCI-CTC scoring systems. Int J Radiat Oncol Biol Phys 55(1):93–98

Denis F, Garaud P, Bardet E et al. (2004) Final results of the 94-01 French Head and Neck Oncology and Radiotherapy Group randomized trial comparing radiotherapy alone with concomitant radiochemotherapy in advanced-stage oropharynx carcinoma. J Clin Oncol 22(1):69–76

Dische S, Saunders M, Barrett A et al. (1997) A randomised multicentre trial of CHART versus conventional radiotherapy in head and neck cancer. Radiother Oncol 44(2):123–136

Dische S, Warburton MF, Jones D et al. (1989) The recording of morbidity related to radiotherapy. Radiother Oncol 16(2):103–108

Eisbruch A, Kim HM, Terrell JE et al. (2001) Xerostomia and its predictors following parotid-sparing irradiation of head-and-neck cancer. Int J Radiat Oncol Biol Phys 50(3):695–704

Ericson S (1969) An investigation of human parotid saliva secretion rate in response to different types of stimulation. Arch Oral Biol 14(6):591–596

Feng FY, Kim HM, Lyden TH et al. (2007) Intensity-modulated radiotherapy of head and neck cancer aiming to reduce dysphagia: early dose–effect relationships for the swallowing structures. Int J Radiat Oncol Biol Phys 68(5): 1289–1298

Grau C, Jensen K, Overgaard J (2007) Risk of severe radiation morbidity in radiotherapy trials: a critical evaluation of the TAME risk classification system. Int J Radiat Oncol Biol Phys 69(2):S140

Grau C, Moller K, Overgaard M et al. (1992) Auditory brain stem responses in patients after radiation therapy for nasopharyngeal carcinoma. Cancer 70(10):2396–2401

Hassan SJ, Weymuller EA Jr. (1993) Assessment of quality of life in head and neck cancer patients. Head Neck 15(6):485–496

Henson BS, Inglehart MR, Eisbruch A et al. (2001) Preserved salivary output and xerostomia-related quality of life in head and neck cancer patients receiving parotid-sparing radiotherapy. Oral Oncol 37(1):84–93

Hughes PJ, Scott PM, Kew J et al. (2000) Dysphagia in treated nasopharyngeal cancer. Head Neck 22(4):393–397

Jellema AP, Doornaert P, Slotman BJ et al. (2005) Does radiation dose to the salivary glands and oral cavity predict patient-rated xerostomia and sticky saliva in head and neck cancer patients treated with curative radiotherapy? Radiother Oncol 77(2):164–171

Jensen K (2007) Measuring side effects after radiotherapy for pharynx cancer. Acta Oncol 46(8):1051–1063

Jensen K, Jensen AB, Grau C (2006) The relationship between observer-based toxicity scoring and patient assessed symptom severity after treatment for head and neck cancer. A correlative cross sectional study of the DAHANCA toxicity scoring system and the EORTC quality of life questionnaires. Radiother Oncol 78(3):298–305

Jensen K, Lambertsen K, Grau C (2007a) Late swallowing dysfunction and dysphagia after radiotherapy for pharynx cancer: frequency, intensity and correlation with dose and volume parameters. Radiother Oncol 85(1):74–82

Jensen K, Lambertsen K, Torkov P et al. (2007b) Patient assessed symptoms are poor predictors of objective findings. Results from a cross sectional study in patients treated with radiotherapy for pharyngeal cancer. Acta Oncol 46(8):1159–1168

Jensen K, Overgaard M, Grau C (2007c) Morbidity after ipsilateral radiotherapy for oropharyngeal cancer. Radiother Oncol 85(1):90–97

Jones RE, Takeuchi T, Eisbruch A et al. (1996) Ipsilateral parotid sparing study in head and neck cancer patients who receive radiation therapy: results after 1 year. Oral Surg Oral Med Oral Pathol Oral Radiol Endod 81(6):642–648

Jung H, Beck-Bornholdt HP, Svoboda V et al. (2001) Quantification of late complications after radiation therapy. Radiother Oncol 61(3):233–246

Langmore SE (2003) Evaluation of oropharyngeal dysphagia: which diagnostic tool is superior? Curr Opin Otolaryngol Head Neck Surg 11(6):485–489

Lazarus CL (1993) Effects of radiation therapy and voluntary maneuvers on swallow functioning in head and neck cancer patients. Clin Commun Disord 3(4):11–20

Levendag PC, Teguh DN, Voet P et al. (2007) Dysphagia disorders in patients with cancer of the oropharynx are significantly affected by the radiation therapy dose to the superior and middle constrictor muscle: a dose–effect relationship. Radiother Oncol 85(1):64–73

Miller AB, Hoogstraten B, Staquet M et al. (1981) Reporting results of cancer treatment. Cancer 47(1):207–214

Navazesh M, Christensen CM (1982) A comparison of whole mouth resting and stimulated salivary measurement procedures. J Dent Res 61(10):1158–1162

Overgaard J, Hansen HS, Specht L et al. (2003) Five compared with six fractions per week of conventional radiotherapy of squamous-cell carcinoma of head and neck: DAHANCA 6 and 7 randomised controlled trial. Lancet 362(9388):933–940

Parise JO, Miguel RE, Gomes DL et al. (2004) Laryngeal sensitivity evaluation and dysphagia: hospital Sirio-Libanes experience. Sao Paulo Med J 122(5):200–203

Parliament MB, Scrimger RA, Anderson SG et al. (2004) Preservation of oral health-related quality of life and salivary flow rates after inverse-planned intensity-modulated radiotherapy (IMRT) for head-and-neck cancer. Int J Radiat Oncol Biol Phys 58(3):663–673

Pauloski BR, Rademaker AW, Logemann JA et al. (1998) Speech and swallowing in irradiated and nonirradiated postsurgical oral cancer patients. Otolaryngol Head Neck Surg 118(5):616–624

Pavy JJ, Denekamp J, Letschert J et al. (1995) EORTC Late Effects Working Group. Late effects toxicity scoring: the SOMA scale. Radiother Oncol 35(1):11–15

Roesink JM, Schipper M, Busschers W et al. (2005) A comparison of mean parotid gland dose with measures of parotid gland function after radiotherapy for head-and-neck cancer: implications for future trials. Int J Radiat Oncol Biol Phys 63(4):1006–1009

Rubin P, Constine LS, III, Fajardo LF et al. (1995) EORTC Late Effects Working Group. Overview of late effects normal tissues (LENT) scoring system. Radiother Oncol 35(1):9–10

Shaker R, Easterling C, Kern M et al. (2002) Rehabilitation of swallowing by exercise in tube-fed patients with pharyngeal dysphagia secondary to abnormal UES opening. Gastroenterology 122(5):1314–1321

Skladowski K, Maciejewski B, Golen M et al. (2006) Continuous accelerated 7-days-a-week radiotherapy for head-and-neck cancer: long-term results of phase III clinical trial. Int J Radiat Oncol Biol Phys 66(3):706–713

Stephens RJ, Hopwood P, Girling DJ et al. (1997) Randomized trials with quality of life endpoints: are doctors' ratings of patients' physical symptoms interchangeable with patients' self-ratings? Qual Life Res 6(3):225–236

Trotti A, Colevas AD, Setser A et al. (2003) CTCAE v3.0: development of a comprehensive grading system for the adverse effects of cancer treatment. Semin Radiat Oncol 13(3):176–181

Trotti A, Pajak TF, Gwede CK et al. (2007) TAME: development of a new method for summarising adverse events of cancer treatment by the Radiation Therapy Oncology Group. Lancet Oncol 8(7):613–624

Tylenda CA, Ship JA, Fox PC et al. (1988) Evaluation of submandibular salivary flow rate in different age groups. J Dent Res 67(9):1225–1228

van Acker F, Flamen P, Lambin P et al. (2001) The utility of SPECT in determining the relationship between radiation dose and salivary gland dysfunction after radiotherapy. Nucl Med Commun 22(2):225–231

Velikova G, Booth L, Smith AB et al. (2004) Measuring quality of life in routine oncology practice improves communication and patient well-being: a randomized controlled trial. J Clin Oncol 22(4):714–724

Wu CH, Hsiao TY, Chen JC et al. (1997) Evaluation of swallowing safety with fiberoptic endoscope: comparison with videofluoroscopic technique. Laryngoscope 107(3):396–401

Wu CH, Hsiao TY, Ko JY et al. (2000) Dysphagia after radiotherapy: endoscopic examination of swallowing in patients with nasopharyngeal carcinoma. Ann Otol Rhinol Laryngol 109(3):320–325

Effects of Radiotherapy on Swallowing Function:

Evaluation, Treatment, and Patient-Reported Outcomes

MOLLY KNIGGE, RACHAEL KAMMER, and NADINE P. CONNOR

CONTENTS

23.1 Patient-Reported Outcomes *260*

23.2 Swallowing Dysfunction of Radiotherapy *260*

23.3 Dysphagia-Specific Quality of Life Measures *261*

23.4 Impact of Age on Swallowing Outcomes *262*

23.5 Swallowing Evaluation for Patients with Head and Neck Cancer *262*

23.6 Swallowing Evaluation and Treatment during Radiotherapy *264*

23.7 Recommendations for Improving Comfort During Oral Intake *265*

23.8 Evaluation and Treatment of Postradiotherapy Dysphagia *265*

23.9 Use of Patient-Reported Outcomes in Clinical Practice *266*

23.10 Conclusions *266*

References *267*

MOLLY KNIGGE, MS
RACHAEL KAMMER, MS
The first two authors contributed equally to this chapter.
Division of Otolaryngology-Head and Neck Surgery, University of Wisconsin, 600 Highland Avenue K4/711, Madison, WI 53792-7375, USA
NADINE P. CONNOR, PhD, Associate Professor
Division of Otolaryngology-Head and Neck Surgery, University of Wisconsin, Clinical Science Center, Room K4/711, Madison, WI 53792-7375, USA

KEY POINTS

- Evolution of radiotherapy techniques has included an increased focus upon survival weighted by health-related quality of life following treatment.
- Radiotherapy can cause significant changes in swallowing function.
- Involvement of speech-language pathologists before, during, and after radiotherapy will help to maximize oral intake and maintain swallowing function.
- Skilled speech-language pathologists use instrumental swallowing evaluations to accurately evaluate for aspiration, characterize swallowing physiology, and identify patients for whom respiratory complications and risk for poor nutritional intake may threaten treatment outcomes.
- Standardized quality-of-life inventories can provide general health-related, disease-specific and dysphagia-specific patient-reported outcomes measurements with which to compare treatment approaches during and following radiotherapy.
- Patient perspectives captured through patient-reported outcomes measures combined with objective measures of swallowing function provide a comprehensive profile of swallowing dysfunction following radiotherapy for head and neck cancer.

23.1
Patient-Reported Outcomes

Health-related quality of life (HR-QOL) is a multidimensional, subjective concept that broadly describes an individual's well-being and satisfaction with their health and related functioning in daily life (FDA GUIDANCE 2006). For measurement purposes, HR-QOL is generally partitioned into conceptual domains that include physical, emotional, functional, or other factors. These conceptual domains are evaluated with the use of valid and reliable "instruments," which are the questionnaires or interview methods used to derive the HR-QOL assessments. The Food and Drug Administration (FDA) has recently described measures of HR-QOL as a subset of those appropriate for measurement of "patient reported outcomes (PRO)" (FDA GUIDANCE 2006). PROs are defined as measures of "any aspect of a patient's health that comes directly from the patient (i.e., without the interpretation of the patient's responses by a physician or anyone else)" (FDA GUIDANCE 2006).

PRO measures can be used in conjunction with more traditional measures of health and disease as additional and important clinical end points, and to evaluate the extent to which a treatment has affected the status of a patient's health (WIKLUND 2004). The use of measures that incorporate the patient's perspective is particularly useful for dimensions of health in which the individual is the only person who can truly appreciate the condition (e.g., pain or dry mouth). PRO measures are important in the care of patients with head and neck cancer because a patient's perspective of disease-related or treatment-related changes in speech, swallowing, hearing, and respiration can influence treatment planning. In addition, research including PRO measures can provide a benchmark for evaluation of new technologies in comparison with conventional or traditional treatments.

Historically, as with other cancers, the primary measure of treatment success in head and neck cancer has been survival rate, but this is now changing to also include an appreciation of PROs. Because the disease in the head and neck must be eradicated within an anatomic environment that contains many critical tissues, it is well-known that there are serious acute and chronic toxicities associated with treatment. These toxicities are well-described in other chapters within this volume and can affect the quality of life in the head and neck cancer patient and survivor (TERRELL et al. 1997; BJORDAL et al. 1999; RAMPLING et al. 2003; MORTON 2003; LIST and BILIR 2004). In head and neck cancer patients, scores on health-related quality-of-life instruments are typically lower after treatment than prior to, but gradually improve over the course of 6–12 months (LIN et al. 2003; RAMPLING et al. 2003). Few significant gains in HR-QOL have been reported after 1 year posttreatment (HAMMERLID et al. 2001).

23.2
Swallowing Dysfunction of Radiotherapy

Among the toxicities associated with radiotherapy, disruption in swallowing function can have a substantial effect on HR-QOL (LARSSON et al. 2003). In a prior study, the inability to chew and swallow was identified only after 2–3 weeks of treatment, and increased in severity as treatment progressed (LARSSON et al. 2003). Eating problems following radiotherapy had a significant impact on patients' quality of life because of pain, swelling, and dryness in the mouth and throat. Patients reported difficulty in chewing and swallowing, which negatively affected their desire to eat, and thus, these patients experienced a loss in togetherness with family in sharing meals (LARSSON et al. 2003). Accordingly, preservation or rehabiliation of swallowing function is an important consideration in the posttreatment management of patients with head and neck cancer.

The main danger of dysphagia is aspiration, leading to increased risk for pneumonia and death (LANGMORE et al. 1998; LUNDY et al. 1999; SMITH et al. 1999), and dysphagia has been found with all modalities of treatment for head and neck cancer. Following radiation treatment and chemotherapy, radiographic changes were found in the pharyngeal constrictor muscles and the supraglottic and glottic larynx and were associated with dysphagia and aspiration (EISBRUCH et al. 2002). These structures were therefore called the "dysphagia/aspiration-related structures," and it was recommended that doses to these areas be minimized and studied to determine the potential clinical benefits (EISBRUCH et al. 2002). Organs at risk are shown graphically in Fig. 23.1 (from JENSEN et al. (2007a)). Postradiation impairments in oral intake and swallowing are also likely due to changes in oral and pharyngeal mucosa caused by the radiation (LAZARUS et al. 2000).

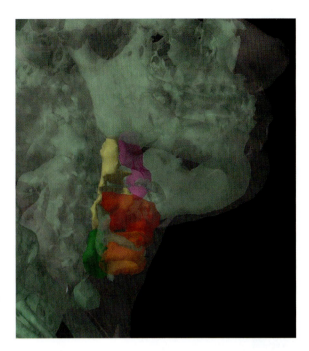

Fig. 23.1. Organs at risk for swallowing impairment due to radiation therapy (Reproduced with permission from JENSEN et al. (2007a, b))

The specific components of abnormal swallowing function after postoperative radiotherapy have been described (EKBERG & NYLANDER 1983; LAZARUS et al. 1996; MURRY et al. 1998; PAULOSKI and LOGEMANN 2000; CHEN et al. 2001; EISBRUCH et al. 2002; CARRARA-DE-ANGELIS et al. 2003; CAMPBELL et al. 2004). For example, after completion of radiotherapy, reduced mobility of oral and pharyngeal structures that contribute to the swallow has been reported, including reduced posterior tongue base movement, reduced laryngeal elevation, and reduced inversion of the epiglottis (PAULOSKI and LOGEMANN 2000; EISBRUCH et al. 2002). Difficulty with pharyngeal clearance during the swallow has also been found, in addition to delayed initiation of swallows and longer swallowing durations, leading to compromised swallowing efficiency overall and increased risk of aspiration (PAULOSKI and LOGEMANN 2000; EISBRUCH et al. 2002). Silent aspiration was reported, in which delayed cough following aspiration, or no cough at all, was observed with videofluoroscopy (EISBRUCH et al. 2002). Accordingly, occult aspiration can occur in a clinical setting when not being monitored via fluoroscopy, and it is therefore important for videofluoroscopic swallow studies to be performed in this population by skilled speech-language pathologists.

23.3
Dysphagia-Specific Quality of Life Measures

Several validated instruments are available for assessing quality of life in head and neck cancer, from overall HR-QOL to dysphagia-specific quality of life. The measures obtained from these instruments are PROs that can be used in combination with quantitative measures made before and after radiotherapy to obtain perspective on the effect of treatment on the patient's perception of swallowing functioning. The global health-related quality-of-life inventories, such as the Medical Outcomes Trust SF-36 (WARE et al. 1992), which measures perception of general health quality, or EORTC QLQ-C30 (AARONSON et al. 1993) for cancer-related health, address function contributing to physical and emotional (mental) health. Scores from these inventories have been found to correspond with swallowing function in head and neck cancer patients treated with conventional three-beam shrinking field radiotherapy at 1 and 6 months posttreatment (CONNOR et al. 2006). Disease-specific quality of life and function scales, including the EORTC QLQ-H&N35 (BJORDAL et al. 1999), PSS-HN (LIST et al. 1990), and FACT-H&N (CELLA et al. 1993), endeavor to measure PROs related to swallowing function, among other treatment-specific outcomes, after head and neck cancer treatment. Associations among aspiration identified during videofluoroscopic swallowing studies and patient ratings on the PSS-HN "normalcy of diet" scale and FACT-H&N "additional concerns" scale have been documented (CAMPBELL et al. 2004). Following conventional radiotherapy, need for diet adjustments as measured by the PSS-HN "normalcy of diet" scale has been found to be as high as 70% at 1 month posttreatment and persisting at levels below baseline at 6 months posttreatment (CONNOR et al. 2006). In addition to swallowing dysfunction, salivary dysfunction, dysgeusia, and nausea also impact diet adjustments following treatment for head and neck cancer.

The EORTC QLQ-H&N35 offers disease-specific measures for swallowing symptoms associated with head and neck cancer. Reduced QOL scores on the "swallowing" symptom scale have been associated with impaired swallowing function as identified using videofluoroscopic swallowing assessment at 1 month posttreatment (CONNOR et al. 2006). Objective measures of swallowing function, like those obtained via videofluoroscopic evaluation, are critical in acquiring detailed characterization of functional impairments contributing to aspiration or weight loss during or following treatment, especially as radiation treatment techniques evolve. Inadequate sensitivity, specificity, and predictive values of patient self-reporting with the EORTC QLQ-H&N35 scales have been identified in comparisons to the objective findings of aspiration or penetration in patients undergoing fiberoptic endoscopic evaluation of swallowing (JENSEN et al. 2007b). Thus, self-reported quality-of-life measures serve to illuminate patient profiles of perceived life impact but can be limited in their ability to specifically characterize swallow function. Accordingly, PROs are only part of a complete swallowing evaluation and cannot be used in isolation.

The MD Anderson Dysphagia Inventory (MDADI) (CHEN et al. 2001) and the SWAL-QOL (MCHORNEY et al. 2000a, b, 2002) represent validated dysphagia-specific PRO instruments. The MDADI questionnaire features three subscales for functional, emotional, and physical aspects of swallowing, intended as supplemental scales for gathering detailed quality-of-life measures to reflect facets of swallowing dysfunction. Focused questions relate patient experience with problems that may result from swallowing dysfunction, including special meal preparation, extended duration of meals, and eating in social situations. Validation of the inventory demonstrated correlations with PSS-HN and SF-36 subscales (CHEN et al. 2001). The latter finding was corroborated in a study where lower scores on the SF-36 Mental Health Subscale were related to lower MDADI scores measured greater than 12 months following completion of conventional radiation treatment with chemotherapy or following surgical resection (GILLESPIE et al. 2004). In contrast, the SWAL-QOL instrument comprises a 44-item swallow-specific PRO tool developed with a broader patient sample with underlying mechanical or neurologic etiologies for dysphagia (MCHORNEY et al. 2000a, b). Correlations were also demonstrated with SF-36 subscales (MCHORNEY et al. 2002), but to date no correlations with disease-specific PROs have been published. Variables that may influence an individual's perception of swallowing function following radiation treatment have been studied little. As noted previously, EISBRUCH et al. (2002) have identified dysphagia/aspiration-related structures that appear to be related to dysphagia postradiation treatment. In examining the tumor site impact, chemotherapy with conventional radiation for oropharyngeal tumor sites has been shown to result in statistically higher MDADI emotional and functional scores, indicative of better function, than postoperative radiation, though no significant advantage was evident for hypopharyngeal or laryngeal tumor sites (GILLESPIE et al. 2004). This study also revealed a relationship between NPO status for greater than 2 weeks and lower scores on the MDADI, reflecting a lower function, at 12 months or more following completion of treatment (GILLESPIE et al. 2004). Strategies for managing swallowing and nutritional decline during treatment remain controversial, and research of swallowing function and quality-of-life outcomes related to each is needed. The role of swallowing exercises performed concurrent with radiation treatment has been shown to benefit patients' swallowing physiology (KULBERSH et al. 2006; CARROLL et al. 2008), and its impact upon posttreatment quality of life is promising but requires further study.

23.4
Impact of Age on Swallowing Outcomes

The impact of aging upon swallowing outcomes after head and neck cancer represents a significant variable that will only increase in importance with the growing elderly patient population. Measurable differences in swallowing physiology with preservation of overall swallowing safety and efficiency in individuals over 70 years of age have been established (ROBBINS et al. 1995). In general, elderly people swallow more slowly and this results in a greater opportunity for penetration or aspiration of a bolus (ROBBINS et al. 1995). A sample of 107 geriatric patients, aged 65 years and older, in an assisted living setting, were administered the MDADI and produced lower scores than the general population on swallowing-related quality of life (CHEN et al. 2008). These findings underscore not only the importance of pretreatment screening for swallowing function in patients facing radiation treatment, but also suggest that caution must be exercised in comparing PROs related to swallowing across the age spectrum.

23.5
Swallowing Evaluation for Patients with Head and Neck Cancer

Speech-language pathologists use several different evaluation procedures to assess swallowing function, and familiarity with the distinctions among them is important for the radiation oncologist to understand. Regardless of the specific procedure used, review of medical and surgical history, patient interview, and clinical evaluation are needed to establish baseline swallow ability. This collective information will help to identify those at risk for developing dysphagia or malnutrition.

The clinical swallowing evaluation, also referred to as the "bedside" assessment, is easily performed within the clinic setting or at a patient's bedside, and does not require special instrumentation or radiography. It comprises a thorough review of medical history and symptoms, oral sensorimotor assessment, and skilled observation of swallowing behaviors. Patients are presented gradations of liquid and solid consistencies that allow assessment of feeding behaviors, mastication efforts, and general oral manipulation. External palpation of hyoid bone and thyroid cartilage range of movement provides a basis for judging pharyngeal swallowing function. The clinical swallowing evaluation is easily accessed and economical. However, it is limited in its ability to accurately identify aspiration (LINDEN et al. 1993) or characterize pharyngeal function to guide intervention planning. Audible signs of aspiration such as coughing or throat clearing do not allow clinicians to differentiate between penetration of bolus material above the vocal folds vs. aspiration. A similar lack of sensitivity has been shown with swallowing screening procedures utilizing blue dye in foods and liquids presented to patients with tracheostomy (BRADY et al. 1999; PERUZZI et al. 2001). Caution must be taken to consider risks for silent aspiration, defined as aspiration without clinical signs of laryngeal effort to eject penetrated material. If dysphagia is suspected, an instrumental evaluation (videofluoroscopy or endoscopy, as described below) may be necessary to determine the safety of oral intake during radiotherapy or to identify compensatory strategies that may make oral intake easier or safer.

Videofluoroscopy has emerged as a reliable assessment for determining the presence or absence of aspiration (KUHLEMEIER et al. 1998; McCULLOUGH et al. 2001). This method allows for visualization of all phases of swallowing, providing a means for assessing the effectiveness of therapeutic maneuvers or postures. Both lateral and anteroposterior viewing under videofluoroscopy offer opportunities to assess patency of the upper esophageal sphincter and cervical esophagus. Figure 23.2 contains a still image taken from a videofluoroscopic swallow study, which is also called a modified barium swallow. The procedure offers sensitivity to silent aspiration and can differentiate among

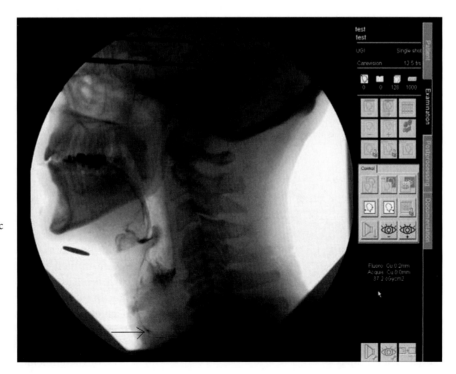

Fig. 23.2. Videofluoroscopic swallow study (VFSS): shown here is a still image of a videofluoroscopic swallow study revealing aspiration of thin liquid (*arrow*). Additionally, stasis can be appreciated in the pyriform sinuses, indicating poor bolus clearance

levels of penetration or aspiration. Standard protocol for videofluoroscopic swallowing studies involves presentation of barium contrasts in gradations of liquid and solid consistencies. The videofluoroscopic examination mandates more controlled conditions for feeding than the clinical swallowing evaluation, and therefore it may be less sensitive to authentic feeding variables that impact swallowing safety or efficiency. The invasive nature of radiographic imaging must be acknowledged, and thus the use of videofluoroscopic imaging requires judicious patient selection by a skilled speech-language pathologist who specializes in swallowing evaluation and treatment.

An instrumental alternative to the videofluoroscopic swallowing study is the fiberoptic endoscopic evaluation of swallowing, or FEES (Fig. 23.3). This examination requires passage of an endoscope nasally to view the pharynx and larynx before and after swallowing. The FEES procedure has demonstrated equal sensitivity to videofluoroscopy for identification of aspiration and penetration (MADDEN et al. 2000), and has been used to identify dysphagia in patients with pharyngeal cancer following radiation therapy (JENSEN et al. 2007a, b). Notably, reduced sensitivity was observed in 94% of patients, residue in 88%, penetration in 59%, and aspiration in 18%, with doses less than 60 Gy to the supraglottic region, larynx, and esophagus representing a low risk of aspiration (JENSEN et al. 2007a).

During the swallow, however, base of tongue contact to the posterior pharyngeal wall obliterates the endoscopic view of the larynx during FEES, but only momentarily. The speech-language pathologist can view bolus entry to the pharynx, clearance of bolus volumes after the swallow, and signs of penetration or aspiration. Direct visualization also allows for assessment of laryngeal function. An option exists for FEES with sensory testing, or FEESST. During this examination, a calibrated pulse of air is introduced to the laryngopharynx to assess for a reflexive response, and thus provides an assessment of sensory integrity of airway protective mechanisms. The absence of a response is associated with risk for silent aspiration (AVIV et al. 1998).

During the initial meeting with the speech-language pathologist, counseling and education are stressed. Patients must be educated on side effects of radiotherapy that can affect oral intake, including xerostomia, mucositis, and dysgeusia. Patients will be introduced to range of motion exercises designed to maintain mobility, including actions of pharyngeal constriction and laryngeal rise, and discourage fibrosis of soft tissues associated with the jaw and base of tongue. Improved global measures of swallowing function at 3 months posttreatment with use of exercises has been shown (LOGEMANN et al. 1997). Finally, the importance of daily oral intake, if safe, should be stressed despite primary gastrostomy feeding. Swallowing even small amounts of soft foods and liquids may help to maintain the range of motion of oropharyngeal structures and muscles, and discourage disuse phenomena.

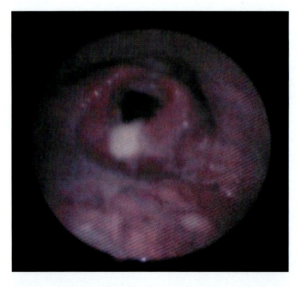

Fig. 23.3. Fiberoptic endoscopic evaluation of swallowing (FEES): A still image from a FEES. A pudding consistency was observed to penetrate the larynx, and the patient is at risk for aspiration of this material. Stasis is also observed in the left pyriform sinus

23.6
Swallowing Evaluation and Treatment during Radiotherapy

Radiotherapy and chemotherapy may be associated with a decline in swallowing function, and patients who were initially tolerating microaspirations may evidence frank aspiration during and following radiotherapy. In their deconditioned treatment state, they are at a higher risk for aspiration pneumonia. Accordingly, involvement of the speech-language pathologist is integral before, during, and after radiotherapy. The role of the clinician will evolve as needs of the head and neck cancer patient change during stages of treatment. An initial clinical evaluation is necessary to establish baseline swallow function. Some patients may already be experiencing oral or pharyngeal dysphagia due to the site of their tumor (PAULOSKI et al. 2000). For example, a tumor at the base of tongue may result in poor bolus propulsion, pharyngeal stasis, and subsequent aspiration. Laryngeal masses may cause vocal fold paralysis, which may lead to decreased airway protection and aspiration. Increased tumor staging correlates with more significant dysphagia (PAULOSKI et al. 2000).

Patients treated primarily with surgery may evidence changes to their swallowing function, depending upon extent and site of surgery. At many institutions, oral cavity cancers are treated primarily with resection of the tumor, followed by possible postoperative radiation or chemoradiation. For example, a tumor of the oral tongue will often require partial glossectomy and may need reconstruction if there is a large defect. These patients will likely have difficulty with bolus transit and oral residual; swallowing efficiency tends to decrease as volume of resection and reconstruction increases (PAULOSKI et al. 2004). Some laryngeal tumors are also treated primarily with surgery, by partial laryngectomy. This surgery will result in decreased airway protection and will put patients at high risk for aspiration. Patients will require early instrumental evaluation and swallow rehabilitation to learn exercises and compensatory strategies (RADEMAKER et al.1993). Severity of postsurgical dysphagia is dependent on the site of tumor and the extent of resection and reconstruction. Many postsurgical patients can learn to compensate but rarely return to preoperative swallow status (PAULOSKI et al. 1993, 1994; LOGEMANN et al. 1993; RADEMAKER et al. 1993).

23.7
Recommendations for Improving Comfort During Oral Intake

Oral intake will often become challenging because of acute side effects of radiotherapy. The importance of water sips will need to be impressed on the patients. Water sips are soothing, will reduce sensation of dryness, and may serve to moisturize mucosa. Soft, moist foods will be easier to swallow, and a liquid wash is often beneficial in clearing oral or pharyngeal residue. Biotene (Laclède Incorporated

Healthcare Products, Gardena, CA) is a product made of three enzymes and one protein found in human saliva, and is often beneficial in relieving mucositis and xerostomia, and decreasing bacteria (EPSTEIN et al.1999). A combination of water, salt, and baking soda has been found to aid in the formation of granulation tissue and promote healing of mucosa (DAEFFLER 1981). Salt and soda rinses will also dissolve mucus and loosen debris (MAUER 1977). Administration of topical or oral analgesics can also enable oral intake. Dygeusia is an issue many patients battle, although there has been no significant investigation regarding treatment. This issue is therefore difficult to predict and challenging to treat. Clinicians should encourage patients to be observational in order to determine what foods are best tolerated. Nursing is also involved in treating the above side effects, and a team approach is desirable to reinforce recommendations.

Patients should be continually reminded of the importance of the range of motion exercises and daily oral intake. Speech-language pathologists can be helpful in downgrading diets, for example to mechanical soft or puree, so that patients may continue oral intake as long as possible. Postural strategies may also become integral. For example, if pain or irritation is unilateral, a head turn to the affected side will guide the bolus through the opposite of the pharynx (RADEMAKER et al. 1993). If patients become completely gastrostomy-tube-dependent, a minimum of a daily puree snack is optimal, and continued water sips. The increased effort needed to swallow the puree consistency may be beneficial for maintenance of swallowing function.

23.8
Evaluation and Treatment of Postradiotherapy Dysphagia

Following completion of radiation, patients will typically continue to experience acute side effects for 2–4 weeks posttreatment. As a result, they may continue to have challenges with oral intake and meeting nutritional requirements. Management strategies for xerostomia, mucositis, dysgeusia, and dysphagia used during radiation therapy should be continued during this transition period. PAULOSKI et al. (2006) has documented reduced oral intake or a nonnormal diet at 1 month postradiotherapy, but improving at 12 months postradiotherapy.

Although acute side effects will likely improve, there may be persistent side effects. Owing to radiation of unilateral or bilateral parotid glands, xerostomia will likely never completely resolve. Patients with xerostomia report dysphagia; they often complain of pharyngeal stasis or slow bolus transit. Interestingly, LOGEMANN et al. (2001) did not find a correlation between xerostomia and physiological swallow changes. Therefore, xerostomia causes patients to perceive dysphagia that may not be manifested in actual reductions in swallowing ability. As a result, patients have been found to change their diet choices. Specifically, crunchy foods may be avoided (LOGEMANN et al. 2003). In response to these complaints, speech-language pathologists can recommend soft, moist foods and a liquid wash. Dysgeusia can also be particularly limiting in patients' transition back to oral intake. Decreased taste function, especially sour taste, postradiotherapy has been documented (MIRZA et al. 2008). Again, this problem is difficult to treat; caregivers and health-care professionals can only suggest the patient keep trying foods on a daily basis.

It is important to discriminate those patients who have true dysphagia from those who continue to be affected by side effects. As previously discussed, it has been well documented that some patients will experience dysphagia as a result of their radiotherapy. There are some options for treatment of radiotherapy-induced dysphagia. Mild dysphagia, characterized by decreased bolus propulsion and minimal pharyngeal residue, may be helped simply with liquid wash or diet alteration. However, moderate to severe dysphagia with aspiration necessitates more intervention. Traditional therapy from speech-language pathologists is pharyngeal exercise, which is intended to improve the range of motion and strength of pharyngeal muscles and structures. As previously referenced, exercises have been found to improve swallowing measures in head/neck cancer patients (LOGEMANN et al. 1997). Oral tongue strengthening exercise has been shown to increase tongue strength in normal and other patient populations that carries over to improved swallowing and swallowing-related quality of life (ROBBINS et al. 2005, 2007; KAYS and ROBBINS 2006) but benefit has not been documented in head and neck cancer patients to date. Other medical assessments and procedures, such as esophagoscopy and dilation, may also be beneficial (LAWSON et al. 2008).

Some patients with dysphagia prior to or during radiotherapy will require a gastrostomy tube because difficulty clearing a bolus through the pharynx requires more effort to eat and often leads to malnutrition and weight loss (SCHATTNER 2003). Interestingly, scores on a health-related quality-of-life instrument specific for head and neck cancer (EORTC) in the areas of fatigue, loss of appetite, global health status, sticky saliva, and swallowing were more impaired at diagnosis in patients who later evidenced severe weight loss (PETRUSON et al. 2005). The authors suggested that administration of a health-related quality-of-life instrument at diagnosis might be useful in predicting those patients who might require special management.

23.9
Use of Patient-Reported Outcomes in Clinical Practice

PROs may be underutilized in clinical practice. In a study that addressed the issue of PRO use in clinical practice, senior oncologists were asked about their perceived value of health-related quality-of-life measures and the role in cancer care (MORRIS et al. 1998). Results indicated that HR-QOL was considered the third most important consideration when cancer cure was the treatment goal, after considerations of tumor response to treatment and potential side effects. However, when palliation was the goal, HR-QOL was the primary concern of physicians. Accordingly, even in situations where cure of a disease is the foremost concern, HR-QOL is regarded as a very important consideration. However, although 80% of physicians questioned thought that HR-QOL was important to measure, only 50% incorporated these measures into their clinical practice (MORRIS et al. 1998). As such, there is a mismatch between perceived need and usefulness of health-related quality-of-life measures and the ability of practitioners to collect the information. It is clear that new approaches to data collection are needed to facilitate ease of use of these measures in clinical care.

23.10
Conclusions

Eating represents a critical balance between physiological efficiency and perceived pleasure, upon which radiation treatments may inflict impairments that threaten respiratory health, nutritional intake, and quality of life. Forthcoming studies examining the advantages of new therapies, such as IMRT and tomotherapy, must define both swallowing function via objective measures and the perceived impact of swallowing dysfunction upon daily life. Establishing treatment protocols based upon relationships among curative intent and these variables will contribute to improved treatment selection, swallowing intervention, and nutritional management for optimizing treatment outcomes for head and neck cancer.

References

Aaronson NK, Ahmedzai S, Bergman B et al. (1993) The European Organization for Research and Treatment of Cancer QLQ-C30: a quality-of-life instrument for use in international clinical trials in oncology. J Natl Cancer Inst 85:365–376

Aviv JE, Kim T, Sacco RL et al. (1998) FEESST: a new bedside endoscopic test of the motor and sensory components of swallowing. Ann Otol Rhinol Laryngol 107:378–387

Bjordal K, Hammerlid E, Ahlner-Elmqvist M et al. (1999) Quality of life in head and neck cancer patients: validation of the European Organization for Research and Treatment of Cancer Quality of Life Questionnaire-H & N35. J Clin Oncol 17:1008–1019

Brady SL, Hildner CD, Hutchins BF (1999) Simultaneous videofluoroscopic swallow study and modified Evans blue dye procedure: an evaluation of blue dye visualization in cases of known aspiration. Dysphagia 14:146–149

Campbell BH, Spinelli K, Marbella AM et al. (2004) Aspiration, weight loss, and quality of life in head and neck cancer survivors. Arch Otolaryngol Head Neck Surg 130: 1100–1103

Carrara-de-Angelis E, Feher O, Barros APB et al. (2003) Voice and swallowing in patients enrolled in a larynx preservation trial. Arch Otolaryngol Head Neck Surg 129:733–738

Carroll WR, Locher JL, Canon CL et al. (2008) Pretreatment swallowing exercises improve swallow function after chemoradiation. Laryngoscope 118:39–43

Cella DF, Tulsky DS, Gray G et al. (1993) The functional assessment of cancer therapy scale: development and validation of the general measure. J Clin Oncol 11:570–579

Chen AY, Frankowski R, Bishop-Leone J et al. (2001) The development and validation of a dysphagia-specific quality-of-life questionnaire for patients with head and neck cancer. Arch Otolaryngol Head Neck Surg 127:870–876

Chen PH, Golub JS, Hapner ER et al. (2008) Prevalence of perceived dysphagia and quality-of-life impairment in a geriatric population. Dysphagia

Connor NP, Cohen SB, Kammer RE et al. (2006) Impact of conventional radiotherapy on health-related quality of life and critical functions of the head and neck. Int J Radiation Oncology Biol Phys 65:1051–1062

Daeffler R (1981) Oral hygiene measures for patients with cancer. Cancer Nurs 4(1):29–35

Eisbruch A, Lyden T, Bradford CR et al. (2002) Objective assessment of swallowing dysfunction and aspiration after radiation concurrent with chemotherapy for head-and-neck cancer. Int J Radiat Oncol Biol Phys 53:23–28

Ekberg O, Nylander G (1983) Pharyngeal dysfunction after treatment for pharyngeal cancer with surgery and radiotherapy. Gastroint Radiol 8:97–104

Epstein JB, Emerton S, Le ND et al. (1999) A double-blind crossover trial of oral balance gel and biotene toothpaste versus placebo in patients with xerostomia following radiation therapy. Oral Oncol 35(2):132–137

Food and Drug Administration, Center for Drug Evaluation and Research (CDER), Center for Biologics Evaluation and Research (CBER), Center for Devices and Radiographic Health (CDRH) (2006) Guidance for industry patient-reported outcome measures: use in medical product development to support labeling claims: draft guidance. Health Qual Life Outcomes 4:79

Gillespie MB, Brodsky MB, Day TA et al. (2004) Swallowing-related quality of life after head and neck cancer treatment. Laryngoscope 114:1362–1367

Hammerlid E, Silander E, Hornestam L et al. (2001) Health-related quality of life three years after diagnosis of head and neck cancer – a longitudinal study. Head Neck 23:113–125

Jensen K, Lambertsen K, Grau C (2007a) Late swallowing dysfunction and dysphagia after radiotherapy for pharynx cancer: frequency, intensity and correlation with dose and volume parameters. Radiother Oncol 85(1):74–82

Jensen K, Lambertsen K, Torkov P et al. (2007b) Patient assessed symptoms are poor predictors of objective findings. Results from cross sectional study in patients treated with radiotherapy for pharyngeal cancer. Acta Oncologica 46:1159–1168

Kays S, Robbins J (2006) Effects of sensorimotor exercise on swallowing outcomes relative to age and age-related disease. Semin Speech Lang 27:245–259

Kuhlemeier KV, Yates P, Palmer JB (1998) Intra- and interrater variation in the evaluation of videofluorographic swallowing studies. Dysphagia 13:142–147

Kulbersh BD, Rosenthal EL, McGrew BM et al. (2006) Pretreatment, preoperative swallowing exercises may improve dysphagia quality of life. Laryngoscope 116:883–886

Langmore SE, Terpenning MS, Schork A et al. (1998) Predictors of aspiration pneumonia: how important is dysphagia? Dysphagia 13:69–81

Larsson M, Hedelin B, Athlin E (2003) Lived experiences of eating problems for patients with head and neck cancer during radiotherapy. J Clin Nurs 12:562–570

Lawson JD, Otto K, Grist W et al. (2008) Frequency of esophageal stenosis after simultaneous modulated accelerated radiation therapy and chemotherapy for head and neck cancer. Am J Otolaryngol 29(1):13–19

Lazarus CL, Logemann JA, Pauloski BR et al. (1996) Swallowing disorders in head and neck cancer patients treated with radiotherapy and adjuvant chemotherapy. Laryngoscope 106:1157–1166

Lazarus CL, Logemann JA, Pauloski BR et al. (2000) Swallowing and tongue function following treatment for oral and oropharyngeal cancer. J Speech Lang Hear Res 43:1011–1023

Lin A, Kim HM, Terrell JE et al. (2003) Quality of life after parotid sparing IMRT for head and neck cancer: a prospective longitudinal study. Int J Radiat Oncol Biol Phys 57:61–70

Linden P, Kuhlemeier KV, Patterson C (1993) The probability of correctly predicting subglottic penetration from clinical observations. Dysphagia 8:170–179

List MA, Bilir SP (2004) Functional outcomes in head and neck cancer. Semin Radiat Oncol 14:178–189

List MA, Ritter-Sterr C, Lansky SB (1990) A performance status scale for head and neck cancer patients. Cancer 66: 564–569

Logemann JA, Pauloski BR, Rademaker AW et al. (1993) Speech and swallow function after tonsil/base of tongue resection with primary closure. J Speech Hear Res 36(5):918–926

Logemann JA, Pauloski BR, Rademaker AW et al. (1997) Speech and swallowing rehabilitation for head and neck cancer patients. Oncology 11(5):651–656, 659; discussion 659, 663–664

Logemann JA, Pauloski BR, Rademaker AW et al. (2003) Xerostomia: 12-month changes in saliva production and its relationship to perception and performance of swallow function, oral intake, and diet after chemoradiation. Head Neck 25(6):432–437

Logemann JA, Smith CH, Pauloski BR et al. (2001) Effects of xerostomia on perception and performance of swallow function. Head Neck 23(4):317–321

Lundy DS, Smith C, Colangelo L et al. (1999) Aspiration: cause and implications. Otolaryngol Head Neck Surg 120: 474–478

Madden C, Fenton J, Hughes J et al. (2000) Comparison between videofluoroscopy and milk-swallow endoscopy in the assessment of swallowing function. Clin Otolaryngol Allied Sci 25:504–506

Maurer J (1977) Providing optimal oral health. Nurs Clin North Am 12(4):671–685

McCullough GH, Wertz RT, Rosenbek JC et al. (2001) Inter- and intrajudge reliability for videofluoroscopic swallowing evaluation measures. Dysphagia 16:110–118

McHorney CA, Bricker DE, Kramer AE et al. (2000a) The SWAL-QOL outcomes tool for oropharyngeal dysphagia in adults: I. Conceptual foundation and item development. Dysphagia 15:115–121

McHorney CA, Bricker DE, Robbins J et al. (2000b) The SWAL-QOL outcomes tool for oropharyngeal dysphagia in adults: II. Item reduction and preliminary scaling. Dysphagia 15:122–133

Mcttorney CA, Robbins J, Lomax K et al. (2002) The SWAL-QOL and SWAL-CARE Outcomes Tool For Oropharyngeal dysphagia in adults: III. Documentation of reliability and validity. Dysphagia 17:97–114

Mirza N, Machtay M, Devine PA et al. (2008) Gustatory impairment in patients undergoing head and neck irradiation. Laryngoscope 118(1):24–31

Morris J, Perez D, McNoe B (1998) The use of quality of life data in clinical practice. Qual Life Res 7:85–91

Morton RP (2003) Studies in the quality of life of head and neck cancer patients: results of a two-year longitudinal study and a comparative cross-sectional cross-cultural study. Laryngoscope 113:1091–1103

Murry T, Madasu R, Martin A et al. (1998) Acute and chronic changes in swallowing and quality of life following intraarterial chemoradiation for organ preservation in patients with advanced head and neck cancer. Head Neck 20:31–37

Pauloski BR, Logemann JA (2000) Impact of tongue base and posterior pharyngeal wall biomechanics on pharyngeal clearance in irradiated postsurgical oral and oropharyngeal cancer patients. Head Neck 22:120–131

Pauloski BR, Logemann JA, Rademaker AW et al. (1993) Speech and swallowing function after anterior tongue and floor of mouth resection with distal flap reconstruction. J Speech Hear Res 36(2):267–276

Pauloski BR, Logemann JA, Rademaker AW et al. (1994) Speech and swallowing function after oral and oropharyngeal resections: one-year follow-up. Head Neck 16(4):313–322

Pauloski BR, Rademaker AW, Logemann JA et al. (2000) Pretreatment swallowing function in patients with head and neck cancer. Head Neck 22:474–482

Pauloski BR, Rademaker AW, Logemann JA et al. (2004) Surgical variables affecting swallowing in patients treated for oral/oropharyngeal cancer. Head Neck 26(7):625–636

Pauloski BR, Rademaker AW, Logemann JA et al. (2006) Relationship between swallow motility disorders on videofluorography and oral intake in patients treated for head and neck cancer with radiotherapy with or without chemotherapy. Head Neck 28:1069–1076

Peruzzi WT, Logemann JA, Currie D et al. (2001) Assessment of aspiration in patients with tracheostomies: comparison of the bedside colored dye assessment with videofluoroscopic examination. Respir Care 46:243–247

Petruson KM, Silander EM, Hammerlid EB (2005) Quality of life as predictor of weight loss in patients with head and neck cancer. Head Neck 27:302–310

Rademaker AW, Logemann JA, Pauloski BR et al. (1993) Recovery of postoperative swallowing in patients undergoing partial laryngectomy. Head Neck 15(4):325–334

Rampling T, King H, Mais KL et al. (2003) Quality of life measurement in the head and neck cancer radiotherapy clinic: is it feasible and worthwhile? Clin Oncol 15:205–210

Robbins J, Kays SA, Gangnon RE et al. (2007) The effects of lingual exercise in stroke patients with dysphagia. Arch Phys Med Rehabil 88:150–158

Robbins J, Levine R, Wood J et al. (1995) Age effects on lingual pressure generation as a risk factor for dysphagia. J Gerontol A Biol Sci Med Sci 50(5):M257–M262

Robbins JA, Gangnon RE, Theis SM et al. (2005) The effects of lingual exercise on swallowing in older adults. J Am Geriatr Soc 53:1483–1489

Schattner M (2003) Enteral nutritional support of the patient with cancer: route and role. J Clin Gastroenterol 36(4):297–302

Smith CH, Logemann JA, Colangelo LA et al. (1999) Incidence and patient characteristics associated with silent aspiration in the acute care setting. Dysphagia 14:1–7

Terrell JE, Nanavati KA, Esclamado RM et al. (1997) Head and neck cancer-specific quality of life: instrument validation. Arch Otolaryngol Head Neck Surg 123:1125–1132

Ware JE, Jr, Sherbourne CD (1992) The MOS 36-Item Short-Form Health Survey (SF-36): I. Conceptual framework and item selection. Med Care 30:473–483

Wiklund A (2004) Assessment of patient-reported outcomes in clinical trials: the example of health-related quality of life. Fundam Clin Pharmacol 18:351–363

Dental Prophylaxis and Care

24

Pamela Sandow, D. M. D.

CONTENTS

24.1   Pretreatment Oral Evaluation   *270*

24.2   Oral Care During and After
       Treatment   *272*

References   *276*

KEY POINTS

- All patients, dentate and edentulous, should receive an oral examination by a dentist prior to head and neck radiotherapy. Direct communication between the dentist and radiation oncologist is essential to provide optimal care for the patient.
- Prior to radiotherapy, teeth with unfavorable prognoses should be extracted if they are located in the proposed high-dose treatment field.
- A minimum of 14–21 days is an acceptable length of time for healing after extraction and before the initiation of radiotherapy.
- Permanent hyposalivation results when salivary glands receive doses greater than 35 Gy, but radiation caries can result from even lower doses.
- Fluoride carriers should be fabricated and delivered before the onset of mucositis. Sodium fluoride gel (1.1%) or stannous fluoride gel (0.4%) should be applied daily in the carriers for the remainder of the patient's life in order to reduce the risk of radiation caries.

Pamela Sandow, DMD, Clinical Professor and Director
Department of Oral & Maxillofacial Surgery and Diagnostic
Sciences, Oral Medicine Clinic, University of Florida, JHMHC,
Box 100416, Gainesville, FL 32610-0416, USA

- Fluconazole (200 mg the first day and 100 mg daily for 6–13 days) has been proven to be effective and safe for treatment of oral candidiasis.
- Hyperbaric oxygen therapy (20 dives before extraction and 10 dives after extraction) may be indicated when removing teeth from bone having received radiation doses greater than 60 Gy.
- Systemic sialagogues such as pilocarpine (5 mg tablets; 5–10 mg t.i.d.) or cevimeline (30 mg tablets; 30–60 mg t.i.d.) may increase the production of saliva in patients with some remaining measurable salivary production.
- Excellent communication between health-care providers is imperative to minimize the negative effects of head and neck cancer therapy and to improve the patient's quality of life.

Preservation of the dentition and its supporting structures is imperative to optimize masticatory function and quality of life in head and neck cancer patients. These objectives are best achieved through communication and coordination of care using a multidisciplinary approach involving surgeons, oncologists, and dentists.

Postradiation oral complications are common when the oral cavity and salivary glands are within the field of radiation. Each complication can initiate a cascade of other adverse sequelae. Mucositis, dysgeusia, and permanent changes in the quality and quantity of saliva are oftentimes unavoidable. Radiation-induced damage to salivary glands reduces the ability of saliva to remineralize teeth, compromises cleansing and buffering capability of the oral cavity, and increases colonization of cariogenic bacteria. The loss of salivary function also predisposes the patient to painful bacterial and fungal infections that inhibit proper nutrition, oral hygiene, and fluoride application. In turn, poor compliance with daily oral hygiene and fluoride use will increase the risk of rampant caries, pain, and eventual tooth loss.

Radiation-induced reduction in the vasculature of bone and soft tissues can lead to trismus, soft tissue necrosis, and osteoradionecrosis (ORN). These possible long-term complications are often interrelated and difficult to predict. Over time, trismus can limit proper access for the dentist to restore teeth and for the patient to properly care for their dentition. Consequently, decreased oral hygiene can initiate or promote existing caries and/or periodontal disease. In addition, teeth in irradiated areas have a greater susceptibility to a loss of periodontal attachment, secondary to radiation-induced hypovascularity and hypocellularity of the periodontal tissues. The loss of tooth attachment from supporting bone can result in irreversible tooth mobility and the need for extraction. As a result of removal of carious or periodontally compromised teeth from irradiated bone, impaired healing or ORN can occur. Therefore, it is extremely important that dentists and radiation oncologists, in a cooperative effort, educate patients and provide reinforcement of measures to prevent interdependent radiation-induced complications.

24.1
Pretreatment Oral Evaluation

All patients should receive an oral examination by a dentist prior to head and neck radiotherapy. Many patients do not have an established general dentist. Even when they do, many general dentists are not familiar with head and neck radiotherapy techniques nor have the training to manage posttreatment complications. The radiation oncologist should establish a professional relationship with at least one dentist in the community for referral of head and neck cancer patients when these situations arise. The oncologist should communicate directly with the dentist to whom the patient is referred in order to ensure that the dentist is knowledgeable in the care of head and neck cancer patients. The oncologist should inform the dentist of the urgency of pretreatment dental care, the proposed radiation dose and treatment field, anticipated level of salivary gland dysfunction, prognosis, and any other information needed to adequately evaluate the patient.

The risk of ORN is greatest in bone receiving doses greater than 64–65 Gy (KOGA et al. 2008a).

The dentist should be advised of any areas of the mandible or maxilla that will be exposed to doses in this range. Extraction of teeth outside of the field of radiation can usually be accomplished with minimal risk of ORN. Therefore, the dentist should carefully evaluate teeth in the proposed high-dose areas to determine the presence of advanced dental disease and need for pretreatment extraction.

There are varying opinions on guidelines for retaining or extracting teeth prior to the initiation of radiotherapy. The ultimate goal of pretreatment extraction is to reduce the lifelong risk of ORN; however, some reports have concluded that the incidence of ORN is essentially the same with pretreatment extraction when compared with the extraction of teeth after radiation (CHANG et al. 2007; KOGA et al. 2008a, b). Despite these inconsistencies, it is generally accepted to extract teeth with an unfavorable long-term prognosis prior to radiotherapy (SULAIMAN et al. 2003). Assessment of the health of the teeth in the proposed high-dose field of radiation, patient age, and anticipated life expectancy is necessary to determine whether extractions are prudent. For example, a 40-year-old patient with an anticipated favorable outcome from cancer therapy and with generalized bone loss from periodontal disease would be at greater risk for eventual tooth loss than a 75-year old with similar periodontal disease status. Therefore, a recommendation for pretreatment extraction may be more likely in the younger patient. It is not advisable to extract asymptomatic teeth, regardless of age, in patients with advanced cancer or end-stage disease.

Each pretreatment oral evaluation should begin with a thorough medical and dental history. Bruxism, tobacco use, and systemic diseases such as diabetes can contribute to poor periodontal health and are risk factors for the progression of dental disease. A caries risk assessment and dietary counseling are advisable to promote good dental health and nutrition. It is very important that all patients be evaluated to determine their current oral hygiene and motivation to maintain a high level of oral hygiene after treatment. Physical or other limitations preventing meticulous oral care should be taken into consideration when formulating a proper treatment plan. The dentist should establish the patient's ability and desire to follow-up with periodic dental care and cleanings. If the patient is unable or unlikely to maintain optimal oral hygiene or follow-up dental care, for any reason, then consideration should be given to extraction of teeth within the proposed high dose field of radiation.

At a minimum, a panoramic radiograph is necessary for evaluation of the dentition prior to the initiation of radiotherapy. This radiograph is helpful in allowing the dentist to quickly visualize the general condition of the dentition, the periodontal bone level, and the presence of root tips or impacted teeth. Additional intraoral radiographs can be taken to establish the extent of periodontal disease, periapical pathology, and caries. The clinical examination should include the recording of periodontal probing depths, assessment of gingival health, and the documentation of tooth mobility and caries in each tooth.

Teeth in the proposed treatment field that have nonrestorable fractures, extensive caries, indications for root canals, or symptoms of irreversible pulpitis should usually be extracted prior to the initiation of radiotherapy. Root tips and teeth with symptomatic periapical pathology or periapical abscesses should also be eliminated. Nonfunctional teeth, such as those which are unopposed in occlusion, should be considered for removal. Teeth that contribute to mucosal irritation are common in some oral cancer patients, and therefore, it may be advisable to extract teeth that are otherwise healthy but could be a potential source of chronic irritation to delicate irradiated tissues. Retained teeth and dentures with sharp or irritating areas should be smoothed to reduce soft tissue trauma.

Extraction of fully impacted teeth prior to radiotherapy can initiate a non-healing extraction site. Most asymptomatic, impacted teeth without pathology should not be extracted due to the high risk of ORN. If a partially impacted tooth is exposed to saliva or the oral cavity or if pathology is associated with the tooth, it is usually advisable to consider pretreatment extraction. In that event, the radiation oncologist should be consulted prior to the extraction and informed that additional time for healing may be necessary.

Periodontal disease is a chronic process with periods of progression and stabilization. It is often difficult to predict the course of periodontal disease progression, especially in postradiation patients. The radiation-induced decrease in vascularity of the tooth-supporting tissues can lead to periodontal disease progression and loss of periodontal attachment (Epstein et al. 1998) (Fig. 24.1). In most cases, a tooth with deep periodontal sulcular depths, advanced root furcation involvement, or mobility should be extracted prior to radiotherapy. Otherwise, teeth with chronic, stabile, generalized beginning to moderate bone loss may be retained with the patient's understanding that meticulous oral hygiene must be maintained. Patients must also accept that despite preventive measures, periodontal bone loss can progress after radiation, resulting in increased risk of tooth loss and ORN.

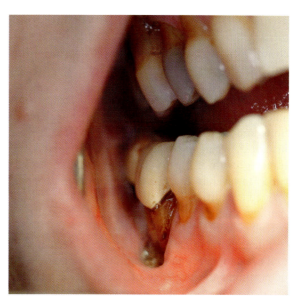

Fig. 24.1. Postradiation patient with loss of periodontal attachment that eventually progressed to ORN

The dentist and the radiation oncologist should be involved in a thorough explanation of the risks, benefits, and possible outcome of retaining or extracting teeth prior to radiotherapy. This is especially important since there is a potential risk of ORN with any pretreatment decision. If the patient comprehends the interrelationship between head and neck radiotherapy and oral complications, he or she is more likely to comply with proper oral hygiene regimens, including long-term daily fluoride use. An assessment of the patient's attitude toward dental issues and likely level of compliance is critical in the pretreatment extraction discussion. Retention of teeth in proposed irradiated areas may be ill-advised in patients who demonstrate a history of poor dental awareness and compliance. All discussions with the patient should be thoroughly documented in the medical and dental records.

If extractions are indicated, they should be performed with careful tissue manipulation. Irradiated bone has diminished ability to remodel, a phenomenon that is necessary for patients to wear dentures comfortably. An increased risk of bone exposure and ORN from denture trauma can develop when sharp bony projections are not properly smoothed at the time of pretreatment extraction. Therefore, preprosthetic surgery or alveoloplasty should be performed during the extraction procedure. Primary closure should be achieved, when feasible, without stretching the tissue beyond its physiologic limitation.

A minimum of 14–21 days is usually an acceptable length of time to allow for healing after extractions and before radiotherapy is initiated. In rare instances, when the patient is experiencing rapid tumor growth, it may be necessary to shorten this time. However, in most cases, if extractions are performed expeditiously, the delay in the start of radiotherapy should not adversely affect the patient's overall outcome.

Edentulous patients should receive a pretreatment oral evaluation. A panoramic radiograph is useful in determining the presence of root tips or partially erupted teeth, especially when they are difficult to visualize with an oral examination. This visit will also allow the dentist to make necessary denture adjustments and discuss proper denture cleansing techniques. Edentulous patients should be advised that oral soft tissues should be brushed daily with a soft toothbrush to remove bacteria and necrotic cells that accumulate during and after radiotherapy.

Dentate patients should have a dental cleaning no later than the second week of radiotherapy, prior to the development of mucositis. Dentists may also remove decay and restore dentition with amalgam or composite restorations during this time. It is prudent to delay the fabrication of dentures, crowns, and bridges until after the full course of radiotherapy.

Impressions for fluoride carriers should be made at the initial pretreatment dental visit. Fluoride carriers should be fabricated and delivered before the onset of mucositis. Bleaching trays should not be used for fluoride application because they do not extend to include the marginal gingival tissues. Radiation caries occurs at the gumline and occlusal surfaces, therefore these areas need to be adequately covered by the carriers (Fig. 24.2). The permanent alteration in the salivary composition after radiotherapy is difficult to quantify. Therefore, fluoride carriers along with clear, concise verbal and written instructions should be delivered to every patient scheduled to receive radiation to any salivary glands, regardless of the dose. It is far easier and less costly for the patient to prevent, rather than restore, rampant tooth decay. Radiation oncologists should be familiar with proper fluoride application so that they are able to reinforce its use at subsequent treatment and follow-up visits.

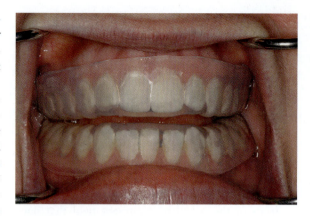

Fig. 24.2. Fluoride carriers

24.2
Oral Care During and After Treatment

Mucositis, presenting as inflammation and ulceration of the oral mucosa, occurs as a result of damage to the epithelial basement membrane and appears in the second to third week of radiotherapy. A neutral rinse comprising quarter teaspoon each of salt and baking soda in one quart of water is soothing to irritated tissues and can be used periodically throughout the day during and after therapy. Topical anesthetics, including lidocaine, benzocaine, and tetracaine, can be helpful in managing mild to moderate pain from mucositis. Patients should use caution when topical anesthetics are utilized while eating to prevent aspiration from a decreased gag reflex. They should avoid trauma to anesthetized tissues. Nonsteroidal anti-inflammatory drugs are also beneficial for relief of pain from mild to moderate mucositis. Opioids are usually necessary for control of moderate to severe pain.

Good oral hygiene can be challenging when experiencing pain from oral mucositis. Extra soft toothbrushes are available for use when tissues are sensitive or ulcerated. The burning sensation from toothpastes can be minimized by using those that are specifically formulated for children or sensitive tissues. Patients should refrain from wearing dentures as much as possible for the duration of radiotherapy and whenever oral tissues are ulcerated or erythematous. Dentures should be disinfected daily to reduce the microbial colonization of the denture surface and to minimize the transfer of organisms, especially Candida species, to the oral cavity.

Xerostomic patients should be continually monitored for candidiasis during and after radiotherapy. The incidence of oropharyngeal candidiasis in head and neck radiotherapy patients has been reported to be as high as 62% during treatment and 75% at subsequent posttreatment visits (RAMIREZ-AMADOR et al. 1997). As radiotherapy progresses, there tends to be a shift in the prevalence of Candida species from *C. albicans* to those which include *C. glabrata*, *C. tropicalis*, *C. parapsilosis*, and *C. krusei* (REDDING et al. 1999). It is often difficult to differentiate between candidiasis and radiation mucositis, but the infection should be suspected in patients with symptoms of burning mouth or tongue, regardless of clinical signs. A cytologic smear can be a valuable tool in diagnosing this common fungal infection. To perform the procedure, epithelial cells are spread on a glass microscope slide, fixed, and stained with periodic acid-Schiff. The stained specimen is examined under a microscope for the presence of *Candida* hyphae and spores (SKOGLUND et al. 1994) (Fig. 24.3).

Various antifungal medications are available for treatment of candidiasis. Patients may not be compliant with the frequent dosing that is required with nystatin or clotrimazole troches. Pastilles or troches are difficult to dissolve with less saliva and can be irritating to delicate irradiated tissues. Fluconazole (200 mg the first day and 100 mg daily for 6–13 days) has been proven to be effective and safe for treatment of oral candidiasis and its single daily dosing promotes compliance (REDDING et al. 1999; YOUNG et al. 1999). Resistance to fluconazole can occur, therefore it is necessary to take measures to prevent repopulation of the Candidal organisms. Chlorhexidine gluconate (2%) oral rinse can be formulated without alcohol and has been shown to inhibit the growth of Candidal organisms. When Candidal infections recur, dentures, toothbrushes, and fluoride carriers should be disinfected daily in 0.12% chlorhexidine, available commercially by prescription or in a diluted sodium hypochlorite solution (2–3 teaspoons bleach in a cup of water). Daily ingestion of yogurt with active cultures may also inhibit the growth of oropharyngeal Candidal populations.

Permanent hyposalivation results when salivary glands receive doses greater than 35 Gy (EISBRUCH et al. 2001). Radiation-induced xerostomia is a major cause of diminished quality of life after head and neck radiotherapy. Severely xerostomic patients are often unable to masticate and swallow food, suffer from sleep disturbances, have difficulty in wearing dentures, and have an increased susceptibility to oral infections and caries. Patients must be periodically counseled by both dentist and radiation oncologist on the relationship between xerostomia and oral complications. They must acknowledge and accept their role in good oral health through meticulous oral hygiene, use of fluoride, and follow-up dental care. This is especially true in patients who have retained teeth in areas of high dose radiation.

There are numerous commercially available saliva substitutes in the form of rinses and gels. None are universally accepted by patients because of differing individual taste or consistency preferences and because of their short duration in providing relief from dry mouth. Sugar-free gum and mints containing xylitol, with its antimicrobial effect, are beneficial in relieving mild xerostomia in some patients. Most patients prefer moistening their mouth with water throughout the day. Systemic sialagogues such as pilocarpine (5 mg tablets; 5–10 mg t.i.d.) or cevimeline (30 mg tablets; 30–60 mg t.i.d.) may increase the production of saliva in patients with some remaining measurable salivary production. Pilocarpine is approved by the FDA for use in radiotherapy patients; however, cevimeline is reported to provide longer duration of action (Fox et al. 2004). There are common side effects from both medications: increase in

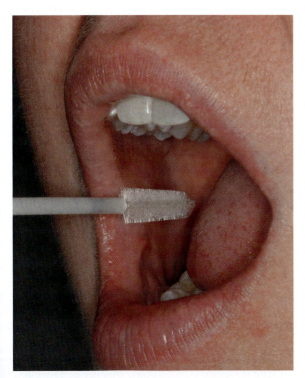

Fig. 24.3. Cytologic smear used for diagnosis of candidiasis

sweating, blurred vision, and gastrointestinal upset. Caution is advised when prescribing systemic sialagogues in patients with cardiovascular disease.

The use of fluoride during radiotherapy can cause discomfort; therefore fluoride in carriers can be initiated no later than 1 week after the completion of radiotherapy. The initiation of fluoride use shortly after the conclusion of treatment also prevents some patients' misinterpretation that the use of fluoride can be discontinued after radiotherapy is completed. Fluoride should be applied daily for the remainder of the patient's life in order to reduce the risk of radiation caries. The daily regimen should include proper brushing and flossing to remove plaque and food debris. All interior surfaces of the carriers should be coated with a thin layer of fluoride gel. The carriers should be placed on the teeth for 5–10 min and then removed. The residual fluoride gel should be expectorated, but not rinsed from the mouth. It is very important that the patient refrain from eating, drinking, or rinsing the mouth for at least 30 min. The best time for fluoride application is at bedtime. However, it is more important that a convenient time of day be selected for the procedure.

The most effective fluoride regimen for xerostomic patients is either 1.1% sodium fluoride gel/toothpaste or 0.4% stannous fluoride gel, delivered in fluoride carriers. Both fluoride preparations have been proven to be successful in the prevention of caries; however, the more acidic stannous fluoride preparation may cause extrinsic staining of enamel surfaces or etch porcelain restorations. Application of fluoride gel with a toothbrush is less effective than fluoride carrier application, but may be advisable in noncompliant patients. Fluoride gels are more effective than fluoride rinses in adhering to tooth surfaces, allowing a longer time for penetration of fluoride into the enamel.

Without proper preventive measures, radiation caries affecting multiple tooth surfaces can develop rapidly within weeks or months after the completion of radiotherapy (Fig. 24.4). Dental radiographs should be taken regularly at follow-up visits because they are necessary to detect restorable caries in its early stages. Without radiographs, it can be especially difficult to detect early caries in patients with crowns or bridges. If the patient develops multiple areas of decay, the dentist and radiation oncologist should determine whether the patient is complying with the daily fluoride regimen. Prior to extensive dental restorations, the patient should be encouraged to use fluoride in the carriers, as directed, for several weeks

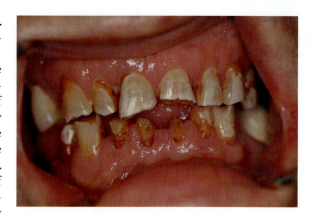

Fig. 24.4. Radiation caries

to allow enamel remineralization to occur. After this time, cavities in posterior teeth should be restored with amalgam restorations, whenever possible. Crowns should not be considered for patients until they demonstrate compliance with daily fluoride and decay is no longer active.

When patients develop rampant, nonrestorable decay, the decision for extraction of teeth should be made by the dentist and radiation oncologist after reviewing the radiotherapy treatment records. Hyperbaric oxygen therapy (HBO) may be indicated prior to extraction to increase oxygen tension and promote angiogenesis in bone having received doses greater than 60 Gy (Koga et al. 2008b). The benefit of HBO in the prevention of ORN has been controversial due in part, to a scarcity of randomized prospective trials (Wahl 2006). Patients in need of extraction of teeth in high-dose areas should be informed of HBO as a treatment option until definitive evidence proves that it is not beneficial in preventing ORN. The HBO protocol for prevention of ORN is 20 sessions or dives before tooth removal/surgery and 10 dives after tooth removal/surgery, with 100% oxygen at 2.4–2.5 atm absolute pressure administered once daily for 90 min (Marx et al. 1985). There is lack of consensus concerning the benefit of adjunctive antibiotic therapy in the prevention of ORN.

When a course of HBO therapy is not a viable option, nonsurgical root canals may be performed, when technically feasible, on nonrestorable teeth that would have a high risk of ORN if extracted. In these situations, the root structure of teeth can be preserved in the irradiated bone, thereby eliminating traumatic removal of the roots and reducing the risk of ORN. The preventive HBO protocol should be considered for surgical endodontic therapy or periodontal surgery in irradiated areas.

Differentiating between a bone sequestrum and early stages of ORN is often difficult (Fig. 24.5). The most common area of bone exposure is the medial surface of the posterior mandible. The patient often complains of an irritated or ulcerated tongue secondary to abrasion from rough, exposed bone. It is reasonable to treat small, asymptomatic bone exposures with conservative therapy that consists of close monitoring and measurement of the bone exposure. Patients should be encouraged to frequently lubricate oral tissues to reduce trauma to the area. When necessary for patient comfort, careful removal of loose bone or smoothing rough, devitalized bone should be accomplished without traumatizing soft tissues. When there is an established ORN, a bone exposure increases in size, persists for more than 3–6 months, becomes symptomatic, or radiographic changes develop, then 30 dives of HBO should be considered. If the wound shows no clinical evidence of improvement after 30 dives, debridement of necrotic bone and 10–30 additional dives of HBO are indicated using this protocol. Additional randomized, placebo-controlled, double-blinded trials are needed to further validate the effectiveness of HBO in patients with established ORN (ANNANE et al. 2004).

Atrophic and chronically irritated mucosal tissues can persist for months to years after the completion of treatment. It is important to reduce or eliminate potential sources of irritation in the oral cavity, such as fractured teeth or restorations and rough areas on removable prostheses. Care should be taken when wearing dentures after radiotherapy. Lack of lubrication and hyposalivation make dentures less retentive and can lead to denture sores that can progress to ORN. Postradiation denture patients often rely on denture adhesives to assist in retention and improve comfort. Patients should be informed of the importance of removing dentures and notifying their dentist immediately if denture sores develop. New dentures should be fabricated when oral tissues have returned to a state of good health, usually 3–4 months after radiotherapy.

Dental implants replace missing teeth, increase retention of removable prostheses, and improve function. They have been placed successfully in head and neck radiotherapy patients, with or without the preventive HBO protocol. Overall success rates are dependent on the radiation dose, fractionation, field, technical ease of implant placement, and tissue health. There are very few randomized controlled clinical trials that have assessed the benefit of HBO in increasing osseointegration of implants in irradiated patients (COULTHARD et al. 2003; ESPOSITO et al. 2008). As with any surgery in an irradiated area, the dentist and radiation oncologist should confer prior to the procedure. The risks vs. benefits of the surgical procedure, with alternative treatment options, should be thoroughly described to the patient and appropriately documented in the medical and dental records.

Trismus often occurs months to years after the completion of radiotherapy due to fibrosis of the muscles of mastication and other soft tissues. The decrease in mouth opening can create a challenge in maintaining oral hygiene and prohibit access by the dentist to restore teeth. In the early stages of trismus, patients should use a device specially designed to slowly increase the vertical dimension with daily use. Tongue depressors taped together and placed between the anterior teeth can also accomplish stretching of the muscle fibers. Warm compresses and anti-inflammatory or muscle relaxant drug therapy may also be required to supplement daily mouth opening and closing exercises.

In the years following radiotherapy, routine dental treatment, including nonsurgical root canal therapy, placement of fixed crowns or bridges, dental cleanings,

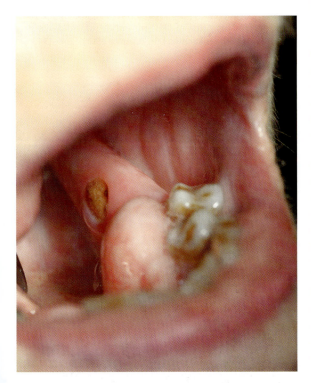

Fig. 24.5. Postradiation patient with mandibular bone exposure that progressed to ORN

restorations, and radiographs can be accomplished safely without antibiotics or HBO.

Radiation-induced complications can be debilitating and last lifelong. Excellent communication between health-care providers is imperative to minimize the negative effects of head and neck cancer therapy and improve the patient's overall quality of life.

References

Annane D, Depondt J, Aubert P et al. (2004) Hyperbaric oxygen therapy for radionecrosis of the jaw: a randomized, placebo-controlled, double-blind trial from the ORN96 Study Group. J Clin Oncol 22:4893–4900

Chang DT, Sandow PR, Morris CG et al. (2007) Do pre-irradiation dental extractions reduce the risk of osteoradionecrosis of the mandible? Head Neck 29(6):528–536

Coulthard P, Esposito M, Worthington HV et al. (2003) Therapeutic use of hyperbaric oxygen therapy for irradiated dental implant patients: a systematic review. J Dent Educ 67(1):64–68

Eisbruch A, Ship JA, Kim HM et al. (2001) Partial irradiation of the parotid gland. Semin Radiat Oncol 11(3):234–239

Epstein JB, Lunn R, Le N et al. (1998) Periodontal attachment loss in patients after head and neck radiation therapy. Oral Surg Oral Med Oral Pathol Oral Radiol Endod 86(6):673–677

Esposito M, Grusovin MG, Patel A et al. (2008) Interventions for replacing missing teeth: hyperbaric oxygen therapy for irradiated patients who require dental implants. Cochrane Database Syst Rev 23(1):CD003603

Fox PC (2004) Salivary enhancement therapies. Caries Res 38(3): 241–246

Koga DH, Salvajoli JV, Alves FA (2008a) Dental extractions and radiotherapy in head and neck oncology: review of the literature. Oral Dis 14(1):40–44

Koga DH, Salvajoli JV, Kowalski LP et al. (2008b) Dental extractions related to head and neck radiotherapy: ten-year experience of a single institution. Oral Surg Oral Med Oral Pathol Oral Radiol Endod 105(5):e1–e6

Marx RE, Johnson RP, Kline SN (1985) Prevention of osteoradionecrosis: a randomized prospective clinical trial of hyperbaric oxygen versus penicillin. J Am Dent Assoc 111(1):49–54

Ramirez-Amador V, Silverman S, Jr, Mayer P et al. (1997) Candidal colonization and oral candidiasis in patients undergoing oral and pharyngeal radiation therapy. Oral Surg Oral Med Oral Pathol Oral Radiol Endod 84(2):149–153

Redding SW, Zellars RC, Kirkpatrick WR et al. (1999) Epidemiology of oropharyngeal *Candida* colonization and infection in patients receiving radiation for head and neck cancer. J Clin Microbiol 37(12):3896–3900

Skoglund A, Sunzel B, Lerner UH (1994) Comparison of three test methods used for the diagnosis of candidiasis. Scand J Dent Res 102(5):295–298

Sulaiman F, Huryn JM, Zlotolow IM (2003) Dental extractions in the irradiated head and neck patient: a retrospective analysis of Memorial Sloan-Kettering Cancer Center protocols, criteria, and end results. J Oral Maxillofac Surg 61: 1123–1131

Wahl MJ (2006) Osteoradionecrosis prevention myth. Int J Radiat Oncol Biol Phys 64(3):661–669

Young GA, Bosly A, Gibbs DL et al.; for Antifungal Prophylaxis Study Group. (1999) A double-blind comparison of fluconazole and nystatin in the prevention of candidiasis in patients with leukaemia. Eur J Cancer 35(8):1208–1213

Smoking Cessation

25

Douglas E. Jorenby

CONTENTS

25.1	**Health Consequences of Smoking**	*277*
25.2	**Evidence-Based Treatment Overview**	*278*
25.2.1	Smoking Cessation Counseling	*278*
25.2.2	Smoking Cessation Medications	*279*
25.2.2.1	Nicotine Gum	*279*
25.2.2.2	Nicotine Inhaler	*279*
25.2.2.3	Nicotine Lozenge	*279*
25.2.2.4	Nicotine Nasal Spray	*281*
25.2.2.5	Nicotine Patch	*281*
25.2.2.6	Bupropion SR	*281*
25.2.2.7	Varenicline	*281*
25.2.2.8	Combination Therapy	*281*
25.2.3	Other Treatments	*282*
25.2.4	Treatment in Patients with Head and Neck Cancer	*282*
25.3	**Motivational Interventions**	*283*
25.4	**Benefits of Smoking Cessation**	*283*
25.4.1	Benefits for Treatment and Beyond	*283*
25.4.2	Quality of Life Benefits	*284*
25.5	**Summary**	*284*
Abbreviations		*284*
References		*284*

Douglas E. Jorenby, PhD, Professor of Medicine
Department of Medicine, University of Wisconsin School of Medicine and Public Health, Center for Tobacco Research and Intervention, 1930 Monroe St., Suite 200, Madison, WI 53711, USA

KEY POINTS

- Smoking is the leading cause of premature death, and a significant risk factor for cancers of the head and neck.
- Evidence-based treatments, including counseling and medication, can significantly increase rates of smoking cessation.
- Treatments found to be effective in the general population have also proven effective in populations of patients with head and neck cancer.
- Continued smoking has negative effects on response to treatment, future health status, and quality of life.

25.1

Health Consequences of Smoking

Smoking is a major public health problem in the United States of America, where ~21% of adults are current smokers (CENTERS FOR DISEASE CONTROL AND PREVENTION 2007a). This results in more than 435,000 deaths each year from heart disease, stroke, chronic obstructive pulmonary disease, cancer at a variety of sites, as well as other diseases (CENTERS FOR DISEASE CONTROL AND PREVENTION 2007a). Among cancers, smoking is most strongly associated in the public's mind with lung cancer, but it also has a powerful relationship to cancers of the head and neck. The Surgeon General's Report (U.S. DEPARTMENT OF HEALTH AND HUMAN SERVICES 2004) concluded that there was sufficient evidence to conclude a causal relationship between smoking and cancers of the esophagus and larynx, and in the case of cancers of the oral cavity and pharynx, to estimate the increased risk at ten times for men and five times for women (compared with never smokers). Along with the increased risk of developing cancer at sites in the head or neck, patients who smoke (especially those smoking more than 20 cigarettes/day) may delay in seeking out medical care, which results in larger tumors at the time of diagnosis (Brouha et al. 2005). Among those diagnosed with head or neck cancer, nearly half may quit smoking in the first year postdiagnosis (Duffy et al. 2007). This is a higher rate than the 5% unassisted cessation rate observed in the general population (Hughes 2003) but still leaves significant room for improvement.

25.2
Evidence-Based Treatment Overview

The United States Public Health Service Clinical Practice Guideline *Treating Tobacco Use and Dependence* (Fiore et al. 2008) was updated in 2008 to reflect advances in smoking cessation treatment since the previous edition in 2000. The Clinical Practice Guideline presents practice recommendations based on meta-analyses conducted upon a base of over 8,700 peer-reviewed, randomized controlled trials that provided at least 5 months of follow-up. As a guide to clinical intervention, the Clinical Practice Guideline utilizes the "5As"mnemonic: (1) that all patients should be *asked* about tobacco use; (2) those who currently use tobacco should be *advised* in a clear, strong, and personalized manner to quit; (3) patient willingness to make a quit attempt should then be *assessed*; (4)for patients willing to make an attempt, *assist* by providing evidence-based treatments; and finally, (5) to *arrange* for follow-up care. In tandem with the clinical intervention framework, the Clinical Practice Guideline meta-analyses identified effective elements of smoking cessation treatment, including counseling and medication. Treatment elements in the Clinical Practice Guideline meta-analyses were evaluated by pooling results from relevant studies and calculating odds ratios (OR) for the treatment in relation to a reference group (typically those who did not receive the treatment) with a fixed OR = 1. Each OR had a 95% confidence interval calculated; confidence intervals that overlaped 1.0 indicated treatments that were not significantly different from the reference group. The presentation convention used by the Clinical Practice Guideline was (OR = X (95% confidence interval)).

25.2.1
Smoking Cessation Counseling

Smoking cessation counseling may be provided in a number of different ways. At the most basic, clinicians conducting the second of the 5As (Advise) provide brief advice that typically requires less than 3 min, conveying the importance of quitting smoking. Brief physician advice has been shown to increase quit rates significantly, relative to no advice (OR = 1.3 (1.1–1.6); Fiore et al. 2008). Thus, even brief advice increases smoking cessation rates, and represents a minimum standard of care. A reliable dose–response relationship was also found, both in terms of total amount of counseling time (OR = 3.2 (2.3–4.6) for 91–300 min of counseling time) and number of counseling sessions (OR = 2.3 (2.1–3.0) for eight or more sessions; Fiore et al. 2008). Although not all patients would be interested in the most intensive treatments, nor would all clinics be able to provide them, the trend is such that any increases in frequency and/or duration beyond brief advice are likely to increase patients' chances of long-term smoking cessation.

Counseling has traditionally been delivered face-to-face, either on an individual basis, or in a group format. Both of these formats are quite effective, with ORs = 1.7 (1.4–2.0) and 1.3 (1.1–1.6), respectively (Fiore et al. 2008). Either may be selected based upon patient preference and available resources. In recent years, counseling has become more widely available because of the emergence of telephone-based proactive tobacco quitlines. Within the United States, any resident may access such services through a uniform toll-free number, 1-800-QUIT-NOW. The evaluation of such quit lines as stand-alone interventions (as opposed to being used with other counseling formats) was a particular focus of the 2008 Clinical Practice Guideline update. A meta-analysis of nine such studies concluded that quitlines were effective, with an OR = 1.6 (1.4–1.8), comparable with face-to-face counseling formats (Fiore et al. 2008). Quitlines have the advantage of being accessible to anyone with a telephone, even those in geographically remote or underserved areas. They also offer clinicians an opportunity to increase the intensity of interventions without requiring additional clinic time or staff members with specialized smoking cessation training. In theory, Internet-based treatments may offer similar advantages, but there is at present an insufficient evidence base to evaluate them.

Effective smoking cessation counseling embraces two elements: problem-solving skills and social support.

The former involves helping patients identify triggers for smoking (e.g., upon waking, after meals, when experiencing stress) and then developing coping skills to either avoid those triggers or cope with the urge to smoke (e.g., deep breathing, distraction). Social support provided by clinicians includes encouraging patients to discuss their quitting experience, expressing a willingness to help with the quit attempt, and communicating belief in the patient's ability to quit smoking.

25.2.2
Smoking Cessation Medications

As of 2008, the United States Food and Drug Administration has approved seven smoking cessation medications. Five of these are nicotine replacement therapies (gum, inhaler, lozenge, nasal spray, and patch), while the other two have non-nicotine mechanisms of action (bupropion SR (sustained release), varenicline). All seven significantly increase smoking cessation rates, relative to placebo. Table 25.1 presents a summary of all seven FDA-approved smoking cessation medications, including dosing regimens, contraindications, and cost estimates.

All five nicotine replacement therapies trade upon the paradox that while nicotine is the psychoactive agent that maintains dependence upon cigarettes and other forms of tobacco, with a very small number of exceptions (e.g., pregnant women), the negative health outcomes described in Sect. 25.1 are not caused by nicotine, but by the carbon monoxide, tar, carcinogens, and other toxins present in cigarette smoke (U.S. DEPARTMENT OF HEALTH AND HUMAN SERVICES 1988). By providing nicotine alone, the therapeutic goals are to (1) break the association between nicotine delivery and smoking, (2) to reduce aversive withdrawal symptoms that may promote relapse to smoking, and (3) to help the patient transition within a matter of months to a lifestyle free of both tobacco and nicotine. Each of the five nicotine replacement delivery systems has advantages and disadvantages, and these may vary from patient to patient.

25.2.2.1
Nicotine Gum

The first nicotine replacement therapy to be approved in the United States, nicotine gum is available over-the-counter in a variety of flavors. The available doses are 2 or 4 mg/piece. The former is recommended for patients smoking fewer than 25 cigarettes/day. Because the nicotine in the gum is absorbed through the oral mucosa, it is important that patients learn to "chew and park" the gum to maximize absorption. The process is also pH-dependent, so consumption of acidic beverages (coffee, cola, citrus juice) will diminish the therapeutic effect. The Clinical Practice Guideline meta-analysis of nicotine gum use for up to 14 weeks produced an OR = 1.5 (1.2–1.7) (FIORE et al. 2008). Side effects of treatment for head and neck cancer may make nicotine gum a less appealing treatment option.

25.2.2.2
Nicotine Inhaler

The nicotine inhaler consists of a cartridge containing nicotine in a fibrous plug. When placed in a plastic mouthpiece, the cartridge is pierced at both ends, delivering a small amount of nicotine to the mouth when the patient puffs. There is no combustion involved, so there is no carbon monoxide or environmental tobacco smoke produced. A single cartridge delivers ~4 mg of nicotine over the course of 80 puffs. Although the puffing has some similarity to smoking behavior (and therefore may be appealing to some patients), the nicotine is absorbed through the oral mucosa, not the lungs. Therefore, the same caveats about acidic beverages that apply to nicotine gum also apply to the inhaler. In the Clinical Practice Guideline meta-analysis, an OR = 2.1 (1.5–2.9) was observed, relative to placebo (FIORE et al. 2008).

25.2.2.3
Nicotine Lozenge

Because some patients find it difficult to master the "chew and park" technique necessary to maximize the therapeutic effect of nicotine gum, a nicotine lozenge was developed. The patient simply places the lozenge in his or her mouth and allows it to dissolve. Because the nicotine is absorbed through the oral mucosa, the same cautions regarding use of acidic beverages just before lozenge use apply. Just as with nicotine gum, lozenges are available in 2- and 4-mg doses. Rather than dosing by number of cigarettes smoked, time to first cigarette upon waking is the metric, with 2-mg lozenges preferred for

Table 25.1. Summary of all FDA-approved smoking cessation medications, including cautions, suggested dosing regimens, and cost estimates

Medication	Cautions	Side effects	Dosage	Use	Availability	Average cost (check insurance)
Bupropion SR 150	Not for use if you: Currently use amonoamine oxidase (MAO) inhibitor; Use bupropion in any other form (Zyban/Wellbutrin); Have a history of seizures; Have a history of eating disorders	Insomnia; dry mouth	Days 1–3: 150 mg each morning; days 4–end: 150 mg twice daily	Start 1–2 weeks before quit date; use 2–6 months	Prescription only:Zyban Wellbutrin SR; Generic SR	One box of 60 tablets, 150 mg = $70–$100/month (generic); $100–$150 (Wellbutrin SR $160 to $210/month (Zyban)
Nicotine gum; (2 or 4 mg)	Caution with dentures. Do not eat or drink 15 min before or during	Mouth soreness; stomach ache	One piece every 1–2 h; 6–15 pieces/day; 2 mg: If smoke < 25 cigarettes per day; 4 mg: If smoke >= 25 cigarettes per day	Up to 12 weeks or as needed	OTC only: Nicorette; generic	2 mg box of 170 pieces = $50–$70; 4 mg box of 170 pieces = $60–$80 (lasts 2–3 weeks)
Nicotine inhaler	May irritate mouth/throat at first (but improves with use)	Local irritation of mouth & throat	6–16 cartridges/day. Inhale 80 times/cartridge. May save partially-used cartridge for next day	Up to 6 months; taper at end	Prescription only: Nicotrol inhaler	One box of 168 10 mg cartridges = $136–$280 (1-month supply)
Nicotine lozenge (2 or 4 mg)	Do not eat or drink 15 min before or during one lozenge at a time. Limit 20 in 24 h	Hiccups Cough Heartburn	2 mg: If smoke / chew ≥30 min after waking; 4 mg: If smoke/ chew ≤30 min after waking; weeks 1–6: 1 every 1–2 h; weeks 7–9: 1 every 2–4 h; weeks 10–12: 1 every 4–8 h	Up to 12 weeks	OTC only: Commit; generic (Nicabate)	72 lozenges = $34 (generic) to $50 (name brand) (lasts 1–2 weeks)
Nicotine nasal spray	Not for patients with asthma. May irritate nose (improves over time). May cause dependence	Nasal irritation	1 "dose" = 1 squirt per nostril; 1–2 doses/h; 8–40 doses/day. Do not inhale	3–6 months; taper at end	Prescription only: Nicotrol NS	$140 a month to $280 a month
Nicotine patch	Do not use if you have severe eczema or psoriasis	Local skin reaction; insomnia	One patch per day. If ≥10 cigarettes/day: 21 mg 4 weeks, 14 mg 2 weeks, 7 mg 2 weeks. If <10/day: 14 mg 4 weeks, then 7 mg 4 weeks	6–8 weeks	OTC: Nicoderm CQ; nicotrol. Generic prescription: Generic (legend)	Box of 14: 14 mg: $20–$40; 21 mg: $36–$50 (2-week supply)
Varenicline	Use with caution in patients: With significant renal impairment. With serious psychiatric illness undergoing dialysis	Nausea; insomnia; abnormal dreams; psychiatric symptoms	Days 1–3: 0.5 mg every morning; days 4–7: 0.5 mg twice daily; day 8 to end: 1 mg twice daily	Start 1 week before quit date; use 3–6 months	Prescription only: Chantix	$70–$120/month ($2.25–$3.87/day)

those who wait more than 30 min for their first cigarette. Because only one treatment outcome study with nicotine lozenges was available (SHIFFMAN et al. 2002), the Clinical Practice Guideline was unable to conduct a meta-analysis as with the other medications. Calculated ORs = 2.0 (1.4–2.8) for 2-mg lozenge and 2.8 (1.9–4.0) for 4-mg lozenge (FIORE et al. 2008). As with the gum, side effects of head and neck cancer treatment may limit the use of nicotine lozenges.

25.2.2.4
Nicotine Nasal Spray

Nicotine nasal spray delivers a nicotine solution through the nose, with a dose consisting of a squirt to each nostril delivering a total of 1 mg of nicotine. It is recommended that patients not exceed 40 doses/day. Because nasal delivery produces more rapid peak concentration than oral or transdermal delivery of nicotine does, there is more potential for development of dependence on the nasal spray. It also may produce significant irritation in the nasal passages, which may have implications for its use in patients receiving cancer treatment in the nasal cavity, nasopharynx, or related areas. When tolerated, the nicotine nasal spray produces significant quit rates. The Clinical Practice Guideline meta-analysis found an OR = 2.3 (1.7–3.0) (FIORE et al. 2008).

25.2.2.5
Nicotine Patch

Partly as a result of the difficulties patients experienced using ad libitum nicotine replacement therapies, nicotine patches were developed to simplify dosing and improve patient adherence. Because nicotine is absorbed readily through the skin, patients could apply a single patch in the morning that would deliver a dose of 21, 14, or 7 mg over a 24-h period, quickly establishing stable blood levels of nicotine to reduce withdrawal symptoms. In the Clinical Practice Guideline meta-analysis, use of the nicotine patch for up to 14 weeks produced an OR = 1.9 (1.7–2.2) (FIORE et al. 2008). Because the nicotine patch is usually applied to the arms or trunk, it may be a more viable option for patients quitting smoking while receiving head or neck cancer treatment.

25.2.2.6
Bupropion SR

Bupropion SR, an atypical antidepressant, was the first non-nicotine therapy approved by the FDA for smoking cessation. With nicotine replacement therapies, patients begin use on their quit day, whereas patients begin taking bupropion SR 1–2 weeks prior to their quit date, tapering up to a target dose of 150 mg twice a day. With data from 26 study arms, the Clinical Practice Guideline found an OR = 2.0 (1.8–2.2) for bupropion SR, relative to placebo (FIORE et al. 2008). Because the medication was originally developed to treat depression, it should be given particular consideration in patients with comorbid depression (DUFFY et al. 2006).

25.2.2.7
Varenicline

The most recent medication to be approved by the FDA for smoking cessation is varenicline, an $\alpha4\beta2$ nicotinic acetylcholine receptor partial agonist. As with bupropion SR, treatment with this non-nicotine medication involves tapering up to a target dose of 1 mg twice a day over a week. Varenicline exhibits a mixture of agonist and antagonist properties. Like the other FDA-approved smoking cessation medications, it reduces the severity of withdrawal symptoms and craving; at the same time, it appears to have unique effects in reducing the rewarding aspects of smoking (GONZALES et al. 2006; JORENBY et al. 2006). The meta-analysis of the recommended varenicline dose in the Clinical Practice Guideline produced an OR = 3.1 (2.5–3.8) (FIORE et al. 2008). The most common side effects reported with varenicline included nausea, abnormal dreams, and sleep disruption. In February 2008, the FDA issued a postapproval warning regarding drowsiness, changes in behavior, and suicidal thoughts in patients using varenicline, recommending that clinicians monitor patients for changes in mood and behavior.

25.2.2.8
Combination Therapy

As of 2008, the FDA has given approval to only one combination of smoking cessation medications: bupropion SR and nicotine patch. The literature reviewed by the Clinical Practice Guideline identified a number of combinations that have been evaluated in randomized controlled trials. Most of these involved adding a form of ad libitum nicotine replacement therapy to nicotine patch. Adding nicotine gum or nasal spray to nicotine patch was shown to increase cessation rates (OR = 3.6 (2.5–5.2); FIORE et al. 2008).

With 83 studies on smoking cessation medications available for analysis, the Clinical Practice Guideline conducted a further meta-analysis that compared both monotherapies and combination therapies to a reference treatment of nicotine patch (the medication with the largest number of study arms available). Table 25.2 presents a sample of these relative effectiveness comparisons.

25.2.3
Other Treatments

A number of additional smoking cessation treatments exist. Some of these may be attractive because they seem to offer the possibility of cessation with little or no motivation on the part of the patient. Hypnosis is one such option. The Guideline was unable to find a sufficient number of studies meeting methodological criteria to evaluate hypnosis (FIORE et al. 2008), while an independent Cochrane Review concluded that hypnosis did not have a greater effect

Table 25.2. Effectiveness of selected smoking cessation therapies and combination therapies referenced to nicotine patch (after FIORE et al. 2008)

Medication(s)	Number of arms	Estimated odds ratio (95% confidence interval)
Nicotine patch (reference)	32	1.0
Varenicline (2 mg/day)	5	1.6 (1.3–2.0)
Nicotine nasal spray	4	1.2 (0.9–1.6)
Nicotine inhaler	6	1.1 (0.8–1.5)
Bupropion SR	26	1.0 (0.9–1.2)
Nicotine gum	15	0.8 (0.6–1.0)
Nicotine patch (>14 weeks) + nicotine gum or nasal spray	3	1.9 (1.3–2.7)

on cessation than no treatment (ABBOT et al. 2002). Acupuncture was not found to differ from a control procedure in a Guideline meta-analysis of five studies (OR = 1.1 (0.7–1.6); FIORE et al. 2008). A Cochrane Review of 24 studies found a marginally significant short-term treatment effect attributable to a single study, but found no long-term difference when compared with no treatment (WHITE et al. 2006). The same Cochrane Review also found no support for the efficacy of the more recent laser treatment, in which lasers (rather than needles) are used to stimulate acupuncture meridians.

25.2.4
Treatment in Patients with Head and Neck Cancer

As noted above (25.1), while smoking cessation rates among patients diagnosed with head and neck cancer are higher than in the general population, significant room for improvement exists. GRITZ et al. (1999) followed a group of 186 newly-diagnosed patients for 12 months. Those who relapsed during the first year were more likely to have attempted to quit using gradual reduction of the number of cigarettes smoked. They also experienced significantly more craving and anxiety (nicotine withdrawal symptoms) during the first week of their initial quit attempt. The increased withdrawal severity may reflect a greater degree of nicotine dependence, as those who relapsed were more likely to smoke less than 30 min after waking in the baseline assessment. Gritz and colleagues found that patients who received total laryngectomy treatment were more likely to quit smoking than those who received only radiation treatment, replicating a result reported by VANDER ARK et al. (1997; however, see CHAN et al. 2004). A limitation of these studies is that they either did not report methods used to attempt smoking cessation, or they were conducted prior to many effective evidence-based treatments being available in clinical practice.

A recent study by DUFFY et al. (2006) made use of an integrated package of evidence-based treatments in a randomized controlled trial of 184 patients with head and neck cancer. Participants were assigned randomly to either "enhanced usual care" (referral to specialized treatment) or an intervention that provided a workbook and 9–11 telephone-based counseling sessions along with medication. The study selected patients who screened positive for smoking, alcohol use, and/or depression. The heterogeneous population introduces a degree of interpretive complexity. However, there is significant comorbidity between the three conditions in real-world populations and the intervention condition contained all the evidence-based elements recommended by the Clinical Practice Guideline. Two positive findings emerged from the study. First, patients who smoked were significantly more likely to participate in the study than were nonsmokers, indicating that this population is interested in clinical assistance with smoking cessation. Second, the counseling and medication intervention increased quit rates by 50% when compared with usual care (47 vs. 31% at 6 months). Alcohol use and depression did not differ significantly from baseline at the 6 month follow-up. This suggests that the same treatment elements found to be effective in the general population of smokers are also effective with head and neck cancer patients, even those with significant comorbidities.

25.3
Motivational Interventions

While there is solid evidence that both the general population of smokers (CENTERS FOR DISEASE CONTROL AND PREVENTION 2007b) and patients with head and neck cancer who smoke (DUFFY et al. 2006) are interested in quitting, not all patients will be willing to make a quit attempt at any given point in time. In recognition of this, the Clinical Practice Guideline advocates use of the "5Rs" intervention: *Relevance, Risks, Rewards, Roadblocks,* and *Repetition.* Relevance refers to personal reasons for quitting. Although it may be tempting to assume that a diagnosis of cancer automatically becomes a reason for quitting, it is important to ask the patient why quitting is relevant to them. In some cases, wanting to protect the health of others (e.g., not exposing grandchildren to environmental tobacco smoke) may be more salient than the patient's own health status. *Risks* and *Rewards* of continued tobacco use are opposite sides of the same coin. Some examples specific to patients with head and neck cancer are discussed in Sect. 25.4. Again, it is important to ask the patient what risks and rewards are important to them. *Roadblocks* are specific barriers to making a quit attempt, such as fear of severe withdrawal symptoms, or lack of knowledge regarding effective treatment options. Clinicians may be able to provide information that helps surmount these barriers. *Repetition* reflects the fact that it is

important to repeat motivational interventions with patients not yet ready to make a quit attempt. Especially among patients with head and neck cancer, many will have made previous quit attempts (CHAN et al. 2004), and it is important to normalize that most people who smoke make multiple attempts before they quit for good.

The 5Rs are largely derived from the principles of Motivational Interviewing (MILLER AND ROLLNICK 2002). A fundamental aspect of Motivational Interviewing is to allow the patients to express their ambivalence about smoking. The clinician then expresses empathy ("Quitting smoking is not an easy thing"), highlights the discrepancies in the patient's behavior in a nonaccusatory way ("You have made some very positive changes in your diet and exercise – how does smoking fit in with that?") while actively supporting the patient's ability to change (i.e., self-efficacy). It is possible for clinicians to obtain specialized training in Motivational Interviewing, but use of the 5Rs can also increase the chance of future quit attempts (CARPENTER et al. 2004).

25.4
Benefits of Smoking Cessation

For the patient with head and neck cancer, there are benefits to smoking cessation above and beyond those experienced by quitters in the general population. These may be grouped into treatment benefits and beneficial effects on quality of life. As discussed in Sect. 25.3, these may be of use in motivating patients who are not yet ready to make a quit attempt.

25.4.1
Benefits for Treatment and Beyond

Smoking status has implications for treatment even before treatment begins, particularly with surgical treatment. In a study of 188 patients receiving reconstructive head and neck surgery, KURI et al. (2005) observed that wound healing was improved when patients quit smoking more than 21 days before the surgery. This remained true even when controlling for a variety of factors, including age, history of diabetes, chemotherapy, and radiation therapy. Entering pack-years of smoking (a measure of cumulative exposure) into their multivariate model did not change the results, suggesting that even among very heavy smokers, quitting smoking even 3 weeks prior to surgery can produce significant benefits. For patients receiving radiation therapy for stage III or IV squamous cell cancer of the head and neck, smoking during therapy was associated with significantly lower rates of complete response, as well as increased mortality within 2 years (BROWMAN et al. 1993). As with surgical treatment, the greater the interval of being smoke-free prior to treatment, the better the outcome. Some evidence suggests that higher expression of epidermal growth factor receptor in continuing smokers may be a mechanism for poorer treatment outcomes (KUMAR et al. 2007).

25.4.2
Quality of Life Benefits

The impact of smoking or smoking cessation upon quality of life is more complex than simple survival analysis, in part because variations in treatment can exert significant influence over quality of life. As an example, a large study of 1 year quality of life outcomes conducted by RONIS et al. (2008) reported that major changes on the 36-item Short-Form Health Survey were related to feeding tube placement, chemotherapy, and radiation therapy. This group found that patients who smoked had poor quality of life at the baseline assessment; smoking was also predictive of poorer quality of life 1 year later, although the magnitude of the effect was less than that of having a feeding tube. Because the general trend was for physical function measures to decrease and mental health measures to improve over the study period, it is noteworthy that patients who smoked not only experienced lower physical functioning, but also scored low in social, emotional, and mental health. The authors did not provide an analysis of patients who quit smoking during the study period, so the specific time course of improvements is uncertain.

Two recent Scandinavian studies provide additional useful information. Both utilized standardized quality of life measures developed by the European Organization for Research and Treatment of Cancer for cancer in general and specific items for head and neck cancer. The Danish study (JENSEN et al. 2007) confirmed the pervasive negative impact of smoking on quality of life. It also found that previous smokers had quality of life scores that were in between those of never smokers and those who continued to smoke after their diagnosis. While this only captures a single timepoint, it is strongly suggestive of a gradual

improvement in quality of life following smoking cessation. The study conducted in Norway (AARSTAD et al. 2007) with a more heterogeneous population replicated the finding of decreased quality of life in terms of function and symptoms among those patients who smoked. A unique contribution of this study was an examination of possible coping styles among the sample. Smoking had a modest ($r = 0.26$, $p < 0.05$) association with "drinking to cope." Because the synergistic head and neck cancer risk resulting from smoking and alcohol use is well-established, it would be useful to determine in future research whether this coping style is common among other populations.

25.5
Summary

Smoking is a major risk factor for development of cancers of the head and neck. It may delay patients seeking treatment, and for those who continue to smoke during treatment there are negative consequences in terms of immediate response to treatment as well as long-term survival. Recent advances in evidence-based treatment of smoking provide a number of options for both patients and clinicians. Smoking cessation counseling is now available through effective telephone-based quit lines. There are seven FDA-approved smoking cessation medications available, with both nicotine and non-nicotine mechanisms of action. These treatments, particularly combining counseling and medication, have been proven effective in patients with head and neck cancer. Clear benefits to cessation for both treatment response and quality of life may help motivate patients initially unwilling to make a quit attempt.

Abbreviations

FDA   Food and Drug Administration
OR   Odds ratio
SR   Sustained release

References

Aarstad AKH, Aarstad HJ, Olofsson J (2007) Quality of life, drinking to cope, alcohol consumption and smoking is successfully treated HNSCC patients. Acta Otolaryngol 127:1091–1098

Abbot NC, Stead LF, White AR et al. (2002) Hypnotherapy for smoking cessation. Cochrane Database Syst Rev (2):CD001008

Brouha X, Tromp D, Hordijk GJ et al. (2005) Role of alcohol and smoking in diagnostic delay of head and neck cancer patients. Acta Otolaryngol 125:552–556

Browman GP, Wong G, Hodson I et al. (1993) Influence of cigarette smoking on the efficacy of radiation therapy in head and neck cancer. NEJM 328:159–163

Carpenter MJ, Hughes JR, Solomon LJ et al. (2004) Both smoking reduction with nicotine replacement therapy and motivational advice increase future cessation among smokers unmotivated to quit. J Consult Clin Psychol 72:371–381

Centers for Disease Control and Prevention (2007a) Cigarette smoking among adults – United States, 2006. MMWR 56:1157–1161

Centers for Disease Control and Prevention (2007b) State-specific prevalence of cigarette smoking among adults and quitting among persons aged 18–35 years – United States, 2006. MMWR 56:993–996

Chan Y, Irish JC, Wood SJ et al. (2004) Smoking cessation in patients diagnosed with head and neck cancer. J Otolaryngol 33:75–81

Duffy SA, Khan MJ, Ronis DL et al. (2007) Health behaviors of head and neck cancer patients the first year after diagnosis. Head Neck 30:93–102

Duffy SA, Ronis DL, Valenstein M et al. (2006) A tailored smoking, alcohol, and depression intervention for head and neck cancer patients. Cancer Epidemiol Biomarkers Prev 15:2203–2208

Fiore MC, Jaen CR, Baker TB et al. (2008) Treating tobacco use and dependence: 2008 update. Clinical practice guideline. Rockville, MD: U.S. Department of Health and Human Services and Public Health Service

Gonzales D, Rennard SI, Nides M et al. (2006) Varenicline, an α4β2 nicotinic acetylcholine receptor partial agonist, vs sustained-release bupropion and placebo for smoking cessation: a randomized controlled trial. JAMA 296:47–55

Gritz ER, Schacherer C, Koehly L et al. (1999) Smoking withdrawal and relapse in head and neck cancer patients. Head Neck 21:420–427

Hughes JR (2003) Motivating and helping smokers to stop smoking. J Gen Intern Med 18:1053–1057

Jensen K, Jensen AB, Grau C (2007) Smoking has a negative impact upon health related quality of life after treatment for head and neck cancer. Oral Oncol 43:187–192

Jorenby DE, Hays JT, Rigotti NA et al. (2006) Efficacy of varenicline, an α4β2 nicotinic acetylcholine receptor partial agonist, vs placebo or sustained-release buropion for smoking: a randomized controlled trial. JAMA 296:56–63

Kumar B, Cordell KG, Lee JS et al. (2007) Response to therapy and outcomes in oropharyngeal cancer are associated with biomarkers including human papillomavirus, epidermal growth factor receptor, gender, and smoking. Int J Radiation Oncology Biol Phys 69:S109–S111

Kuri M, Nakagawa M, Tanaka H et al. (2005) Determination of the duration of preoperative smoking cessation to improve wound healing after head and neck surgery. Anesthesiology 102:892–896

Miller WR, Rollnick S (2002) Motivational interviewing: preparing people for change, 2nd edn. Guilford Press, New York

Ronis DL, Duffy SA, Fowler KE et al. (2008) Changes in quality of life over 1 year in patients with head and neck cancer. Arch Otolaryngol Head Neck Surg 134:241–248

Shiffman S, Dresler CM, Hajek P et al. (2002) Efficacy of a nicotine lozenge for smoking cessation. Arch Intern Med 162:1267–1276

U.S. Department of Health and Human Services (1988) The health consequences of smoking: nicotine addiction. Atlanta, GA, U.S. Department of Health and Human Services, Centers for Disease Control and Prevention, National Center for Chronic Disease Prevention and Health Promotion, Office on Smoking and Health

U.S. Department of Health and Human Services (2004) The health consequences of smoking: a report of the Surgeon General. Atlanta, GA, U.S. Department of Health and Human Services, Centers for Disease Control and Prevention, National Center for Chronic Disease Prevention and Health Promotion, Office on Smoking and Health

Vander Ark W, DiNardo LJ, Oliver DS (1997) Factors affecting smoking cessation in patients with head and neck cancer. Laryngoscope 107:888–892

White AR, Rampes H, Campbell JL (2006) Acupuncture and related interventions for smoking cessation. Cochrane Database Syst Rev (1):CD000009

Supportive Therapy Including Nutrition

26

Jørgen Johansen and Jørn Herrstedt

C O N T E N T S

26.1 **Introduction** *288*

26.2 **Mucositis** *288*

26.3 **Prevention and Treatment of Oral or Pharyngeal Mucositis** *288*
26.3.1 Oral Care *289*
26.3.2 Chlorhexidine *289*
26.3.3 Benzydamine *289*
26.3.4 Sucralfate *290*
26.3.5 Antibiotics *290*
26.3.6 Growth Factors *290*
26.3.7 Amifostine *290*

26.4 **Pain** *291*

26.5 **Taste Alterations** *291*

26.6 **Tobacco** *291*

26.7 **Candidiasis** *292*

26.8 **Skin Toxicity** *293*

26.9 **Nutrition** *294*
26.9.1 Evaluation Strategies *294*
26.9.2 Intervention Strategies *294*
26.9.3 Tube Feeding *295*

26.10 **Conclusion** *296*

References *296*

KEY POINTS

- Radiation treatment causes significant acute morbidity due to affection of normal tissues such as skin, mucosa, salivary glands, teeth, bony structures, and muscles.
- Radiation dermatitis, mucositis, pain, mucosal infections, taste loss, dysphagia, and xerostomia are common side effects to radiation treatment.
- Morbidity is aggravated by surgery, altered fractionation, and concomitant chemotherapy.
- Oral mucositis has previously been reported in 45% of patients receiving radiation treatment. With accelerated or hyperfractionated schedules combined with chemotherapy, 80–90% will experience severe mucositis. This may hamper the effectiveness of treatment because of dose reductions, dose delay, and hospitalization.
- Poor nutrition, weight loss, and fatigue affect quality of life and possibly recovery.
- Preventive measures are important, including the use of intensity-modulated radiation therapy to spare normal tissues.
- Few clinical trials have documented superiority of various preventive treatment schedules, emphasized by the many different supportive care initiatives.
- Supportive care during radiation treatment aims at alleviating mucositis, pain control, preservation of adequate nutrition, and elimination of infections.

Jørgen Johansen, MD, PhD
Jørn Herrstedt, MD, DMSci, Professor
Department of Oncology, Odense University Hospital, Sdr. Boulevard 29, 5000 Odense C, Denmark

26.1
Introduction

Modern head and neck cancer treatment, including accelerated and hyperfractionated fractionation schedules, are known to increase acute side effects to radiation. Furthermore, concurrent chemoradiation aggravates acute mucosal reaction (BRIZEL et al. 1998), which now has become the limiting factor in radical head and neck cancer treatment. For this reason, supportive care strategies are necessary to prevent, treat, and alleviate discomfort and to maintain nutrition and compliance to treatment.

Highly variable study designs, small sample sizes, and lack of consistent results do not allow strictly evidence-based recommendations for basic oral care and prevention and treatment of side effects, including mucositis (RUBENSTEIN et al. 2004; SUTHERLAND and BROWMAN 2001). Consequentially, institutional strategies and oral care programs are based on guidelines with low levels of evidence or on clinical experience only.

This chapter will focus on preventive strategies and treatment of major problems during treatment for head and neck cancer, such as oral mucositis, pain, and nutrition.

26.2
Mucositis

Mucositis of the mouth and pharynx is the most distressing side effect in radiation treatment of head and neck cancer patients. Many factors play an important role in its manifestation. The radiation-induced damage to the mucosa induces a significant problem for the patient because of consequential pain and eating and swallowing difficulties. Mucositis presents initially as erythema but as cell destruction proceeds, the epithelium will present as a pseudo membranous desquamation, often mimicking candidiasis. Complete denudation and ulceration may evolve. Besides the discomfort for the patient, these symptoms may also compromise nutrition.

Incidence rates of mucositis are dependent on tumor location, use of concomitant chemotherapy, fractionation schedules, and physical aspects (HENK 1997; TROTTI et al. 2003; LALLA et al. 2008) such as total dose (WALDRON et al. 2008), dose intensity (GRAU et al. 2006; OVERGAARD et al. 2003), and

treatment volumes (POULSEN et al. 2008; MIRABELL et al. 1999). Furthermore, use of concurrent chemotherapy such as 5-fluorouracil may aggravate oral mucositis and induce intestinal mucositis and leucopenia as well, thereby increasing the risk of systemic infection.

Oral mucositis of any degree occurs in ~90%, while confluent mucositis occurs in about 50% of patients undergoing radiotherapy for head and neck cancer (SUTHERLAND and BROWMAN 2001; TROTTI et al. 2003; OVERGAARD et al. 2003). However, very accelerated radiation schedules have shown incidence rates of confluent mucositis as high as 90% (POULSEN et al. 2001) while chemoradiation schedules induce grade 3–4 mucositis in 51–66% of the patients (VAN DEN BROEK et al. 2006; ELTING et al. 2007) often accompanied by leucopenia (VAN DEN BROEK et al. 2006).

26.3
Prevention and Treatment of Oral or Pharyngeal Mucositis

Owing to the immense clinical problems related to oropharyngeal mucositis, prevention is a very important issue. However, the evidence of benefit from various preventive actions is scarce.

SUTHERLAND and BROWMAN (2001) published a meta-analysis on clinical randomized trials investigating prophylactic interventions of oral mucositis induced by radiotherapy. The overall outcome of severe oral mucositis, as assessed by the patients themselves, showed only a trend towards a benefit from prophylactic treatments. Using the clinicians' assessments, only 1 out of 13 trials was able to demonstrate a significant benefit from prophylaxis; however, the overall analysis did show a significant risk reduction of severe mucositis by 36% corresponding to an absolute benefit of 9% from all preventive strategies.

The Multinational Association for Supportive Care (MASCC) and the International Society for Oral Oncology (ISOO) Mucositis Study Group have developed evidence-based guidelines reviewing the literature between 1966 and 2002 (RUBENSTEIN et al. 2004) and these were recently updated (KEEFE et al. 2007b). Positive and negative recommendations for the treatment of mucositis were given.

Numerous studies have been conducted to improve preventive strategies and treatment of oral mucositis. In the MASCC/ISOO guidelines update, the panel retrieved 3,974 papers published from January 2002 until May 2005. Of these, 622 were considered of sufficient quality and relevance to be included in the final recommendation (KEEFE et al. 2007b).

The recommendations can be grouped according to the target of intervention (Table 26.1), and some of the most important physical and medical interventions are described here.

26.3.1
Oral Care

Dental examination and management of oral disease are important before the initiation of radiation treatment. During radiotherapy, regular assessment of oral pain and of the degree of mucositis should be done using validated scales (KEEFE et al. 2007b). Optimum oral hygiene is recommended. This may be carried out in collaboration with in-hospital dentists. Patients are generally advised to omit irritating factors such as spicy meals, acidic drinks, or alcohol.

Table 26.1. Treatment and preventive measures of mucositis

Reducing exposure to normal tissues	IMRT
	Optimized target definition
Epithelial protection	Sucralfate
	Amifostine
Parotid cell protection	Pilocarpine
Enhancement of epithelial maturation	Keratinocyte growth factor
	GM-CSF/G-CSF
	Low energy laser therapy
Anti-inflammatory agents	Steroids
	Nonsteroidal anti-inflammatory drugs
	Benzydamine
Antimicrobials	Topical, systemic antifungal and antibacterial drugs
	Benzydamine
	Chlorhexidine
Analgesics	Topical, systemic formulations

Moistening fluids, mouthwashes, or sprays are necessary to prevent or reduce dryness of the mucosa and lips during treatment but the effect on the occurrence of radiation-induced mucositis is questionable. Lubrication using self-made (one part water, one part glycerin and optional flavoring) or commercial products is encouraged.

Because the viscous saliva from the parotid glands is reduced in the early phase of radiotherapy, many patients tend to complain of sticky, mucous saliva. Consequential gagging, nausea, and even vomiting may occur. With the risk of exacerbating xerostomia, anticholinergic drugs may be prescribed to reduce salivary problems.

26.3.2
Chlorhexidine

The value of oral disinfectants, such as chlorhexidine or benzydamine, in the prevention and treatment of mucositis is uncertain. In a study by FOOTE et al. (1994), substantially more toxicity was noted during radiotherapy in the chlorhexidine-treated patients, compared with the control arm regarding mouthwash-induced discomfort, taste alteration, and teeth staining – and even a trend to more mucositis on the chlorhexidine arm. It should be kept in mind that various commercial products contain up to 10% alcohol which in itself my cause irritation. Preventive use of chlorhexidine is not recommended by guidelines (WORTHINGTON et al. 2008; KEEFE et al. 2007b).

26.3.3
Benzydamine

Benzydamine is a cytoprotectant with anti-inflammatory, analgesic, and antimicrobial activity, which has been found to prevent mucositis in a small placebo-controlled trial in patients undergoing radiotherapy with or without chemotherapy for head and neck cancer (PRADA and CHIESA 1987). This was confirmed in a large placebo-controlled trial in patients receiving moderate-dose radiation therapy (EPSTEIN et al. 2001). The latter trial led the MASCC guidelines to recommend benzydamine for prevention of radiation-induced mucositis in patients with head and neck cancer receiving moderate-dose (up to 50 Gy) radiation treatment (KEEFE et al. 2007b). The Cochrane Collaboration analysis on prevention did not include the above study (EPSTEIN et al. 2001) in their analysis (the study did not fit the analysis criteria, reason not specified), and based on the small study of PRADA and CHIESA (1987) only, they considered the evidence of a preventive benefit weak and unreliable (WORTHINGTON et al. 2008). Also, the Cochrane Collaboration meta-analysis on intervention for treating oral mucositis has considered benzydamine ineffective (CLARKSON et al. 2007).

Overall, the value of benzydamine seems limited because the total radiation dose in head and neck cancer most often exceeds 50 Gy.

26.3.4
Sucralfate

Sucralfate has been approved for treating gastric and duodenal ulcers as well as for gastroesophageal reflux. Unlike other drugs used for peptic ulcers, sucralfate binds to the hydrochloric acid in the stomach as well as to proteins of the denudated mucosa to form a cytoprotective layer.

Several randomized trials have studied the preventive or therapeutic effect of sucralfate on oral and pharyngeal radiation-induced mucositis. Generally, sucralfate mouthwash plus swallow was tested against placebo and doses varied between 1 and 2 g, 4–6 times/day. Unfortunately, the investigations have produced conflicting results and this includes both the effect on radiation-induced mucositis, pain, and consumption of analgesics (KWONG 2004).

The randomized studies are generally small, with only two studies including more than 100 patients. No statistically significant differences were found in a meta-analysis using mucositis at different levels as the end point after either radiation treatment or chemotherapy and it was concluded that there is insufficient evidence to support or refute that sucralfate is more or less effective than placebo in preventing or alleviating symptoms (KEEFE et al. 2007b; WORTHINGTON et al. 2008; CLARKSON et al. 2007).

26.3.5
Antibiotics

Various antibiotics and antifungal medications have been investigated to reduce mucositis by a selective elimination of Gram-negative bacteria and yeasts. A meta-analysis (SUTHERLAND and BROWMAN 2001) indicated that narrow-spectrum antibacterial lozenges containing polymyxin E, tobramycin, and amphotericin

B were effective in preventing mucositis. However, in subsequent randomized studies, this finding was not confirmed (STOKMAN et al. 2003; EL-SAYED et al. 2002), and antibiotic lozenges are not recommended for routine use (KEEFE et al. 2007b; WORTHINGTON et al. 2008).

26.3.6
Growth Factors

Palifermin is a recombinant form of human keratinocyte growth factor (rHuKGF) which has been approved for preventing and reducing the incidence and duration of oral mucositis in patients with hematological malignancies undergoing stem cell transplantation. The receptor – a tyrosine kinase – is expressed exclusively in epithelial cells, including the oral and pharyngeal mucosa. KGF stimulates epithelial proliferation, migration, and differentiation (RUBIN et al. 1995). Theoretically, KGF may stimulate tumor cell growth because epithelial tumor cells often express the KGF receptor (FINCH and RUBIN 2006). Besides from a small positive trial in patients receiving chemotherapy for colorectal cancer (ROSEN et al. 2006), palifermin has not yet been established in treatment of solid tumors (other than lymphomas) and its use in head and neck cancer patients should be limited to clinical trials (MCDONNELL and LENZ 2007). The common adverse effects of palifermin seem to be rash, pruritus, cough, and taste alterations.

GM-CSF stimulates proliferation and differentiation of hematopoietic cells, increasing the number of circulating neutrophils and monocytes which may improve the immune response to local infections in the oral and pharyngeal mucosa during radiotherapy. GM-CSF may also exert a direct effect on oral epithelial cells. Subcutaneous or locally applied GM-CSF has demonstrated some benefit in preventing severity and duration of mucositis after chemotherapy, while the evidence of an effect of GM-CSF has been less impressive during radiation treatment, and so far, GM-CSF cannot be recommended for either prevention or treatment of radiation-induced mucositis (KWONG 2004; FUNG and FERRILL 2002; CLARKSON et al. 2007).

26.3.7
Amifostine

Amifostine is an organic thiophosfate that acts through its metabolite as a free-radical scavenger to protect normal tissues during irradiation. It is approved for preventing xerostomia after radio-therapy.

The two largest randomized studies to date, with more than 400 patients, evaluated amifostine in head and neck cancer and found no reduction of amifostine on acute mucositis (BRIZEL et al. 2000; BUENTZEL et al. 2006). A subset analysis (BUENTZEL et al. 2006) in patients receiving "smaller fields" demonstrated less mucositis in the amifostine arm and it was speculated whether the effect of amifostine would benefit from an increase in dose.

The Cochrane Collaboration (WORTHINGTON et al. 2008) concluded that amifostine does provide a minimal benefit in preventing mild and moderate mucositis (risk reductions of 5 and 12%, respectively). However, generally, amifostine has been evaluated in small studies and the findings have been inconsistent (KEEFE et al. 2007b; ANDREASSEN et al. 2003).

Owing to the toxicity profile of amifostine, it is not clear whether mucositis can be prevented within a dose range that does not cause unacceptable side effects during weeks of radiation treatment (BUENTZEL et al. 2006; ANDREASSEN et al. 2003).

26.4

Pain

Pain is inevitably associated with head and neck cancer either because of local destructive and ulcerating tumors or severe tissue reactions to aggressive treatment. Pain may arise from complications to surgery, chemotherapy, radiation, or a combination.

Irritating and pain-aggravating factors should be omitted and preventive oral strategies should be carried out as described elsewhere, but only rarely will the patients go through treatment without additional pain management, often including opioid analgesics.

When denudation of the mucosa or even ulcerations are prevalent, topical lidocaine gel (2%) may alleviate the painful, burning sensations. Swallowing is often compromised and a combination of topical lidocaine and morphine mixture may be advantageous, probably because of binding to peripheral opioid receptors (DONNELLY et al. 2002).

The classical World Health Organization (WHO) three-step ladder of cancer pain relief is a basic strategy for pain management. This consists of nonopioid antiprostaglandins such as aspirin or paracetamol. However, if an anti-inflammatory actions is requested,

then nonsteroidal anti-inflammatory drugs may be used every 4–6 h, supplemented with paracetamol for breakthrough pain. WHO recommends mild opioids such as codeine as the next step (DONNELLY et al. 2002), but because codeine is a prodrug of morphine with a limited analgesic effect when given in therapeutic doses, low doses of morphine may be used as well. Morphine is suitable for the treatment of pain in head and neck cancer patients with mucositis, because it can be administered as a mixture (which is appropriate for feeding tubes) or as a suppository.

It has been suggested that methadone might be superior to morphine in the treatment of neuropathic pain which is common in head and neck cancer because of erosive lesions in the rich innervated region, but this could not be confirmed by a Cochrane meta-analysis (NICHOLSON 2007).

If long-lasting pain problems are expected, sustained release analgesics can be useful for continuous pain relief in head and neck cancer patients. Fentanyl patches have become increasingly popular and often relevant to use when swallowing becomes difficult, but because of costs, morphine mixtures are to be preferred, unless patients suffer from concomitant nausea or vomiting.

26.5

Taste Alterations

Alteration in taste often affects food intake. Patients may complain about lack of flavor and loss of taste. Taste alterations are among the first symptoms to radiation treatment, occurring within the first 2 weeks, and often precede objective signs of mucositis.

Loss of taste is related to reduced saliva, but despite significant xerostomia, loss of taste is transient and one of the first signs of recovery after radiation treatment.

26.6

Tobacco

Smoking has been shown to exert an adverse effect on survival rates and quality of life after treatment of patients with head and neck cancer (BROWMAN et al. 2002; JENSEN et al. 2007). The impact on acute side effects from tobacco is less clear (BROWMAN et al.

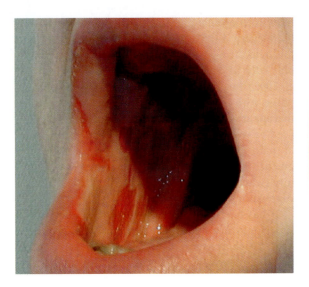

Fig. 26.1. Radiation-induced confluent, oral mucositis

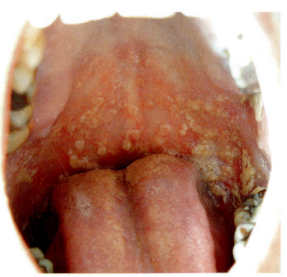

Fig. 26.2. Oral candidiasis

1993; RUGG et al. 1990). It has been hypothesized that hypoxic conditions such as those inflicted by smoking might reduce radiation response in normal tissues (FRANZÉN et al. 1989), but so far, tobacco has not been shown to reduce acute mucosal reactions. Owing to the risk of decreased effect of radiation, patients should be encouraged to quit smoking, before initiation of radiotherapy.

26.7
Candidiasis

Fungal infections are frequent during radiation treatment. When dietary changes are instituted, due to radiotherapy-induced painful mucositis, patients tend to eat softer foods or even blended food or fluids, whereby the mechanical rinse of the mucosa ceases.

The pseudomembranous mucositis, which is observed during radiation treatment, is often mistaken as candidiasis and treated as such (Figs. 26.1 and 26.2). Because *Candida* species belong to the normal mucosal flora of the oropharynx, it should be emphasized that only verified infections should be treated.

Positive isolates can be recovered in about one third of head and neck cancer patients before treatment without clinical signs of a fungal infection, but during radiotherapy up to 80% of patients may have positive cultures (RAMIREZ-AMADOR et al. 1997; BELAZI et al. 2004). Isolation of yeast before commencement of radiotherapy may rise to 55% in patients receiving concomitant medications at screening (CORVÒ et al. 2008).

It seems obvious to treat fungal infections when clinically apparent. To avoid treating nonfungal lesions, positive cultures should be obtained before initiation of antifungal therapy. Since resistance is quite common to antifungal medications, such as the popular azoles, the resistance pattern should preferably be determined in the local uptake area of the head and neck clinic to qualify antifungal treatment.

It should also be noted that the general use of antifungal treatment, whether prophylactic or therapeutic, exerts a significant change to the normal mucosal flora with an increase in bacterial species such as streptococcus species and lactobacillus.

Treatment must be based on sufficient microbiological culturing, though empirical decisions are often made. In this case, sufficient investigations must be performed to support the clinical decisions and fiber or videoscopy must be compulsory to qualify the clinical decision whether the mucositis is caused by radiation, mucosal infection by bacteria or yeast, or a combination.

Continuous cultures to support candidiasis can be obtained easily by inoculation on Nickerson's medium

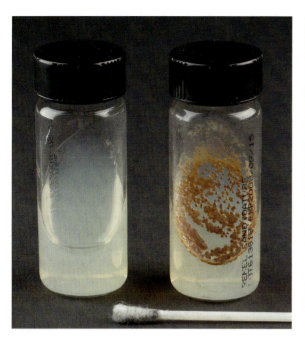

Fig. 26.3. Nickerson's medium overgrown with *Candida*

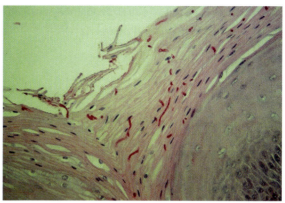

Fig. 26.4. *Candida* species in the upper epithelial layers of the oral mucosa

which will be overgrown within days if positive (Fig. 26.3). Negative cultures on the other hand will exclude *Candida* as the cause of the epithelial desquamation in which case it is important to abstain from treatment to prevent resistance to antifungal treatment. Alternatively, cultures can be obtained by gently scraping the affected areas and the patient does a mouth swish with 10 ml of saline, which is then inoculated.

Localized painful erythema may harbor *Candida*, which can be diagnosed by cytopathology from mucosal smears. Because *Candida* is located in the upper epithelial layers (Fig. 26.4), a topical application of antifungal gels is recommended. If the application of a gel is painful and inconvenient, it may be replaced by mixtures QID for 2 weeks. Treatment with azoles should not be extended to more that 1–2 weeks to prevent resistance.

In a randomized study, prophylactic treatment with fluconazole (100 mg) in patients treated with radiotherapy for head and neck tumors significantly reduced the rate and the time to development of oropharyngeal candidiasis, compared with placebo. However, no statistically significant differences were found between the groups regarding worsening in RTOG acute toxicity scores (Corvò et al. 2008). Positive yeast cultures were caused by *Candida* in 85% of the cases.

26.8
Skin Toxicity

Acute radiation-induced skin toxicity is common and varies from slight erythema to wet, ulcerative desquamation. Modern treatment strategies such as intensity-modulated radiation therapy (IMRT) which often uses odd angles compared with conventional portals may cause tangential irradiation to the skin and increase the likelihood of severe reactions. In addition, concomitant chemoradiation and the introduction of epidermal growth receptor inhibitors has accentuated this problem (Budach et al. 2007).

A number of wet and dry skin care regimens to be used during and after radiotherapy (Momm et al. 2003) exists. In other cancer diseases, several studies have evaluated various medications and creams to postpone and reduce acute skin reactions to radiation treatment. Most studies have shown little if any benefit when compared with standard skin care; however, steroids seem to offer some relief in alleviating acute radiation-induced dermatitis (Boström et al. 2001).

In a retrospective study of head and neck patients, urea lotion was compared in 43 hospitalized patients plus 20 outpatients to a dry skin care of 25 outpatients (Momm et al. 2003). Less grade 3 reactions and a delay in acute skin toxicity were obtained with the urea lotion. Owing to the lack of well-executed clinical trials no firm conclusions about skin care can be made. Sufficient skin hydration, to preserve elasticity, may be recommended as well as avoidance of inflammation, infections, scratching, and irritating factors such as perfumes and sun exposure.

26.9
Nutrition

26.9.1
Evaluation Strategies

The pretreatment nutritional status of head and neck cancer patients varies considerably. Furthermore, it should be noticed that a number of functional and perceptive disturbances may affect food intake (Table 26.2). Except for glottic cancer, most head and neck cancer patients are diagnosed in advanced stages often associated with mechanic obstruction impeding food intake. Low social status with poor dietary habits and high alcohol consumption are risk factors for poor nutritional condition. Additionally, poor dentition as unfitted dentures in relation to pretreatment dental management affect normal food consumption as well.

A pretreatment assessment of the nutritional status of the head and neck patient is mandatory. This should preferably be done using a validated nutrition assessment tool and, various screening guidelines have been proposed (ISENRING et al. 2008,

Table 26.2. Functional and perceptive disturbances affecting food intake

Erosive tumor lesions
    pain
    obstruction

Muscle edema
Appetite
Reduced saliva
Trismus
Nausea/vomiting during chemotherapy
Taste loss
Loss of teeth
Dentures unfitted after surgery
Viscous saliva
Cracked lips

KONDRUP et al. 2003). From the risk screening procedure, one should be able to identify undernourished patients and to predict whether a patient needs additional counseling by a dietician or even a prophylactic feeding tube or gastrostomy. Patients should be encouraged to begin a high-protein/high-calorie diet with nutritional supplements if necessary.

During radiotherapy patients should be monitored weekly by measurement of weight, hemoglobin, albumin, hydration, and performance status, and a consultation should explore whether food and energy requirements are being met. Constipation, nausea, and pain should be managed. The risk of insufficient food intake leading to malnutrition, and inevitable weight loss, is increased by concomitant chemotherapy and surgery to the masticatory organs.

The reduction in salivary flow-rate, which is observed early after the start of radiation treatment, makes the normal fluent salivary turn into white viscous salivary. This is unpleasant and may provoke cough or even vomiting.

26.9.2
Intervention Strategies

The goal of nutritional support is to minimize weight loss and to prevent specific nutrient deficiencies (KEEFE et al. 2007a). Intervention with dietary counseling and addition of nutritional supplements in cancer patients in general have produced superior results, compared with oral diet alone regarding quality of life, improved food and energy intake, nutritional status, functional recovery, complication rates, and mortality (ISENRING et al. 2008; ARENDS et al. 2006; STRATTON and ELIA 2007). However, these findings are generalizations from surgical and nonsurgical studies of different cancer diseases and opposing arguments against the guidelines on enteral feeding has been put forward (KORETZ 2007), especially regarding nutritional interventions and survival rates (DAVIES et al. 2006). At present, the evidence of a benefit from enteral feeding in head and neck cancer and radiation treatment is limited. Therefore, it must be cautioned not to extrapolate data from surgical series and different cancer diseases to head and neck cancer patients, especially regarding survival estimates.

It has been indicated that individual dietary counseling may have a more pronounced effect on sustained intake of protein and calories in head and neck cancer patients than in patients with or without supplements (RAVASCO et al. 2005). This should encourage head and neck teams to focus on counseling as well as monitoring changes in nutritional status. On the other hand, data have indicated that patients having nutrition support before radical radiation treatment may even have a poorer locoregional control as well as a poorer survival probability than other patients (RABINOVITCH et al. 2006). Therefore, clinicians should report the dose-fractionation factors which impact on acute toxicity and nutrition, as described above, to be able to discern the effect of nutrition compared with other factors associated with radiation treatment.

Weight loss before commencing treatment has been described to occur in as many as 60% of head and neck cancer patients (LEES 1999). TROTTI et al. (2003) reported weight loss in 34% during radiotherapy with a mean incidence of $\geq 10\%$ weight loss of 17% derived from three studies (range 5–70%). As shown in Table 26.3, weight loss >10% was reported in 23–26% of 1,420 patients undergoing standard fractionation or slightly accelerated radiotherapy without chemotherapy.

Weight loss before radiation is a more relevant measure of nutritional status than weight or body

mass index (BMI). In high economic countries, where overweight and obesity are common problems, head and neck patients will often present with BMIs above the upper normal range (>25). In a small study of 35 consecutive patients undergoing IMRT, we observed that overweight patients were commonly seen, with a median BMI of 25.9, and only two patients had a BMI below 20 (JOHANSEN et al. 2008). High BMIs may apply to patients eligible for curative strategies only; however, when looking at 619 patients referred to our university clinic for either curative or palliative treatment, we found a median BMI of 24.3 (13.1–47.8) with just 2.1% below a BMI of 20 (unpublished data).

26.9.3
Tube Feeding

If oral intake is insufficient before or during radiation treatment or if a patient has difficulties swallowing his medicine a feeding tube should be inserted.

In large randomized studies, the number of patients needing a feeding tube amounts to 15–35% after receiving conventional fractionation, but this number may vary considerably since the likelihood of receiving a feeding tube is closely associated with tumor stage, tumor localization, performance status, and the clinician's preference. The latter may raise tube feeding in up to 92% of cases (POULSEN et al. 2001).

In 672 patients, in our institution, who underwent accelerated RT with a hypoxic radiosensitizer, tube placement was significantly related to tumor site. Patients with treatment volumes covering the pharynx, such as pharyngeal or supraglottic carcinomas, were much more likely to obtain a feeding tube when compared with patients being treated to the oral cavity or glottic larynx only. Patients with stage III–IV disease had a threefold higher tube rate than stage II patients (unpublished data).

Supplementation has been shown to be associated with a decrease from 31 to 6% in the need for a percutaneous endoscopic gastrostomy (PEG) tube placement in patients treated with radiotherapy (LEE et al. 2008). The benefits of a feeding tube should be weighed against the discomfort and side effects. A nasogastric tube is preferable for short-term interventions, but if tube placement time is expected to last weeks, a patient may benefit from a PEG. PEG should also be the first choice when cosmetic or

Table 26.3. Peak incidence of acute morbidity in week 0–14 of radiation treatment in 1,420 patients from the DAHANCA 6&7 trials of 5 vs. 6 fractions/week (Modified from GRAU et al. (2006))

Acute reaction	5 fractions/ week (%)	6 fractions/ week (%)	p-value
Confluent mucositis	33	53	0.001
Use of opioids	56	65	0.001
Significant dysphagia	38	47	0.001
Moderate/severe edema	52	59	0.04
Moist skin desquamation	16	19	NS
Severe xerostomia	22	26	NS
Complete loss of taste	27	30	NS
Weight loss >10%	23	26	NS

NS nonsignificant

social considerations are important. It should be noticed that PEG tubes can increase diarrhea (KEEFE et al. 2007a), which is often a problem in patients receiving concomitant chemotherapy inducing intestinal mucositis. Both types of tubes have proven effective in achieving adequate protein and energy intakes and weight maintenance in head and neck cancer patients undergoing radiation therapy compared with oral intake alone (ISENRING et al. 2008).

The rate of complications after endoscopic placement of enteral feeding tubes is estimated to be 8–30%, and depends on the different definitions of what actually constitutes a complication. Serious complications, requiring treatment, occur in ~1–4% of cases (LÖSER et al. 2005).

Poor nutritional status may bring the patient into a vicious cycle. With reduced food intake, the probability of weight loss and fatigue in itself will render the patient less likely to take care of the necessary intake of nutrients, fluids, and vitamins. It is unknown, however, whether maintenance of nutritional status facilitates the recovery of mucositis.

During a period dominated by radiation-induced symptoms, the consciousness of having to eat and not being able to do so sufficiently can be very stressful for the patient. An insufficient diet will inevitably lead to fatigue and compromise the ability to overcome the necessity to eat. Moreover, the well-intentioned help and advices from family and friends may cause an overwhelming situation for the patient. In this case a feeding tube may be a relief to the patient and a means of breaking the vicious cycle.

The question about prophylactic vs. therapeutic tube and nasogastric vs. gastrostomy placement is still unsettled, because studies have been small and predominantly retrospective. Persistent tube-feeding at 12 months after hyperfractionated and accelerated radiotherapy seems to be associated with poorer quality of life (RINGASH et al. 2008). Also, prolonged tube feeding may be a risk factor of long-term dysphagia, since prolonged nothing-by-mouth (more than 2 weeks) has an impact on swallowing (GILLESPIE et al. 2004).

It is often argued that patients with prophylactic tube placement experience less weight loss than patients receiving delayed PEG (BEER et al. 2005), and that patients who require a therapeutic feeding tube, due to significant weight loss during radiotherapy, suffer greater morbidity than do patients who receive tubes prophylactically (CADY 2007). This may seem as a circular reasoning because dysphagia and weight loss during radiation treatment is the principal indication for tube placement. So far, no difference in time from tube insertion to removal has been found between the prophylactic and the therapeutic strategy (RINGASH et al. 2008).

Well-designed clinical trials to confirm these observations, considering weight changes per se and with corrections for confounders such as tumor stage, radiation dose, treatment volume, age, and comorbidity, are highly warranted.

It is unknown whether nutrition status is a prognostic factor. No prospective studies have been conducted properly with disease-specific survival or overall survival as end points. Questions about the impact of nutritional interventions on disease-specific end points have been raised. So far, no clear evidence exists from many retrospective or small prospective studies that dietary counseling as such impacts on treatment response or survival.

26.10
Conclusion

Despite intense investigation in radiation-induced mucositis of the head and neck, only few therapeutic interventions have proven effective in preventing or alleviating treatment-related mucosal symptoms from the oral cavity or throat. Numerous drugs and oral care strategies have been applied in head and neck cancer patients with limited success. Therefore, great efforts should be exerted to obtain optimal dose plans for sparing of normal tissues during radiotherapy.

It must be emphasized that care of head and neck cancer patients during radiation treatment has a supportive approach and while only few therapeutic interventions are available, continuous care must be undertaken to recognize and treat adverse symptoms and reactions to prevent dehydration and weight loss as a result of pain, inflammation, and infections.

References

Andreassen CN, Grau C, Lindegaard JC (2003) Chemical radioprotection: a critical review of amifostine as a cytoprotector in radiotherapy. Semin Radiat Oncol 13:62–72

Arends J, Bodoky G, Bozzetti F et al. (2006) ESPEN guidelines on enteral nutrition: non-surgical oncology. Clin Nutr 25:245–259

Beer KT, Krause KB, Zuercher T et al. (2005) Early percutaneous endoscopic gastrostomy insertion maintains nutritional state in patients with aerodigestive tract cancer. Nutr Cancer 52:29–34

Belazi M, Velegraki A, Koussidou-Eremondi T et al. (2004) Oral *Candida* isolates in patients undergoing radiotherapy for head and neck cancer: prevalence, azole susceptibility profiles and response to antifungal treatment. Oral Microbiol Immunol 19:347–351

Boström Å, Lindman H, Swartling C et al. (2001) Potent corticosteroid cream (mometasone furoate) significantly reduces acute radiation dermatitis: results from a double-blind, randomized study. Radiother Oncol 59:257–265

Brizel DM, Albers ME, Fisher SR et al. (1998) Hyperfractionated irradiation with or without concurrent chemotherapy for locally advanced head and neck cancer. N Engl J Med 338:1798–1804

Brizel DM, Wasserman TH, Henke M et al. (2000) Phase III randomized trial of amifostine as a radioprotector in head and neck cancer. J Clin Oncol 18:3339–3345

Browman GP, Mohide EA, Willan A et al. (2002) Association between smoking during radiotherapy and prognosis in head and neck cancer: a follow-up study. Head Neck 24:1031–1037

Browman GP, Wong G, Hodson I et al. (1993) Influence of cigarette smoking on the efficacy of radiation therapy in head and neck cancer. N Engl J Med 328:159–163

Budach W, Bolke E, Homey B (2007) Severe cutaneous reaction during radiation therapy with concurrent cetuximab. N Engl J Med 357:514–515

Buentzel J, Micke O, Adamietz IA et al. (2006) Intravenous amifostine during chemoradiotherapy for head-and-neck cancer: a randomized placebo-controlled phase III study. Int J Radiat Oncol Biol Phys 64:684–691

Cady J (2007) Nutritional support during radiotherapy for head and neck cancer: the role of prophylactic feeding tube placement. Clin J Oncol Nurs 11:875–880

Clarkson JE, Worthington HV, Eden OB (2007) Interventions for treating oral mucositis for patients with cancer receiving treatment. Cochrane Database Syst Rev (2):CD001973

Corvò R, Amichetti M, Ascarelli A et al. (2008) Effects of fluconazole in the prophylaxis of oropharyngeal candidiasis in patients undergoing radiotherapy for head and neck tumour: results from a double-blind placebo-controlled trial. Eur J Cancer Care 17:270–277

Davies AA, Smith GD, Harbord R et al. (2006) Nutritional interventions and outcome in patients with cancer or pre-invasive lesions: systematic review. J Natl Cancer Inst 98:961–973

Donnelly S, Davis MP, Walsh D et al. (2002) Morphine in cancer pain management: a practical guide. Support Care Cancer 10:13–35

El-Sayed S, Nabid A, Shelley W et al. (2002) Prophylaxis of radiation-associated mucositis in conventionally treated patients with head and neck cancer: a double-blind, phase III randomized, controlled trial evaluating the clinical efficacy of an antimicrobial lozenge using a validated mucositis scoring system. J Clin Oncol 20:3956–3963

Elting LS, Cooksley CD, Chambers MS et al. (2007) Risks, outcomes and costs of radiation-induced oral mucositis among patients with head-and-neck malignancies. Int J Radiat Oncol Biol Phys 68:1110–1120

Epstein JB, Silverman S Jr, Paggiarino DA et al. (2001) Benzydamine HCl for prophylaxis of radiation-induced oral mucositis: results from a multicenter, randomized, double-blind, placebo-controlled clinical trial. Cancer 92:875–885

Finch PW, Rubin JS (2006) Keratinocyte growth factor expression and activity in cancer: implications for use in patients with solid tumors. JNCI 98:812–824

Fung SM, Ferrill MJ (2002) Granulocyte macrophage-colony stimulating factor and oral mucositis. Ann Pharmacother 36:517–520

Foote RL, Loprinzi CL, Frank AR et al. (1994) Randomized trial of a chlorhexidine mouthwash for alleviation of radiation-induced mucositis. J Clin Oncol 12:2630–2633

Franzén L, Bjermer L, Henriksson R et al. (1989) Does smoking protect against radiation-induced pneumonitis? Int J Radiat Biol 56:721–724

Gillespie MB, Brodsky MB, Day TA et al. (2004) Swallowing-related quality of life after head and neck cancer treatment. Laryngoscope 114:1362–1367

Grau C, Hansen HS, Specht L et al. (2006) Morbidity of accelerated radiotherapy for head and neck caner: prevalence and peak incidence of acute and late morbidity endpoints in the DAHANCA 6 & 7 randomized trial. Radiother Oncol 81(suppl 1):S130

Henk JM (1997) Controlled trials of synchronous chemotherapy with radiotherapy in head and neck cancer: overview of radiation morbidity. Clin Oncol (R Coll Radiol) 9:308–312

Isenring E, Hill J, Davidson W et al. (2008) Evidence based practice guidelines for the nutritional management of patients receiving radiation therapy. Nutr Diet 65(Suppl 1):S1–S20

Jensen K, Jensen AB, Grau C (2007) Smoking has a negative impact upon health related quality of life after treatment for head and neck cancer. Oral Oncol 43:187–192

Johansen J, Bertelsen A, Hansen CR et al. (2008) Setup errors in patients undergoing image guided radiation treatment. Relationship to body mass index and weight loss. Acta Oncologica 47(7):1454–1458

Keefe DM, Rassias G, O'Neil L et al. (2007a) Severe mucositis: how can nutrition help? Cur Opin Clin Nutrit Metab Care 10:627–631

Keefe DM, Schubert MM, Elting LS et al. (2007b) Updated clinical practice guidelines for the prevention and treatment of mucositis. Cancer 109:820–831

Kondrup J, Allison SP, Elia M et al. (2003) ESPEN guidelines for nutrition screening. Clin Nutr 22:415–421

Koretz RL (2007) Should patients with cancer be offered nutritional support: does the benefit outweigh the burden?. Eur J Gastroenterol Hepatol 19:379–382

Kwong KK (2004) Prevention and treatment of oropharyngeal mucositis following cancer therapy: are there new approaches? Cancer Nurs 27:183–205

Lalla RV, Sonis ST, Peterson DE (2008) Management of oral mucositis in patients who have cancer. Dent Clin N Am 52:61–77

Lee H, Havrila C, Bravo V et al. (2008) Effect of oral nutritional supplementation on weight loss and percutaneous endoscopic gastrostomy tube rates in patients treated with radiotherapy for oropharyngeal carcinoma. Support Care Cancer 16:285–289

Lees J (1999) Incidence of weight loss in head and neck cancer patients on commencing radiotherapy treatment at a regional oncology centre. Eur J Cancer Care (Engl) 8: 133–136

Löser C, Aschl G, Hébuterne X et al. (2005) ESPEN guidelines on artificial enteral nutrition – percutaneous endoscopic gastrostomy (PEG). Clin Nutr 24:848–861

McDonnell AM, Lenz KL (2007) Palifermin: role in the prevention of chemotherapy- and radiation-induced mucositis. Ann Pharmacother 41:86–94

Mirabell R, Allal AS, Mermillod B et al. (1999) The influence of field size and other radiotherapy parameters on acute toxicity in pharyngolaryngeal cancer. Strahlenther Onkol 175:74–77

Momm F, Weissenberger C, Bartelt S et al. (2003) Moist skin care can diminish acute radiation-induced skin toxicity. Strahlenther Onkol 179:708–712

Nicholson AB (2007) Methadone for cancer pain. Cochrane database Syst Rev (4):CD003971

Overgaard J, Hansen HS, Specht L et al. (2003) Five compared with six fractions per week of conventional radiotherapy of squamous-cell carcinoma of head and neck: DAHANCA 6 and 7 randomised controlled trial. Lancet 362(9388):933–940

Poulsen MG, Denham JW, Peters LJ et al. (2001) A randomised trial of accelerated and conventional radiotherapy for stage III and IV squamous carcinoma of the head and neck: a Trans-Tasman Radiation Oncology Group Study. Radiother Oncol 60:113–122

Poulsen MG, Riddle B, Keller J et al. (2008) Predictors of acute grade 4 swallowing toxicity in patients with stages III and IV squamous carcinoma of the head and neck treated with radiotherapy alone. Radiother.Oncol 87:253–259

Prada A, Chiesa F (1987) Effects of benzydamine on the oral mucositis during antineoplastic radiotherapy and/or intra-arterial chemotherapy. Int J Tissue React 9:115–119

Rabinovitch R, Grant B, Berkey BA et al. (2006) Impact of nutrition support on treatment outcome in patients with locally advanced head and neck squamous cell cancer treated with definitive radiotherapy: a secondary analysis of RTOG trial 90-03. Head Neck 28:287–296

Ramirez-Amador V, Silverman S, Jr., Mayer P et al. (1997) Candidal colonization and oral candidiasis in patients undergoing oral and pharyngeal radiation therapy. Oral Surg Oral Med Oral Pathol Oral Radiol Endod 84:149–153

Ravasco P, Monteiro-Grillo I, Marques VP et al. (2005) Impact of nutrition on outcome: a prospective randomized controlled trial in patients with head and neck cancer undergoing radiotherapy. Head Neck 27:659–668

Ringash J, Lockwood G, O'Sullivan B et al. (2008) Hyperfractionated, accelerated radiotherapy for locally advanced head and neck cancer: quality of life in a prospective phase I/II trial. Radiother Oncol 87:181–187

Rosen LS, Ehtesham A, Davis ID et al. (2006) Palifermin reduces the incidence of oral mucositis in patients with metastatic colorectal cancer receiving fluorouracil-based chemotherapy. J Clin Oncol 24:5194–5200

Rubenstein EB, Peterson DE, Schubert M et al. (2004) Clinical practice guidelines for the prevention and treatment of cancer therapy-induced oral and gastrointestinal mucositis. Cancer 100(Suppl 9):2026–2046

Rubin JS, Bottaro DP, Chedid M et al. (1995) Keratinocyte growth factor. Cell Biol Int 19:399–411

Rugg T, Saunders MI, Dische S (1990) Smoking and mucosal reactions to radiotherapy. Br J Radiol 63:554–556

Stokman MA, Spijkervet FK, Burlage FR et al. (2003) Oral mucositis and selective elimination of oral flora in head and neck cancer patients receiving radiotherapy: a double-blind randomised clinical trial. Br J Cancer 88:1012–1016

Stratton RJ, Elia M (2007) Who benefits from nutritional support: what is the evidence? Eur J Gastroenterol Hepatol 19:353–358

Sutherland SE, Browman GP (2001) Prophylaxis of oral mucositis in irradiated head-and-neck cancer patients: a proposed classification scheme of interventions and meta-analysis of randomized controlled trials. Int J Radiat Oncol Biol Phys 49:917–930

Trotti A, Bellm LA, Epstein JB et al. (2003) Mucositis incidence, severity and associated outcomes in patients with head and neck cancer receiving radiotherapy with or without chemotherapy: a systematic literature review. Radiother Oncol 66(3):253–262

Van den Broek GB, Balm AJM, van den Brekel MWM et al. (2006) Relationship between clinical factors and the incidence of toxicity after intra-arterial chemoradiation for head and neck cancer. Radiother Oncol 81:143–150

Waldron J, Warde P, Irish J et al. (2008) A dose escalation study of hyperfractionated accelerated radiation delivered with integrated neck surgery (HARDWINS) for the management of advanced head and neck cancer. Radiother.Oncol 87:173–180

Worthington HV, Clarkson JE, Eden OB (2008) Interventions for preventing oral mucositis for patients with cancer receiving treatment. Cochrane Database Syst Rev (4):CD000978

Communication and Palliative Care in Head and Neck Cancer

27

Toby C. Campbell and James F. Cleary

CONTENTS

27.1 Introduction *299*

27.2 The Palliative Care Comprehensive Assessment *300*

27.3 Maintaining Hope While Negotiating Goals of Care *300*
27.3.1 Setting *303*
27.3.2 Perception *303*
27.3.3 Invitation *303*
27.3.4 Knowledge *303*
27.3.5 Emotions and Empathic Responses *304*
27.3.6 Summary and Strategize *304*

27.4 Dealing with Emotion *305*

27.5 Summary *305*

References *306*

KEY POINTS

- Cancer care is a journey for the patient, family, and oncologist from the time of diagnosis.
- The palliative care comprehensive assessment is a specialized diagnostic and therapeutic interview.
- Using a defined set of skills, such as SPIKES (setting, perception, invitation, knowledge, emotions and empathetic responses, summary and strategize and summarize) and NURSE (naming, understanding, respecting, supporting, exploring), helps the oncologist communicate effectively with patients and deal with emotions.

Toby C. Campbell, MD, MSCI
James F. Cleary, MBBS
Department of Medicine, Division of Hematology-Oncology,
K6/546 CSC, 600 Highland Avenue, Madison, WI 53792, USA

- Maintaining hope while setting clear goals of care starts with orienting the patient to his or her situation, making clear plans and using a "hope for the best but plan for the worst" communication tool.

27.1

Introduction

Head and neck cancer is a particularly morbid malignancy because of the accumulation of physical and emotional losses patients and their families suffer. Many of these patients are destined to have recurrent malignancy, second malignancies, or life-threatening complications from their disease or other illness. Providing palliative medical care to the dying cancer patient requires expertise in several key areas: antitumor therapy, symptom management, and communication. Patients rely on his or her physician to provide accurate information on the most effective chemotherapy, radiation therapy, and surgical options to treat their underlying disease. Patients, and their support system, also benefit from excellent symptom management through the expert use of a broad range of medications, cognitive and behavior therapies, and symptom-relieving procedures. Patients and families have a right to understand their disease and the dying process and have this information presented in a way they can understand. As patients near the end of life, their need for responsive, compassionate, *aggressive* medical care often increases because of worsening symptom burden from the disease and its treatment. We undervalue ourselves when we think just because a patient is done with active therapy, that there is "nothing more we can do." In this chapter we will focus primarily on the communication issues related to the care of patients with head and neck cancer, especially as they near the end of life.

Each patient is on his or her own cancer journey from the moment they receive their diagnosis until they die. We are a sometime-guide, sometime-passenger, and sometime-cheerleader on this journey. Just as we would want to know anyone traveling with us, palliative care medicine starts with an intimate, comprehensive interview to begin a relationship and identify the patient's priorities for life and medical care.

27.2
The Palliative Care Comprehensive Assessment

Effective end-of-life care depends upon the open exchange of information between the physician, patient, and family. To provide comprehensive medical care in dying patients, providers need to be sensitive to the concept of *total pain*, a term first used by Dame Cicely Saunders to describe the complex etiology of pain, including its physical, emotional, social (including economic), and spiritual components. Total pain provides a fundamental framework for patient assessment at the end of life. As we begin the cancer journey, the comprehensive assessment guides the telling of a wide range of life experiences in an effort to help the patient tell their life story. This life history helps the provider understand the patient and their perspective on life and illness but also, in the telling, may be therapeutic for the patient. Armed with this information, physicians are poised to effectively negotiate medical goals of care in a way that respects the individual patient's priorities.

A variety of comprehensive assessment tools are available to facilitate the comprehensive assessment and evaluate patients' preferences, symptoms, and causes of suffering (EMANUEL et al. 2001; OKON et al. 2004; STEINHAUSER et al 2002). In general, these assessment tools, such as the PEACE Tool (OKON et al. 2004), assess various domains: physical symptoms, emotional and cognitive symptoms, autonomy-related issues, communication and closure of life projects, economic concerns, and transcendent and existential issues. Sample questions for each of the domains in the PEACE Tool are included in Table 27.1.

27.3
Maintaining Hope While Negotiating Goals of Care

As we travel with the patient on the cancer journey, our role at the beginning is to serve as a guide, providing the patient an overview, including describing the most likely outcome, the chances of an ideal outcome, and any anticipated hurdles and detours. The orientation we provide can reduce anxiety and help maintain hope by clearly establishing treatment goals, setting milestones to reach for, and providing a sense of the future. In times of crisis, most people cope, in part, by planning and acting in small ways: a "one step at a time" mentality. The very action of moving forward with a plan allows for patients to expect – hope – for good things to happen along the way. Throughout the treatment relationship, especially at times of transition (e.g., second-line chemotherapy after progression), re-orienting the patient to their location on this metaphorical map clears up confusion and allays fears of the unknown. With this method, when the time comes for the transition to end-of-life care, the patient, while disappointed, is not surprised and is often intellectually prepared for the final leg of the journey.

At the time of transition to purely palliative or end-of-life care, providers often worry about patients and families losing hope. Hope, however, is a complicated emotion not necessarily related to survival. Hope can be defined as a cherished desire or anticipated outcome. Patients and families may hope for quality time with loved ones, good symptom management, a final meal, or other outcomes. EVANS et al. (2006) suggest we help maintain hope by facilitating the exploration of realistic goals and objectives for the limited time remaining by using a "hope for the best but plan for the worst" phrase as a communication technique allows patients to maintain hope of an ideal outcome. "I know that you're hoping for a complete remission from the cancer. While I'm hoping for that too, we both need to make plans in case the cancer does not respond to treatment."

The transition between antitumor therapy and supportive care only is also smoother when the two have been integrated throughout the journey. Figure 27.1 shows a model describing the interaction between palliative care and traditional antitumor therapy with a graduated increase in the need for supportive care punctuated with exacerbations of

Table 27.1. PEACE tool, example of the domains and sample questions in a comprehensive palliative care assessment tool

PEACE tool		
Domain	**Symptom**	**Question**
Physical	Pain	Are you in pain?
	Anorexia	How is your appetite?
	GU	Do you have control of your bladder?
	GI	Nausea? vomiting? diarrhea? constipation?
	Respiratory	Are you short of breath?
		Do you have a cough?
	Skin	Any irritation, rash, bruises, ulcers, or infection?
	Level of function	Do you take a nap each day? For how long?
		Are you able to prepare your own meals?
		How far can you walk without taking a break?
	Treatment side effects	Are you having side effects from you medicine?
Emotional	Sad	Are you sad?
	Anxiety	Are you anxious?
	Depression	How is your mood? Are you depressed?
Autonomy	Control	Do you feel in control of your care?
		Are we doing only the things you want?
		Do you know what to expect from treatment?
	Decision making	Do you feel we are listening to you?
		Are your preferences being followed?
		Do you have a health care power of attorney?
		Have you told your decision maker how you feel about…?
Communication and closure	Closure, life review, hopes	What do you hope for?
		What are your dreams and goals?
		What things do you still want to complete?
		What do you still enjoy doing?
		Are there any people you have not seen in a long time whom you wish to contact?
	Legacy	How would you like to be remembered?
		What are you especially proud of?
	Support	Who are you closest to?
	Relationships	What brings you joy?
	Resilience and self-efficacy	When times are difficult, what gives you strength?
		What do you do to help yourself?
Economic		Are you worried about money?
		Has your illness created a financial strain?
		Do you worry you may become a burden to your family?
Transcendent and existential		Are you at peace?
		Are you suffering?
		Do you think about dying?
		Is faith important to you?

Okon et al., 2004

symptoms requiring a temporary increase in symptom management.

In contrast to the model, many oncologists perceive supportive care as distinctly different from antitumor therapy. The oncologist may mention that "while more therapy is possible, my concern is it will be too toxic and my recommendation is we focus on symptom control alone and potentially work with palliative care and hospice." In this case, the discussion with patients at the time of transition is similar to an informed consent conversation about a procedure. It is relevant to consider how most patients weigh information when making decisions. Patient preferences for therapies are heavily influenced by the *most likely outcome* of any given procedure rather than the acknowledged risks and benefits presented during the typical consent discussion (PATRICK et al. 1994; FRIED et al. 2002). When weighing options, patients consider the overall burden of treatment, including the estimated length of time in the hospital, invasiveness of the procedure, the need for additional testing; the *perceived* benefit of the ideal outcome; and the likelihood of the *ideal* outcome (FRIED et al. 2002). Therefore, if patients are presented with options, they are most likely to elect a given option if the most likely outcome matches their perceived benefit and burden of treatment. A patient may consider some conditions as worse than death, leading them away from therapy, because of the risk of such unacceptable conditions as coma, persistent vegetative state, or severe dementia (PATRICK et al. 1994).

Doctor: An example of how to approach this difficult crossroad could be phrased: "Because of how weak the cancer and chemotherapy have made you, I think more chemotherapy at this point is most likely to make you very sick, worsen your quality of life, or potentially even make you die faster. I think there is little chance for chemotherapy to accomplish your goal of spending more time with your family. Okay? My suggestion is that we focus instead on your symptoms directly and aggressively treat any suffering to try and maximize your quality of life and your time at home."
Patient: Does this mean I'm dying?
Doctor: I think so. I wish there were more time. I want you to know I will be with you until the end.

Considering that words can be as sharp as scalpels, one should approach transition conversation carefully, as if performing a procedure. ZACHARIAE et al. (2003), for example, demonstrated that oncologists' communication style and physical behaviors directly impacted patient satisfaction, distress, and perceived control over their disease. As a patient realizes the significance of the news – that his or her life is nearing its end – emotional reactions are common: sadness, fear, anger, loss, anxiety, frustration, denial, etc. We will discuss how to deal with emotion in the next section.

First, there is another set of communication tools one can use for goal setting in the clinic setting while maintaining hope (BAILE et al. 2000; VON ROENN and VON GUNTEN 2003). Maintenance of hope in the face of lethal and debilitating illness assumes that an oncologist has more to offer patients than chemotherapy. We can be a guide and witness, confidant and symptom reliever, counselor and signpost on a winding road. One mechanism for helping maintain

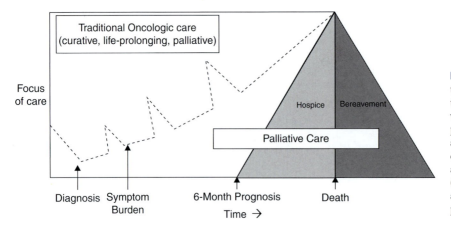

Fig. 27.1. A model describing the intersection of antitumor therapy and palliative care with the increasing role of palliative care over time and periodic symptom exacerbations requiring aggressive supportive care (as published in CAMPBELL and VON ROENN (2007, pp 376)

hope is the very task of setting goals and intentionally making plans for the future.

BAILE et al. (2000) described a six-step protocol for conveying bad news using the mnemonic SPIKES. While SPIKES is a very helpful tool for delivering bad news in the cancer clinic, the principles apply to multiple settings, including transitions in care and negotiating goals of care.

27.3.1
Setting

The clinical or hospital setting can be manipulated to enhance our ability to explore and respond to emotion and effectively communicate important information. Setting refers to the environmental factors and set-up factors for the conversation. The physician or team should discuss their objectives for the conversation in advance and mentally rehearse the plan and strategies for dealing with emotion. It is helpful to arrange for privacy, involve significant friends and family members, sit down, and to reduce potential interruptions. In fact, the simple act of sitting down when delivering news has been shown to significantly increase the patient's perception of compassion (BRUERA et al. 2007).

27.3.2
Perception

The most important assessment to gain is the patient's understanding of his or her condition. "I want to make sure you and I are on the same page. Can you tell me what you understand about what is happening now?" or "What is your understanding of why we did the CT scan?" The few minutes spent assessing their understanding gains important information about their perceptions and misconceptions as well as any unrealistic expectations. For example, it is easy to see that the conversations with the following patients, each with newly diagnosed metastatic disease, will be very different:

Doctor: What are you hoping for?
Patient 1: I know the cancer is bad. I'm just hoping you can buy me some time.
Patient 2: I'm a fighter and there is no way this is going to get me, doc.

Often, by seeking first to understand, one finds the patient already knows, or suspects, most of the new information. Or, one may discover they have a great deal of ground to cover but both conversations are more easily managed by knowing upfront what needs to be accomplished.

27.3.3
Invitation

Is this an okay time to go over the results of your CT scan?

The invitation may be obvious if the patient has returned to clinic for CT results or more subtle: "How much information do you want about the test results when they come back? Is there anyone else you want present if we have to discuss bad news?" While most patients desire complete disclosure of information, some patients do not. The invitation respects the patient's autonomy by ensuring the timing is convenient for them to have a serious conversation.

27.3.4
Knowledge

By providing test results and recommendations, we intend to give the patient knowledge about his or her life and health. Knowledge is a higher cognitive order than information because knowledge means they are able to understand the information, incorporate it into their mental framework, and then use the information to make decisions and act. The first step in helping patients be ready to receive information is by warning them bad news is coming. This lessens the shock and improves information processing (MAYNARD 1997). For example, "I'm afraid I have some bad news," or "The results from the CT scan are not good."

Strategically, there are several verbal skills to use to continue to build a relationship with the patient even when bad news is being delivered, including avoiding the use of medical jargon (see common translations in Table 27.2) and giving a maximum of three pieces of information before checking in with the patient for understanding. For example, "The CT shows that the cancer has spread to the liver. This means the cancer is not curable though we can certainly treat both your symptoms and the cancer with medicines. Do you understand?"

Emphasize what can be done: "while we cannot treat your cancer directly with chemotherapy or radiation, we can be very aggressive in our attempts

Table 27.2. Translating medical terms to lay terms. A similar table exists in this reference.

Medical jargon	Suggested Lay Language
Cure	The cancer is gone and it is not coming back
Control	We are hoping to slow or the stop the growth for a while
Remission, complete response	There is no visible evidence of cancer but we expect it to come back
Partial response	The cancer is smaller, but still there
Stable disease	The cancer is still present and has remained the same size
Progressive disease	The cancer is worse

Von Roenn, 2003

to control your pain and shortness of breath. You need not suffer."

Try to avoid using negative phrasing such as "there is nothing more we can do."

27.3.5
Emotions and Empathic Responses

Physicians receive little training in dealing with emotion. Oncologists routinely face the prospect of breaking bad news. Without adequate training in dealing with emotion this may create a sense of anxiety or dread for the physicians, further jeopardizing an effective interaction. There are a few straightforward strategies for dealing with emotion that may powerfully change the dynamic in the clinic room when breaking bad news.

— After breaking bad news, allow the patient to have the next word even if seconds or minutes pass. This gives them space and time to consider the information and reflect and react to it.
— Observe the patient's reaction and note any emotions you see. Simply try and identify or name what you think they are feeling: "You must be sad."
— Explore the emotion to give patients permission to express themselves and avoid presuming their emotion is due to the news itself. "You seem angry, can you tell me about it?"
— Allow the emotion to pass before moving on to the next steps. If one rushes ahead before patients are emotionally ready, they frequently do not process or remember the next pieces of information. In effect, you save time at a later appointment by not having to repeat information.
— Any NURSE statement may be appropriate at this time (see Table 27.3).

27.3.6
Summary and Strategize

When patients are ready to proceed, summarize the information again and then move forward into your diagnostic and therapeutic recommendations. Continue to limit the amount of information into manageable pieces and check for understanding. Emphasize your ongoing relationship with the

Table 27.3. NURSE – a mnemonic for empathic statements

Naming	State the patient's emotion	I can see you're sad
		This must be a shock
Understanding	Empathizing with and legitimizing patient emotion	It's completely reasonable to feel scared and angry, this is not the news we were hoping for
Respecting	Praise patient	I'm so impressed with the courage you have shown at every turn
Supporting	Show support	I want you to know we are in this together until the end
Exploring	Ask the patient to elaborate on their feelings	Can you tell me more about what's going through your mind right now?

patient to try and allay fears of abandonment and further loss. Finally, set a time to meet again.

27.4 Dealing with Emotion

Cancer, and all that word implies, induces a host of emotional reactions in a patient and family often causing a "cancer crisis" (Baile 2008). When patients receive bad news, face transitions in goals of care, or deal with other unanticipated events, they often experience emotional crises. Patients, for a variety of reasons, hesitate to express these emotions to their oncologist and, in turn, oncologists infrequently address emotions with their patients (Pollak et al. 2007). Panagopoulou et al. (2008) showed that oncologists who are ill-equipped to handle emotional reactions may even alter or intentionally conceal information to minimize the patient's emotional reaction.

In addition to a lack of training in dealing with emotion, another reason oncologists struggle using clear ("blunt") language is insufficient practice simply saying the words out loud: "cancer, incurable, relapse, remission, dying." While these words can help us transmit knowledge, save time and frustration, and avoid the disillusionment of failed false hopes, they are hard to say without practice. As a result, we may try to find ways of breaking bad news without actually using the word. For example, euphemisms for "cancer" include the words spot, nodule, shadow, lesion, mass, abnormality, fullness, growth. In another example, "hospice" becomes symptom management experts, a team approach to your care, supportive oncology, symptom directed therapy, etc. The use of these euphemisms inhibits the transfer of knowledge because the words do not change the facts at hand but allow the meaning to be lost. If patients and families do not understand, or can misinterpret the meaning of the words, it unwittingly forces both parties (doctor and patient) to continue the cancer journey alone because they are now traveling in different cars. The doctor thinks the patient understands that the cancer has returned, while the patient may think that he or she probably has an infection. Clear, direct, and compassionate communication offers the advantage of quickly transferring knowledge.

- "There is an abnormal nodule in your lung, I'm concerned it could be *cancer* but I cannot be certain until we use a needle to get a piece of it and then look at it under the microscope."
- "When head and neck cancer has spread from where it started to somewhere else in the body it means it is *metastatic* and cannot be cured. That means that while we can treat your cancer, hopefully lengthening your life and controlling symptoms, we can never make it go away completely. And because you are otherwise healthy, it means it's likely you will one day *die* from this cancer."
- "I'm afraid you are *dying*."

Using these words or statements takes practice alone and with patients. These are examples of words that transfer knowledge quickly and easily. How the oncologist reacts after the patient ingests this knowledge is the key to compassion and maintenance of hope: attend to the fragile human receiving this devastating news, honor his or her emotion, whatever it is, in that moment with your silence. Then, allow and encourage his or her fear/anger/sadness/regret/grief/joy to have space and depth and time. By giving that emotion a few minutes all its own, a stronger relationship emerges and empowers the patient with the knowledge to play a part in the coming decisions.

Dealing with emotion starts with a toolkit called NURSE (see Table 27.3) (Pollak et al. 2007).

NURSE statements work for a variety of technical reasons. When we state back a patient's emotional condition it is clear we are trying to understand and the patient feels that his or her experience is being honored. By seeking to clarify and explore their concerns and emotions we promote continued expansion of their own knowledge. Respecting the patient's experience decreases anxiety, improves optimism, and explicitly acknowledges his or her effort. In providing space and time for emotional exploration, the physician cements strong relationships with patients, which enables them to move beyond the emotion and back to a cognitive connection where they can now take in additional technical information.

27.5 Summary

Cancer care is a journey for patient, family, and oncologist from the time of diagnosis. Palliative care should be a component of patients' care throughout the illness. By using a variety of communication tools, the oncologist can help prepare patients for the future, maintain hope, set appropriate goals for care, and deal with emotion all while staying on time and providing excellent comprehensive care of the patient.

References

Baile WF (2008) Supporting the patient and family through the cancer crisis. J Support Oncol 6:132–133

Baile WF, Buckman R, Lenzi R et al. (2000) SPIKES-a six-step protocol for delivering bad news: application to the patient with cancer. Oncologist 5:302–311

Bruera E, Palmer JL, Pace E et al. (2007) A randomized, controlled trial of physician postures when breaking bad news to cancer patients. Palliat Med 21:501–505

Campbell T, Von Roenn J (2007) Palliative care for interventional radiology: an oncologist's perspective. Semin Intervent Radiol 24:375–381

Emanuel LL, Alpert HR, Emanuel EE (2001) Concise screening questions for clinical assessments of terminal care: the needs near the end-of-life care screening tool. J Palliat Med 4:465–474

Evans WG, Tulsky JA, Back AL et al. (2006) Communication at times of transitions: how to help patients cope with loss and re-define hope. Cancer J 12:417–424

Fried TR, Bradley EH, Towle VR et al. (2002) Understanding the treatment preferences of seriously ill patients. N Engl J Med 346:1061–1066

Maynard D (1997) How to tell patients bad news: the strategy of "forecasting". Cleve Clin J Med 64:181–182

Okon TR, Evans JM, Gomez CF et al. (2004) Palliative educational outcome with implementation of PEACE tool integrated clinical pathway. J Palliat Med 7:279–295

Panagopoulou E, Mintziori G, Montgomery A et al. (2008) Concealment of information in clinical practice: is lying less stressful than telling the truth? J Clin Oncol 26:1175–1177

Patrick DL, Starks HE, Cain KC et al. (1994) Measuring preferences for health states worse than death. Med Decis Making 14:9–18

Pollak KI, Arnold RM, Jeffreys AS et al. (2007) Oncologist communication about emotion during visits with patients with advanced cancer. J Clin Oncol 25:5748–5752

Steinhauser KE, Bosworth HB, Clipp EC et al. (2002) Initial assessment of a new instrument to measure quality of life at the end of life. J Palliat Med 5:829–841

Von Roenn JH, von Gunten CF (2003) Setting goals to maintain hope. J Clin Oncol 21:570–574

Zachariae R, Pedersen CG, Jensen AB et al. (2003) Association of perceived physician communication style with patient satisfaction, distress, cancer-related self-efficacy, and perceived control over the disease. Br J Cancer 88:658–665

Organized Head and Neck Cancer Care

28

Peggy A. Wiederholt

C O N T E N T S

28.1   Introduction   *307*

28.2   **Step 1: Recognize Challenges of HNC Treatment**   *308*

28.3   **Step 2: Form a Multidisciplinary Team**   *308*

28.4   **Step 3: Identify Barriers to Team Performance**   *308*

28.5   **Step 4: Define Patient-Centered Treatment Goals**   *309*

28.6   **Step 5: Provide Patient Navigation Assistance**   *309*

28.7   **Step 6: Describe the Nurse Coordinator Role**   *309*

28.8   **Step 7: Coordinate the Plan of Care**   *311*
28.8.1   Phase I: Access to Care   *312*
28.8.2   Phase II: Pretreatment   *312*
28.8.3   Phase III: Treatment   *312*
28.8.4   Phase IV: Posttreatment   *312*

28.9   **Step 8: Address Patient Needs**   *313*
28.9.1   Airway   *313*
28.9.2   Pain   *313*
28.9.3   Nutrition   *313*
28.9.4   Dysphagia   *313*
28.9.5   Dental   *314*
28.9.6   Skin Care   *314*
28.9.7   Psychosocial   *314*
28.9.8   Tobacco and Alcohol   *314*
28.9.9   Patient/Family Education   *314*

28.10   **Conclusion**   *315*

Abbreviations   *315*

References   *315*

Peggy A. Wiederholt, RN
Department of Radiation Oncology, University of Wisconsin
Paul P. Carbone Comprehensive Cancer Center, University of
Wisconsin Hospital & Clinics, 600 Highland Ave K4/B100 CSC,
Madison, WI 53792, USA

KEY POINTS

- Advanced head and neck cancers and their complex treatments can significantly impact morbidity, functional abilities, physical appearance, and health-related quality of life.
- The physical and emotional challenges confronting head and neck cancer patients and the multimodality treatment regimens they must endure require the expertise of a multidisciplinary team.
- An eight-step process is presented as a means of organizing, communicating, and implementing comprehensive care across the continuum.
- The oncology nurse coordinator role has emerged as a critical core component to organizing and providing quality, patient-centered, multidisciplinary head and neck cancer care.

28.1

Introduction

Advanced head and neck cancer (HNC) treated with curative intent is often managed with a combination approach that may include surgery, radiation, and chemotherapy (FORASTIERE et al. 2001). While these options offer the potential for better patient outcomes, they create complex organizational challenges and are associated with significant toxicities that can complicate the treatment course, threaten long-term functionality, and adversely affect health-related quality of life (HRQL). This chapter presents an eight-step process for organized HNC care (Fig. 28.1).

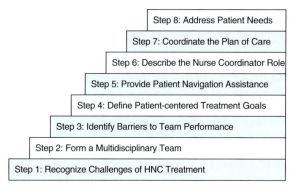

Fig. 28.1. Eight steps to organized head and neck cancer care

targeted therapy to radiation has shown improvement in locoregional control and survival but is associated with skin and other toxicities (Bonner et al. 2006).

The logistics of multimodality therapy present organizational challenges in the scheduling of appointments, procedures, and treatments across the continuum. More important, novel developments for the treatment of HNC, the serious side effects associated with these regimens, and the consequences they can have on functional ability and HRQL demand a specialized multidisciplinary approach to HNC care (Licitra et al. 2006; Dingman et al. 2008).

28.2
Step 1: Recognize Challenges of HNC Treatment

Surgical resection and reconstruction for tumors of the head and neck may result in life-changing structural and functional impairments that can have profound effects on body image and quality of life (Dropkin 1999). Patients may require intense postoperative rehabilitation and life-style changes due to disfigurement, dependence on a tracheal stoma to breathe, mechanical or prosthetic devices to speak, or a gastrostomy tube to administer life-sustaining liquids and nutrition.

Radiation to the upper aerodigestive tract is also associated with significant toxicities intensified by concomitant, radiosensitizing cytotoxic agents. Acute treatment-related side effects include radiation dermatitis, mucositis-induced pain, xerostomia (dry mouth), dysgeusia (altered taste), and dysphagia (difficulty swallowing). These toxicities place patients at risk for nutritional compromise, weight loss, dehydration, treatment interruptions, and hospitalization (Beaver et al. 2002). Long-term adverse effects of radiation can cause structural and functional problems as well, resulting in a documented or perceived decrease in swallow function, dry mouth due to diminished saliva production, and a subsequent decrease in quality of life (Connor et al. 2006; Logeman et al. 2003).

Protocols for induction, concurrent, or adjuvant chemotherapy partnered with radiation may improve treatment outcomes in advanced HNC but they are accompanied by an increase in treatment-related adverse effects (Choong and Vokes 2008). Likewise, the addition of concurrent molecularly

28.3
Step 2: Form a Multidisciplinary Team

The multidisciplinary HNC team is composed of numerous health-care professionals. The otolaryngologist, head and neck surgeon, radiation oncologist, and medical oncologist serve as team leaders to guide treatment. A neuroradiologist and surgical pathologist assist with interpretation of diagnostic testing. Team members also include dentists, oral surgeons, prosthodondists, nurses, nurse practitioners, physician assistants, pharmacists, nutritionists, speech-language pathologists, social workers, psychologists, radiation therapists, physical therapists, and occupational therapists. Other disciplines may be consulted as well to address individualized needs. In addition, the primary care physician plays a pivotal role in providing supportive and general medical care in collaboration with the multidisciplinary team.

28.4
Step 3: Identify Barriers to Team Performance

Multidisciplinary cancer care is very complex and at risk for potential disorganization and miscommunication between disciplines. Although it is assumed that multidisciplinary teams should improve coordination, communication, and collaborative decision-making between providers and patients, research in this area remains scarce (Fleissig et al. 2006).

Interpersonal and professional disagreements can have a negative effect on team interactions and cohesiveness, but barriers within the health system itself can also hamper communication and team performance. Obstacles may include the time constraints of a busy clinical practice, scheduling conflicts, and different clinic locations between colleagues that limit or prohibit team meetings. Centralized multidisciplinary clinics and tumor board conferences may facilitate some discussions but even then representation of all multidisciplinary team members is usually impossible. In addition, inabilities for ongoing interactions as new events occur may result in a potential disconnect over the course of treatment. Once identified, steps should be taken to overcome barriers to team performance. One possible solution to improving communication is a team coordinator (see Sect. 28.7).

28.5

Step 4: Define Patient-Centered Treatment Goals

The development of good communication skills by providers is an important part of comprehensive cancer care, especially at times of crisis such as diagnosis, disease recurrence, and transition to palliative care (BAILE and AARON 2005). Patient–provider communication is essential to achieve patient-centered care focused on understanding the patient as a unique person and ensuring that their individual needs, values, and preferences guide clinical decision-making and define treatment goals (MEAD and BOWER 2000). These concepts are especially important when therapy options involve *imperfect trade-offs* with variable risks and benefits, serious treatment-related toxicities, and potential long-term sequalae that can significantly affect HRQL (CHEWNING et al. 2001).

The impact of HNC and associated treatments on speech, swallow, breathing, and cosmesis may be more frightening to some patients than the fear of death. This may in turn influence treatment goals based on functionality and quality of life rather than cure or prolonged survival. Understanding and respecting a patient's beliefs and wishes must be the foundation for building effective and empathetic patient–provider communication and the cornerstone for developing an organized, patient-centered plan of care.

28.6

Step 5: Provide Patient Navigation Assistance

Cancer patients must not only cope with a life-threatening illness, they must do so while navigating through a maze of appointments and procedures within the architecture of a fragmented medical infrastructure. The concept of a patient navigator, someone to communicate with and help cancer patients and their families navigate the complex health-care system, has emerged as an important aspect of cancer care. Originally developed to address health-care disparities and access to care in the underserved (FREEMAN et al. 1995), navigation programs have expanded over the past decade to address needs in a much broader cancer patient population (SEEK and HOGLE 2008). The profile of the patient navigator is very diverse from one program to another with different variations of responsibilities. They may be community volunteers or organization employees with no formal health-care education, professional nurses, or social workers (INSTITUTE FOR ALTERNATIVE FUTURES 2007).

Given the broad spectrum of multidisciplinary specialists involved and the complex treatment regimens required for their care, HNC patients can clearly benefit from navigation services to bring a sense of order to a world spinning out of control (Fig. 28.2). However, the multiplicity and severity of problems associated with their treatment demand a professional level of oncology nursing expertise. Although the title of *navigator* is well established, the diversity of the position across community settings is confusing. Therefore, this chapter will use the title *Head and Neck Oncology Nurse Coordinator* (HNONC) to more clearly identify the role of an oncology nurse clinician specializing in this unique role.

28.7

Step 6: Describe the Nurse Coordinator Role

The HNONC functions as the multidisciplinary team coordinator and partners with the patient as an advocate and gatekeeper to restore order and control and to bridge gaps in patient–provider and provider–provider communication (WIEDERHOLT et al. 2007).

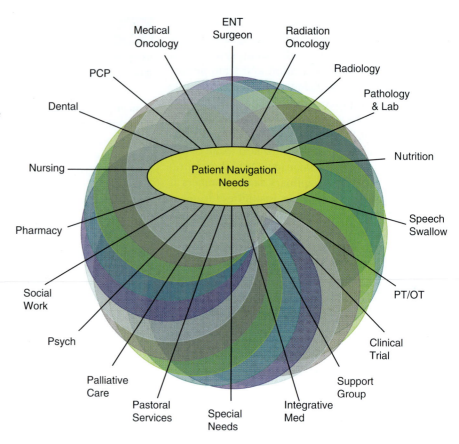

Fig. 28.2. Navigating multidisciplinary head and neck cancer care. *ENT* ear, nose, throat (otolaryngology); *Psych* psychology/psychiatry; *PT* physical therapy; *OT* occupational therapy; *PCP* primary care provider

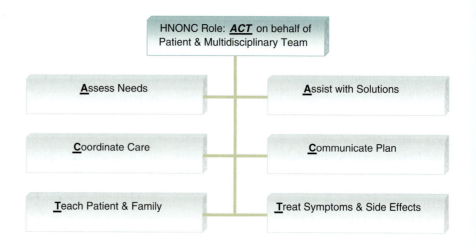

Fig. 28.3. Role of the Head Neck Oncology Nurse Coordination (HNONC)

The role of the nurse coordinator is to *act* as a catalyst on behalf of the patient and health-care team to enhance multidisciplinary patient-centered care, improve HRQL, and achieve better treatment outcomes. The term "act" can be used as an anagram. Responsibilities are to (1) *assess* the needs of the patient and the multidisciplinary team and *assist* with viable solutions to meet those needs; (2) *coordinate* the plan of care and *communicate* the plan to the patient and the health-care team; (3) *teach* the patient and their family about health, disease, and symptom management, and help *treat* symptoms and side effects (Fig. 28.3).

28.8
Step 7: Coordinate the Plan of Care

Coordination of HNC care begins when a patient or referring physician contacts the clinic to schedule a consultation and continues throughout the pretreatment, treatment and posttreatment phases. Patient assessments are performed during each phase to identify physical and psychosocial needs and assist with appropriate referrals (Fig. 28.4).

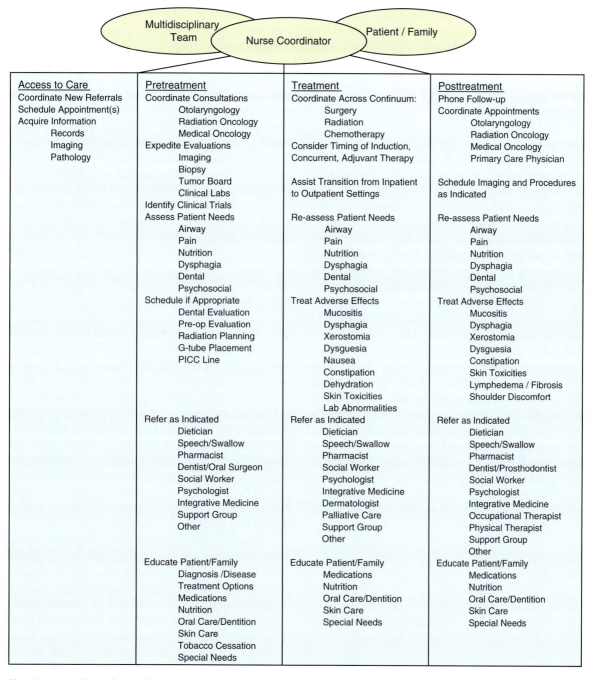

Fig. 28.4. Coordinated multidisciplinary HNC care

28.8.1
Phase I: Access to Care

An organized plan must have a well-defined point of contact that allows patients to access the health-care system in a timely, nonobstructive manner. Appointments should be scheduled with the appropriate specialist(s) and with the urgency expected in the setting of a new cancer diagnosis. If available, medical records and diagnostic studies should be acquired from the referral source prior to the consult.

28.8.2
Phase II: Pretreatment

The pretreatment phase focuses on gathering information and performing diagnostic procedures and tests required to guide clinical decision-making. Biopsies and radiology scans identify histopathology and better define the extent of disease for accurate staging. Laboratory tests determine candidacy for chemotherapy regimens. Access to pathology slides and radiology films for tumor board review fosters collaborative team efforts. Identifying potential clinical trial subjects triggers screening for study eligibility. Expediting appointments, tests, and procedures and initiating urgent consultations activates the multidisciplinary team so that the plan of care can move forward quickly.

The coordinator's presence during initial consultation serves the interests of both the patient and provider. Often during a physician encounter, patients and families are overwhelmed, and it is not until after the physician has left that information is processed and questions are asked (PENSON et al. 2006). An awareness of how and what information was shared during an encounter prepares the coordinator to answer questions with consistency, and to communicate this information to the multidisciplinary team.

28.8.3
Phase III: Treatment

Organized care during the treatment period is important for patients undergoing definitive combination therapy. Coordination of treatments avoids conflicting appointments across clinical settings and accommodates patient scheduling needs which may result in better compliance and increased satisfaction. Neo-adjuvant or adjuvant therapies must be scheduled in a specific time frame to achieve maximum therapeutic outcomes. Examples include induction chemotherapy, postoperative radiation, and postchemoradiation neck dissection and associated imaging. Transitions from inpatient to outpatient settings must be addressed for hospitalized patients to maintain continuity of care whether discharged to home or to a skilled nursing facility. Patients with metastatic or recurrent disease treated with palliation may require the services of a palliative care team or hospice.

Treatment-related side effects present significant challenges to the multidisciplinary team. Frequent assessments and communication among disciplines are necessary for managing toxicities such as radiation-induced mucositis. Establishing an evidence-based treatment protocol or algorithm provides a coordinated approach to side effect management across the trajectory (BENZINGER et al. 2008). Similar strategies can be applied to other adverse effects such as nausea, constipation, and skin toxicities. Collaboration with the professional pharmacist is helpful in these endeavors.

28.8.4
Phase IV: Posttreatment

The immediate posttreatment period can be the most difficult time for those who have undergone HNC treatment. Patients recovering from extensive surgery or aggressive chemoradiation often find themselves and their caregivers overwhelmed, exhausted, and fearful of being home alone while dealing with the peak effects of their treatment. This mandates careful discharge planning for the hospitalized patient, and thoughtful scheduling of posttreatment clinic appointments to provide safe supportive care during the early recovery period. Interim phone assessments can be very beneficial during this time.

Treatments for advanced HNC can significantly affect *long-term* function and quality of life as well (LIST and BILIR 2004). Adverse effects from surgery or radiation may include trismus and impairments of speech, mastication, salivary and swallow function. Lymphedema, subcutaneous fibrosis, and post neck dissection shoulder pain may also present posttreatment challenges that require intervention. In addition, chemotherapy-induced fatigue, neuropathies, and chronic pain from cancer treatment can lead to long-term disability (TAYLOR et al. 2004).

Not uncommonly, patients may experience depression or anxiety. Involvement of multidisciplinary specialists (e.g., speech-language pathologist, physical therapist, occupational therapist, psychologist) is critical during posttreatment rehabilitation as patients struggle to deal with the physical and emotional scars of their treatment and strive to reach a new normal.

28.9
Step 8: Address Patient Needs

Patient-focused care addresses the physical, social, emotional, and spiritual needs of patients. An organized plan includes a comprehensive evaluation of patient needs in partnership with collaborative interactions with multidisciplinary team members.

28.9.1
Airway

Tumors of the upper aerodigestive tract as well as laryngeal edema and increased tracheal secretions secondary to surgery or radiation can place patients at risk for aspiration or suffocation. Airway assessment across clinical settings must be performed before and throughout treatment to identify the need for emergent or elective intervention with a tracheotomy.

28.9.2
Pain

Appropriate pain management is associated with a more rapid recovery, shorter hospital stays, fewer readmissions, and improved quality of life (PHILLIPS 2000). Pain should be assessed at every visit. A unified approach to treating pain in the multidisciplinary setting may be best accomplished by having a single provider assume the responsibility for pain management when possible to prevent underprescribing, overprescribing, or drug abusive behavior. The oncology nurse coordinator is also a good resource to identify pain management needs and to monitor response to therapy across the continuum of care. Referral to a pain specialist or palliative care may be indicated for chronic pain or end-of-life care.

28.9.3
Nutrition

Nutrition and hydration are especially challenging for patients undergoing HNC treatment. Patients often have a history of significant weight loss at the time of initial presentation and may lose 10% or more of their pretherapy weight during the course of treatment (LEES 1999). Height, weight, and basic metabolic needs should be evaluated prior to treatment with consultation by a certified dietician and guidelines provided on how to achieve nutritional goals. Patients receiving concurrent chemoradiation should be weighed and evaluated weekly during treatment to assure they are meeting minimum caloric and fluid requirements. Odynophagia, nausea, gastroesophageal reflux, and food intolerance must be assessed and strategies introduced to overcome nutritional barriers. Elective administration of intravenous fluids may be necessary.

The prophylactic use of a gastrostomy tube (G-tube) for select patients receiving intense chemoradiation may decrease the need for hospitalization to treat dehydration and malnutrition (LEE et al. 1998). Although there are no established criteria to determine what patients will benefit from elective G-tube placement, clinicians may be able to identify higher risk patients based upon performance status, the intensity of planned treatment, and the anatomical site of disease (CADY 2007). Once decided, the G-tube should be placed prior to or early in treatment to avoid crisis intervention later in therapy.

28.9.4
Dysphagia

Dysphagia is a well-recognized, often debilitating, and potentially life-threatening consequence of concurrent chemoradiation for HNC (NGUYEN et al. 2004) that can significantly impact quality of life and lead to social isolation. Involvement of the speech–language pathologist before, during, and after treatment, and initiation of preventive exercises and rehabilitative measures can potentially reduce or eliminate long-term swallowing dysfunction and optimize feeding (MITTAL et al. 2003).Further information concerning the role of the speech-language pathologist in swallowing evaluation and treatment can be found in Chap. 25 of this volume. Collaboration with the multidisciplinary team to keep patients swallowing throughout treatment is critical to achieve better long-term outcomes. Patients presenting with symptoms suggestive of aspiration or at high risk for aspirating should undergo an instrumental evaluation with a formal swallow study to guide therapy (ROSENTHAL et al. 2006).

28.9.5
Dental

Dental prophylaxis for patient's undergoing head and neck radiation is essential to prevent dental caries, periodontal infections, and the most severe complication of osteoradionecrosis. Pretreatment referral to a dentist is important to evaluate dental and periodontal health, and the need for extraction of unrestorable or at-risk teeth (MILLER and QUINN 2006). Communication with the dental professional can expedite procedures to prevent treatment delays and assure adequate healing time prior to starting radiation. Fluoride treatments, strategies to manage xerostomia, and close surveillance by the dentist are also an important part of long-term postradiation care.

28.9.6
Skin Care

The introduction of epithelial growth factor (EGFR) inhibitors for the treatment of HNC has mandated a new approach to skin care across clinical settings, particularly in the irradiated patient. Treatment guidelines should be established to prevent and treat possible complications of EGFR skin-related toxicities (EABY et al. 2008). Consultations with a dermatologist may also be beneficial.

28.9.7
Psychosocial

A comprehensive care plan must address the psychosocial needs of each patient, recognize how those needs impact decision-making and compliance, and identify resources to provide assistance and support. Assessments include evaluation of insurance coverage, living situation, personal relationships, employment, benefits, finances, transportation needs, and addictive behaviors. Early interaction with a social worker can help overcome barriers that may otherwise delay treatment or influence patient compliance. All patients are encouraged to review the Power of Attorney for Health Care.

Mental distress in HNC patients with associated anxiety, depression, and a decreased sense of well-being are well documented and may occur at the time of diagnosis, during treatment, or after therapy has been completed (HAMMERLID et al. 1999). Although counseling by physicians and nurses may result in some improvements, patients should be referred to a professional psychologist (or psychiatrist) with expertise in evidence-based assessment and intervention strategies (HUMPHRIS 2008).

Adjunctive psychosocial therapy associated with spirituality, patient support groups, and integrative medicine may positively influence HRQL for some patients. Although understudied and often overlooked, religion and spirituality can help patients cope with a cancer diagnosis and may be associated with a better quality of life (BALBONI et al. 2007). Likewise, benefits of patient support group participation include potential improvements in emotional state, adaption to illness, relationships, and HRQL (ZABALEGUI et al. 2005; VAKHARIA et al. 2007). Patients who use complimentary and alternative medicine report the need to feel hopeful and to have more control over their medical care with the expectation that they will experience an improvement in quality of life with therapies they may consider beneficial and less toxic. The growing interest in these therapies emphasizes the importance of improved patient–provider communication to offer reliable information and guidance (RICHARDSON et al. 2000).

28.9.8
Tobacco and Alcohol

Tobacco and alcohol are known risk factors in HNC. Recent data suggest that while cigarettes and alcohol have multiplicative effects when used in combination with one another, they are also independent risk factors in the development of cancers of the head and neck (HASHIBE et al. 2007). Informing patients of these risks and providing appropriate counseling and resources for tobacco cessation and alcohol abstinence must be part of standard HNC care.

28.9.9
Patient/Family Education

Patient education is integrated as needs are identified to teach patients and their families about their disease, treatment options, the plan of therapy, and side effect management.

Providing information and instructions about medications, nutrition, oral hygiene, dentition, and skin care prepares the patient for what lies ahead, may improve compliance with recommended treatment, and may prevent or limit the intensity of some treatment-related toxicities. Special needs such as the care of a tracheotomy or G-tube must also be addressed as those needs arise. The use of diaries or tracking calendars may be implemented to help patients organize, record, and report information about symptoms, side effects, medications, and nutrition during encounters with their providers. This can potentially improve communication, identify patient needs, and help guide therapy (WIEDERHOLT and WIEDERHOLT 1997).

28.10
Conclusion

A step-by-step process has been presented to assist with the development and implementation of organized HNC care. The oncology nurse coordinator role is a critical core component to organizing and promoting multidisciplinary team efforts to achieve excellence in patient-centered care, enhance long-term functional outcomes, and improve HRQL for HNC patients.

Abbreviations

ENT	Ear, nose, throat (otolaryngology)
G-tube	Gastrostomy tube
HNC	Head and neck cancer
HNONC	Head and neck oncology nurse coordinator
HRQL	Health-related quality of life
OT	Occupational therapy
PCP	Primary Care Provider
Psych	Psychology/psychiatry
PT	Physical therapy

References

Baile WF, Aaron J (2005) Patient-physician communication in oncology: past, present, and future. Curr Opin Oncol 17:331–335

Balboni TA, Vanderwerker LC, Block SD et al. (2007) Religiousness and spiritual support among advanced cancer patients and associations with end-of-life treatment preferences and quality of life. J Clin Oncol 25(5):555–560

Beaver ME, Matheny KE, Roberts DB et al. (2002) Predictors of weight loss during radiation therapy. Otolaryngol Head Neck Surg 125:645–648

Benzinger W, Schubert M, Ang K et al. (2008) NCCN task force report: prevention and management of mucositis in cancer care. J Natl Compr Canc Netw 6(Suppl 1):S1–S24

Bonner JA, Harari PM, Giralt J et al. (2006) Radiotherapy plus cetuximab for squamous cell carcinoma of the head and neck. N Eng J Med 354:567–578

Cady J (2007) Nutritional support during radiotherapy for head and neck cancer: the role of prophylactic feeding tube placement. Clin J Oncol Nurs 11:875–880

Chewning B, Wiederholt J, Boh L et al. (2001) Does the concordant framework serve medicine management? Int J Pharm Prac 9:71–79

Choong N, Vokes E (2008) Expanding role of the medical oncologist in the management of head and neck cancer. CA Cancer J Clin 58:32–53

Connor NP, Cohen SB, Kammer RE et al. (2006) Impact of conventional radiotherapy on health-related quality of life and critical functions of the head and neck. Int J Radiat Oncol Phys 65(4):1051–1062

Dingman C, Hegedus P, Likes C et al. (2008) A coordinated, multidisciplinary approach to caring for the patient with head and neck cancer. J Support Oncol 6:125–131

Dropkin MJ (1999) Body image and quality of life after head and neck surgery. Cancer Pract 7(6):309–313

Eaby B, Culkin A, Lacouture ME (2008) An interdisciplinary consensus on managing skin reactions associated with human epidermal growth factor receptor inhibitors. Clin J Oncol Nurs 12:283–290

Fleissig A, Jenkins V, Catt S et al. (2006) Multidisciplinary teams in cancer care: are they effective in the UK? Lancet Oncol 7:935–943

Forastiere A, Koch W, Trotti A et al. (2001) Head and neck cancer. N Engl J Med 345(26):1890–1900

Freeman HP, Muth BJ, Kerner JF (1995) Expending access to cancer screening and clinical follow-up among the medically underserved. Cancer Pract 3:19–30

Hammerlid E, Ahlner-Elmqvist M, Bjordal K et al. (1999) A prospective multicentre study in Sweden and Norway of mental distress and psychiatric morbidity in head and neck cancer patients. B J Cancer 80:766–774

Hashibe M, Brennan P, Benhamou S et al. (2007) Alcohol drinking in never users of tobacco, cigarette smoking in never drinkers, and the risk of head and neck cancer: pooled analysis in the international head and neck cancer epidemiology consortium. J Natl Cancer Inst 99:777–789

Humphris GM (2008) The missing member of the head and neck multidisciplinary team: the psychologist. Why we need them. Curr Opin Otolaryngol Head Neck Surg 16:108–112

Institute for Alternative Futures (2007) Patient navigator program overview: a report for the Disparity Reducing Advances (DRA) Project. pp 3–11

Lee JH, Machtay M, Unger LD et al. (1998) Prophylactic gastrostomy tubes in patients undergoing intensive irradiation for cancer of the head and neck. Arch Otolaryngol Head Neck Surg 124(8):871–875

Lees J (1999) Incidence of weight loss in head and neck cancer patients on commencing radiotherapy treatment at a regional oncology centre. Eur J Cancer Care 8:133–136

Licitra L, Bossi P, Locati LD (2006) A multidisciplinary approach to squamous cell carcinomas of the head and neck: what is new? Curr Opin Oncol 18:253–257

List MA, Bilir SP (2004) Functional outcomes in head and neck cancer. Semin Radiat Oncol 14:178–189

Logeman JA, Pauloski BR, Rademaker AW et al. (2003) Xerostomia: 12-month changes in saliva production and its relationship to perception and performance of swallow function, oral intake, and diet after chemoradiation. Head Neck 25(6):432–437

Mead N, Bower P (2000) Patient-centredness: a conceptual framework and review of the empirical literature. Soc Sci Med 51:1087–1110

Miller EH, Quinn AI (2006) Dental considerations in the management of head and neck cancer patients. Otolaryngol Clin North Am 39(2):319–329

Mittal BB, Pauloski BR, Haraf DJ et al. (2003) Swallowing dysfunction – preventive and rehabilitation strategies in patients with head-and-neck cancers treated with surgery, radiotherapy, and chemotherapy: a critical review. Int J Radiat Oncol Biol Phys 57:1219–1230

Nguyen NP, Moltz CC, Frank C (2004) Dysphagia following chemoradiation for locally advanced head and neck cancer. Ann Oncol 15:383–388

Penson RT, Kyriakou H, Zuckerman D et al. (2006) Teams: communication in multidisciplinary care. Oncologist 11:520–526

Phillips DM (2000) JCAHO pain management standards are unveiled. JAMA 284:428–429

Richardson MA, Sanders T, Palmer JL et al. (2000) Complimentary/alternative medicine use in a comprehensive cancer center and the implications for oncology. J Clin Oncol 18:2505–2514

Rosenthal DI, Lewin JS, Eisbruch E (2006) Prevention and treatment of dysphagia and aspiration after chemoradiation for head and neck cancer. J Clin Oncol 24:2636–2643

Seek AJ, Hogle WP (2008) Modeling a better way: navigating the health care system for patients with lung cancer. Clin J Oncol Nurs 11(1):81–85

Taylor JC, Terrell JE, Ronis DL et al. (2004) Disability in patients with head and neck cancer. Arch Otolaryngol Head Neck Surg 130:764–769

Vakharia KT, Ali MJ, Wang SJ (2007) Quality-of-life impact of participation in a head and neck cancer support group. Otolaryngol Head Neck Surg 136:405–410

Wiederholt J, Wiederholt P (1997) The patient! our teacher and friend. Am J Pharm Ed 61:415–423

Wiederholt PA, Connor NP, Hartig GK et al. (2007) Bridging gaps in multidisciplinary head and neck cancer care: nursing coordination and case management. Int J Radiat Oncol Biol Phys 69(2 Suppl):S88–S91

Zabalegui A, Sanchex S, Sanchex PD et al. (2005) Nursing and cancer support groups. J Adv Nurs 51:369–381

Subject Index

A

Acute toxicity, 22–23, 37, 39, 70, 156, 164, 207–210, 212, 255, 260, 293, 295
Adaptation strategies, 183, 184, 187–189
Adaptive image-guided radiotherapy, 183–189
Adenoid cystic carcinoma, 75, 76, 90, 92, 96–97, 158, 197
Adjuvant radiation, 34–35
Age, 4, 6–8, 16, 57–59, 68, 91–93, 95, 111, 113, 120–123, 126, 137, 138, 210, 211, 262, 270, 283, 296
Aggressive histology lymphoma, 104, 113
Alcohol, 4–6, 16, 32, 44, 89, 93, 247, 273, 282–284, 289, 294, 314
Altered fractionation, 19, 31, 34, 37, 46, 139–140, 209, 228
Amifostine, 23, 148, 210, 227, 233, 289–291
Analytical end points, 253
Anaplastic thyroid cancer, 117, 118, 122–123
Antibiotics, 220, 274–276, 290
Anxiety, 37, 244, 282, 300–302, 304, 305, 312–314
Atrophy, 95, 228, 253
Aurora kinase, 219

B

Benzydamine, 289–290
Betel quid chewing, 5
Bevacizumab, 112, 216, 218, 221
Bone necrosis, 89, 92, 96
Bone sarcomas, 103–109, 112, 158
Brachytherapy, 11, 12, 23, 37, 63, 68, 83, 84, 108, 135–143, 150, 236, 237
Bragg peak, 156
Bupropion SR, 279–282

C

Candidiasis, 269, 273, 288, 292–293
Carcinogens, 4–6, 32, 59, 279
CBCT. *See* Cone-beam CT
Cervical lymph node metastases, 125–131
Cetuximab, 20, 34, 206–207, 210, 216–218, 220–221
Chemoradiotherapy, 19, 57, 60, 65, 67, 125, 191–192, 199, 203–205, 211, 247
Chest X-ray, 33, 119–120
Chlorhexidine, 273, 289
Chondrosarcoma, 105–112, 197

CO_2 laser resection, 195, 197
Comorbidity, 39, 80, 89, 92–94, 121, 210, 211, 247, 282–283, 296
Concomitant chemotherapy, 34, 43, 45–47, 75, 136, 139, 227–228, 254, 287–288, 294–296
Cone-beam CT (CBCT), 184–186, 188–189
Conformal radiation therapy, 21–22, 26, 80–81, 131, 136, 139, 145–152, 157–158, 183–184, 256
Cranial irradiation, 113

D

3DCRT. *See* 3-Dimensional conformal radiation therapy
Deafness, 63, 68
Dealing with emotion, 303–305
Deformable registration, 186–189
Delineation of primary tumor GTV, 170–172
Dental care, 269–276
Dental implants, 84, 194, 275
Dental prophylaxis, 269–276
Dental rehabilitation, 35–36, 84
Dermatofibrosarcoma protruberans, 104–105
Diet, 6, 16, 37, 59, 137–139, 141, 142, 150,151, 193,195, 234, 236, 246, 261, 265–266, 270, 283, 292,294, 296, 311, 313
3-Dimensional conformal radiation therapy (3DCRT), 21–22, 26, 97, 136, 137, 139, 141, 146, 147, 157–158
Doxorubicin, 83, 111, 122, 123
Dysphagia, 23, 32, 33, 39, 63, 69, 118, 135–143, 145–147, 149–152, 207–209, 234–236, 246, 248, 252, 253, 259–266, 287, 295, 296, 308, 311, 313–314
Dysphagia-related quality of life, 135–143
Dysphagia-specific QOL instrument, 246

E

EBV. *See* Epstein-Barr virus
EGFR. *See* Epidermal growth factor receptor
EGFR blockade, 216–218
En-bloc resection, 198
End-of-life care, 300, 313
Epidemiology, 3–8, 15–26, 31–32, 43–53, 57–60, 70, 76, 90
Epidermal growth factor receptor (EGFR), 20, 26, 123, 206, 215–222, 314

Epstein-Barr virus (EBV), 57, 59, 64, 127
Ethmoidectomy, 197
Etiology, 6, 32, 33, 57, 59, 92–93, 95, 253, 300
European Organization for the Research
  and Treatment of Cancer (EORTC)
– H&N35 QOL, 135, 142–143
– QLQ-32, 38, 245
– SF-38, 151
Ewing's sarcoma, 104–105
Extracapsular nodal extension (ECE), 20–21, 26

F

Facial nerve function, 89, 93–94
FACT-G. *See* Functional assessment of cancer therapy
FACT-head and neck (FACT-H&N), 70, 245, 261
FACT head and neck symptom index (FHNSI), 246
FDG-PET, 33, 35, 78, 84, 105, 125–127, 131, 164,
  170–172, 195, 199
Fiberoptic endoscopic evaluation of swallowing
  (FEES), 234, 236, 253, 255, 264
Fiberoptic endoscopic evaluation of swallowing
  with sensory testing (FEEST), 253, 264
Fibrosis, 63, 256, 306
Fibular free flap, 193–194
Fine-needle aspiration (FNA), 118–119, 123
Fluconazole, 269, 273
Fluoride carriers, 269, 272
[18]Fluoro deoxy-glucose, 17–18
5-Fluoruracil (5-FU), 19–20, 23, 26, 34, 83, 84,
  204–206, 208, 209
Free tissue transfer, 191–195, 197, 199
Frontal craniotomy, 197–198
Functional assessment of cancer therapy
  (FACT-G), 245, 247
Functional endoscopic sinus surgery (FESS), 79, 84
Function sparing operation, 107

G

Gastrointestinal toxicity, 220–221
Gastrostomy tube (PEG), 195–196, 207, 235, 237,
  265, 266, 295–296, 308, 313, 315
GM-CSF, 289, 290

H

Head and neck radiotherapy questionnaire, 246
Health-related quality of life (HRQOL), 36–38,
  227–231, 234, 237, 259–261, 266, 307, 315
Hearing loss, 89, 92, 94–95, 98, 99, 155, 156, 210
Hemorrhagic toxicity, 221
Histology, 16, 65, 83–84, 90, 91, 96–97, 103–105,
  108, 110, 113, 118, 158, 221
HLA-A2, 59
HN-specific QOL, 32, 36, 38–39, 151, 246

Human keratinocyte growth factor (KGF), 23, 207, 290
Human papillomavirus (HPV), 5, 6, 15–17, 26, 32, 127
Hyperbaric oxygen therapy, 269, 274
Hypersensitivity reactions, 220
Hypopharyngeal cancer, 31–32, 34, 35, 37–39, 186, 206
Hypopharynx, 21, 31–39, 94, 128, 150, 165, 196, 205, 209
Hypopituitarism, 63

I

Image-guided RT (IGRT), 13, 184, 188
Imatinib, 112, 220–221
Implants, 84, 194, 275
Indolent lymphoma, 104, 105, 112–113
Induction chemotherapy, 20, 34, 45, 60, 204–206, 312
In-room image-guidance, 184–185
Insulin-like growth factor, 219
Intensity-modulated proton therapy (IMPT),
  81, 155–160
Internal carotid artery pseudo-aneurysm, 69
Intra-arterial infusion, 83
Ipsilateral irradiation, 127–128

L

Laryngeal cancer, 5, 36, 43–53, 206
Laryngectomy, 33, 35, 36, 43–53, 107, 108, 191, 196,
  205–206, 265
Larynx, 21–23, 31–39, 44–53, 82, 94, 105, 107, 108,
  120, 122, 127–131, 149–150, 164, 165, 185, 196,
  198, 203, 205, 206, 209, 227, 230, 236, 260,
  264, 277–278, 295
Larynx preservation, 35–37, 44, 47–50
Laser excision, 45–49, 51, 53, 195
Late toxicity, 23, 26, 57, 63, 68–69, 96, 110–111, 150, 210
Lymphoma, 7, 8, 103–113, 118, 245, 290

M

Magnetic resonance imaging (MRI), 17, 18, 26,
  33, 75, 76, 78, 81–82, 84, 120, 123, 126, 129,
  131, 163–172, 184
Maintaining hope, 299, 300, 302
Malignant fibrous histiocytoma, 104–105
MALT. *See* Mucosa-associated lymphoid tissue
Mastoiditis, 89, 95–96, 98
Maxillectomy, 157, 197
Measurement of QOL, 244–246
Medullary thyroid cancer, 118, 119, 123
Molecular targeted agents, 34, 220
MRI. *See* Magnetic resonance imaging
Mucosa-associated lymphoid tissue (MALT)
  lymphoma, 105, 112–113
Mucositis, 22, 23, 159, 203, 206–210, 228, 253, 264, 265,
  269–270, 272, 273, 287–292, 295, 296, 308, 311, 312

Subject Index **319**

Multidisciplinary, 15, 18, 22, 39, 75, 79–81, 107, 191–192, 197–198, 204, 206, 215, 269, 307–313, 315

N

Nasal cavity, 75–84, 157, 203, 281
Nasal vestibule, 84
Nasopharyngeal cancer, 32, 39, 58, 70, 95, 148, 150–151, 186, 187, 210
Nasopharynx, 32, 57–70, 77, 82, 90, 94, 126, 165, 205, 209, 281
Neck dissection, 11, 12, 18–19, 23–24, 31, 35, 39, 44, 48, 120–121, 123, 125, 127, 129–131, 135, 137, 140–142, 165, 173, 191, 198, 199, 312–313
Nerve-sparing surgery, 93–94
Neuroendocrine carcinoma, 76, 83
Nicotine
– gum, 279–282
– inhaler, 279, 282
– lozenge, 279–281
– nasal spray, 280–282
– patch, 280–282
Nodal CTV, 164–169
NPC-9901, 61, 66, 68
NPC-9902, 61, 67
Nurse coordinator, 307–311, 313, 315
Nutrition, 5, 21, 22, 32, 39, 259, 262, 265–267, 269–270, 287–296, 308, 310, 311, 313, 315

O

OARs. *See* Organs at risk
Objective signs, 253, 291
Observer-scored subjective symptoms, 252–254
Optical tracking, 175–181
Oral analgesics, 265
Oral cavity cancer, 3–13, 265
Oral disinfectants, 289
Oral hygiene, 6, 16, 210, 269–273, 275, 289, 315
Organized care, 312
Organs at risk (OARs), 61, 64, 75–77, 82, 150, 156, 176–179, 184, 228, 236, 260–261
Oropharyngeal cancer, 95–96, 136, 139–141, 148, 151, 159–160, 237
Oropharynx, 3, 6, 15–26, 33, 36–38, 93–94, 99, 127–128, 130, 131, 135–143, 165, 172, 194–195, 209, 292
Osteoradionecrosis (ORN), 11, 95–96, 210, 211, 270–271, 274–275, 314

P

Pain, 22, 33, 36–39, 76, 82, 92, 93, 151, 203, 220, 244–246, 260, 265, 269, 270, 272, 287–294, 296, 300, 301, 304, 308, 311–313
Palfermin, 23, 207, 290

Palliative care, 299–306, 309–313
Paranasal sinus, 75–84, 113, 146–147, 157, 170, 191, 197–198
Parotid gland, 19, 21, 38, 82, 89, 90, 92–97, 145, 147–149, 158, 164–166, 169, 185–187, 230–232, 234, 253, 266
Partial laryngectomy, 43–47, 49, 196, 265
Particle therapy, 82–83
Pathology, 94–95, 104, 105, 125, 191–192, 198–199, 271, 293, 310–312
Patient
– education, 243, 247, 314–315
– motion, 175–179, 181, 185
– needs, 294, 308, 311, 313, 315
Patient-assessed symptoms, 254
Patterns of spread, 33
Pectoralis major myocutaneous (PMC) transfer, 192
PEG. *See* Gastrostomy tube
Performance status scale (PSS), 37, 137–139, 141–142, 234, 236, 246, 247
Perineural invasion, 20, 46, 47, 92, 93, 96–97
Periodontal disease, 270–271
PET. *See* Positron emission topography
PET/CT, 17–18, 26, 75, 76, 78, 81, 84
Photons, 80–82, 96–97, 106, 107, 110–111, 155–160
Pilocarpine, 23, 210, 227, 233–234, 269, 273–274, 289
Plan of care, 308–312
Platinum, 20, 129, 204, 207, 210, 218, 220
Positron emission topography (PET), 17–18, 123, 127, 163–172, 228, 253
Postoperative radiation, 20, 26, 34–36, 39, 157, 262, 265, 312
Pretreatment oral evaluation, 270–272
Prevention, 6, 22, 233, 237, 274, 277–278, 283, 288–290
Prostheses, 194, 275
Protons, 75, 81, 82, 96, 110–111, 146, 149, 155–160
PSS. *See* Performance status scale
Psychosocial, 35, 69–70, 220, 243–246, 248, 311, 314

Q

QOL-RT instrument, 246
Quality of life instruments, 158, 237, 243–248, 260, 266

R

Radial forearm free flap (RFFF), 33, 192–193, 195
Radiation
– caries, 269, 272, 274
– fractionation, 19
Radiation therapy technique, 21–22
Radioactive iodine scanning, 120
Radioiodine ablation, 121, 122
Radio-protective agents, 233–234
Recombinant human TSH (rhTSH), 121
Rehabilitation, 35, 36, 84, 136, 192, 195–196, 237, 265, 308, 312–313
Re-optimization, 183, 187–189

Subject Index

Reporting toxicity, 251–256
Retinal vasculopathy, 158
RET mutations, 123
RFFF. *See* Radial forearm free flap
Robotic surgery, 195, 198
RTOG-0615, 61

S

Salivary gland tumors, 76, 78–79, 89–93, 95, 97, 98
Saliva substitutes, 210, 273
Sarcoma, 7, 8, 103–113, 158, 197
Segmentation of structures, 183
Selective neck dissection (SND), 18–19, 47, 123, 165, 198
Sentinel node, 191, 199
SFKs. *See* Src family kinases
Sino-nasal cancer, 80–84, 158
Sinonasal undifferentiated carcinoma (SNUC),
    75, 76, 83, 84, 197
Skin
– creams, 293
– toxicity, 208–209, 220, 293–294, 311–312
Smokeless tobacco, 4–5
Smoking cessation, 15, 16, 22, 32
– medications, 277, 279–282, 284
SND. *See* Selective neck dissection
SNUC. *See* Sinonasal undifferentiated carcinoma
Social functioning, 33, 93, 94, 231, 245, 246
Soft tissue sarcoma (STS), 104–112, 158
Speech, 206, 262, 265, 310, 311
Squamous cell carcinoma (SCC), 6, 15, 16, 18, 24,
    26, 32, 38, 44, 76, 81–82, 84, 93, 126–129, 131,
    136, 158, 160, 165, 203, 207–215
Src family kinases (SFKs), 219
Staging, 13, 17, 32, 43–45, 51, 61, 64, 66, 75–78, 121, 122,
    126–127, 136, 164, 166, 199, 228, 265, 312
Sucralfate, 23, 289, 290
Supportive care, 210, 211, 287, 288, 300–303
Supraglottic laryngeal cancer, 43–53
Swallow dysfunction, 155, 156, 207, 211, 227–231,
    234–237, 259–262, 266–267, 313, 450
Swallow exercises, 237, 262
Systemic therapy, 13, 60, 83

T

Target
– definition, 163–172
– volumes, 18, 22, 60, 61, 78, 80–82, 84, 96, 97, 106, 108, 109,
    127–128, 158, 163–166, 172, 176, 177, 181, 185–187

Targeted therapy, 13, 18, 20, 26, 92, 131, 308
Taste alterations, 290, 291
Taxane, 20, 204
Teeth extraction, 270–272, 274, 314
Temporal lobe necrosis, 60, 68, 69
Three-dimensional conformal radiation
    therapy, 21–22, 26, 97, 136, 137, 139,
    141, 146, 147, 157–158
Thyroid cancer, 117–123
Thyroidectomy, 117, 120–123
Tobacco smoking, 4–5, 32, 291–292
Tonsillectomy, 98, 126
Topical analgesics, 22, 265, 289
Transoral microscopic laser techniques, 195
Treatment-related toxicities, 15, 22–25, 155, 156, 203,
    207–211, 309
Trismus, 210, 270, 275, 294, 312
Tube feeding, 23, 140, 295–296
Tyrosine kinase inhibitors (TKI), 83, 216–218

U

UICC/AJCC classification, 76, 77, 138
Ultrasound, 23, 118–120, 136, 176, 184
University of Michigan Head and Neck Quality-of-
    Life-Questionaire (HNQOLQ), 226
University of Washington QOL (UW-QOL)
    questionnaire, 69, 245–246
Unknown primary tumors, 125–131

V

Varenicline, 279–282
Vascular endothelial growth factor, 112, 123, 215,
    216, 218
Veterans affairs larynx study group, 35
Videofluoroscopy, 39, 149, 234–237, 253, 263
Viral infection, 5–6
Visual toxicity, 157, 158
Vocal cord carcinoma, 45–46, 48
Voice quality, 46, 47
Voice-related QOL measure (V-RQOL), 246
Volumetric imaging, 176, 183–185, 188

W

Weight loss, 22, 32, 33, 183–185, 187, 188,
    207, 208, 236, 255, 262, 266, 287,
    294–296, 308, 313

List of Contributors

Robert J. Amdur, MD
Department of Radiation Oncology
University of Florida College of Medicine
P.O. Box 100385
Gainesville, FL 32610-0385
USA

Athanassios Argiris, MD
Division of Hematology-Oncology
University of Pittsburgh School of Medicine
UPMC Cancer Pavilion, 5th Floor
5150 Centre Avenue
Pittsburgh, PA 15232
USA

Email: argirisae@upmc.edu

Hendricus P. Bijl, MD
Department of Radiation Oncology
University Medical Centre Groningen
University of Groningen
P.O. Box 30.001, 9700
RB Groningen
The Netherlands

Toby Campbell, MD
Department of Medicine
Division of Hematology-Oncology
University of Wisconsin
K6/546 CSC, 600 Highland Avenue
Madison, WI 53792
USA

Email: tcc@medicine.wisc.edu

Scott Chaiet, MD
Otolaryngology-Head and Neck Surgery
UW Health, 600 Highland Ave., Madison
WI 53792
USA

Email: schaiet@uwhealth.org

Annie W. Chan, MD
Department of Radiation Oncology
Massachusetts General Hospital
Francis H. Burr Proton Therapy Center
Harvard Medical School, 55 Fruit Street, Boston
MA 02114-2622
USA

Email: awchan@partners.org

Herbert Chen, MD, FACS
Department of Surgery
Section of Endocrine Surgery
University of Wisconsin, H4/750 CSC, 600 Highland
Avenue, Madison, WI 53792
USA

Email: chen@surgery.wisc.edu

James F. Cleary, MD
Department of Medicine
Division of Hematology-Oncology
University of Wisconsin, K6/546 CSC, 600 Highland
Avenue, Madison, WI 53792
USA

Email: jfcleary@wisc.edu

Nadine P. Connor, PhD
Associate Professor, Division of Otolaryngology-Head
and Neck Surgery, University of Wisconsin
Clinical Science Center, Room K4/711, 600 Highland
Avenue Madison, WI 53792-7375
USA

Email: connor@surgery.wisc.edu

Avraham Eisbruch, MD
Department of Radiation Oncology
University of Michigan Health System
UH B2C490, 1500 E. Medical Center
Dr. SPC 5010, Ann Arbor, MI 48109
USA

Email: eisbruch@umich.edu

ULRIK VINDELEV ELSTROEM, MSc
Department of Oncology
Aarhus University Hospital
44 Nøerrebrogade, Building 5
DK-8000 Aarhus C
Denmark

Email: ulrielst@rm.dk

EDITH FILION, MD
Department of Radiation Oncology
Stanford University Cancer Center
875 Blake Wilbur Drive, Stanford
CA 04305-5847
USA

XAVIER GEETS, MD
Radiation Oncology Department and
Center for Molecular Imaging and Experimental
Radiotherapy, Université Catholique de
Louvain, St-Luc University Hospital, 10 Avenue
Hippocrate, 1200 Bruxelles
Belgium

Email: xavier.geets@imre.ucl.ac.be

MICHAEL K. GIBSON, MD
Division of Hematology-Oncology
University of Pittsburgh School of Medicine
UPMC Cancer Pavilion, 5th floor
5150 Centre Avenue, Pittsburgh
PA 15232
USA

CAI GRAU, MD, DMSC
Department of Oncology
Aarhus University Hospital
44 Nøerrebrogade, Building 5
DK-8000 Aarhus C
Denmark

Email: caigrau@dadlnet.dk

VINCENT GRÉGOIRE, MD, PhD
Radiation Oncology Department and
Center for Molecular Imaging and
Experimental Radiotherapy, Université Catholique de
Louvain, St-Luc University Hospital
10 Avenue Hippocrate, 1200 Bruxelles
Belgium

Email: vincent.gregoire@uclouvain.be

PAUL M. HARARI, MD
Department of Human Oncology
University of Wisconsin School of Medicine
600 Highland Avenue, K4/332, Madison
WI 53792
USA

Email: harari@humonc.wisc.edu

GREG HARTIG, MD
Otolaryngology-Head and Neck Surgery
Department of Surgery, H4/750 CSC
University of Wisconsin School of Medicine
600 Highland Avenue, Madison
WI 53792
USA

Email: hartig@surgery.wisc.edu

JØRN HERRSTEDT, MD, DMSci
Department of Oncology
Odense University Hospital
Sdr. Boulevard 29, 5000 Odense C
Denmark

Email: herrstedt@ouh.regionsyddanmark.dk

RUSSELL W. HINERMAN, MD
Department of Radiation Oncology
University of Florida College of Medicine
P.O. Box 100385, 2000
SW Archer Road, Gainesville
FL 32610-0385
USA

TIEN HOANG, MD
Department of Medicine
University of Wisconsin School of Medicine and
Public Health, 600 Highland Avenue, K4/319 CSC
Madison, WI 53792
USA

Email: txh@medicine.wisc.edu

JONATHAN IRISH, MD, FRCPC
Department of Department of Surgical Oncology
Princess Margaret Hospital
University of Toronto
610 University Avenue
Toronto, ON M5G 2M9
Canada

Kenneth Jensen, MD, PhD
Department of Oncology
Aarhus University Hospital
Noerrebbrogade 44, 8000 Aarhus C
Denmark

Email: kennethjensen@dadlnet.dk

Jørgen Johansen, MD, PhD
Department of Oncology
Odense University Hospital
Sdr. Boulevard 29, 5000 Odense C
Denmark

Douglas E. Jorenby, PhD
Department of Medicine
University of Wisconsin School of Medicine
and Public Health
Center for Tobacco Research and Intervention
1930 Monroe Street, Suite 200
Madison
WI 53711
USA

Email: dej@ctri.medicine.wisc.edu

Rachael Kammer, MS
Division of Otolaryngology-Head
and Neck Surgery
University of Wisconsin Medical School
600 Highland Avenue K4/711, Madison
WI 53792-7375
USA

Michalis V. Karamouzis, MD
Division of Hematology-Oncology
University of Pittsburgh School of Medicine
UPMC Cancer Pavilion, 5th floor
5150 Centre Avenue
Pittsburgh, PA 15232
USA

Email: mihkaram@hotmail.com

Molly Knigge, MS
Division of Otolaryngology, Head and
Neck Surgery, University of Wisconsin
600 Highland Avenue K4/711, Madison
WI 53792-7375
USA

Claus Andrup Kristensen, MD, PhD
Department of Oncology 5073
The Finsen Centre, Rigshospitalet
Blegdamsvej 9, 2100 Copenhagen
Denmark

*Email: claus.andrup.kristensen@rh.regionh.dk;
cak@dadlnet.dk*

Johannes A. Langendijk, MD
Department of Radiation Oncology
University Medical Centre Groningen
University of Groningen
P.O. Box 30.001, 9700 RB Groningen
The Netherlands

Email: j.a.langendijk@rt.umcg.nl

Quynh-Thu Le, MD
Department of Radiation Oncology
Stanford University Cancer Center
875 Blake Wilbur Drive, Stanford
CA 04305-5847
USA

Email: qle@stanford.edu

Anne W. M. Lee, MD
Department of Clinical Oncology, Pamela
Youde Nethersole Eastern Hospital
3, Lok Man Road, Chai Wan, Hong Kong
China

Email: awmlee@ha.org.hk

Peter C. Levendag, MD, PhD
Department of Radiation Oncology
Erasmus MC, Daniel den Hoed Cancer Center
Groene Hilledijk 301, 3075 EA Rotterdam
The Netherlands

Email: p.levendag@erasmusmc.nl

Norbert Liebsch, MD
Department of Radiation Oncology
Massachusetts General Hospital, Francis
H. Burr Proton Therapy Center
Harvard Medical School
55 Fruit Street, Boston
MA 02114-2622
USA

Marcy A. List, PhD
University of Chicago, Cancer Research Center
5841 S Maryland, MC 1140, Chicago
IL 60637
USA

Email: mlist@medicine.bsd.uchicago.edu

William M. Mendenhall, MD
Department of Radiation Oncology
University of Florida Health Science Center
P.O. Box 100385, 2000 SW Archer Road
Gainesville, FL 32610-0385
USA

Email: mendwm@shands.ufl.edu

Inge Noever, RTT
Department of Radiation Oncology
Erasmus MC, Daniel den Hoed Cancer Center
Groene Hilledijk 301, 3075 EA Rotterdam
The Netherlands

Wai Tong Ng, MD
Department of Clinical Oncology
Pamela Youde Nethersole Eastern Hospital
3, Lok Man Road, Chai Wan, Hong Kong
China

Li Ning, MD
Department of Surgery, H4750 CSC
University of Wisconsin, 600 Highland Avenue
Madison, WI 53792
USA

Email: ning@surgery.wisc.edu

Department of Surgery
Peking Union Medical College Hospital
1 Shuaifuyuan, Wanfujing Avenue
Beijing 100730
China

Brian O'Sullivan, MD, FRCPC
Department of Radiation Oncology
Princess Margaret Hospital
University of Toronto
610 University Avenue
Toronto, ON M5G 2M9
Canada

Email: brian.osullivan@rmp.uhn.on.ca

Gregory M. Richards, MD
Department of Human Oncology
University of Wisconsin School of Medicine
600 Highland Avenue, Madison, WI 53792
USA

Email: richards@humonc.wisc.edu

Pamela Sandow, MD
Department of Oral & Maxillofacial Surgery and
Diagnostic Sciences, Oral Medicine Clinic
University of Florida, JHMHC, Box 100416, Gainesville
FL 32610-0416
USA

Email: psandow@dental.ufl.edu

Paul I. M. Schmitz, PhD
Department of Biostatistics, Erasmus MC, Daniel den
Hoed Cancer Center, Groene Hilledijk 301, 3075 EA
Rotterdam, The Netherlands

Rebecca S. Sippel, MD
Department of Surgery, University of Wisconsin
H4/755 CSC, 600 Highland Avenue
Madison, WI 53792
USA

Email: sippel@surgery.wisc.edu

David N. Teguh, MD
Department of Radiation Oncology, Erasmus MC
Daniel den Hoed Cancer Center, Groene Hilledijk
301, 3075 EA Rotterdam
The Netherlands

Chris Terhaard, MD, PhD
Department of Radiotherapy, UMC Utrecht
Huispost D01.213, Postbus 85500, 3508 GA Utrecht
The Netherlands

Email: c.h.j.terhaard@umcutrecht.nl

Wolfgang A. Tomé, PhD
Department of Human Oncology
University of Wisconsin School of Medicine and
Public Health, K4/314 CSC, 600 Highland Ave., Madison
WI 53705
USA

Email: tome@humonc.wisc.edu

ALEXEI TROFIMOV, MD
Department of Radiation Oncology
Massachusetts General Hospital
Francis H. Burr Proton Therapy Center
Harvard Medical School
55 Fruit Street, Boston, MA 02114-2622
USA

RICHARD TSANG, MD, FRCPC
Department of Radiation Oncology
Princess Margaret Hospital
University of Toronto, 610 University Avenue
Toronto, ON M5G 2M9
Canada

HENRIE VAN DER EST, RTT
Department of Radiation Oncology
Erasmus MC, Daniel den Hoed Cancer Center
Groene Hilledijk 301, 3075 EA Rotterdam
The Netherlands

PETER VAN ROOIJ, MSc
Department of Radiation Oncology
Erasmus MC, Daniel den Hoed Cancer Center
Groene Hilledijk 301, 3075 EA Rotterdam
The Netherlands

MIKHAIL VAYSBERG, MD
Department of Otolaryngology
University of Florida College of Medicine
P.O. Box 100264, 1600
SW Archer Road Room M228
Gainesville, FL 32610-0264
USA

PETER VOET, RTT
Department of Radiation Oncology
Erasmus MC, Daniel den Hoed Cancer Center
Groene Hilledijk 301, 3075 EA Rotterdam
The Netherlands

JOHN W. WERNING, MD
Department of Otolaryngology
University of Florida College of Medicine
P.O. Box 100264, 1600
SW Archer Road Room M228
Gainesville, FL 32610-0264
USA

DERIC L. WHEELER, PhD
Department of Human Oncology
University of Wisconsin School of Medicine and
Public Health, 600 Highland Avenue
K4/319 CSC, Madison
WI 53792
USA

Email: dlwheeler@wisc.edu

PEGGY A. WIEDERHOLT, RN
Department of Human Oncology
University of Wisconsin Paul P. Carbone
Comprehensive Cancer Center
University of Wisconsin Hospital
& Clinics, 600 Highland Avenue
K4/B100 CSC, Madison
WI 53792
USA

Email: wiederholt@humonc.wisc.edu

REBECCA M. W. YEUNG, MD
Department of Clinical Oncology
Pamela Youde Nethersole Eastern Hospital
3, Lok Man Road, Chai Wan
Hong Kong
China

WEINING (KEN) ZHEN, MD
987521 Nebraska Medical Center
Omaha, NE 68198
USA

Email: wzhen@unmc.edu

MEDICAL RADIOLOGY Diagnostic Imaging and Radiation Oncology

Titles in the series already published

DIAGNOSTIC IMAGING

Innovations in Diagnostic Imaging
Edited by J. H. Anderson

Radiology of the Upper Urinary Tract
Edited by E. K. Lang

The Thymus - Diagnostic Imaging, Functions, and Pathologic Anatomy
Edited by E. Walter, E. Willich, and W. R. Webb

Interventional Neuroradiology
Edited by A. Valavanis

Radiology of the Lower Urinary Tract
Edited by E. K. Lang

Contrast-Enhanced MRI of the Breast
S. Heywang-Köbrunner and R. Beck

Spiral CT of the Chest
Edited by M. Rémy-Jardin and J. Rémy

Radiological Diagnosis of Breast Diseases
Edited by M. Friedrich and E. A. Sickles

Radiology of Trauma
Edited by M. Heller and A. Fink

Biliary Tract Radiology
Edited by P. Rossi. Co-edited by M. Brezi

Radiological Imaging of Sports Injuries
Edited by C. Masciocchi

Modern Imaging of the Alimentary Tube
Edited by A. R. Margulis

Diagnosis and Therapy of Spinal Tumors
Edited by P. R. Algra, J. Valk and J. J. Heimans

Interventional Magnetic Resonance Imaging
Edited by J. F. Debatin and G. Adam

Abdominal and Pelvic MRI
Edited by A. Heuck and M. Reiser

Orthopedic Imaging
Techniques and Applications
Edited by A. M. Davies and H. Pettersson

Radiology of the Female Pelvic Organs
Edited by E. K. Lang

Magnetic Resonance of the Heart and Great Vessels
Clinical Applications
Edited by J. Bogaert, A. J. Duerinckx, and F. E. Rademakers

Modern Head and Neck Imaging
Edited by S. K. Mukherji and J. A. Castelijns

Radiological Imaging of Endocrine Diseases
Edited by J. N. Bruneton
in collaboration with B. Padovani and M.-Y. Mourou

Radiology of the Pancreas
2nd Revised Edition

Edited by A. L. Baert. Co-edited by G. Delorme and L. Van Hoe

Trends in Contrast Media
Edited by H. S. Thomsen, R. N. Muller, and R. F. Mattrey

Functional MRI
Edited by C. T. W. Moonen and P. A. Bandettini

Emergency Pediatric Radiology
Edited by H. Carty

Liver Malignancies
Diagnostic and Interventional Radiology
Edited by C. Bartolozzi and R. Lencioni

Spiral CT of the Abdomen
Edited by F. Terrier, M. Grossholz, and C. D. Becker

Medical Imaging of the Spleen
Edited by A. M. De Schepper and F. Vanhoenacker

Radiology of Peripheral Vascular Diseases
Edited by E. Zeitler

Radiology of Blunt Trauma of the Chest
P. Schnyder and M. Wintermark

Portal Hypertension
Diagnostic Imaging and Imaging-Guided Therapy
Edited by P. Rossi.
Co-edited by P. Ricci and L. Broglia

Virtual Endoscopy and Related 3D Techniques
Edited by P. Rogalla, J. Terwisscha van Scheltinga and B. Hamm

Recent Advances in Diagnostic Neuroradiology
Edited by Ph. Demaerel

Transfontanellar Doppler Imaging in Neonates
A. Couture, C. Veyrac

Radiology of AIDS
A Practical Approach
Edited by J. W. A. J. Reeders and P. C. Goodman

CT of the Peritoneum
A. Rossi, G. Rossi

Magnetic Resonance Angiography
2nd Revised Edition
Edited by I. P. Arlart, G. M. Bongartz, and G. Marchal

Applications of Sonography in Head and Neck Pathology
Edited by J. N. Bruneton
in collaboration with C. Raffaelli, O. Dassonville

3D Image Processing
Techniques and Clinical Applications
Edited by D. Caramella and C. Bartolozzi

Imaging of the Larynx
Edited by R. Hermans

Pediatric ENT Radiology
Edited by S. J. King and A. E. Boothroyd

Imaging of Orbital and Visual Pathway Pathology
Edited by W. S. Müller-Forell

Radiological Imaging of the Small Intestine
Edited by N. C. Gourtsoyiannis

Imaging of the Knee
Techniques and Applications
Edited by A. M. Davies and V. N. Cassar-Pullicino

Perinatal Imaging
From Ultrasound to MR Imaging
Edited by F. E. Avni

Diagnostic and Interventional Radiology in Liver Transplantation
Edited by E. Bücheler, V. Nicolas, C. E. Broelsch, X. Rogiers and G. Krupski

Imaging of the Pancreas
Cystic and Rare Tumors
Edited by C. Procacci and A. J. Megibow

Imaging of the Foot & Ankle
Techniques and Applications
Edited by A. M. Davies, R. W. Whitehouse and J. P. R. Jenkins

Radiological Imaging of the Ureter
Edited by F. Joffre, Ph. Otal and M. Soulie

Radiology of the Petrous Bone
Edited by M. Lemmerling and S. S. Kollias

Imaging of the Shoulder
Techniques and Applications
Edited by A. M. Davies and J. Hodler

Interventional Radiology in Cancer
Edited by A. Adam, R. F. Dondelinger, and P. R. Mueller

Imaging and Intervention in Abdominal Trauma
Edited by R. F. Dondelinger

Radiology of the Pharynx and the Esophagus
Edited by O. Ekberg

Radiological Imaging in Hematological Malignancies
Edited by A. Guermazi

Functional Imaging of the Chest
Edited by H.-U. Kauczor

Duplex and Color Doppler Imaging of the Venous System
Edited by G. H. Mostbeck

Multidetector-Row CT of the Thorax
Edited by U. J. Schoepf

Radiology and Imaging of the Colon
Edited by A. H. Chapman

Multidetector-Row CT Angiography
Edited by C. Catalano and R. Passariello

Focal Liver Lesions
Detection, Characterization, Ablation
Edited by R. Lencioni, D. Cioni, and C. Bartolozzi

Imaging in Treatment Planning for Sinonasal Diseases
Edited by R. Maroldi and P. Nicolai

Clinical Cardiac MRI
With Interactive CD-ROM
Edited by J. Bogaert, S. Dymarkowski, and A. M. Taylor

Dynamic Contrast-Enhanced Magnetic Resonance Imaging in Oncology
Edited by A. Jackson, D. L. Buckley, and G. J. M. Parker

Contrast Media in Ultrasonography
Basic Principles and Clinical Applications
Edited by E. Quaia

Paediatric Musculoskeletal Disease
With an Emphasis on Ultrasound
Edited by D. Wilson

MR Imaging in White Matter Diseases of the Brain and Spinal Cord
Edited by M. Filippi, N. De Stefano, V. Dousset, and J. C. McGowan

Imaging of the Hip & Bony Pelvis
Techniques and Applications
Edited by A. M. Davies, K. Johnson, and R. W. Whitehouse

Imaging of Kidney Cancer
Edited by A. Guermazi

Magnetic Resonance Imaging in Ischemic Stroke
Edited by R. von Kummer and T. Back

Diagnostic Nuclear Medicine
2nd Revised Edition
Edited by C. Schiepers

Imaging of Occupational and Environmental Disorders of the Chest
Edited by P. A. Gevenois and P. De Vuyst

Virtual Colonoscopy
A Practical Guide
Edited by P. Lefere and S. Gryspeerdt

Contrast Media
Safety Issues and ESUR Guidelines
Edited by H. S. Thomsen

Head and Neck Cancer Imaging
Edited by R. Hermans

Vascular Embolotherapy
A Comprehensive Approach
Volume 1: *General Principles, Chest, Abdomen, and Great Vessels*
Edited by J. Golzarian. Co-edited by S. Sun and M. J. Sharafuddin

Vascular Embolotherapy
A Comprehensive Approach
Volume 2: *Oncology, Trauma, Gene Therapy, Vascular Malformations, and Neck*
Edited by J. Golzarian.
Co-edited by S. Sun and M. J. Sharafuddin

Vascular Interventional Radiology
Current Evidence in Endovascular Surgery
Edited by M. G. Cowling

Ultrasound of the Gastrointestinal Tract
Edited by G. Maconi and G. Bianchi Porro

Parallel Imaging in Clinical MR Applications
Edited by S. O. Schoenberg, O. Dietrich, and M. F. Reiser

MRI and CT of the Female Pelvis
Edited by B. Hamm and R. Forstner

Imaging of Orthopedic Sports Injuries
Edited by F. M. Vanhoenacker, M. Maas and J. L. Gielen

Ultrasound of the Musculoskeletal System
S. Bianchi and C. Martinoli

Clinical Functional MRI
Presurgical Functional Neuroimaging
Edited by C. Stippich

Radiation Dose from Adult and Pediatric Multidetector Computed Tomography
Edited by D. Tack and P. A. Gevenois

Spinal Imaging
Diagnostic Imaging of the Spine and Spinal Cord
Edited by J. Van Goethem, L. van den Hauwe and P. M. Parizel

Computed Tomography of the Lung
A Pattern Approach
J. A. Verschakelen and W. De Wever

Imaging in Transplantation
Edited by A. Bankier

Radiological Imaging of the Neonatal Chest
2nd Revised Edition
Edited by V. Donoghue

Radiological Imaging of the Digestive Tract in Infants and Children
Edited by A. S. Devos and J. G. Blickman

Pediatric Chest Imaging
Chest Imaging in Infants and Children
2nd Revised Edition
Edited by J. Lucaya and J. L. Strife

Color Doppler US of the Penis
Edited by M. Bertolotto

Radiology of the Stomach and Duodenum
Edited by A. H. Freeman and E. Sala

Imaging in Pediatric Skeletal Trauma
Techniques and Applications
Edited by K. J. Johnson and E. Bache

Image Processing in Radiology
Current Applications
Edited by E. Neri, D. Caramella, C. Bartolozzi

Screening and Preventive Diagnosis with Radiological Imaging
Edited by M. F. Reiser, G. van Kaick, C. Fink, S. O. Schoenberg

Percutaneous Tumor Ablation in Medical Radiology
Edited by T. J. Vogl, T. K. Helmberger, M. G. Mack, M. F. Reiser

Liver Radioembolization with ^{90}Y Microspheres
Edited by J. I. Bilbao, M. F. Reiser

Pediatric Uroradiology
2nd Revised Edition
Edited by R. Fotter

Radiology of Osteoporosis
2nd Revised Edition
Edited by S. Grampp

Gastrointestinal Tract Sonography in Fetuses and Children
A. Couture, C. Baud, J. L. Ferran, M. Saguintaah and C. Veyrac

Intracranial Vascular Malformations and Aneurysms
2nd Revised Edition
Edited by M. Forsting and I. Wanke

High-Resolution Sonography of the Peripheral Nervous System
2nd Revised Edition
Edited by S. Peer and G. Bodner

Imaging Pelvic Floor Disorders
2nd Revised Edition
Edited by J. Stoker, S. A. Taylor, and J. O. L. DeLancey

Coronary Radiology
2nd Revised Edition
Edited by M. Oudkerk and M. F. Reiser

Integrated Cardiothoracic Imaging with MDCT
Edited by M. Rémy-Jardin and J. Rémy

Multislice CT
3rd Revised Edition
Edited by M. F. Reiser, C. R. Becker, K. Nikolaou, G. Glazer

MRI of the Lung
Edited by H.-U. Kauczor

Imaging in Percutaneous Musculoskeletal Interventions
Edited by A. Gangi, S. Guth, and A. Guermazi

Contrast Media. Safety Issues and ESUR Guidelines
2nd Revised Edition
Edited by H. Thomsen, J.A. W. Webb

Inflammatory Diseases of the Brain
Edited by S. Hähnel

Imaging of Bone Tumors and Tumor-Like Lesions - Techniques and Applications
Edited by A.M. Davies, M. Sundaram, and S.J. James

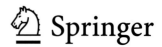

MEDICAL RADIOLOGY Diagnostic Imaging and Radiation Oncology
Titles in the series already published

Radiation Oncology

Lung Cancer
Edited by C. W. Scarantino

Innovations in Radiation Oncology
Edited by H. R. Withers and L. J. Peters

Radiation Therapy of Head and Neck Cancer
Edited by G. E. Laramore

Gastrointestinal Cancer – Radiation Therapy
Edited by R. R. Dobelbower, Jr.

Radiation Exposure and Occupational Risks
Edited by E. Scherer, C. Streffer, and K.-R. Trott

Interventional Radiation
Therapy Techniques – Brachytherapy
Edited by R. Sauer

Radiopathology of Organs and Tissues
Edited by E. Scherer, C. Streffer, and K.-R. Trott

Concomitant Continuous Infusion
Chemotherapy and Radiation
Edited by M. Rotman and C. J. Rosenthal

Intraoperative Radiotherapy – Clinical Experiences and Results
Edited by F. A. Calvo, M. Santos, and L. W. Brady

Interstitial and Intracavitary Thermoradiotherapy
Edited by M. H. Seegenschmiedt and R. Sauer

Non-Disseminated Breast Cancer
Controversial Issues in Management
Edited by G. H. Fletcher and S. H. Levitt

Current Topics in Clinical Radiobiology of Tumors
Edited by H.-P. Beck-Bornholdt

Practical Approaches to Cancer Invasion and Metastases
A Compendium of Radiation Oncologists' Responses to 40 Histories
Edited by A. R. Kagan with the Assistance of R. J. Steckel

Radiation Therapy in Pediatric Oncology
Edited by J. R. Cassady

Radiation Therapy Physics
Edited by A. R. Smith

Late Sequelae in Oncology
Edited by J. Dunst, R. Sauer

Mediastinal Tumors. Update 1995
Edited by D. E. Wood, C. R. Thomas, Jr.

Thermoradiotherapy and Thermochemotherapy
Volume 1: *Biology, Physiology, and Physics*

Volume 2: *Clinical Applications*
Edited by M. H. Seegenschmiedt, P. Fessenden and C. C. Vernon

Carcinoma of the Prostate
Innovations in Management
Edited by Z. Petrovich, L. Baert, and L. W. Brady

Radiation Oncology of Gynecological Cancers
Edited by H. W. Vahrson

Carcinoma of the Bladder
Innovations in Management
Edited by Z. Petrovich, L. Baert, and L. W. Brady

Blood Perfusion and Microenvironment of Human Tumors
Implications for Clinical Radiooncology
Edited by M. Molls and P. Vaupel

Radiation Therapy of Benign Diseases
A Clinical Guide
2nd Revised Edition
S. E. Order and S. S. Donaldson

Carcinoma of the Kidney and Testis, and Rare Urologic Malignancies
Innovations in Management
Edited by Z. Petrovich, L. Baert, and L. W. Brady

Progress and Perspectives in the Treatment of Lung Cancer
Edited by P. Van Houtte, J. Klastersky, and P. Rocmans

Combined Modality Therapy of Central Nervous System Tumors
Edited by Z. Petrovich, L. W. Brady, M. L. Apuzzo, and M. Bamberg

Age-Related Macular Degeneration
Current Treatment Concepts
Edited by W. E. Alberti, G. Richard, and R. H. Sagerman

Radiotherapy of Intraocular and Orbital Tumors
2nd Revised Edition
Edited by R. H. Sagerman and W. E. Alberti

Modification of Radiation Response
Cytokines, Growth Factors, and Other Biolgical Targets
Edited by C. Nieder, L. Milas and K. K. Ang

Radiation Oncology for Cure and Palliation
R. G. Parker, N. A. Janjan and M. T. Selch

Clinical Target Volumes in Conformal and Intensity Modulated Radiation Therapy
A Clinical Guide to Cancer Treatment
Edited by V. Grégoire, P. Scalliet, and K. K. Ang

Advances in Radiation Oncology in Lung Cancer
Edited by B. Jeremi´c

New Technologies in Radiation Oncology
Edited by W. Schlegel, T. Bortfeld, and A.-L. Grosu

Multimodal Concepts for Integration of Cytotoxic Drugs and Radiation Therapy
Edited by J. M. Brown, M. P. Mehta, and C. Nieder

Technical Basis of Radiation Therapy
Practical Clinical Applications
4th Revised Edition
Edited by S. H. Levitt, J. A. Purdy, C. A. Perez, and S. Vijayakumar

CURED I · LENT
Late Effects of Cancer Treatment on Normal Tissues
Edited by P. Rubin, L. S. Constine, L. B. Marks, and P. Okunieff

Radiotherapy for Non-Malignant Disorders
Contemporary Concepts and Clinical Results
Edited by M. H. Seegenschmiedt, H.-B. Makoski, K.-R. Trott, and L. W. Brady

CURED II · LENT
Cancer Survivorship Research and Education
Late Effects on Normal Tissues
Edited by P. Rubin, L. S. Constine, L. B. Marks, and P. Okunieff

Radiation Oncology
An Evidence-Based Approach
Edited by J. J. Lu and L. W. Brady

Primary Optic Nerve Sheath Meningioma
Edited by B. Jeremi´c, and S. Pitz

Function Preservation and Quality Life in Head and Neck Radiotherapy
Edited by P.M. Harari, N.P. Connor, and C. Grau

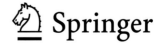

Printing and Binding: Stürtz GmbH, Würzburg